A MANUAL

OF

PHARMACODYNAMICS.

A MANUAL

OF

PHARMACODYNAMICS.

SIXTH EDITION.

BY

RICHARD HUGHES,

L.R.C.P., ED.

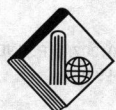

B. Jain Publishers (P) Ltd.
USA — Europe — India

A MANUAL OF PHARMACODYNAMICS

6th Impression: 2016

Published by Kuldeep Jain for
B. JAIN PUBLISHERS (P) LTD.
B. Jain House, D-157, Sector-63, NOIDA-201307, U.P. (INDIA)
Tel.: +91-120-4933333 • Email: info@bjain.com
Website: www.bjain.com

Printed in India by
JJ Imprints Pvt. Ltd.

ISBN: 978-81-319-1962-0

PREFACE TO THE SIXTH EDITION.

THE Publishers are glad to find that there is need for another edition of this valuable work, the last one (consisting of two thousand copies) having met with such a rapid sale—proving by this incontestable fact that the author has given the readers of " Pharmacodynamics " a key to an intelligent study of Materia Medica which had not existed heretofore. An eminent practitioner, in reviewing this work, writes : " The volume is cast in the form of lectures on the remedies, and presents the subject of the lecture in a pleasantly personal fashion ; carefully but succinctly stating the history of the plant, or mineral, or what not, its current use or abuse, its preparation for our school, and the general lines along which its most important remedial measures have been proved. Thus by a system of historical narration the reader, be he practitioner, student, or layman, finds an image of the remedy forming in his mind—a picture which being once ' seen ' is endowed with greater permanency of existence than pages upon pages of laboured verbal description of isolated non-associated symptoms. * * * One hundred and five pages of the ' Pharmacodynamics ' are devoted to a splendid exposition of homœopathy, the sources of its Materia Medica, the general principles of drug action, and other interesting data to the homœopath ; while the appendix gives Hahnemann's dosage from 1796 to his death. This appendix is an unique and interesting paper, and cannot fail to dispel some of the extravagant notions prevalent at this day concerning Hahnemann's potencies. In the present (the last) edition the volume contains nearly 1,000 pages, is handsomely and strongly bound, and ought to be on the library table of every Materia Medica student who has ever grumbled because of the difficulty of comprehending the Materia Medica of our school."

September, 1893.

PREFACE TO THE FOURTH EDITION.

WHEN publishing (in 1875-6) the third edition of this Manual, I introduced it in the following words :—

"This work originally appeared in 1867, as the first part of a 'Manual of Homœopathic Practice for students and beginners.' It was couched in the form of letters to an enquiring friend. A second edition was published in 1870. The additions rendered necessary by the progress of knowledge were, for the convenience of those who possessed the volume in its original form, placed between brackets or affixed as notes.

"When, in 1874, I was called upon to prepare a third edition, it seemed desirable that the work should assume a homogeneous and as it were primary character; and that the matter of the first two editions, together with such additions as I might have to make, should be welded together in one consecutive whole. But I found, on consideration, that more than this would be necessary. I had by this time become painfully conscious of the limited range of the information with which I had previously worked, especially as regards original provings and French and German literature. The endeavours I now made to extend my knowledge showed me that the work must be, to a great extent, not only re-cast but re-written, if it was to satisfy my present sense of what was required of it.

"While I was planning and initiating the undertaking, the circumstances arose which led to my being requested by the British Homœopathic Society to deliver a course of lectures in London on Materia Medica and Therapeutics. The form

of my work was thus determined for me ; and an additiona}
motive supplied for making its substance as full and accurate
as possible. The lectures were delivered between February
and June, 1875, and again from October to January, 1875-6.
The present volume contains them. I have added the minor
medicines omitted in my course, and some re-arrangement
has been necessitated hereby. With this exception, the lectures
stand here substantially as they were given.

" In my introductory discourse I have stated fully the scope
and method of my procedure ; and need not dwell upon them
in this preface. On one feature of the work only I would
make a remark. While I had hitherto been content to say—
the proving of such and such a drug is in the *Materia Medica
Pura*, or *Chronic Diseases*, or elsewhere, I have now thought
it advisable to give a brief analytic account of each pathogenesis, stating the sources from which it is derived, and the
proportion in which they have contributed to it ; and also,
where possible, the manner in which the symptoms were
obtained. I have reason to think that a very vague conception exists in most minds (I know it once did in my own) as
to the nature of the pathogenetic materials of Homœopathy.
This imperfect knowledge is apt to lead, on the one side to
superstitious veneration, on the other to sceptical neglect—
both being, I conceive, unwarranted towards the Materia
Medica as a whole, and either being generally misplaced in its
own reference. I have accordingly done my best (though I
have yet more to do in the same field) to ascertain and exhibit
the general character of such pathogenetic collections as we
possess, so that a reference to them may carry its own
meaning with it. And I have also examined each constituent
member of these, and each separate contribution of the kind,
on its own 'merits, and stated the results ; so that the student
may know in each case the nature of the material with which
he is working, and esteem and use it accordingly."

In 1877, the London School of Homœopathy was founded,
and I was appointed to fill the chair of Materia Medica and
Therapeutics therein. My Manual naturally became the text-

book of my course, and the groundwork of the lectures I delivered. Such fresh matter as from time to time I have brought before my class, and such improvements in presentation as have occurred to me while going on, I have incorporated into the substance of the book which is now offered to the profession in its fourth edition.

I have described this as " revised and augmented." It is not, as was the third edition, " mainly re-written :" the framework on which that was constructed will be found here substantially unaltered. But it has been filled in with a liberal hand, so as to make the volume more than one-fourth larger than its predecessor, and—I hope—proportionately more satisfying to the student. There is hardly an article which has not received some fresh touch ; and those on most of the polychrests, and on Chamomilla, Gelsemium, Iris, Plumbum and others have been much enlarged. Supplementary lectures on some minor and recently-introduced medicines are appended ; while several of those which occupied such rank in the former edition find place in the main series, in which also will be found new sections on the picric and salicylic acids, on chlorine and its derivatives, and on Œnanthe crocata.

Following upon the introductory lecture will be found six new ones. The two on the sources of the Homœopathic Materia Medica contain the substance of the little book I have published under that title. Those on the general principles of drug-action bear the same relation to the lectures I delivered at the London Homœopathic Hospital in 1877, and which appeared in the earlier numbers of the *Monthly Homœopathic Review* of that year. That entitled " Homœopathy— what it is " is a similar reproduction of the paper on " The Two Homœopathies " which I had the honour of reading at the British Homœopathic Congress held at Liverpool in 1877; and that on " Homœopathic Posology " has already appeared in the *British Journal of Homœopathy* for January, 1879. By including these materials in my present volume, I have made it contain all work I have hitherto been able to do in the field to which it belongs; and I hope that it may continue to be useful to the class which I am no longer able to conduct in person.

My third edition, at its appearance in two parts, in 1875 and 1876 respectively, received very full notice in the *Monthly Homœopathic Review*. Of the general tone and bearing of my reviewer's criticism I have nothing to express but sincere acknowledgment; and I have shown my sense of the weight of such exceptions as he has taken to my work by the large consideration I have given them, both here and elsewhere. His remarks on my treatment of certain medicines I have had before me in my revision of the articles upon them for the present edition. His challenge of my ignoring or rejecting the doctrine of the opposite action of large and small doses I have fully met in the pages of the *Review* itself, and (to some extent) in the fifth lecture of my present series. The only points raised by him which yet remain for notice are my large employment of the results of experimentation on animals, and my copious reference to and quotation of the works of Drs. Ringer and Phillips. As to the first, I would remark that the main object of my work is to illuminate the symptom. atology of our medicines by aid of such side-lights as can be thrown upon it; and of these none are more important than the experiments of the physiological laboratory. They are necessarily excluded from our ordinary pathogenetic collections: it is all the more important that they should find large place in commentary and interpretation such as this. My object in making so much employment of the treatises mentioned was that, lecturing, as I always have done, to auditors trained in the schools of traditional medicine, it was a clear gain to be able to support my arguments as to the homœopathicity of certain practices by evidence accredited therein. Drs. Ringer and Phillips were both Professors of Materia Medica in recognised colleges. It was for them to account for the unusual amount of homœopathic matter contained in their pages: I, finding it there, turned it to the advantage of my position.

PREFACE.

I have only now, in presenting this fourth edition of my book to the profession, to repeat my hope that the kind appreciation it has hitherto received, both in its own language, and in French, German and Spanish translation, will continue to be extended to it.

36, SILLWOOD ROAD, BRIGHTON.
June, 1880.

CONTENTS.

xii

CONTENTS xiii

LECTURE I.

GENTLEMEN,—

We are met to-day to inaugurate a course of instruction upon Materia Medica and Therapeutics, *i.e.*, upon the materials used in the practice of medicine, with their properties, and of the application of these to the art of healing. It will be well, at the outset, to indicate and define our field of study.

1. There are agents employed and measures prescribed in the treatment of disease which are roughly classed under the term *hygienic*. These include the diet and regimen of the patient, the choice of his climate, the regulation of his habits. Again, there are ways in which the various forces and elements of nature can be pressed into therapeutic service, as the use of water in its various forms, the bringing to bear of heat and cold in due proportions, and the application of electricity.   In systematic treatises on Materia Medica many of these agents are discussed, and they cannot be denied a title to the name. If I exclude them from our consideration here, it is not from their being undervalued. It is simply because I have nothing to say about them which is not better said elsewhere ; and because I wish to devote our entire attention to the action of *drugs*.

2. Drugs—that is, substances which have the power of affecting the animal body in health and disease—are the Materia Medica of which I propose to speak. And of these, again, solely as they affect the body. Taken from the animal, vegetable, and mineral kingdoms, they have characters and relations which belong to the sciences dealing with those departments of nature. In the treatises of which I have spoken, such features of drugs often occupy a large space ; and to them I must refer you for all detailed information of the kind. I shall use it only so far as may be necessary to identify the drug before us, and to ensure a concrete concep-

B

tion of its origin and character in your minds ; for which purpose the specimens contained in our museum will come in aid. This done, it will be discussed as a drug and nothing else.

3. Such discussion, as I have said, will embrace the action of each substance upon the organism in health and disease,—its action physiological (or pathogenetic), and its action therapeutical. Of the former little needs now to be said. There is no question but that our knowledge on this head should be as full and accurate as possible. The only limitation is on the side of Toxicology. Our subject is pharmacodynamics ; but it is the δυνάμεις of φάρμακα as medicines, not as poisons. We require to know their poisonous action for the purpose of using them as curative agents : in as far as it comes within the range of Forensic Medicine—in all that relates to diagnosis, tests, antidotes, and such like—it is beyond the range of our present inquiry.

4. A far more important qualification of our task arises from the therapeutic side of the action of drugs. These lectures are delivered as part of the course of instruction of the London School of *Homœopathy*. How far do the principles indicated by this name modify the teaching of Materia Medica ?

It is not my province to expound to you in any detail the nature of homœopathy : this task belongs to my colleague occupying the chair of the Practice of Medicine. The only assumption regarding it needful for my present purpose is that it is a therapeutic method, and a legitimate one. It is nevertheless entirely ignored in the common text-books on Materia Medica, the few known applications of medicines which come within its range finding place there as empirical uses only. It accordingly becomes the duty of a teacher of this subject in a School of Homœopathy to give, in the therapeutic part of his task, the foremost rank to such uses of his medicines as result from the rule *similia similibus curentur*—let likes be treated by likes. He will not neglect to glance at and estimate other modes of employing them, but he will give his main strength to these : these he will do, and not leave the others undone.

But the avowed recognition of homœopathy in this place will have further effects.

First, it will influence the range of the Materia Medica we shall have to consider. Homœopathy presses into its service a far greater number of natural products than traditional medicine employs. It has revived many valuable agents from the unmerited oblivion into which they had fallen, and is continually adding new remedies to its stock by means of the organon it possesses in the law of similars ; for it has but to ascertain the pathogenetic action of any substance, and its medicinal use is indicated forthwith. The Materia Medica we shall study will be that of Homœopathy, which embraces all the ordinary medicines, and adds many another thereto.

Secondly, our homœopathic standpoint will greatly enrich the materials on which we can draw for the knowledge of the pathogenetic action of drugs. The practical carrying out of our therapeutic rule has necessitated extensive and minute "proving" upon the healthy body. The record of such experimentation constitutes the distinctive Materia Medica Homœopathica. Passed by in the ordinary lectures and treatises, this record will take special prominence here. We may use as freely as others can the observations of poisoning and over-dosing, and the experiments on animals, which constitute the bulk of the pathogenetic material generally available. But we shall add to these, and rank above them in importance, the pure proving on the healthy which, though not unknown previously, has been in an especial manner the (confessedly meritorious) endeavour of the disciples of Hahnemann. Such experimentation on the human organism is now gladly welcomed in the old school of medicine, but only when its conductors and subjects are of the orthodox creed. We, having no such prejudices, shall be free to use all material of the kind, estimating it simply on its own merits.

Once more, the homœopathic character of our therapeutics will give a special direction to our study of pathogenetics. There are three recognised kinds of action possessed by drugs, which are commonly called mechanical, chemical, and dynamic respectively. The first is that which they exert in virtue of their bulk, weight, or character of surface, as when mercury used to be given to force a passage through obstructed bowels, or the mucuna pruriens to detach intestinal parasites. The second is the action of acid substances on alkalies and alkalies on acids, and such like, whereby the re-actions of the laboratory are reproduced as far as may be possible in the interior of the organism. The third or dynamic operation of drugs embraces all effects of theirs which cannot be accounted for by physical and chemical laws, and which—unlike those of the two former classes—are only produced in the *living* body. It is this last class of the actions of drugs which will chiefly occupy us, as it is by means of this alone that homœopathy works its rule. If we avail ourselves of the mechanical or chemical properties of the substances we employ, we do so on mechanical or chemical principles. *Similia similibus* belongs to the living organism only, and to the re-actions of drugs which are peculiar thereto.

The sum of what has now been said is this. It will be my duty to discourse from this chair on the Homœopathic Materia Medica,—embracing, that is, all the substances which homœopathy uses as medicines; setting forth, in addition to other information, the peculiar knowledge which homœopathy possesses as to their pathogenetic properties; and, while omitting no known actions or uses which belong to them, dwelling especially on those which homœopathy employs in its treatment of disease. These lectures will not attempt to supersede, but only to supplement, the instruction on the subject elsewhere given, and which you have already received or will be receiving. They belong, not to a School of Medicine in general, but to a School of Homœopathy. Of course, if the time should ever come when the lectures given here should be officially recognised as substitutes for corresponding courses delivered elsewhere, I should not assume any previous knowledge, but should treat my subject *ab initio.* As it is, it will economize time and strength on your part and mine to confine ourselves within the limits just laid down.

I have now to introduce you to that which, in a more limited and technical sense, homœopathy calls its "Materia Medica," viz.: the record of the pathogenetic effects of the medicines it uses. The primary sources of our information on this head, and the compilations of pathogenesy which are available for us, I shall bring before you in the next two lectures. It will also be my duty to refer you, for each medicine, to the original records of its provings, and to any special work in the way of study or arrangement which has been done upon it. The means of following up such references are to a large and increasing extent provided by the library of our School. I must now tell you what, in this so-called "Materia Medica" itself, you must expect to find.

Let us take as an example the section on Arnica in the first volume of Hahnemann's *Materia Medica Pura.* After a short preface, speaking of some of its therapeutic uses, we have a list of symptoms, 638 in number, purporting to be observed pathogenetic effects of the drug. Of these, 280 have no name attached, and are to be understood as contributed by Hahnemann himself. Of the remainder, 311 are marked with the abbreviated names of the fellow-observers acknowledged by him in his preface, seven in all; and 47 are credited to certain authors, reference being given to the place where the observation may be found. The symptoms are arranged in an order mainly anatomical, proceeding from those of the head to those of the extremities, and ending with generalities and psychical phenomena. No information is given as to the subjects on whom they were observed, the doses by which they were produced, or the connection and sequence in which they occurred.

This description, with slight variations, will hold good for all Hahnemann's medicines, and for a great many of those furnished by his followers. The first impression made upon the mind by the symptom-lists it characterises is one of utter confusion and discouragement. As has been said (in allusion to the order of the schema)—the reader begins with vertigo, and ends with rage. But let us inquire why Hahnemann originated, and others imitated, such a mode of presenting the pathogenetic effects of drugs ; and what use was intended to be made of the symptoms furnished. Then, perhaps, we shall understand the rationale of the form adopted.

Now it is obvious to any one who considers the subject, that there are two conceivable modes of working the homœopathic method—of following the rule, "let likes be treated by likes." The one may be called the *à priori* mode, the other the *à posteriori*. The former infers from the pathogenetic action of any substance what will be the morbid conditions in which it should prove curative. The latter begins with disease instead of drugs : it is the course we adopt when, having examined a case, we turn to our pathogenetic records to see what medicine has caused similar symptoms in the healthy.

That the latter was Hahnemann's ideal plan seems to me incontestably proved by his *Organon*. There is no trace there of wish on his part that the homœopathic practitioner should make any study of medicines in themselves · prior to their application to practice. Their pathogenetic effects having been ascertained and recorded, we have but to refer to such record, after we have examined our patient, to discover the *similimum* to his case. Hence the arrangement of the pathogeneses in the form of a schema of disconnected symptoms. If every case is to be treated by writing down its phenomena in anatomical order, and finding what medicine has produced all, or the greatest number, or the most characteristic of them, then the form adopted answers every purpose. That it is impossible to form any *à priori* notion of the medicine, or to see in its effects any true pictures of disease, is, upon this system, of no consequence.

That this is the explanation of the form of the Homœo-pathic Materia Medica is, I think, unquestionable. Nor is it doubtful but that provision must be made for this mode of homœopathising. So many morbid states are known to us only as an assemblage of phenomena, that there is no other way of treating them than by comparing them at the time with our pathogenetic records, and fitting drug symptoms to those of disease. Hence the pathogenesis of every medicine must be arranged in schema form for our purposes, and the only change to be desiderated is the improvement of the arrangement. But were this the whole of homœopathy, the function of a lecturer on Materia Medica would have no existence. The only knowledge required would be the whereabouts of the pathogeneses; the only faculty to be exercised upon them would be that of memory, and even this would be superseded by the employment of the indices we call repertories.

The fact of my delivering this course of lectures in the London School of Homœopathy shows that in the judgment of its conductors previous knowledge of medicines *is* necessary and desirable. Even to use the Materia Medica aright upon the *à posteriori* plan, it is very helpful to know the significance of the several symptoms as fully as may be, and to be acquainted with the general sphere and character of the medicine. Mere mechanical symptom-covering is as likely to miss as to hit the mark. Still more important is it that you should be furnished for what I have described as the *à priori* method of homœopathising, that as far as possible you should go forth ready equipped for your work without cumbersome apparatus of books of reference. So to inform, and so to furnish you, is the task I have undertaken. Let me say a few words upon the ποῦ στῶ which a lecturer has for this purpose.

First, in nearly all the new provings which have appeared since the death of Hahnemann, it has been recognised as essential that the daily records of the experiments should be furnished, and not merely a schema of the results. These records are invaluable, both for illuminating the individual symptoms, and for revealing the morbid states to which the drug-effects are similar. For the provings of Hahnemann and his immediate followers we have no such aids, so far as their own symptoms are concerned. But those cited from authors, which in some pathogeneses constitute an important element, can in most cases be examined in their originals, and thus their meaning and value be ascertained. This work has been done for some of the medicines by Drs. Roth, Langheinz, and others; and I have myself completed it for the whole Hahnemannic series. Dr. Allen's *Encyclopædia*, and also the new translation of Hahnemann's *Materia Medica Pura* now in progress, embody my results.

Secondly, we have the facts brought forward in the ordinary treatises on Toxicology and Materia Medica. They want the fulness and minuteness required for the application of the law of similars; yet in their measure they are extremely helpful. To know that a poison is narcotic, narcotico-irritant, or irritant only is knowledge sufficiently vague; but it is a clue. It indicates the relative importance of various symptoms, and the class of diseases to which the drug corresponds. The revelations of morbid anatomy carry us a step onward yet. They show the organs and tissues upon which the poison exerts its influence, and in a broad way the character of that influence. The classifications of manuals of therapeutics—which study drugs as cathartics, diuretics, expectorants, and so forth—help us still further to localise the sphere of the influence of each; and of late the physiological side of the action of medicines has received much greater attention in these works, to our corresponding profit.

It is perhaps supererogatory to point out the best books of this kind. Christison and the first edition of Taylor *On Poisons*, with Orfila's *Toxicologie*, have made any later works on the subject needless at present. Of the older treatises on Materia Medica, the English Pereira, the French Trousseau and Pidoux, and the American Wood may be named as excellent in their way. The modern books of Phillips,* Ringer,† and the younger Wood ‡ are of a different stamp. The first is rather the record of what the writer learned during the twenty years in which he avowedly practised homœopathy, than the result of his observations since he only did so in secret: it is of interest to us mainly as showing how much he could retain and put forward under another name. Dr. Ringer's book, when it first appeared, was an incorporation with the traditional uses of medicines of such knowledge as he could obtain of their employment in the school of Hahnemann. The facts of this latter class it contained (stated always without reference to their source) made it like a stream of fresh air to practitioners of the old system; and it rapidly attained great popularity. In subsequent editions, the author has spoken

---

* *Materia Medica and Therapeutics. Vegetable Kingdom.* By Charles D. F. Phillips, M.D., F.R.C.S.E. 1874.

† *A Handbook of Therapeutics.* By Sydney Ringer, M.D. 7th Edition. 1879.

‡ *A Treatise on Therapeutics.* By H. C. Wood, junr., M.D. 3rd Edition. 1879.

more frankly as to the authorities for his novel statements;
and has himself both supplied many fresh provings on the
human subject, and enlarged the therapeutic sphere of several
medicines by using them according to the law of similars in
the large field of practice at his command. His seventh
edition—which I shall cite here—is thus a work of great
value. The *Treatise on Therapeutics* of Dr. Horatio Wood
has a usefulness of another kind. Himself a diligent worker
in the physiological laboratory, he has made it his business to
keep *au courant* with all that is done of this sort elsewhere.
He can thus present to us a summary of all experimentation
that has been carried on with any drug down to the date of
his publication, and has done so with very satisfying fulness.
His book is as necessary for our knowledge of the pathogenetics of the old school, as they now are, as Dr. Ringer's
for its therapeutics, and throws many a side-light on our own
Materia Medica. Besides these works, I may name with much
commendation the elaborate, and indeed exhaustive treatise of
Dr. Stillé,* and the later American contribution on the
subject by Dr. Bartholow.†

Thirdly, we are materially aided in our studies of pharmacology by clinical experience, by what we are accustomed
to call the *usus in morbis*. As soon as this has become sufficiently extensive, it avails to stamp the character of the
various medicines, and to show in what part of the body and
in what kinds of derangement they have real energy. Light
is thus thrown back on the pathogeneses, and their characteristic features and fundamental phenomena become manifest.
In these, each medicine seems to affect more or less every
organ or function of the body; but from the *usus in morbis* we
learn which are the primary seats of its influence, and which
the merely subordinate and sympathetic.

A great mass of clinical experience with medicines used
after the homœopathic method has now accumulated in our
periodical literature. Collections of it have been made from
time to time, as those of Rückert in German and Beauvais (a
pseudonym for Roth) in French. But for your introduction
to the subject, and for our present purpose, I can commend to
you no more excellent books than the *Applied Homœopathy*
of the honoured founder of this School, Dr. Bayes, and the
Hints for the Practical Study of the Homœopathic Method of

* *Therapeutics and Materia Medica.* By Alfred Stillé, M.D. 4th
Edition. 1874.
† *A Practical Treatise on Materia Medica* and *Therapeutics.* By
Robert Bartholow, M.A., M.D. 1877.

Dr. Chepmell; both of which are in our library. The former by stating his own experience with our leading remedies, the latter by a series of typical clinical records with observations, stamps indelibly on the mind of the student the leading features of the drugs he specifies. But it is not on avowed homœopathic experience only that we can draw for this object. All treatment by single medicines used for their direct effects upon the disease is truly of this kind, though it knows or acknowledges it not. Hence such collections as those of Frank's *Magazin* * are of great value to us. This exists only in German; but in M. Teste's *Systématisation pratique de la matière médicale homœopathique* (1853), which we have also in English, copious use is made of the experience of the older medical writers as illuminative of the special properties of our remedies.

Taking his stand upon the ground thus described, the lecturer on Materia Medica will survey for his hearers the field of pathogenetic phenomena he has to characterise. My main object will be to set forth the *sphere of action* of each drug. Every medicine, even though it be one of those great polychrests which seem to embrace nearly the whole organism within the circle of their influence, has one or more centres of action. What these centres are we learn, sometimes from the pathogenetic, sometimes from the clinical side. When we have learnt them, they become all-important stand-points for the understanding and the remembrance of the medicine. These centres I shall endeavour, wherever practicable, to reach, and around them to group the several actions and uses of the drugs. There will always be residuary phenomena in such a process; but these I shall not fail to note when their importance demands it.

Besides sphere, moreover, I shall endeavour to set forth the *kind* of action of each drug. Its action upon a certain organ or tissue, a certain physiological function, a certain pathological process, may belong to it in common with several other medicines; and yet there is nearly always something special in the manner of its action which differentiates it from these, and gives it an individual character. Such specialty may sometimes be capable of rational description; but more commonly, perhaps, it will reside in certain symptomatic phenomena which can only be given as they are observed, without attempt at explanations of their meaning. To these belong the facts about drug-action known as " characteristics "

* *Magazin für physiol. und klinisch. Arzneim. und Toxikol.* 4 vols. Leipzig, 1845 – 54.

and "key-notes," which have been largely used in homœopathising of late, especially in America. Their foremost
advocate is Dr. Guernsey, of Philadelphia; and I know no
better exposition of their true place and value than a paper
upon them from his pen contained in the third volume of the
Hahnemannian Monthly. They are shown there to be no
substitutes for the " totality of symptoms " required by Hahnemann in the comparison between drug-action and disease,
but ancillary only thereto, in suggesting the remedy which
shall be found to contain this totality, or in determining
the choice between several candidates for the post of the
similimum. For our present purpose, in giving an *à priori*
view of medicines, these characteristics have been aptly
compared to personal peculiarities which, as much as outline
and feature, conduce to the recognition of any one, and, in
the case of there being others like him, aid in his distinguish-
ment. I shall indeed lay much more stress upon outline and
feature, complexion and manner ; but I shall not neglect any
" trick o' the voice," any habitual working of the lips or twitch
of the eyelids which may serve in cases of difficulty to identify
the individual. Nor may we despise such characteristics
because of their seeming triviality. It may appear a small
thing (the illustration is Dr. Guernsey's) to say that Cina
is indicated in metrorrhagia when the patient is given to
picking the nose ; but when we remember the occasional
dependence of this symptom on the presence of worms in the
intestines, the reality of the indication becomes obvious.

Our method will be as follows :—After defining what it is
that we are administering under the common names of the
drugs—Aconite, Arsenic, and so forth—I shall refer you to
the authorities for our knowledge of each. Under this head
will be mentioned the original provings, and any special
sources of information which may exist. Then I shall proceed to describe the pathogenetic influence, and to indicate
the therapeutic uses of the drug. A list of allied medicines
will next be given, with which the drug under study may be
profitably compared. Lastly, I shall touch upon the question
of dose, but only so far as to state whether the lower or higher
dilutions seem to have been most efficacious in the treatment
of disease. The question of the relative superiority of these
is a moot one among us; and I have no pretensions, nor is
this the occasion, to pronounce upon it. But it is a matter of
fact that certain remedies belong almost exclusively to the
partisans of infinitesimals, while others are in chief favour
among those who prefer appreciable fractions of the drug.

Such facts I shall state for what they are worth. They, together with the individual items of experience on record, are the *data* from which all future generalisations must be drawn ; and in the meantime they are hints for practical use.

Here, as elsewhere, you will desire to know whether homœopathic literature possesses any books which you may profitably study in connection with the present course of instruction. There are two well known among us, the *Traité méthodique et pratique de matière médicale et de thérapeutique* of Dr. Espanet of Paris (1861), and the *New and Comprehensive System of Materia Medica and Therapeutics* of our indefatigable American colleague, Dr. Hempel (2nd ed., 1865). The former is brilliant, but its pathogenetic statements have rather too much assumption about them. The latter contains much information ; and, with pruning of many redundancies, and supplying of more deficiencies,* would be a valuable treatise. No commendation of mine, moreover, is needed in introducing to you the posthumous *Lectures on Materia Medica* of the lamented Carroll Dunham, now just given to the world. A smaller and humbler work, yet one in which I cannot but feel an interest, since it is my own, is the *Manual of Pharmacodynamics*. The third edition of this book, containing the lectures given by me at our Hospital in 1875-6, will be the text-book of our present course, which will embrace all that is contained there, with such additions, modifications, and re-arrangements as the progress of knowledge requires.

And here, as there, I must state that what I shall say in no way professes to be a substitute for the Materia Medica itself. It is rather an introduction at first, and then a guide and companion to it. The pathogeneses of the medicines, given in detail therein, I shall present in the way of descriptive outline, of analysis, or (wherever possible) of physiological expression. But the Materia Medica itself is the mine where the treasure, however rough its form, really lies. To indicate the vein where each mineral may be worked, to estimate the value of its yield, to exhibit such of its products as have been obtained and smelted, and especially such as have been applied to use,—this will be my task. If there are any who cannot or will not work the mine for themselves, the knowledge of what I show them out of it will be better than total ignorance. In most of my hearers I hope that the specimens I exhibit will excite a thirst for research on their own part, rather than a less worthy content with the result of the labour of others.

How best to study the Materia Medica—*i.e.*, the catalogues

* See review in *Brit. Journ. of Hom.*, xxiii.

of pathogenetic symptoms—is a question of importance. I would advise you to read three excellent papers on the subject. The first is by Dr. Constantine Hering, in the second volume of the *British Journal of Homœopathy ;* the second by Dr. Dunham, in his tractate entitled *Homœopathy the Science of Therapeutics*, first published in 1863, and now forming the eponymous essay of the first volume of his collected works ; the third by Dr. Madden, read before our Congress of 1870, and printed in the *Monthly Homœopathic Review* of that year. The methods they respectively advocate may be described as those of simple comparison, of physiological analysis, and of pathological relation. Dr. Hering would have us learn to know our medicines as a forester comes to know every tree within his range. Dr. Dunham would impress each upon our minds by penetrating to its inmost character. Dr. Madden would group them around morbid conditions, and study their pathogenetic effects in reference thereto, so that "the knowledge of the entire action of any medicine should be left as the ultimate result of a completed study of pathological phenomena." All these methods have their value. The two former are best suited to those who are yet students, the last to those who are already in practice. Perhaps the comparative method of Dr. Hering may go best with these lectures, as I shall be myself occupying Dr. Dunham's ground in delivering them.

A few words in conclusion upon the nomenclature and pharmaceutics I shall employ in these lectures, which will necessarily be those of homœopathy.

1. If any of you have read much of homœopathic literature, you must have been surprised at our many singularities in the matter of nomenclature. That the liquid now known as hydrochloric acid we style muriatic might be passed over as of little importance. But it seems strange that we should talk of China and Chininum sulphuricum instead of Cinchona and sulphate of quinine, and of Mercurius instead of Hydrargyrum. Still more strange is our retention of the old names kali and natrum, so long superseded in ordinary parlance by potassa and soda. And the apparent uncouthness is crowned by the phraseology used to designate the chemical salts, *e.g.*, Ammonium carbonicum, Antimonium tartaricum, Argentum nitricum, Calcarea phosphorica, Magnesia muriatica, and Natrum sulphuricum. Perhaps, at a first glance, all may not recognise under these titles their old acquaintances carbonate of ammonia, tartar emetic, nitrate of silver, phosphate of lime, chloride of magnesium, and sulphate of soda.

The *explanation* of this singularity is easy to find. At the time when homœopathy first arose, our present nomenclature prevailed throughout Europe. The medicines were proved, and took their places in the Materia Medica, under their ancient names. In this form the converts to the new doctrine received them : under these titles they spoke and thought of them. It would have seemed little less than sacrilege to alter the familiar names because modern chemistry had rechristened its compounds. Perhaps if Germany, the mother-land of our system, had revised the nomenclature of her drugs, other countries might have followed in her wake. But the German Pharmacopœia of either school still retains the ancient names. And so we also have them unaltered ; and even name our newly proved medicines—*e.g.,* Kali bichromicum—according to their analogy.

But the explanation does not in this case contain in itself the *justification* of the usage. If you should feel disposed to protest against the retention of such obsolete and often cacophonous forms, I cannot but sympathise with you ; for I myself felt of much the same mind in the early days of my homœopathy, and I retain my sentiment still. I have contended myself, however, with things as they are for the following reasons :—

1st. Our nomenclature is of historical value ; it tells of the place of our origin, of the rock whence we were hewn and the pit from which we were dug. The preservation of names involving history is much thought of elsewhere ; one must attach some little importance to it here.

2nd. It affords a bond of union to homœopathists in all parts of the world. It is like the Latin language to the learned in the middle ages. Each country is free to revise its pharmacological nomenclature independently ; and, to a great extent, has done so. If a German or French book is translated into English, many of the names of the drugs have to be explained. It is not so in homœopathic literature : we speak a language universally intelligible.

3rd. It is like the Latin tongue, not to the learned only, but to the Church. While the Roman Empire was one, the public Offices were, as a matter of course, recited in Latin. When it fell to pieces, and separate nations, each with its own language, began to rise out of the ruins, some may have desired that the Service-books should be rendered everywhere into the vernacular. But such a step would have been most unwise. The Church held on to her original and unalterable tongue, and would not commit her prayers to the ever changing and endlessly varying dialects of the nations in her communion. The wisdom of her course is obvious; and the retention of our ancient nomenclature rests on the same grounds. Chemistry is perpetually and necessarily changing her names, and the adoption of her suggestions is not simultaneous in all countries. So, while each national Pharmacopœia speaks a drug-dialect of its own, homœopathy holds on to the changeless mother-tongue, and her words are comprehensible by all alike.

You will have anticipated me in suggesting that this parallel must ultimately tell the other way—that a time did come at last when the demand for vernacular Offices of worship was no longer unwise, but most just and righteous; and that so it must be here. I grant it fully. When chemistry has finally made up her mind as to the nature of the compounds she studies, and when the nomenclature she suggests has met with general acceptance, and has stood firm for many years, then it will be our duty to translate our present language into one understanded of the people. To do so earlier would just be to quit our vantage-ground, and commit ourselves to the waves of change and confusion.

That this time has now come has been maintained with much ability by Dr. Hutchinson, in a paper on " Our Nomenclature" in the twenty-fourth volume of the *British Journal of Homœopathy*. I cannot, however, assent to his conclusions. When the latest edition of the British Pharmacopœia converts calomel and corrosive sublimate into the subchloride and perchloride of mercury, after they had so long been known as the chloride and bichloride respectively, I see no permanence yet in chemical nomenclature. For practical purposes, I think it better to go on calling them Mercurius dulcis and Mercurius corrosivus, as we have done from the beginning.

The principles of our nomenclature of the chemical salts are very simple. Instead of making two substantives of the base and the acid, putting the former into the genitive and the latter into the nominative case, we throw the acid into the adjectival form, with an ending in " ic " or " os." Thus, instead of Magnesiæ carbonas, we have Magnesia carbonica; instead of Potassæ arsenis, Kali arsenicosum. For the haloid compounds we use the termination " at," as in Kali iodatum. The last revision of her nomenclature made by chemistry (in the larger use of the terminations " ous " and " ic " to express different degrees of oxidation), is a return in this direction.

II. So much for our nomenclature; and now a few words upon pharmaceutics. I have no intention of entering into the minute details which belong rather to the chemist than to the physician. I just want you to know what it is you are prescribing when you order this attenuation of a vegetable or that of a mineral substance. We have now an excellent Pharmacopœia :* and to this I refer you for the full information of which here I give you an outline.

The object of homœopathic pharmacy is so to prepare each substance that the whole of its active virtues shall be present in a form suitable for administration. In the case of vegetable substances this is always done, when practicable, by expressing the juice of the whole plant, and mixing it with alcohol in which the residue has been steeped for some hours. When the plant can only be procured in the dry state, or when but little juice is obtainable by pressure, a tincture is made from it by percolation. The resulting tincture in each case is arranged to contain the medicinal substance in the proportion of about one part in ten. This is what is dispensed as the "mother-tincture," and is ordinarily represented by the Greek ϕ or θ. From it are prepared the "dilutions," "potencies," or (as best called) "attenuations." The 1st is made by adding one part of the mother-tincture to nine of alcohol ; the 2nd by mixing one part of the 1st with nine of alcohol ; and so on up to the 6th. These dilutions are on what is called the "decimal scale ; " and the 2nd, 4th, and 6th decimal obviously correspond with the 1st, 2nd, and 3rd of a centesimal scale, *i.e.*, in which the dilutions are prepared in the proportion of one to ninety-nine. This latter being the method originally in use, its nomenclature is preferred when practicable. So that throughout these lectures, when an attenuation is mentioned, you will understand that the centesimal scale is intended. When I mean the decimal, I will say so. The usefulness of this latter scale is that it gives us dilutions intermediate between ϕ and 1, and between 1 and 2, which are written 1^x and 3^x respectively. After 3 such intermediate stages are unnecessary, and the further dilution may always be proceeded with upon the centesimal scale.

The mineral substances used in our practice are differently prepared according as they are soluble or not. In the former case the . dilutions are made with water, which is also the vehicle of the mineral acids. The metals themselves, and their insoluble salts, are prepared by the Hahnemannic process of *trituration*. This consists in rubbing up a grain of the substance with nine grains of sugar of milk to form the first trituration, a grain of this with nine grains more of sugar of

* *British Homœopathic Pharmacopœia,* published by the British Homœopathic Society. 1870. 2nd edition, 1876.

milk for the 2nd, and so on to the 6th.   After the 6th decimal
the further dilution is carried on according to the centesimal
scale, and is commonly effected by solution.   A grain of the
3rd trituration is dissolved in fifty drops of water, and to this
are added fifty drops of alcohol.   A drop of this fourth dilution is mixed with ninety-nine drops of alcohol for the fifth
potency, and so on.   Long ago, however, Dr. Madden advised*
that all the potencies of insoluble substances should be prepared by trituration ; and the recommendation is now very
generally carried into effect.

Struck by the remarkable development of medicinal power
obtained by this process of trituration—even such inert bodies
as the metals becoming actively pathogenetic and curative—
Hahnemann was led to employ it in the preparation of several
vegetable substances, as lycopodium and charcoal, with the
result of elevating them to a high rank as medicines.   The
process of trituration is also resorted to in the case of such
products as coral and sponge, and (as an alternative to a
tincture prepared by percolation) of such dry plants or portions of plants as Ipecacuanha and Nux vomica.

The globules or pilules used in homœopathic practice are
small spheres of sugar of milk, prepared by immersion for
some time in the tincture of the drug they are intended to
represent.   The former were introduced by Hahnemann to
reduce still farther the quantity of the drug administered ;
the latter perform no such office, and are employed simply
for convenience.   Both labour under the objection of being
second-hand preparations ; and we cannot desire to furnish an
additional element of uncertainty to a process already so
perilously delicate as that of attenuation.   Tinctures and
triturations are the form in which our drugs are most generally used, and to my mind are greatly preferable to any
other.   The globule, however, is still a useful form in which
to administer medicines to infants.

* British Journal of Homœopathy, v. 372-3.

LECTURE II.

SOURCES OF THE HOMŒOPATHIC MATERIA MEDICA.

In my introductory lecture I spoke briefly of the distinctive
"Materia Medica"—technically so called—of Homœopathy. I
stated that when this phrase is used in our literature, it is not
to be understood of drugs themselves, but of that collection of
their pathogenetic effects—of the derangements they are capable
of causing in the healthy body, by means of which is worked
the principle, "let likes be treated by likes." Some of these
pathogenetic effects are observations of poisonings and over-
dosings, as recorded in general medical literature; but the
great bulk of them are the result of "provings" of the various
drugs on the healthy human body, or of their side effects (so to
speak) when administered as medicines to the sick. Such
collections of drug-symptoms are called "pathogeneses;" and
they have been appearing from time to time in the school of
Hahnemann ever since 1805. The history of the several
publications containing them, and an analysis of the material
presented in each, will constitute the account of the sources of
the Homœopathic Materia Medica which I now design to
bring before you.

1. The earliest volume of the series is that of Hahnemann's
entitled *Fragmenta de viribus medicamentorum positivis, sive
in sano corpore humano observatis*. It was written in Latin, as
its title implies, and published at Leipsic in 1805. A copy of
the original edition, and another of the more elegant form in
which Dr. Quin edited the work in 1834, lie on the table
before you.

The *Fragmenta de viribus* contains pathogeneses of twenty-
seven drugs, which you will see enumerated in the list I now
hand round, with the number of symptoms in each.

C

I.—*Fragmenta de Viribus.*

	Hahnemann.	Obs. of others.
Aconitum napellus	138	.. 75
Acris tinctura (Causticum) . .	30	.. 0
Arnica montana	117	.. 33
Belladonna	101	.. 304
Camphora	73	.. 74
Cantharides	20	.. 74
Capsicum annuum	144	.. 3
Chamomilla	272	.. 3
Cinchona	122	.. 99
Cocculus	156	.. 6
Copaifera balsamum . . .	12	.. 8
Cuprum vitriolatum . . .	29	.. 38
Digitalis	23	.. 33
Drosera	36	.. 4
Hyoscyamus	45	.. 290
Ignatia	157	.. 19
Ipecacuanha	70	.. 13
Ledum	75	.. 5
Melampodium (Helleborus) . .	32	.. 25
Mezereum	62	.. 34
Nux vomica	257	.. 51
Papaver somniferum (Opium) . .	82	.. 192
Pulsatilla	280	.. 29
Rheum	39	.. 13
Stramonium	59	.. 157
Valeriana	25	.. 10
Veratrum album	161	.. 106

You will notice that some of the symptoms of each drug are " observations of others." This does not mean that Hahnemann had as yet any fellow-observers. The " others " are in every case authors from whose writings he has cited. The symptoms for which he himself vouches are such as had come under his own observation as effects of poisoning or excessive dosing, and (in far larger proportion) those which he had obtained by provings on himself and others. " I have instituted experiments," he writes in the preface, " in chief part on my own person, but also on some others whom I knew to be perfectly healthy and free from all perceptible disease."

He gives no information as to his doses or mode of administration. We can shrewdly infer these, however, from the remarks on the proving of medicines made in his essay entitled *The Medicine of Experience*, which was published in the next year (1806). " In order," he writes, " to ascertain the effects of medicinal agents, we must give only one pretty strong dose to the temperate healthy person who is the subject of the experiment ; and it is best to give it in solution. If we wish to ascertain the remaining symptoms which were not revealed by the first trial, we may give to another person, or to the same individual, but to the latter only after the lapse of several days, when the action of the first dose is fully over, a similar or even a stronger portion, and note the symptoms of irritation thence resulting in the same careful and sceptical manner. For medicines that are weaker we require, in addition to a considerable dose, individuals that are healthy, it is true, but of very irritable delicate constitutions." It would thus appear that the symptoms of the *Fragmenta* obtained from provings were the results of single full doses of the several drugs.

Of the twenty-seven drugs which this volume shows to have received Hahnemann's earliest attentions, twenty-two were carried on into his *Reine Arzneimittellehre.* Two—Cuprum and Mezereum—did not reappear till the second edition of his *Chronischen Krankheiten ;* and three—Cantharis, Copaiba, and Valerian—were not again taken up by himself.*

2. Six years now elapsed before Hahnemann published any more pathogeneses. But all this time he must have been diligently working, both in provings and literary researches; for in 1811 appeared the first volume of his *Reine Arzneimittellehre*, containing twelve medicines, six of which were new, the pathogeneses also of those which had already appeared being considerably increased. In 1816 a second volume was published, containing the pathogenetic effects of eight medicines, together with those ascribed to the magnet. This was followed in 1817 by a third, with eight medicines; in 1818 by a fourth, with twelve ; in 1819 by a fifth, with eleven ; and in 1821 by a sixth, with ten.

The first edition of the *Materia Medica Pura* (so we render *Latiné* Hahnemann's name for his book), which I have now described, is a very rare work. I am glad to be able to lay a copy of it before you to-day ; and the table which I now put into your hands will show you its contents as I have done those of the *Fragmenta de viribus.*

---

* Dr. Waring, in his *Bibliotheca Therapeutica* recently published by the New Sydenham Society, speaks of the *Fragmenta* as " the basis of the homœopathic system. However much," he adds, " one may be inclined to differ from the inferences or conclusions drawn by the author from his facts, all must admire the zeal and labour bestowed by Hahnemann in his investigations, as set forth in this work."

II.—*Reine Arzneimittellehre.* 1st ed.

VOL. I. 1811.

	Hahn.		Others.
Belladonna	176	..	474
Dulcamara	31	..	92
Cina	23	..	15
Cannabis sativa	15	..	54
Cocculus	224	..	6
Nux vomica	908	..	53
Opium	114	..	464
Moschus	0	..	39
Oleander	10	..	18
Mercurius	232	..	110
Aconite	206	..	108
Arnica	175	..	55

VOL. II. 1816.

Causticum	99	..	176
Arsenicum	294	..	368
Ferrum	228	..	36
Ignatia	570	..	54
Magnes	243	..	51
,, , North Pole	236	..	14
,, , South Pole	237	..	48
Pulsatilla	971	..	102
Rheum	79	..	115
Rhus	409	..	334
Bryonia	408	..	102

VOL. III. 1817.

Chamomilla	448	..	33
Cinchona	391	..	691
Helleborus	90	..	108
Asarum	14	..	254
Ipecacuanha	144	..	87
Scilla	85	..	201
Stramonium	83	..	463
Veratrum album	307	..	404

VOL. IV. 1818.

Hyoscyamus	103	..	436
Digitalis	63	..	355
Aurum	110	..	203
Guaiacum	26	..	116
Camphor	104	..	240
Ledum	182	..	130
Ruta	23	..	201
Sarsaparilla	34	..	111
Conium	87	..	286
Chelidonium	23	..	128
Sulphur	112	..	49
Argentum	48	..	152

VOL. V. 1819.

					Hahn.		Others.
Euphrasia	.	.	.	.	25	..	90
Menyanthes	.	.	.	.	28	..	269
Cyclamen	.	.	.	.	3	..	197
Sambucus	.	.	.	.	19	..	97
Calcarea acetica	.	.	.	.	0	..	255
Muriatic acid	.	.	.	.	57	..	217
Thuja	.	.	.	.	222	..	287
Taraxacum	.	.	.	.	0	..	209
Phosphoric acid	.	.	.	.	160	..	411
Spigelia	.	.	.	.	95	..	543
Staphisagria	.	.	.	.	210	..	398

VOL. VI. 1821.

					Hahn.		Others.
Angustura	.	.	.	.	93	..	209
Manganum	.	.	.	.	89	..	242
Capsicum	.	.	.	.	277	..	69
Verbascum	.	.	.	.	32	..	143
Colocynth	.	.	.	.	17	..	210
Spongia	.	.	.	.	89	..	227
Drosera	.	.	.	.	124	..	155
Bismuth	.	.	.	.	4	..	97
Cicuta	.	.	.	.	36	—	205
Stannum	.	.	.	.	95	—	457

There are, you will see, sixty-one medicines contained in
these volumes, besides the magnet. Twenty-two of them are,
as I have said, transferred from the *Fragmenta*, but always
with their pathogeneses enlarged : the remaining thirty-nine
are new. There is an important change now manifest, moreover, in the "observations of others." These had hitherto
consisted entirely of citations from authors ; and the description still holds good of them as they appear in the first volume
of the *Reine Arzneimittellehre*. In the five years, however,
which elapsed before the second was published, Hahnemann—
now in Leipsic, and at the zenith of his fame—had gathered
round him a band of disciples, and enlisted them in the task
of proving. Of the eight medicines which appear in the
second volume, seven have contributions from this source ; and
henceforth their presence becomes the invariable rule, and
they form an increasing proportion of the bulk of the pathogeneses.

It is right that the names of the men who thus combined
with Hahnemann to prove drugs on their own persons, and
so to lay, at the sacrifice of their own ease, the foundation

of the future Materia Medica, should be on record. They
are as follows, arranged alphabetically :—

Ahner.	Hartmann.	Mossdorf.
Anton.	Hartung.	Rosazewsky.
Baehr.	Haynel.	Rückert (two).
Becher.	Hempel.	Stapf.
Clauss.	Herrmann.	Teuthorn.
Cubitz.	Hornburg.	Urban.
Franz.	Kummer.	Wagner.
Gross.	Langhammer.	Wahle.
Günther.	Lehmann (two).	Walther.
Gutmann.	Meyer.	Wenzel.
Fr. Hahnemann.	Michler.	Wislicenus.
Harnisch.	Möckel.	

Of these thirty-seven names, some occur comparatively
rarely among the provers, but some with great frequency. Of
the latter I may specify Franz, Gross, Hahnemann's son
Friedrich, Hartmann, Herrmann, Hornburg, Langhammer,
Rückert the elder, Stapf, Teuthorn, and Wislicenus. From
the accounts we have of these ·men* we seem generally
warranted in full dependence on the symptoms they have
furnished. Of the few exceptions to this rule, the mental and
moral symptoms of Langhammer are the chief. This prover,
deformed in body and unfortunate in his circumstances, is
represented by those who knew him as so depressed and altogether morbid in disposition, that his psychical state could at
no time be fairly ascribed to the medicine he was taking.
His moral symptoms are, as Dr. Roth has shown,† of a very
similar character under every drug he proved ; and they must,
I think, be held as doubtful unless confirmed from purer
sources. It has also been noted that every drug proved by
Stapf and von Gersdorff excited in the former erotic manifestations, in the latter flatuosities ; so that such symptoms in
them are of dubious connection with the medicaments taken.‡

Of the pains taken by Hahnemann to ensure the genuineness
of his symptom-lists we have abundant evidence. He himself writes thus, in the preface to the latest edition of his
first volume :—

"In those experiments which have been made by myself
and my disciples, every care has been taken to secure the

* See *Allg. Hom. Zeit.*, xxxviii and xxxix., and *Brit. Journ. of Hom.*, xxxii., 451.
† See *Brit. Journ. of Hom*. xix, 625.
‡ See also my remarks on F. Hahnemann's contributions to the pathogenesis of Mercurius solubilis.

true and full action of the medicines. Our provings have been made upon persons in perfect health, and living in contentment and comparative ease.

"When an extraordinary circumstance of any kind—fright, chagrin, external injuries, the excessive enjoyment of any one pleasure, or some event of great importance—supervened during the proving, then no symptom has been recorded after such an event, in order to prevent spurious symptoms being noted as genuine.

"When such circumstances were of slight importance, and could hardly be supposed to interfere with the action of the medicine, the symptoms have been placed in brackets, for the purpose of informing the reader that they could not be considered decisively genuine."

To this we may add the testimony of one of the later accessions to the band of disciples—one who still lives, the venerable Constantine Hering, of Philadelphia :—

"Hahnemann's way of conducting provings was the following. After he had lectured to his fellow-workers on the rules of proving, he handed them the bottles with the tincture, and when they afterwards brought him their day-books, he examined every prover carefully about every particular symptom, continually calling attention to the necessary accuracy in expressing the kind of feeling, the point or the locality, the observation and mentioning of everything that influenced their feelings, the time of day, &c. When handing their papers to him, after they had been cross-examined, they had to affirm that it was the truth and nothing but the truth to the best of their knowledge, by offering their hands to him— the customary pledge at the universities of Germany instead of an oath. This was the way in which our master built up his Materia Medica."

Of the doses used and the mode of administration employed in these later provings, we have no more information than we had as to those of the *Fragmenta*. From the few glimpses we get here and there it seems probable that insoluble substances were proved in the first trituration, and vegetable drugs in the mother tincture—repeated small doses being taken until some effect was produced.

3. In 1822 Hahnemann began to issue a "second, augmented edition" of his *Arzneimittellehre*. It appeared volume by volume, like the first, in the years 1822, 1824, 1825 (two), 1826, and 1827 respectively. Each contained the same list of medicines as before, save that in the sixth Ambra and Carbo animalis and vegetabilis were introduced for the first time.

Of the extent to which the augmentation has been carried you will best form an estimate by looking at the table I now pass round.

III.—*Reine Arzneimittellehre.*

Medicine.	1st Edition.		2nd Edition.	
	Hahn.	Others.	Hahn.	Others.
Acidum muriaticum . . .	57	217	61	218
Acidum phosphoricum . .	160	411	268	411
Aconite	206	108	246	183
Ambra	—	—	141	349
Angustura	93	209	96	203
Argentum	48	152	64	175
Arnica	175	55	278	314
Arsenicum	294	368	431	517
Asarum	14	254	16	254
Aurum	110	203	173	205
Belladonna	176	474	380	1042
Bismuth	4	97	11	97
Bryonia	408	102	537	244
Calcarea acetica . . .	0	255	34	236
Camphor	104	240	105	240
Cannabis	15	54	42	266
Capsicum	277	69	275	69
Carbo animalis	—	—	159	32
Carbo vegetabilis . . .	—	—	276	447
Causticum	99	176	106	201
Chamomilla	448	33	461	33
Chelidonium	23	128	28	128
Cicuta	36	205	36	205
Cina	33	15	40	247
Cinchona	391	691	427	716
Cocculus	224	6	330	224
Colocynthis	17	210	26	224
Conium	87	286	89	286
Cyclamen	3	197	5	197
Digitalis	63	355	73	355
Drosera	124	155	132	155
Dulcamara	31	92	52	297
Euphrasia	25	90	37	90
Ferrum	228	36	249	41
Guaiacum	26	116	29	116
Helleborus	90	108	92	196
Hepar sulphuris . . .	182	24	282	24
Hyoscyamus	103	436	104	478
Ignatia	570	54	620	54
Ipecacuanha	144	87	146	87
Ledum	182	130	186	152
Magnes—*sud* und *nord* . .	716	113	861	372

Medicine.	1st Edition.		2nd Edition.	
	Hahn.	Others.	Hahn.	Others.
Manganum	89	242	89	242
Menyanthes	28	269	28	267
Mercurius	232	110	663	761
Moschus	0	39	2	150
Nux vomica	908	53	1198	69
Oleander	10	18	16	336
Opium	114	464	119	519
Pulsatilla	971	102	1046	117
Rheum	79	115	94	115
Rhus	409	334	575	361
Ruta	23	201	26	262
Sambucus	19	97	20	99
Sarsaparilla	34	111	34	111
Scilla	85	201	86	202
Spigelia	95	543	130	542
Spongia	89	227	156	235
Stannum	95	457	204	456
Staphisagria	210	398	283	438
Stramonium	83	463	96	473
Sulphur	112	49	755	62
Taraxacum	0	209	0	264
Thuja	222	287	334	300
Veratrum	307	404	315	401
Verbascum	32	143	32	141

It will be noticed that the chief increase has taken place in the medicines of the first volume, and here mainly in the "observations of others." This is easily accounted for. In the first edition, as we have seen, this volume contains no contributions from fellow-provers. But when its medicines reappear in the second edition, their pathogeneses have been freely supplied from this source, and are largely augmented accordingly.

Hahnemann's own additions, moreover, occur most largely in the medicines of the earlier volumes of the series. Four only of those contained in the fifth volume, and two only of the sixth, have their pathogeneses notably increased in his section of the symptoms. We may be glad that it is so, for Hahnemann had now been driven from Leipsic, and since 1821 had been living in solitude and obscurity at Cœthen. Entering upon the eighth decade of his life, he was too old for further experimentation on his own person; and he had no other material at hand. We shall see, when we come to the pathogeneses of the *Chronic Diseases*, that his main source of symptoms at this time was the supposed effect upon the sick of the medicines he administered to cure their chronic maladies. We shall see, moreover, that his avowed prepossessions and actual mode of practice in this matter make all symptoms so obtained by him of dubious value. We are glad, therefore, that most of his additions to the second edition are referable to the Leipsic instead of the Cœthen period, and may be counted as homogeneous with the unmistakeably genuine matter of the first edition.

It is time now that I should speak of the citations from authors, which occupy so large a space in many of the pathogeneses, and are entirely absent from but very few. This table will exhibit the number of symptoms due to such sources in the various pathogeneses of the *Reine Arznei-mittellehre*.

IV.—*Citations from Authors.*

Acidum muriaticum	22	Helleborus	54
Aconite	110	Hepar sulphuris	10
Argentum nitricum	8	Hyoscyamus	355
Arnica	47	Ignatia	15
Arsenicum	382	Ipecacuanha	41
Asarum	6	Ledum	4
Aurum	6	Magnes	195
Belladonna	475	Manganum	1
Camphor	93	Menyanthes	3
Cannabis	47	Mercurius	139
Capsicum	4	Moschus	39
Carbo animalis	3	Nux vomica	48
Chamomilla	3	Oleander	10
Chelidonium	6	Opium	518
Cicuta	37	Pulsatilla	25
Cina	11	Rheum	14
Cinchona	141	Rhus	49
Cocculus	6	Ruta	3
Colocynth	29	Sambucus	1
Conium	155	Sarsaparilla	4
Cyclamen	1	Scilla	30
Digitalis	131	Spigelia	17
Drosera	3	Stannum	5
Dulcamara	83	Stramonium	383
Euphrasia	2	Sulphur	10
Ferrum	37	Veratrum	247
Guaiacum	3		

The medicines which are omitted from the list, as having no citations from authors attached to them, are Acidum phosphoricum, Ambra, Angustura, Bismuth, Bryonia, Calcarea acetica, Carbo vegetabilis, Causticum, Spongia, Staphisagria, Taraxacum, Thuja, and Verbascum—thirteen only. Of the remainder, you will see that many are abundantly supplied from this source, whose value it is therefore of importance to ascertain.

I have said that these symptoms are taken from observations of poisoning or of over-dosing. But it makes a great difference to which of the two classes they belong. If they are from poisoning, their subject will ordinarily be a healthy one, and all is well. If they are from over-dosing—real or supposed—they must have occurred in sick persons who were taking the drugs as medicines ; and here an element of uncertainty comes in. There can be no doubt, indeed, that, with proper precautions, the pathogenetic effects of a drug may be observed upon patients taking it for their ailments almost as well as upon healthy subjects. Some of our best records of the effects of Atropia—as those of Grandi and Michéa—have been made from epileptics treated by it. The disease must be of a definite and limited character, consistent with fair general health ; all symptoms conceivably resulting from it, or occupying the same seat, must be excluded, and likewise all phenomena previously observed in or by the patient during his ill health.

Nor did Hahnemann fail to recognise the necessity of such precautions to obtain even a tolerable result, as is evident from his preface to the first volume of the *Reine Arzneimittellehre*. He there writes :—" Among the observations of others which are mingled with the following symptoms some were obtained from sick persons. However, inasmuch as they were chronic patients, with symptoms well known, these last need not be confounded with the effect produced by the medicines, as Greding has shown and carefully exemplified. Symptoms observed upon such patients, therefore, are not without value, and may at any time serve for corroboration when analogous or identical symptoms appear among the pure effects of the drugs in healthy persons." He also says, in his *Medicine of Experience* (1806) : " how, even in diseases, amid the symptoms of the original disease, the medicinal symptoms may be discovered, is a subject for the exercise of a higher order of inductive minds, and must be left solely to masters in the art of observation." This statement stands unchanged in the last edition of the *Organon* (1833) ; and a note is added to the words " medicinal symptoms," explaining them to be such as " during the whole course of the disease might have been

observed only a long time previously, or never before ; consequently new ones belonging to the medicines."

We, then, acknowledging Hahnemann a " master in the art
of observation," and seeing how sound were the canons he
professed, might have taken without question the symptoms he
has cited in his pathogeneses, even though they were obtained
from the sick. But, unfortunately for our trustfulness, he has
given us by his references the means of testing his practice in
the matter ; and the result is by no means favourable.

Let us first take Greding, as one whom Hahnemann mentions by name as a typical instance of care in distinguishing
between medicinal and morbid symptoms. It is the way of
this writer to give a series of cases of the same disease treated
by a particular drug, recording all the phenomena noticed in
the patient during its administration. He sometimes, but not
always, in summarising the results, indicates which of the
symptoms recorded may or may not be fairly referred to the
drug. Now, when he does so, Hahnemann does not necessarily follow him. When treating some epileptics with Cuprum,
one, immediately after swallowing the pill, lost sense and
thought for a short time ; and another, who suffered from
piles, had hæmorrhage from them for four days together
These, Greding with good sense writes, " huic remedio nequâ-
quam tribui posse videntur." But they appear (S. 15 and 208)
in Hahnemann's pathogenesis as effects of Cuprum. Again,
this author narrates the treatment of twenty-three epileptics
and epilepto-maniacs by Belladonna. One would expect that
any symptoms taken from such a source would steer very
clear of epileptiform and maniacal phenomena. Yet from one
of them we have S. 1322 ("with a sudden cry, he trembles in
the hands and feet "), which Dr. Russell, in his *Clinical Lectures*,
cites as contributing to the evidence for the homœopathicity of
Belladonna to epilepsy ;* and the forms of mental disturbance
standing as S. 1375, 1376, 1377, and 1387 are all taken from
maniacs or melancholics. Once more, Greding treats three
cases of jaundice with Belladonna. Two of them have green
stools during the transition from clayeyness to their natural
tint ; but this phenomenon stands (S. 703, 704) among the
effects of the drug on the healthy. Lastly, I would refer you
to the account I have given in the seventeenth volume of the
Monthly Homœopathic Review of the cases treated by Greding
with Aconite, from which Hahnemann has taken symptoms.
One was a female maniac, and, not unnaturally, showed signs
of her disorder at the monthly period. Hahnemann tells us

* See also S. 1374.

(S. 252) that Aconite causes "rage at the time of the appearance of the menses." Another has, as part of a chronic ailment, a troublesome cough. S. 353 belongs to him, and speaks of "frequent cough" as if a part of the effect of the drug.

I need go no farther to show that the use Hahnemann has made of Greding's records has no countenance from that observer himself, and is of a most questionable character. Let us take another author of the same stamp, the famous Baron Störck. His cases treated by Aconite are summarised in the paper to which I have already referred. In one of these a "considerable tumour in the left iliac region" diminished and finally disappeared under the action of the drug, with an accompanying discharge from the vagina of a viscous yellowish matter in abundance. Hahnemann (S. 251) sets down "profuse, tenacious, yellowish leucorrhœa" as caused by Aconite! But the most curious facts in relation to this author belong to his celebrated reports of the use of Conium in cancer. He repeatedly states that no bad effects were observed from the doses he gave; and his recorded cases, as well as our subsequent knowledge of the drug, seem to bear out the assertion. Hahnemann, however, cannot believe this; and so the pathogenesis of Conium contains thirty-three symptoms, to which the name of Störck is attached. The following are specimens of them. A patient with mammary cancer coughs and brings up pus before she dies. As might have been expected, her lungs are found invaded by the disease; but "purulent expectoration" and "a pain shoots into the ulcers when coughing" are contributions from her to the pathogenesis of Conium. Another sufferer with the same disease gets a chill in the street while selling fruit on a cold, windy day, has colic and purging, and finally dysentery, of which she dies. "Violent belly-ache with chill" and "weakening diarrhœa" are extracted from the narrative as effects of the Conium she was taking. Another had a group of symptoms deemed traceable to overloading of the stomach, and which all disappeared after an emetic; but they swell the pathogenesis of Conium.

I could mention numerous facts of the same order. Most of the cited symptoms of Arnica were observed upon injured persons treated by it, or paralytics recovering under its use, and they belong, as a rule, solely to the bruised or powerless parts. To Antimonium crudum are credited a number of phenomena which are obviously the mechanical effects of the violent vomiting caused by it. All the bad results ascribed to suppressing agues by bark, as dropsy, jaundice, phthisis

and the like, are given us as pure effects of Cinchona, though
they never occurred in any but aguish subjects. The critical
evacuant phenomena with which Dulcamara, in the hands of
Carrére, accomplished the cure of gout, rheumatism, cutaneous
disease, and suppression of the latter or of the secretions—the
eruptions, diarrhœas, sweatings, and urinary depositions which
accompanied the subsidence of the symptoms—are set down
by Hahnemann as pure pathogenetic effects of the drug. It
is needless to go farther. The principles on which he selects
the true medicinal symptoms from among those of the disease
are not such as we can approve at this day.

It has been suggested that Hahnemann must have employed
others in this part of his collection, and hence is not charge-
able with their errors. I wish it could be proved so to have
been ; but there is an entire lack of evidence for the supposition. I believe that the real explanation lies in the exaggerated
notions he was led to entertain of the potency of drugs. In
the later *Organon,* he lays down the canon (§ cxxxviii) that
" all the sufferings, accidents, and changes of the health of the
experimenter during the action of a medicine (provided the
proper conditions are complied with) are solely derived from
this medicine, and must be regarded and registered as belonging peculiarly to this medicine, as symptoms of the medicine,
even though the experimenter had observed, a considerable
time previously, the spontaneous occurrence of similar phenomena in himself." He seems to have entertained the same
principle in his mind as regards the administration of drugs in
disease, and to have considered " all the sufferings, accidents,
and changes of health " of the patient as " solely derived from
the medicine " he was taking.

It is clear, then, that before you can use with any reliance
the symptoms cited by Hahnemann from authors, you must
know whether they are taken from narratives of poisoning of
the healthy, or whether they were observed upon the sick ; and
if of the latter kind, under what circumstances they appeared.
In Dr. Allen's *Encyclopædia,* and in the new translation of the
Reine Arzneimittellehre issued by the Hahnemann Publishing
Society, are contained the results of an examination of the
originals of all Hahnemann's cited symptoms. Under the
head of the authority for each is given all available information
regarding the circumstances under which the observation was
made. The symptoms themselves, thus illuminated to their
utmost, are also corrected, or (in Dr. Allen's work) bracketed
as dubious, whenever required ; so that you will know exactly
what you are about in making use of them.

4. I have only a few words to say upon the two remaining volumes of *Reine Arzneimittellehre* which stand upon the table. They are the commencement of a third edition, and bear the dates of 1830 and 1833 respectively. This new edition was not wanted, and it stopped there.

The two volumes contain the same medicines as before, save that Causticum is omitted from the second, having been transferred to the *Chronic Diseases*, the first edition of which was now published. The pathogeneses are somewhat increased in most instances. When the new symptoms are but thirty or forty in number, they are usually Hahnemann's own, *i.e.,* observed upon the sick. When they are more numerous, they will be the result of some fresh provings, which are mentioned in the preface. But the chief change which has taken place has been the amalgamation of all the symptoms of Hahnemann's own observations with those of others into one continuous schema. This was done, Dr. Hering tells us, under pressure from his disciples, and against his own judgment. However, it continued to characterise all his pathogeneses from this time forward.

5. Our attention is now claimed by another collection of pathogeneses from the same author—those contained in the work entitled *Die chronischen Krankheiten*, that is, Chronic Diseases.

You will remember that in 1821 Hahnemann had been compelled to leave Leipsic, and, in difficulty where to find a place in which he could practise in freedom, had been offered an asylum in the little country town of Cœthen. Thither he repaired, and there he remained till his removal to Paris in 1835. He now ceased to attend acute disease, save in the family of his patron, the reigning Duke. But his fame brought him for consultation chronic sufferers from all parts; and the varied, shifting, and obstinate morbid states under which so many men and women labour were pressed closely upon his attention. It is not my place here to tell you of the facts and reasonings which led him to his celebrated theory of chronic disease, namely, that it was always the outcome of one of three infections—the psoric, the syphilitic, and the sycosic. The point of interest to us at present is, that to meet the multiform disorders induced by the first of these miasms it seemed to him that a new set of remedies were required. For, in the years from 1828 to 1830, there appeared from his pen the four volumes, now before you, of the first edition of the *Chronischen Krankheiten ;* the last three of which (the first being devoted to an exposition of his theory) contained pathogeneses of medicines hitherto strange to his *Reine Arzneimittellehre*, and (in some cases) to any Materia Medica whatever.

These new medicines are seventeen in number, and are as follows :

Ammonium carbonicum.	Natrum carbonicum.
Baryta carbonica.	Natrum muriaticum.
Calcarea carbonica.	Nitri acidum.
Graphites.	Petroleum.
Iodium.	Phosphorus.
Kali carbonicum.	Sepia.
Lycopodium.	Silica.
Magnesia carbonica.	Zincum.
Magnesia muriatica.	

All these, save Kali carbonicum and Natrum muriaticum, are contained in the second and third volumes of the work, and follow in the alphabetical order of their (Latin) names. The fourth volume was evidently an after-thought. It contains—in this succession—Carbo animalis and vegetabilis, Causticum, Conium, Kali carbonicum, Natrum muriaticum, and Sulphur ; five of which medicines will be recognised as having already appeared in the *Reine Arzneimittellehre*.

Another difference, moreover, is manifested in the seven medicines of the fourth volume. The pathogeneses of those of the second and third are introduced without a word of explanation, and no fellow-observers are acknowledged. But of the two new medicines of the fourth volume—Kali carbonicum and Natrum muriaticum—we are told that two persons co-operated in obtaining the pathogenesis of the one and three in that of the other, and that the symptoms of the latter were produced on healthy persons taking globules saturated with the 30th dilution. Fresh associates also are acknowledged in the case of Conium. The difference evidently is that the first list of medicines was compiled, and their symptom-lists completed, as part of the original scheme of the work ; but that their publication brought fellow-workers to Hahnemann's aid, and thus—and through the later recognition of other medicines as " anti-psorics "—evoked the additional volume. This, indeed, bears the date of 1830, while the other three were all published in 1828.

In estimating, then, the character and value of the pathogeneses of the first edition of the *Chronischen Krankheiten*, I must speak of those of the second and third volumes separately from .those of the fourth, as belonging to different categories. The last, indeed, so entirely correspond with the distinctive features of the second edition of the work, that I shall say nothing of them till I come to that.

The pathogeneses of the fifteen drugs contained in the second and third volumes appear (as I have said) without a word of explanation as to how the symptoms were obtained, and without acknowledgment (as there is in the *Reine Arznei-mittellehre*) of fellow-observers. The absence of any co-operation on the part of others is further to be inferred from what we are told of the first announcement of the work. After six years of solitude at Cœthen, Hahnemann "summoned thither his two oldest and most esteemed disciples, Drs. Stapf and Gross, and communicated to them his theory of the origin of chronic diseases, *and his discovery of a completely new series of medicaments for their cure.*" So writes Dr. Dudgeon. This was in 1827. That he should now first reveal these new remedies, and in the following year should publish copious lists of their pathogenetic effects, confirms the inference to be drawn from his position and from his silence as to fellow-observers. He was himself between seventy and eighty years old, and it is hardly likely that he did anything in the way of proving upon his own person. We are compelled to the conclusion that he drew these symptoms mainly—if not entirely—from the sufferers from chronic disease who flocked to his retreat to avail themselves of his treatment.

The prefatory notices to the several medicines still further substantiate this view, and throw some light on the doses with which the symptoms were obtained. He recommends all the medicines to be given in the dilutions from the 18th to the 30th (save Magnesia muriatica and Natrum carbonicum, of which he advises the 6th and 12th respectively); and repeatedly makes some such remark as this :—" For a long time past I have given the 6th, 9th, and 12th potencies, but found their effects too violent." Occasionally, too, he must have used the second and third triturations ; as he speaks of having begun by giving a "small portion of a grain" of these, but, as this was an indefinite quantity, having subsequently dissolved and attenuated them. He mentions cases, moreover, in which he treated itch with Carbo vegetabilis and Sepia of the latter strength.

We conclude, therefore, that it is these "violent effects" of the attenuations from the second to the twelfth, experienced by the sufferers from chronic disease who took them, which make up the bulk—if not the whole—of the symptoms of the first edition of the *Chronischen Krankheiten.*

D

6. The second edition of the work was published in successive parts—five in all—between 1835 and 1839.* Besides the twenty-two medicines of the first edition it contains twenty-five others, of which thirteen are new, and twelve had already appeared in the *Reine Arzneimittellehre.* The new ones are—

Agaricus.	Cuprum.
Alumina.	Euphorbium.
Ammonium muriaticum.	Mezereum.
Anacardium.	Nitrum.
Antimonium crudum.	Platina.
Borax.	Sulphuris acidum.
Clematis.	

The old ones are—

Arsenicum.	Hepar sulphuris.
Aurum.	Manganum.
Colocynth.	Muriatis acidum.
Digitalis.	Phosphori acidum.
Dulcamara.	Sarsaparilla.
Guaiacum.	Stannum.

The ιogeneses appear in one continuous list, as in the third edition of the *Reine Arzneimittellehre.* Those which had already seen the light have (generally) large additions : for all he acknowledges contributions from fellow-observers,† and for many cites symptoms from the extant literature of his day.

The tables I now lay before you exhibit these facts, and enable the history and growth of each medicine to be ascertained at a glance.

* Parts 1 and 2 in 1835 ; parts 3, 4, and 5, in 1837, 1838, and 1839 respectively.

† These associates are fewer than they were in the days of the *Reine Arzneimittellehre,* and are taken from a fresh set of men. Their names are Adam, Apelt, Bethmann, Brunner, Bute, Caspari, Foissac, von Gersdorff, Goullon, Hartlaub, Haubold, Hering, Jahr, Lesquereur, Kretschmar, Nenning, Piepors, Röhl, Rummel, Schönke, Schreter, Schweikert, Seidel, Tietze, Trinks, Wahle, Woost. Many of these names appear only once or twice. Wahle's is the only one found also in the older work.

Name.	Materia Medica Pura.	Chronic Diseases. Ed. I.	Chronic Diseases. Ed. II.
Agaricus	—	—	715
Alumina	—	—	1161
Ammonium carbonicum .	—	159	789
Ammonium muriaticum .	—	—	397
Anacardium . . .	—	—	622
Antimonium crudum . .	—	—	471
Arsenicum	1079	—	1231
Aurum	376	—	461
Baryta carbonica. . .	—	286	794
Borax	—	—	460
Calcarea	269	1090	1631
Carbo vegetabilis. . .	720	930	1189
Carbo animalis . . .	191	191	728
Causticum	307	1014	1505
Clematis	—	—	150
Colocynth	250	—	283
Conium	375	700	912
Cuprum	—	—	397
Digitalis	428	—	702
Dulcamara	401	—	409
Euphorbium . . .	—.	—	281
Graphites	—	590	1144
Guaiacum	145	—	160
Hepar sulphuris . . .	307	—	661
Iodium	—	133	624
Kali carbonicum . . .	—	938	1650
Lycopodium . . .	—	891	1608
Magnesia carbonica . .	—	128	890
Magnesia muriatica . .	—	69	749
Manganum	331	—	469
Mezereum	—	—	610
Muriatic acid . . .	279	—	574
Natrum carbonicum . .	—	306	1082
Natrum muriaticum . .	—	897	1349
Nitric acid	—	803	1424
Nitrum	—	—	710
Petroleum	—	623	776
Phosphorus	—	1025	1915
Phosphoric acid . . .	679	—	818
Platina	—	—	527
Sarsaparilla . . .	145	—	561
Sepia	—	1242	1655
Silica	—	567	1193
Stannum	660	—	648
Sulphur	815	1041	1969
Sulphuric acid . . .	—	—	521
Zincum	—	723	1375

Number of symptoms cited from Authors.

Name.	Total symptoms.	Cited symptoms.
Agaricus	715	21
Anacardium . . .	622	3
Antimonium crudum . .	471	71
Arsenicum	1231	382
Aurum	461	6
Baryta	799	4
Clematis	150	6
Colocynth	283	29
Conium	912	155
Cuprum	397	154
Digitalis	702	131
Dulcamara . . .	409	83
Euphorbium . . .	281	22
Guaiacum	160	3
Hepar sulphuris . .	661	11
Iodium . . .	624	348
Mezereum . . .	610	34
Muriatic acid . . .	574	16
Nitric acid . . .	1424	30
Nitrum . . .	710	122
Phosphorus . . .	1915	84
Sarsaparilla . . .	561	4
Stannum . . .	648	5
Sulphur	1969	10
Sulphuric acid . . .	521	8

There are, it is evident, some fresh features in the pathogeneses of the second edition of the *Chronic Diseases ;* and
there are more than appear on the surface.   Hahnemann was
able, at this time, to draw upon other sources than those I
have hitherto specified.   Hartlaub and Trinks had published
an *Arzneimittellehre* of their own.   Stapf had begun to issue
his journal called the *Archiv ;* and many provings, made
more or less independently of Hahnemann, adorned its pages.
And, while these pathogenetic materials were accumulating
in the homœopathic school, outside of it Professor Joerg, of
Leipsic, was following in Hahnemann's track, and proving
medicines on himself and his students.   Hahnemann availed
himself of all these materials, incorporating them with his
own observations and those of the fellow-observers he acknowledges.   In my future lectures I shall take pains to specify
the proportion in which these several elements exist in the
pathogenesis of each medicine, and of their sources themselves I shall speak at our next meeting.   Hahnemann's own
additions to the second issue of his work must be of the
same character as his contributions to the first, *i.e.*, they must
be collateral effects of the drugs observed on the patients to

whom he gave them. They must all, moreover, be supposed to have resulted from the 30th dilution; for since 1829 Hahnemann had urged the administration of all medicines at this potency. The same thing must be said of the contributions of Hahnemann's friends to this edition. They may fairly be conceived to have been provings on themselves or other healthy persons, save where, as in Wahle's symptoms of Mezereum and Hering's of Arsenic, the internal evidence is strong in the contrary direction. But they must in all cases have been evoked from the 30th dilution; for in the edition of the *Organon* published in 1833 Hahnemann recommends all provings to be made therewith, as yielding the best results. In the preface to Natrum muriaticum in the fourth volume of the first edition of the *Chronic Diseases* he states that the symptoms of that medicine were so obtained; and we may fairly extend the inference to all provings subsequently made.

It thus appears that a large proportion of the symptoms contained in the final recension of the *Chronic Diseases* are effects, real or supposed, of very infinitesimal doses—of the potencies from the sixth to the thirtieth of the centesimal scale. This is an altogether new element of our pathogeneses, one which has not encountered us as we have been studying the *Materia Medica Pura*. It may fairly be demanded what evidence we have in support of the assumption made in these symptom-lists, viz., that infinitesimal portions of drugs, from the billionth to the decillionth of a grain, have the power of affecting the healthy organism.

Now into this question I propose to enter on a subsequent occasion, when I shall discuss the infinitesimals of homœopathy. I shall then adduce evidence which will, I think, satisfy your minds—as it does my own—that there is nothing in the fact that the symptoms before us were chiefly obtained with such doses which need discredit them as genuine effects of the drugs administered; though it does give them a special place and character. But there is another element in Hahnemann's own contributions, at least, to these pathogeneses, which is novel. I have shown that his symptoms must be presumed to have been observed upon patients taking the medicines, and not upon healthy persons proving them. Here, again, you will challenge me, and ask what guarantee we have that such symptoms are not effects of the disease existing rather than of the drug being taken.

And here I regret that I cannot meet your challenge. We saw, when upon the *Reine Arzneimittellehre,* how very unsatisfactory was Hahnemann's mode of proceeding in this matter.

We followed him, by means of the references he has given us, to the authors whose observations he cites, many of which were made upon the sick. Here we saw him, as it were, at work among his patients; we noticed the symptoms he selected as resulting from the drug administered, and not from the disease present; we noted their conformity to his own canons and to common sense. The result was to show that his eager desire for symptoms, and his over-estimation of the activity of drugs, had led him in numerous instances to put down as pathogenetic effects phenomena which were obviously those of the disease or of occasional causes. We can have no confidence, but rather the reverse, that he has not followed the same course in his observations upon his own patients. Hence the thousand symptoms of Calcarea and Phosphorus and the twelve hundred of Sepia—all derived from sick persons during the six or seven years of the Cœthen period. The recent re-proving of the latter medicine in America, in which thirty healthy persons took part, has only yielded 517 symptoms as its result.

There is one source especially on which Hahnemann seems to have relied at this time for pathogenetic effects of drugs. I mean aggravations, real or supposed, of the existing symptoms of patients. In 1813, he had written to Stapf :*—" You are right in supposing that the increase by a medicine of symptoms that had been previously present most probably indicates that the medicine given can of itself also excite similar symptoms. *Still, we must not include such symptoms in the list of the pure, positive effects of the medicine, at least not in writing.*" Ægidi's Colocynth case shows how, in the later time, this salutary caution was dropped. A patient labouring long under neuralgia starting from a nephritic complaint, and suffering several times a day from " agonizing pain proceeding from the region of the left kidney down the corresponding limb as far as the outer malleolus," took at 9 a.m. a drop of Colocynth 6. In the evening the patient had, periodically, " a dreadful cutting in the abdomen, proceeding from the left renal region, spasmodically drawing the left thigh up to the body, and forcing the patient to bend herself completely forward." This, at the utmost, was a medicinal aggravation, but it appears as S. 114 of the pathogenesis of Colocynth in the second edition of the *Chronischen Krankheiten.* This suggests how many of the apparently wonderful effects of drugs which experience has proved of little activity (as Natrum carbonicum) were obtained.

* Dudgeon's *Lectures*, p. 181.

I am compelled, therefore, to draw the conclusion that the great bulk of the pathogeneses of the *Chronischen Krankheiten* are not to be relied upon as genuine physiological effects of the drugs. The fact of their being obtained with infinitesimal doses would not at all disqualify them, however much they would stand in need of clinical verification. But their appearance in the sick, after the revelation we have had of Hahnemann's mode of dealing with such symptoms, puts them (to my thinking) utterly without the pale of genuine drug effects. They *may* be such, but we have no means of knowing that they are; and here pathogenetic verification—the reproduction of the same symptoms on the healthy—is required ere we can use them with any confidence in working the rule *similia similibus*.

It is otherwise with the *Reine Arzneimittellehre*. We have in that work a genuine contribution, and the first made on any large scale, to the ascertainment of the physiological effects of drugs, of their action on the healthy human body. Urged as a necessity by Haller, feebly attempted by Störck and Alexander, no real step was taken towards this end till Hahnemann published that *Fragmenta de viribus*, of which the *Reine Arzneimittellehre* is the flower and fruit. Whatever additions have been made to our knowledge since, whatever improvements have been introduced into our methods of obtaining it, this first essay of the kind can never be superseded, and stands as an imperishable record of the wisdom, devotion, and industry of its author. If I have had to criticise here and there, it is not that I less admire. I cordially subscribe to Dr. Dudgeon's panegyric. "I may safely say" (he writes)* "that in the mere labour of the Materia Medica, Hahnemann's own doings are tenfold as great and important as all the labours of all his predecessors and all his followers; that while we might manage to get on though we were deprived of all the provings of every other contributor to our Materia Medica, were we deprived of Hahnemann's observations, and especially his earlier provings, such as those of Belladonna, Aconite, Bryonia, Nux, Pulsatilla, Rhus, Arnica, Mercurius, &c., we might shut up shop at once. In the matter of the Materia Medica, we must all acknowledge that among them that are born of women there hath not arisen a greater than Samuel Hahnemann."

Lectures, p. 241.

LECTURE III.

SOURCES OF THE HOMŒOPATHIC MATERIA MEDICA.

(Continued.)

In the preceding lecture on the sources of the Homœo-pathic Materia Medica I gave you an account of our chief mines of knowledge on this subject—the *Reine Arzneimittel-lehre* and *Chronischen Krankheiten* of Hahnemann. Before proceeding to speak of the other and later contributions to it which go to make up our wealth, I ought to tell how far Hahnemann's pathogeneses have been rendered available to us in our mother tongue.

It is obvious that such work must come either from Great Britain or from America ; and it is a physician practising in the latter country who has given us the only English version of the master's provings we have hitherto possessed. I refer to Dr. Hempel, from whose pen appeared, in 1846, the four volumes of the *Materia Medica Pura* and the five of the *Chronic Diseases* which now stand before you. You have only to open them to find that they fall very far short of reproduc-ing their original. It is perhaps a small matter that the medicines of the *Materia Medica Pura* are re-arranged accord-ing to the alphabetical order of their Latin names. But you will perceive that all names of authorities are omitted, so that for the medicines where the symptoms from all sources are thrown together we have no clue whatever to their origin, and in no case can we distinguish between the results of provings and the observations cited from authors. The pathogeneses in which Hahnemann has separated his own symptoms from those contributed by others are rarely allowed to stand as he left them ; but sometimes (as with Bryonia) the latter are made to follow the former in each division of the schema, enclosed in square brackets for distinctness, sometimes (as with Argen-tum and Camphor) they are thrown together in one series without distinction. The symptoms are printed continuously, instead of in separate paragraphs ; and are divided into sec-tions, with headings according to their subject.

A closer examination will discover still further and more serious faults. The medicines of the second volume of the *Reine Arzneimittellehre* have been translated from the edition of 1824, not—as they should have been—from the later one of 1833. Ferrum and Verbascum have been omitted from this work, doubtless by accident. But we miss from it a number of other medicines, and find by the translator's preface that these include all those which subsequently appeared in the *Chronischen Krankheiten.* The reasons Dr. Hempel assigns for such omissions are incorrect, and, in my judgment, wholly insufficient ; and English readers have lost materially from not having had the articles on these drugs, with their prefaces and annotations, presented to them in their original forms.

A yet graver objection remains behind ; and that is, that the translation is not a faithful one. Dr. Wilson has abundantly proved this in respect of wholesale omission and careless rendering of symptoms, and I must affirm the same as to the presentation of the introductions and notes. *Il va sans dire* that we can never depend upon the version of the cited symptoms, which often suffer materially in their passage from English, French, or Latin into Hahnemann's German, and thence (in ignorance of the originals) into Dr. Hempel's English. I must regretfully say that I have long ceased to have any reliance on this translation, and never venture now to quote Hahnemann as given by Hempel lest I should misrepresent him.

You will find these facts stated in more detail in an article "On the Translations of Hahnemann's Pathogeneses ; with a plea for a new English version," which I published in · the *British Journal of Homœopathy* in 1877. My plea has since been entertained by the Hahnemann Publishing Society of this country, so far as the *Reine Arzneimittellehre* is concerned ; and Dr. Dudgeon, so favourably known by his rendering of the *Organon* and the lesser writings of the master, has undertaken this work also. I have gladly co-operated with him in revising from the originals the quotations made from authors, and supplying to these from the same sources such illumination as they need. The first volume of the work is now before you, and I am sure that you will find it as true a reproduction in detail as you will see it to be in general outline. I hope that, either here or in America, the *Chronischen Krankheiten* will soon be presented in a similar manner ; so that English readers may feel with confidence that they possess Hahnemann's pathogeneses in their own tongue.

I now proceed to tell you of the later contributions which have been made to the Materia Medica of Homœopathy.

1. The first to appear in the field of drug-proving after Hahnemann had led the way was no follower of his, but a professor of the University of Leipsic, Dr. Johann Christian Gottfried Jörg. His academical position gave him pupils to assist him ; and twenty-one of these, with himself, his two young sons, and three females (aged forty-five, eighteen, and twelve respectively), formed his company of provers. He published at Leipsic in 1825 a first volume of the results obtained, under the title of *Materialien zu einer künftigen Heilmittellehre durch Versuche des Arzneyen an gesunden Menschen.* It contained experiments with the following drugs :

Acidum hydrocyanicum (with aqua laurocerasi and aqua amygdalarum amararum).
Arnica (flowers and root).
Asafœtida.
Camphor.
Castoreum.
Digitalis.

Ignatia.
Iodium.
Moschus.
Nitrum.
Opium.
Serpentaria.
Valerian.

All these substances were taken in moderate doses, repeated (and if necessary increased) until a decided impression was made. The experiments of each prover are related in full, just as they were made and as the symptoms occurred. In the preface a description is given of the age, temperament, and constitution of those engaged in the task, and the assurance afforded that all were in good health.

You will see at once that in the mode of giving these provings to the world, Professor Jörg has greatly improved upon Hahnemann. While the latter leaves us in darkness as to the subjects of the provings, the doses taken, and the order and connection in which the symptoms appeared, here all is clear daylight. Of the intrinsic value of the provings the best evidence is that Hahnemann was glad to incorporate them in his own pathogeneses. He seems to have been ignorant of them up to 1833 ; for in the volume of the *Reine Arznei-mittellehre* then published, he credits Jörg's symptoms of Ignatia to Hartlaub and Trinks, who had simply copied them into the collection of theirs of which I shall speak next. But in the second edition of the *Chronischen Krankheiten* (1835-9) he uses Jörg's pathogeneses of Digitalis, Iodium, and Nitrum, referring them to him by name and work.

You have only, I think, to examine these provings to come to the same opinion of their value. You may see the original work in the library of the College of Surgeons ; or may read its experiments in the fourth volume of Frank's *Magazin*, from which, moreover, many of them have been translated by Dr. Hempel in his *Materia Medica*. It is a pity that a volume so rich in instruction and usefulness has not long ago been rendered into English as it stands ; and I commend the work to any competent person who desires to do service to his fellow-homœopathists of the English speech.

2. The next to take up the work of instituting and publishing drug-provings were two distinguished members of the homœopathic school—Drs. Hartlaub and Trinks. They also named their collection *Reine Arzneimittellehre*, evidently intending it to be a sequel to Hahnemann's work. It was published at Leipsic in three volumes, dated 1828, 1829, and 1831 respectively. Each contains an elaborate pathogenesis of certain new medicines, and shorter contributions to the knowledge of others already familiar to homœopathists. The former, like Hahnemann's, are made up of original provings instituted by them and of citations from authors ; the latter are chiefly single provings or cases of poisoning. All are arranged in the usual schematic order ; and there is a great, though not entire, lack of information as to the circumstances of the experiments.

The first volume contains full pathogeneses of Plumbum, Cantharis, Laurocerasus, Phosphorus, and Antimonium crudum, and shorter additions to the symptomatology of eighteen other drugs.

The second volume gives us, in the first category, Gratiola, Oleum animale, Alumina, and Phellandrium, and fourteen medicines in the second.

The third volume introduces to us Bovista, Kali hydriodicum, Ratanhia, Strontian, and Tabacum, and adds to our knowledge of no less than thirty other substances.

As these volumes came into existence between 1828 and 1831, it was obviously open to Hahnemann to avail himself of them for the third edition of his *Reine Arzneimittellehre* (1830-3), and the second of his *Chronischen Krankheiten* (1835-9). This he has done to the fullest possible extent. He has not only used their new provings, but has transferred to his pages the symptoms they have extracted from authors, and in doing so has frequently omitted the references to the work and page, leaving those curious in the matter to refer to Hartlaub and Trinks. I was much hindered in my work of examining the originals of some of his citations until I discovered this practice of his.

I come now to an important and much-questioned feature of Hartlaub and Trinks' pathogeneses—I mean the provings furnished by the person designated as " Ng." On the first occasion of Hahnemann's using their work in his *Chronischen Krankheiten,* viz., in the section on Alumina, he makes in his preface the following remarks :—" With merely these two letters (anonymousness indeed !) Drs. Hartlaub and Trinks designate a man who has furnished the greatest number of symptoms for their *Annalen,* but these often expressed in a careless, diffuse, and indefinite manner." He goes on to say that he has extracted that which was useful from his contributions, believing that he was a truthful and careful person ; but that it was not to be expected that in so delicate and difficult a matter as drug-proving, the homœopathic public would place confidence in an unknown person designated simply as " Ng." This note of Hahnemann's has led to a good deal of mistrust of the symptoms of the anonymous observer in question, which has been increased by their excessive number,— Dr. Roth having counted more than eleven thousand in the several contributions to the Materia Medica furnished by him between 1828 and 1836. So far has confidence been lacking, that the compilers of the earlier parts of the Cypher Repertory have felt themselves warranted in omitting " Ng.'s " symptoms from the materials they have indexed. But there are important considerations on the other side. Dr. Hering has satisfactorily explained the anonymousness. " Ng.," he writes,[*] " was a surgeon near Budweis, in Bohemia, a candid, upright, well-meaning man, not very learned : his name was Nenning, and everybody knew it. According to the laws of his country he had no right to practise except as a surgeon. A lameness of the right arm disabled him from following his calling. His wife commenced a school and instructed girls in millinery ; she supported the family by this. Nenning became acquainted with homœopathy, and soon was an ardent admirer. He had the grand idea to aid the cause by making provings on the girls in his wife's millinery shop. He succeeded in persuading them. Unluckily enough he came in connection with Hartlaub in Leipzig, instead of with Hahnemann himself. All Austrians were forbidden by a strict law to send anything outside of Austria to be printed ; hence not only Nenning, but all other Austrians, appeared in our literature with only initials." Nenning himself has given, in the *Allgemeine Hom.*

[*] See Allen's *Encyclopædia,* III., 640.

Zeitung for 1839, a similar account, to explain the number of his symptoms. "If I have perchance," so he writes, "made too many provings, for it is remarked that I have furnished too many symptoms, that should, in my opinion, deserve sympathy rather than ridicule. The exhortation of Hahnemann not only to enjoy but to put our hand to the work animated my zeal, and the active support of Hartlaub rendered it possible for me to do that which perhaps strikes Hahnemann as surprising. A number of persons, partly related to me, and partly friendly, were gathered together by me, and, in consideration of board and payment, made experiments. Along with them were also my two daughters, and, with complete reliance on the honesty of them all, I gave one medicine to one and another to another, writing down all that they reported. It was a matter of conscience on my part also not to omit the smallest particular ; and that thereby frequent repetitions have arisen I grant readily, but I thought that just in that way the sphere of action of the medicine could be best recognised."

It seems, then, that Nenning's symptoms were obtained in the true way, viz., by provings on the healthy body ; but that the payment of the provers and the want of discrimination exercised in receiving their reports throw some shade of doubt upon the results. I cannot think, however, that they warrant their entire rejection. The only thing which such symptoms need is "clinical verification," testing, that is, by being used as materials wherewith to work the rule *similia similibus curentur*. If, when submitted to this test, they (as a rule) prove trustworthy, we may safely assume them to be genuine, and admissible into the Materia Medica. Now, we have the testimony of three of the most industrious symptomatologists of our school—Bönninghausen, Hering, and Wilson—that they have found no reason to distrust Nenning's symptoms, and have used them as satisfactorily as those of other observers. No statement to the reverse of this has come from the other side ; so that we may accept Nenning's contributions as at least provisionally established to be good and sound additions to our pathogenetic material.

3. The next name on our list is that of Dr. Ernst Stapf. This physician, one of Hahnemann's oldest and most valued disciples, began in 1822 to publish a journal devoted to the interests of the new method. He called it *Archiv für die homöopathische Heilkunst ;* but it is generally known simply as the *Archiv*, or—very often—Stapf's *Archiv*. To this journal the contributions most urgently called for and most

largely furnished were provings of medicines. By the time that fifteen volumes had been published a considerable number of these had accumulated ; and it became desirable to give them a separate form for practical use. Some of them— notably those of Anacardium, Cuprum, Mezereum, and Platina—Hahnemann (who had himself taken part in many of the experiments) designed to use for the second edition of his *Chronic Diseases;* and these Stapf left alone. But the rest—in all containing twelve medicines—he published in 1836 in a volume entitled *Beiträge zur reinen Arzneimittellehre,* *i.e.,* Additions to the *Materia Medica Pura.* The medicines are—

Agnus castus.	Ranunculus	Sabina.
Clematis.	(bulbosus and sceleratus).	Senega.
Coffea.	Rhododendron.	Teucrium.
Crocus.	Sabadilla.	Valerian.

All those as to which any information is given on the point were proved in Hahnemann's earlier manner, *i.e.,* in moderate but substantial doses, generally taken singly. The results are presented in the usual schema form, but with copious reference to the separate experiments of the provers, when these are specified. The introductions to the several medicines are full and interesting, and contain much information about their former uses and about such homœopathic experience as had been gained with them. The whole makes a very valuable volume ; and, as it has been rendered into English by Dr. Hempel, it is available for all students.

4. I have next to speak of the Austrian provings. By the year 1842 homœopathy had come to number many able and active representatives in Vienna; and it seemed to them (in the words of one of their number) " a shame to be stretching their indolent limbs and lolling lazily upon the couch prepared for them by the laborious toil of the master : " they deter- mined to have " courage to tread bravely in his footsteps, and to pursue, with untiring patience, the path he had opened up to them." They considered the most serious obstacle to the practice and advance of the homœopathic method to be the form in which Hahnemann had given his provings to the world, *i. e.,* as a schema of detached symptoms, without infor- mation as to how, or in what order and sequence, they were obtained. They set therefore before themselves, as their main task, the re-proving of medicines, without excluding occasional original experiments.

In pursuance of this object they gave us re-provings of Aconite, Bryonia, Colocynth, Natrum muriaticum, Sulphur, and Thuja; and primary provings of Argentum nitricum, Coccus cacti, and Kali bichromicum. Each drug was entrusted to one member of the society into which they formed themselves, who undertook and superintended the experiments, and published them in full detail, with an elaborate account of all that was known of the medicine up to the time of writing. From twenty to thirty persons took part in every proving; and, though trials of the attenuations were not neglected, the great aim of the experimenters seems to have been the development of the full physiological action of drugs from repeated and increasing doses of the mother-tincture, which, in the case of Thuja, even reached as much as 1000 drops at a time.

The monographs containing these most valuable provings were chiefly published in the *Œsterreichische Zeitschrift für Homöopathie*, a journal conducted by the Austrian Society, which runs through four years. Wurmb's re-proving of Sulphur is contained in a later periodical, the *Zeitschrift des Vereins der homöopathischen Aerzte Œsterreichs* (vols. i and ii). Most of them have been translated into English* with more or less completeness. They will always be ranked among the chief materials we possess for the construction of the Materia Medica of the future; and the labourers at them, of whom we may mention as pre-eminent Watzke, Huber, Mayerhofer, Wachtel, Wurmb, Arneth, Gerstel, and von Zlatarovich, have written their names indelibly on the roll of the heroes of the homœopathic history.

While thus giving prerogative rank to the Austrian provings, it must be added that they are but one instance of the activity of German homœopathy in this field down almost to the present day. Not only Stapf's *Archiv*, but the other journals published in that country, as Hartlaub and Trinks' *Annalen*, Griesselich's *Hygea*, and, later, the *Allgemeine homöopathische Zeitung* and *Vierteljahrschrift*, teem with provings and re-provings. Among the former may be mentioned those of Berberis, Coca, Colchicum, Hypericum, Kreosote, and Nux moschata; among the latter those of Agaricus, Chamomilla, Cyclamen, Chelidonium, and Euphrasia. The men whose names stand out most prominently as conductors of

* Colocynth, Coccus cacti, and Thuja, in Metcalf's *Homœopathic Provings*, Sulphur in the *British Journal of Homœopathy* (vols. xv. and xvi.), and Argentum nitricum as an appendix to Hempel's translation of Stapf's *Beiträge*.

these experiments are Buchmann, Buchner, Helbig, Hencke, Hoppe, Koch, Lembke, and Reil. The last great contribution to the Materia Medica we have received from this source has been Buchmann's Chelidonium ; but an endeavour to have a thorough re-proving of Cuprum has recently been set on foot by the Central Verein, and we hope it may bear good fruit.

Nor has the old school of medicine in Germany been altogether insensible to the exhortations and example of Jörg. Professor Martin, of the University of Jena, has occasionally proved medicines on his students, and published the results obtained : to this source we owe the pathogenesy of Kali chloricum. In 1848 the Vienna Society of Physicians set itself—in emulation of its homœopathic "double"—to make provings. The medicines selected were Arnica, Belladonna, Chamomilla, and Chelidonium ; and each was tested by from five to twelve persons, taking the drugs after the manner of Jörg. Unfortunately, "the committee" (I quote from Dr. Dudgeon's account) "who had the drawing-up of the report of the results of the trials cut down the symptoms of each prover in a most arbitrary manner, and only recorded such symptoms as were common to all or most of the experimenters." One of these, however—Schneller by name—has given a detailed account of his provings of the above-named drugs, and also of some additional experiments instituted on himself with Aconite, Conium, Hyoscyamus, Rheum, and Stramonium. You will find his communication translated in the sixth volume of the *British Journal of Homœopathy*. Besides these, the followers of Rademacher have made a few provings ; their experiments with Ferrum have been translated in the ninth volume of the same journal. More recently Professor Schroff, though giving his attention mainly to experiments with drugs on animals, has not been unmindful of the value of occasionally instituting them on the human subject, and has given us (especially from Aconite) some valuable provings.

Before passing to the other chief scene of homœopathic provings—the United States of America—let me say a few words as to what has been done of the kind in the rest of the countries into which the method of Hahnemann has penetrated.

The only original pathogenesis of note which *France* has given us is that of Quinine by Dr. Alphonse Noack ; and the two great compilers of Materia Medica in that country have been Drs. Roth and Jahr. All these three names point plainly to the German extraction of their bearers. Some indigenous proving, however, has been done by Pétroz, Ozanam, Teste, Molin, and Imbert-Gourbeyre; and published in the French homœopathic journals.

England has contributed little more to our pathogenetic treasury. The Kali bichromicum of Drysdale, the Naja of Russell, the Cedron of Casanova, the Cotyledon umbilicus of Craig, and the Uranium nitricum of Edward Blake—these are all the provings of any note of which we can boast during the forty and more years in which homœopathy has been practised in this country.

Still less can be said of *Spain* and *Italy*, which have only given us (so far as I know) one medicine each—the Tarantula of Nuñez from the former and the Cactus of Rubini from the latter. From *Brazil* we have received a collection of provings of the plants and animal venoms indigenous to that country instituted by Dr. Mure, of Rio. They are of obscure origin and doubtful value; and hardly one of the substances tested has come into general use. Still more dubious are the *Nouvelles Données* of Dr. Houat, of the French island of Réunion. If you will read the review of his first volume in the twenty-seventh volume of the *British Journal of Homœopathy*, and will then verify the suspicions expressed by looking through a few of his pathogeneses as given by Dr. Allen in his *Encyclopædia*, you will not wonder that the latter generally (I could have wished it had been always) places them in an appendix by themselves, as unworthy to rank with the *bonâ fide* experiments derived from other quarters.

5. I come now to the American sources of the Homœopathic Materia Medica; and the first and most illustrious name on the record is that of Dr. Constantine Hering. I should suppose that the number of medicines in whose proving this physician has taken a more or less principal part is only less than that which we owe to Hahnemann; and though the latter, being first in the field, has given us most of our greatest remedies, yet we cannot forget our debt to Hering for Lachesis, for Apis, and for Glonoin.

I believe that a good many of Dr. Hering's provings remain in manuscript to this day; and I hope that, in spite of his already venerable age, he may live to publish them. Those which have already seen the light are contained in the Transactions of the American Institute or the *American Homœopathic Review*, or they appear in one or other of his two separate publications—the *Amerikanische Arzneiprüfungen* and the first

E

(and as yet only) volume of his *Materia Medica*. The former is written, as its name imports, in the German tongue, Dr. Hering having originally come from that country. He began to issue it, in parts, in 1852 ; and, when discontinued, it had come to contain monographs on twelve medicines—most of them new to homœopathy—embracing clinical observations as well as pathogenetic effects. Among the drugs included I may mention Benzoic acid, Aloes, Apis, Allium Cepa, Glonoin, and Millefolium. The greater number of these have been translated in one or other of our journals. In 1869 Dr. Hering set on foot the *American Journal of Homœopathic Materia Medica*, with the design of appending thereto another series of monographs on medicines. He ceased to do so when sixteen of these had been completed, and then published them separately as the volume of *Materia Medica* which I have mentioned. Besides elaborate arrangements of several of our old remedies—as Cuprum, Spongia, and Stramonium—it gives us the Biniodide of Mercury, Natrum sulphuricum, and Osmium.

I have omitted to mention Dr. Hering's first publication, which dates as far back as 1837. It is his *Wirkungen des Schlangengiftes*—a full collection of the observed phenomena of snake-bites, together with provings on the healthy subject mainly instituted with Lachesis, which great remedy he thus introduced to medicine.

But, while all would give the precedence to this honoured name among the American contributors to our Materia Medica, it is far from standing alone. In the earlier period those of Neidhard, Jeanes, Williamson and Joslin may be named in association with it : in later times those of Dunham, Allen and Conrad Wesselhoeft—not to mention Dr. E. M. Hale, of whose work I must speak separately. The chief instigation and collection of the provings of the United States has proceeded from the American Institute of Homœopathy. This association, at its first meeting (under Dr. Hering's presidency) in 1846, appointed a " bureau " (or committee as we should call it) for the augmentation and improvement of the Materia Medica. The first fruit of its labours was the volume entitled *Materia Medica of American Provings*, whose third edition I now lay before you. It contains the original provings of the Benzoic, Fluoric, and Oxalic acids, of Kalmia, Podophyllum, Eupatorium, Sanguinaria, and several other important drugs. From that time to this, the Transactions of the Annual Assembly of the Institute have rarely failed to contain fresh provings furnished by its Bureau of Materia Medica, down to those of Physostigma and Sepia which constitute its chief labours for 1874 and 1875 respectively. Provings have also formed a prominent feature in many of the American journals. Excellent material for them is now afforded by the students of both sexes who flock to the homœopathic colleges of the States ; and the teachers of Materia Medica therein have not been slack in availing themselves of their opportunities.

6. A new fountain of Materia Medica was opened in 1865 by Dr. E. M. Hale, of Chicago. For some years previously his attention had been drawn to the mine of remedial wealth which existed in the indigenous plants of his country. A few only had been proved and employed in the homœopathic school ; but all around him he found them in constant use by the common people, and by the " botanic" and "eclectic" practitioners—cures often resulting from them where both allopathy and homœopathy had failed. He determined to collect into one volume all pertinent information regarding the principal medicines thus obtained, to reproduce old and institute new provings, and to present all trustworthy recommendations and experiences as to their use. The result was the volume entitled *New Remedies in Homœopathic Practice*. It obtained great success, so that in two years a second edition was demanded. This appeared in 1867, following the same order as the first, but incorporating all fresh facts that had come to light, and adding thirty-five more medicines to the forty-five previously published. In 1873 a third edition was issued, in which (very unwisely, as I think) the materials previously collected were boiled down to a list of (so-called) "characteristic" symptoms. But in the fourth and latest form which the work has assumed this error has been retrieved. The first volume, indeed—entitled *Special Symptomatology*— is of the same character as the third edition. But in the second volume, or *Special Therapeutics*, history, account of provings, testimonies of authors, and narratives of cases have been restored. We only want the detailed provings of the second edition to make the work complete.

I do not hesitate to say that by these publications Dr. Hale has rendered an inestimable service to homœopathy, and thereby to the art of medicine. There has been plenty of severe criticism on his indiscriminate collection of material, his too fond estimates of his new treasures, and the assumptions in which he has sometimes indulged. But these are small matters compared with the actual enrichment of our remedial treasury which has been effected by his means. We really owe to him Actæa, Æsculus, Apocynum, Baptisia, Caulophyllum, Collinsonia, Dioscorea, Eupatorium purpureum,

Gelsemium (as Dr. Allen will have us call it), Hamamelis, Helonias, Hydrastis, Iris, Phytolacca, Sanguinaria, and Veratrum viride. It is no abatement of this obligation to say that some of these had been known previously, and that none have been actually proved by Dr. Hale himself. It was his book that made them current coin, wherever they had been minted before ; and it was he who incited the new provings, though he acted only as their promulgator and expositor. The school of Hahnemann in every country owes him hearty thanks for all this ; and allopathy is beginning to share our gain.

I would advise students, until they can obtain the fifth edition (which I have reason to believe will meet every requirement), to endeavour to procure a copy of the second, supplementing it, if possible, by a perusal of the second volume of the fourth.

7. I have now mentioned all the primary sources of the special Materia Medica of Homœopathy. In doing so I have had to bring before you more than a score of separate volumes, besides referring to whole series of Journals and Transactions. You will naturally ask whether no attempt has been made to bring these multitudinous and scattered provings into one collection, so that they may be accessible to the student and available for use by the practitioner. This brings me to the last name in my list to-day, that of Dr. Allen of New York.

Our only *codices* of symptomatology hitherto had been those of Jahr and of Noack and Trinks. Both date from thirty years ago ; and were at the best abridgements. They were of great use in their time, but have long been superannuated. In 1874, however, a work was commenced which it will take many decades to make obsolete, and which gives us our whole pathogenetic treasury in full. I speak of the *Encyclopædia of Pure Materia Medica*, whose ten volumes are now before you. Here, under the head of each drug, are collected all the symptoms obtained from it by every prover who has tested it, from Hahnemann down to the latest student of the American colleges. All are copied, translated, and arranged afresh ; and every available information is given regarding the circumstances under which they occurred. Nor is this all. Dr. Allen has made a new collection of symptoms observed from poisoning and overdosing, as recorded in medical literature since Hahnemann's day ; and has thereby greatly enriched many of our old pathogeneses, and originated no small number of fresh ones. The work has been improving as it has gone on ; and now that it is completed, it forms a treasury upon which the homœopathic practitioner will thankfully draw for many years to come.

We may partly estimate the value of Dr. Allen's volumes by comparing them with the only work of the kind we have hitherto possessed in English, Jahr's *Manual.* I speak not so much of the greater completeness of the present *Encyclopædia*, as of its manner of presenting its material. Jahr gave us a mind-burdening, a heart-breaking list of bare symptoms, without hint of the manner in which they were obtained or the subjects in whom they appeared. They were themselves but a selection from the original pathogeneses, our sole warrant for the choice made being the judgment of the compiler. Interspersed with them were numerous so-called "clinical symptoms," obtained by breaking up the features of cases reported as cured by the drugs into their component elements, and sowing these in their appropriate plot in the schema. This hideous composition, which has been fitly styled "nonsense made difficult," was, I say, for many years the only general Materia Medica available for homœopathists of the English speech. Contrast it with what we have now. To every symptom Dr. Allen gives us (none but physiological ones being admitted, and none of these omitted) a number is attached, which refers to the observer who warrants it. Appended to his name is a statement, whenever such information is to be had, of the form and dose of the drug used, and the subjects to whom it was administered ; while the thousands of symptoms cited by Hahnemann from authors have received all possible illumination and revision from their originals.

I earnestly recommend all students of homœopathy to possess themselves of Dr. Allen's *Encyclopædia* ; but I do not advise them to content themselves therewith. No collections of symptoms, however thoughtfully made, can convey the same instruction to the mind as the original records of provings. Procure then (I would say), or seek access to as many as possible of the primary sources of our knowledge which I have characterised, and to which Dr. Allen's book will refer you in the case of each drug. Read the day-books of the provers (where we have them), and such narratives of poisoning as are collected in Frank's *Magazin*, in Dr. Hempel's *Materia Medica*, and in the " Pathogenetic Record" which the industry of Dr. Berridge is now giving us as an appendix to the *British Journal of Homœopathy.* You will thus obtain that enlightened general knowledge of the action of medicines ' which, and which alone, will enable you to use the Symptomen-Codex aright.

LECTURE IV.

THE GENERAL PRINCIPLES OF DRUG-ACTION.

I think it well to occupy you, even yet, with considerations of a general and preliminary character. It has occurred to me more than once, when speaking in time past of the action of special drugs, that we ought to have some mutual understanding on the principles of drug-action in general. I propose, therefore, in this and the following lecture, to ask your attention to a brief exposition of my way of looking at this subject, that you may know with what thoughts—whether correct or not—I am wont to analyse the phenomena presented to us by the working of medicines in the organism.

I would begin by reminding you that the basis of all our knowledge on this point must be the science of physiology. Physiology tells us of the healthy substance and functions on which drugs act : we cannot begin to think of the manner in which they disorder unless we understand the order they derange. This, thanks to the unwearied labours of several generations of students, is very largely known. Some portions of it, indeed, are still obscure : some are yet of doubtful significance. But a large tract is fully open to our gaze, and there is substantial agreement as to its general features. It would be quite beyond my province to sketch here, however briefly, the special physiology of the body. But there are certain general principles regarding it which I must recall to your minds ; if for no other purpose, at least to define the basis on which my reasonings about drug-action will rest.

First of all, then, I conceive it must be postulated that this organism of ours is not alive throughout and in every part. I do not know what is the teaching now given in the schools as to the nature of life. For myself, I hold what is called the "protoplasmic theory"; and, whatever modifications may be required in the time to come as to its details, I think there can be no doubt of its substantial truth. Consider the difference between hair and nails at the one extreme, and the amœboid white corpuscle of the blood at the other. It is obvious ; and we may follow either inwards or outwards as the case may be for some distance, ere we come to a region of doubtful import, where there may be gradual transition or a sudden transformation. All on one side is life : on the other, it is non-life. Now this white corpuscle, which I have taken as the type of living matter, is a structureless, transparent, colourless, semi-fluid substance, consisting of minute spherical particles, of very complex chemical constitution, and in continued spontaneous movement. Such is living matter everywhere, whether it be naked, as here, or, as in other parts (the cell for instance), associated with material of another kind. The cell-wall may be taken as a type of this other substance. In it there is the beginning of structure, of rigidity, and perhaps of colour. It is "formed material," and so far has passed from life to death, and has become the subject of chemical and mechanical laws, of which in its living state it was independent. Such formed material constitutes the great bulk of the organism, both of animals and of plants, and determines the manner and fashion of their lives. But that which, in all and everywhere, lives the life is the protoplasm itself, the same whether animal or vegetal, the germinal matter which, like a soul, forms its own body, inhabits, and animates it.

To this protoplasm life belongs, as elasticity belongs to india-rubber. Life is not a force, playing about it only at times, and capable of interchange with other forms of energy : it is its fixed, inherent property, never to leave it as long as it maintains its own integrity. This is the doctrine long ago taught by Fletcher of Edinburgh. It has been—so far as the restriction of vitality to protoplasm goes—re-originated in the present day by Dr. Lionel Beale, and established by him on the basis of physical demonstration. He, however, regards the life here manifested to be an independent entity, a quasi-soul. Dr. Drysdale, from our own school, has taken up the subject; and, while showing the essential harmony of Fletcher and Beale, and the truth of the doctrine on which they agree, has (to my mind) irrefutably argued the preferableness of the position of the former as to the nature of life itself. I would refer you to his works " On Life and the Equivalence of Force" and " The Protoplasmic Theory of Life" for a full exposition of the subject.*

Now this protoplasm, as it is the only vital substance, so does all the vital work of the organism. There is, of course,

* See also what Dr. Drysdale justly calls a " brilliant essay " on this matter, by Dr. Madden, in the fifteenth volume of the *Monthly Homœopathic Review*.

plenty of mechanical and chemical work done there; but with
this we are not at present concerned. It is protoplasm which
effects all those operations which belong peculiarly to living
bodies. It is the formative agent for all their tissues : according to its situation it dies into (to use Dr. Beale's graphic
expression) nerve, muscle, epithelium, areolar tissue, bone.
And, lest by such continuous drain on its material it should
dwindle away, it has the power of taking up fresh pabulum
from the blood, and converting it into its own substance. It
has been itself in other situations the appropriator of the food
from the digestive canal and its elaborator up to the point at
which it reaches the tissues ; and now, by a final act of assimilation, it lays hold of it in its altered form, and absorbs it into
itself, to reappear as the tissue it has to make. Thus the
whole process of *nutrition*, from the time that the mechanical
and chemical acts of digestion are over—the chain of operations consisting of chylification and sanguification, of the
taking up of the blood-plasma by the tissues, and the formation from it of new material—all this is the work of protoplasm. No less is *secretion* performed by it Secretion is but
nutrition under altered conditions. It is merely that the
matter appropriated by the glandular cells is formed by them
into bile, saliva, and so forth, instead of into bone and muscle
and skin. The process is the same, and the proceeder is the
same—the everywhere-present, everywhere-active protoplasm.
And as protoplasm is the agent in nutrition and secretion, so
is it the seat of vital *function*. It is this which, in the gray
substance of the nervous centres, enables us to think and feel,
which receives impressions and conveys volitions. It is this,
in all probability, which contracts in the muscles. Wherever
we have living action—action impossible to the same body
when dead, and unknown in the extra-vital world—there we
have protoplasm at work.

I have said that protoplasm exists alike in the vegetable
and the animal—in either the basis of organic life. But there
is this difference, that in the former it stands as it were on a
common level, while in the latter a portion of it is differentiated
into a system previously unknown,—the nervous. This new
organism (for so we may call it), while it lives its own life and
carries on its own operations of nutrition and function, exerts
a regulating influence over the vegetative processes which were
before it and are beneath it. Though they be for their own
affairs independent of it, yet they all acknowledge its sway.
By its control (through the muscular coats of the arteries) of
the circulation it determines the all-important blood-supply of

the tissues; and if (as is most probable) there are secretory and trophic nerves, ending in the cells themselves, it must influence them still more directly.

This will suffice for our physiological basis. But, before we go on to build upon it any theory of drug-action, we must dwell awhile in the region of pathology. Pathology is physiology altered by the causes of disease in general, as pathogenesy—pharmacology we may call it for analogy's sake—is physiology altered by drugs. Hence the one cannot but throw much light upon the other. Since, moreover, pathology tells of that very disorder which by means of our remedies we seek to restore to physiological order, it is evident that we must have clear conceptions and substantial agreement about its principles ere we advance to the therapeutical side of pharmacodynamics.

Now as we have seen physiology largely concerned with the doings of protoplasm, so also pathology must be. If there are any diseases primarily mechanical or chemical, in these of course it would not come into account. But as most, if not all, of the maladies to which flesh is heir are disorders of vital processes—alterations in nutrition, secretion, or function, protoplasm must be the seat of these also. Let us see how it is in the two most frequent forms of disease, inflammation and fever.

1. The most obvious fact about *inflammation* is the change in the circulation of the affected part; the dilatation of its blood vessels, the throbbing of its afferent arteries, its own redder colour and heightened temperature. It was natural to suppose that this vascular disturbance was the prime factor of the process; that inflammation consisted in increased determination of blood to a part, and consequent functional change. But experiment has shown that such elements do not of themselves constitute inflammation. The circulation of a part may be greatly exaggerated by dividing its vaso-motor nerves, and its colour, temperature, and nutritive and secretory operations enhanced in proportion; but no inflammation need occur. The blood flows through it more rapidly, instead of having its current retarded; and there is an entire absence of exudation, and of swelling or pain. On the other hand, let an irritant be applied to a given spot, or conveyed thither by the circulation. There is the same dilatation of vessels and increased afflux of blood; but at the seat of irritation stasis soon supervenes, and liquor sanguinis and corpuscles begin to be extravasated. If any secretion is carried on there, it is (at least as far as the production of fluid is concerned) diminished even to arrest,

and nutrition, though still exaggerated, is perverted. There is, in Hughes Bennett's words, increased attraction but diminished selection ; and formation is hurried, but imperfect. What can we conclude but that the protoplasm of the part is the seat of the irritation ; that the circulatory changes are subsidiary only, and the real seat of inflammation is (as Lister and Virchow teach) the extra-vascular tissues ? Nor is this less true when division of the vaso-motor nerves of a part *does* cause inflammation ; which obtains when the subject of experiment is already in a weak state, as from partial inanition. The new factor which allows the process to be set up is still the protoplasm of the tissues, which in its feeble state seems unable to bear the stress of the active hyperæmia and its consequences. Here, however, the inflammation is primarily neurotic in origin, while in the case of the application of irritants it begins in the organic cells of the part affected.

2. We have a corresponding series of facts in regard to *fever*, which is—as Fletcher long ago pointed out—inflammation in the system at large. Here, too, the circulatory disturbance is that which arrests the attention, and by which the older observers sought to explain the phenomena. In dilatation of the blood-vessels throughout the frame, preceded or not by their contraction, with quickened action of the heart, they thought they had all the necessary elements of the case. But experiment now proves that we may have these conditions without any fever necessarily being associated with them. They may be induced, for instance, by paralysis of the arteries, brought about by removal of the vaso-motor centres. The result of this proceeding is to make the subject of experiment very sensitive to its environment. If the animal be placed in a hot room, it does become feverish, and probably the same thing would occur if it were in feeble health ; but if the surrounding temperature be lowered, its own bodily heat falls in proportion, and it may readily die from very moderate cold. Clinical observation, moreover, ascertains that increased heat of the blood itself is the real essence of fever ; that the febrile chill, when it occurs, is the first sign that such increase has begun ; and that the subsequent hot period, as also its several common phenomena, depend upon the heightened temperature of the blood stream, and vary with its intensity. Then, going a little farther back to ascertain the cause of the augmented heat of the blood, we find preceding it as well as accompanying it throughout evidence of increased metamorphosis of tissue. That this precedes the rise of temperature shows that it is not caused by it : on the other hand, physiology tells us

that *it* may well be its cause. We can follow Dr. Burdon Sanderson, therefore,* when, after examining all the elements of fever, he comes to the conclusion that at present we must be content to refer it to increased heat-production, and to connect this with the tissue-changes occurring in the proto-plasm. Here, however, as with inflammation, the whole pro-cess may begin in the nervous system, and reach the tissues only secondarily ; or, on the other hand, the tissues themselves may initiate the morbid action. The former is probably the history of the catarrhal fevers, the latter of those of toxæmic origin.

I need hardly tell you that fever and inflammation, in their various forms, lie at the bottom—constitute the proximate cause—of a very large proportion of the diseases we have to treat. The remainder are mostly " functional " disorders—increase, diminution, or irregularity of the action of the various organs of the body. As protoplasm' has been seen to be the seat of function also, we are not beyond its sphere when deal-ing with these disorders. The only difference is that we have now to do with its *vis* rather than its *substantia*, with the energy it puts forth rather than with its own internal opera-tions of appropriation, assimilation, and transformation of pabulum. Inflammation and fever belong to it as the agent of nutrition ; neuroses, spasms, and such like derangements may be connected with its functional duties. And here a word about secretion. This process, though merely nutrition under altered conditions, by this very alteration comes somewhat within the domain of function. It may be altered by inflam-mation or fever, but it is easy to conceive of it as having a *plus* and *minus* of its own, independent of these processes, independent even of the state of its blood-supply. We must bear this in mind when discussing the influence of drugs on glandular organs.

It follows, from what has been said, that every organ of the body is a complex whole, admitting of being reached in various ways. Its own inherent living matter may be affected ; and this either by its nutrition being disordered in the special manner we term inflammation, or by its functional activity being altered in the direction of *plus* or *minus*. Again, all these changes may be effected by the agency of the nervous system. We do not need nervous intervention, indeed, for the sufferings any more than for the actings of protoplasm ; and an exclusive neuro-pathology would be as false as a neuro-physiology. But by the influence of the nervous system of which I have

* See *Practitioner*, vol. xviii.

spoken, certainly upon the blood-supply, and probably also upon the actual substance of the tissues, both nutritive and functional disturbance may be brought about. Yet again, the nervous protoplasm may itself be the seat of trophic change; and its functions, as also those of other parts, may be affected secondarily through altered nutrition, as by the supervention of inflammation or fever.

These, gentlemen, seem to me to be the physiological and pathological *data* required for the construction of a theory of drug-action; and to that task I shall now address myself.

All writers on the subject begin by distinguishing between the mechanical, the chemical, and the dynamic effects of drugs. The distinction is as true as it is obvious, and the ground of it is not far to seek. Drugs can act mechanically and chemically upon the body because a large portion of it, being no longer alive, has come under the dominion of mechanical and chemical laws. And that they have another action over and above these exactly corresponds with that which physiology has shown us, viz.: that there is in every organism, animal or vegetal, a certain proportion of living matter, exempt from the operation of merely physical laws, and subject to actions and re-actions all its own. The dynamic influence of drugs is exerted upon the living matter of the body—upon its proto-plasm. And upon this as such. It does not (as is some-times supposed) affect the nervous system only, for it manifests itself to a large extent in plants, which have no nerves. Nervous protoplasm may be the primary seat of the influence of any drug, and other changes may be secondary to its disorder; but no less may the same living matter anywhere else be attacked in the first instance, and without such medium.

It is with these dynamic effects of medicines that homœo-pathy, as a distinctive method, has to do. Homœopathists —so-called because they acknowledge the rule *similia simili-bus* and its practical corollaries to be by far the most important thing in therapeutics—may have at times to avail themselves of the mechanical and chemical influences which drugs can exert; and they, as well as others, must understand these, and know how to apply them when they are needed. But the method they predominantly follow is concerned with the dynamic actions of medicines only ; and to these, accordingly, my further remarks must be understood exclusively to refer.

Drugs act upon protoplasm; but in so doing they make manifest that which is otherwise ascertained to be true, that all protoplasm is not the same protoplasm. They do not affect all parts of the body indiscriminately and alike, but select one or more organs or tissues or regions, and there expend their power. This *elective* action of drugs is no novelty; it has been made the foundation of a system of practice by Rademacher, who himself traces the thought to Paracelsus.* But it receives very little recognition in the orthodox school of medicine, and even in homœopathic philosophy has hardly taken the place it deserves. We are, in this country, much indebted to Dr. Sharp for his insistance on the truth of the local action of drugs. I hope you are all acquainted with this author's " Tracts," which are about the best exposition and defence of homœopathy we possess. He has in later years devoted himself to an enquiry into the basis of the system; and you will do well to read the volume of *Essays in Medicine* (1874) in which most of his work at the subject is contained. But previous to the appearance of his essays insisting on this point, Dr. Imbert-Gourbeyre had, in his *Lectures Publiques sur l' Homœopathie* (1865), called atten- tion to the same fact, and formulated it as the "law of electivity." Dr. Drysdale also has laid much stress on what he calls "specificity of seat," connecting it with the special irritability displayed by the various parts for their natural stimuli and for causes of disease, and extending it to the minutest localities or nerve-branches which have anything independent and special about them.† In quoting this phys- ician now, I am referring to a series of papers of his extending through the twenty-fifth and two following volumes of the *British Journal of Homœopathy*. They are weighty with solid and original thought; and I commend them to your earnest attention.

In relation to these *Wahlverwandschaften*—these elective affinities existing between drugs and organs, we must observe the caution that we do not infer them from manifestations of topical action only, however strong they may be. A substance when swallowed may inflame the stomach and intestines; when inhaled, it may set up coryza, cough, even bronchitis; when applied to the skin, erythema or eczema may result,— but we cannot therefore infer its specific influence upon these cutaneous or mucous tracts, and give it homœopathically for their corresponding morbid states. We might do so, indeed, if we applied it locally as a remedy also; but not if we administered it by any indirect channel. We can only demon- strate the elective action of a drug on a given part by intro-

* See *Brit. Journ. of Hom.*, viii., 253; *Monthly Hom. Review,* Nov., 1879.

† See *Brit. Journ. of Hom.*, xxvii.. 86

ducing it into the circulation at some other point,—as when gastritis results from Arsenic applied to an ulcer, duodenitis from Podophyllin inserted into the peritoneal cavity (the serous membrane itself being unharmed), bronchitis from Kali bichromicum swallowed, eczema even on covered parts from the emanations of Rhus. We know then that, however taken, it will go to its proper mark,—that it is a bullet which has its billet, and will assuredly find it. We shall have abundant illustration of this distinction between specific and merely topical actions as we proceed.

Special seat of action is the first fact about the behaviour of drugs, and special *kind* of action is the second. Dr. Drysdale has dwelt upon and illustrated what he calls the *qualitative* action of drugs at considerable length. He shows that as there are specific as well as common inflammations, so there must be medicines related to the special quality present as well as to the generic lesion—medicines appropriate to gouty, rheumatic, and syphilitic inflammation in virtue of some peculiar similarity to the element which makes them what they are. He goes on to make some very interesting remarks on the fact of certain remedies being specially indicated by the nature of the exciting cause of the morbid condition to be treated—as Arnica when this is mechanical injury, Dulcamara when it is damp cold, and so forth. He argues that there must be a qualitative difference in the affections produced by these various causes, and a corresponding one in the drugs which thus become their best remedies. He also points out, as others have done, that at the same seat there may be set up very different pathological processes; that the intestines, for instance, may be affected by cholera, common diarrhœa, the typhoid process, tubercular ulceration, and dysentery, and require different remedies accordingly to modify their disorder.

So far I am entirely at one with Dr. Drysdale. But I go on to make another distinction as to the kind of action of drugs which he refuses to recognise. He maintains Fletcher's doctrine that all drugs are stimuli, analogous to the natural agencies so-called—heat, light, &c.—which, acting on the excitability of organic matter, evoke the phenomena of life. Any symptoms of depression which appear in the course of their action he explains as signifying exhaustion following upon over-stimulation. Now I cannot think that this view of drug-action is borne out by facts. Take such a substance as the nitrite of amyl, whose effects when inhaled are immediate. We all know the general flushing of the surface which ensues, and agree to ascribe it to dilatation of the arteries from relaxation of their muscular coats. What is this but primary depression, whether the drug's influence fall (as I think it does) on the vessels directly, or through their nervous supply ? It may be suggested that the amyl really acts as a stimulant to those vaso-dilator nerves which recent research has discovered in connexion with certain vascular areas, and which may exist throughout the circulatory system. But the proof that it is otherwise lies in the fact that, simultaneously with the flushing it excites, the inhalation of the amyl nitrite causes relaxation of any spasm that may exist, as that of angina pectoris or of dysmenorrhœa. As no dilator nerves can be conceived to exist here, the hypothesis of a primary sedative influence seems the only one applicable to the whole group of phenomena. The same thing may be said of the action of Curare, Conium, Physostigma, and Gelsemium upon the musculo-motor nerves and centres. There is ordinarily no trace of excitation here from first to last. Claude Bernard, indeed, laid it down that " every substance which in large doses abolishes the property of an organic element stimulates it if given in small ones ; " and so some evidence of augmented energy may occasionally appear in experiments made with these motor depressants. It is too slight, however, for the subsequent paresis to be ascribed to exhaustion following over-excitement ; and I shall ere long have occasion to argue that it is a reaction of the organism against doses too feeble to induce the direct effect of the drug.

I must maintain, therefore, that while many drugs are primarily stimulant to the tracts they influence, others are primarily depressant. And I must draw a further distinction between stimulants and irritants. Stimulants excite function, irritants inflame tissue. Strychnia is an excellent example of the former class. It powerfully excites nervous tissue, motor or sensory, wherever it finds it : mobility and impressionability are both morbidly heightened, but there is no inflammation. On the other hand, substances like Arsenic, Iodine, and Cantharides have no definite action upon function ; but they inflame tissue wherever they are locally applied or electively attracted. They act (we may suppose) in the latter case like other internal causes of the process. Conveyed in the circulation to the part for which they have affinity, they there act upon the protoplasm, and fret it into that morbid and blind activity in which I apprehend inflammation to consist.

There are three things, then, which drugs can do with protoplasm. They can affect its functional operations simply, and this either by exciting or depressing them ; or they can induce that morbid change in its work of nutrition and tissue-making, which (in its full development) locally we call inflammation, and generally fever. The function-modifiers are those drugs which, from their giving rise to nervous phenomena chiefly or solely, we call neurotics; and I should add to them the myotics, which seem to influence directly the unstriped muscular fibre, as Secale does, and perhaps some direct excitants of certain secretions, like Jaborandi. The modifiers of nutrition form a still larger collection. To this belong all those substances which Toxicology classes as irritants, so far as their irritation is not a mere chemical effect, as with the strong mineral acids. That they act topically only, and not when introduced into the circulation, would not disqualify them for this place ; but they must be used topically as remedies also. There are many true irritants, however, of which Toxicology knows nothing ; for they produce no dangerous effects. Nor would they be discovered by the method which has recently come into so much favour—of experiments on the lower animals with large single doses. In this sphere they can only be recognised by persistent administration over a length of time, as carried out by Wegner with Phosphorus, and by our colleague, Dr. Eugéne Curie, with Bryonia and Drosera. But the main source of knowledge regarding them is proving on the healthy human subject. It is thus that we get a number of drug effects which are not explicable on the supposition of a *plus* or *minus* state of any function, but which, if not inflammatory or febrile in the full sense of the words, at least show signs enough of these morbid conditions to evidence a power on the part of the drugs of causing them, if pushed far enough, and to lead us, on the principle of similarity, to give such remedies for their cure. There is many a feverish condition in childhood which yields to Calcarea, and many a smouldering inflammation put out by Sulphur.

I would divide drugs, then, in their influence upon protoplasm—in other words, their dynamic operation—into two classes, those which affect its performance of function, and those which disorder its nutritive processes. There are, of course, many drugs which belong to both classes, as Toxicology recognises in naming some poisons acro-narcotics. Each substance must be separately studied, and examined on its own merits. But the classification I have proposed, whether affect-.ing the whole or only a part of the actions, is no less valid. It fits in, moreover, with an important distinction in the dynamic effects of drugs which has been much insisted upon both by Dr. Drysdale and Dr. Madden. The latter, regarding chiefly the fact that some properties are common to a number of drugs—as emesis, purgation, and the like—and others peculiar to individuals, has named them *genico-dynamic* and *idio-dynamic* respectively.* The former, pointing out that the common dynamic effects of medicines are producible at will, while the peculiar ones depend for their production on the presence of a special susceptibility in the subject, would call the one *absolute* and the other *contingent*. Now I think that if these generic actions of drugs, producible at will, be examined, they will all be found to belong to functional excitation or depression; while the peculiar effects, which require special susceptibility, are nearly, if not quite, always disorders of nutrition. The subcutaneous injection of atropia, for instance, will always dilate the pupil, always depress the inhibitory influence exerted upon the heart by the pneumogastric. But it is only in this individual or in that that it produces a scarlatinal rash or an inflamed throat, that it induces neuralgic pain or excites fever. Dr. Drysdale has forcibly pointed out that it is the contingent effects of medicines which we chiefly use in applying the law of similars, their absolute actions being often entirely incongruous therewith. " For example," he writes, " if we are watching a group of chest symptoms produced by Tartar emetic, or the characteristic pustular eruption on the skin, and suddenly a large emetic dose is given, though the whole action is certainly that of Tartar emetic, yet if we admit the vomiting as a part of either morbid picture, we should be unable to comprehend it." Trousseau and Pidoux, viewing the matter from Dr. Madden's stand-point, make a similar remark upon the relation of the two orders of symptoms to those of disease. " In special medicines, in medicines properly so called, above all in poisons, we find two elements. They enjoy properties which belong to the whole genus; these are their common properties, which scarcely excite in the organism more than common and general action, as to stimulate, irritate, weaken, calm, etc. But they possess, beyond this, special properties peculiar to each, *and which excite in the organism morbid actions more or less resembling the symptoms of disease*." Dr. Imbert-Gourbeyre, without distinguishing between the absolute and contingent effects of drugs, lays much stress on the latter, and adds *contingenter* to the *similiter* and *elective* in which he formulates homœopathic action.

He also adds *omni dosi*. Dr. Drysdale agrees with him, and

* See *Brit. Journ. of Hom.*, viii., 13,

shows that herein lies another distinction between absolute and contingent symptoms, the former requiring the drug to be given in a certain quantity for their production, the latter being singularly independent thereof. You may, in proving a medicine, reduce the dose until its recognised physiological effects cease to appear ; but, unless the subject of experiment be insusceptible to its action, he will manifest one or more of the peculiar phenomena which belong to it. Trousseau and Pidoux, also, say of the " special effects " of drugs which they recognise, that " if we wish to obtain them, small doses must generally be administered, for then the common effects are very little perceived." Dr. Drysdale believes that the same independence of quantity holds good in disease ; and that, where a condition resembling the contingent effects of a drug is present, you can hardly (within certain limits) give so small a dose as to fail to benefit, or (and this is a new point) so large a dose as to aggravate. Everything depends on the special susceptibility of the part ; and, this once exhausted, the medicine has no longer any influence upon it. He illustrates this view by a case in which Glonoin, given for a neuralgia because of the presence of some of its characteristic physiological effects, caused its well-known throbbing headache, without aggravation—and rather with amelioration—of the troubles for which it was administered. He thus extends the *omni dosi* of Dr. Imbert-Gourbeyre's formula to the other extreme also of the scale. A similar thing appears in provings. You will see ever and anon in Hahnemann's pathogeneses the term " curative effect " applied to a symptom. This does not mean (save sometimes in the quotations from authors, as under Iodium) the result of the administration of the drug in disease. It means that the prover who took it, though otherwise in good health, was morbid in this particular, and that the medicine, while causing pathogenetic effects elsewhere, finding disorder already present here, reduced it to order. To take an indisputable instance. One of the most constant effects of iodism, as observed in the sensitive Genevese patients, is palpitation ; but " in a case altogether exceptional," Trousseau writes, " M. Rilliet has seen palpitation cease, instead of appearing or increasing, under iodism ; *the patient was one habitually subject to it.*"

This mention of dose brings me to yet one other feature of the kind of action of drugs, in which it plays an important part. But I will reserve this portion of the subject for another lecture.

LECTURE V.

THE GENERAL PRINCIPLES OF DRUG ACTION.

(Continued.)

Upon the last occasion of our meeting, we discussed several of the features of the *kind* of action produced by various drugs. To-day I have to bring before you those modifications of their influence—real or supposed—which are brought about by difference of dosage.

You will find Dr. Sharp, in his later essays, insisting much on a fact which he denominates "antipraxy," by which he means that large and small doses of drugs exert a precisely opposite effect. He does not mean merely that they do this in health and in disease respectively, which would only be describing the apparent working of the law of similars; but he affirms that the opposition holds good in health, so that, whatever be the effect of a large dose, a small dose may be found whose action shall be of a precisely contrary kind. It was early pointed out* that, so far as this double action of medicines existed, it belonged to those primary and secondary effects long ago discovered in them by Hahnemann, and employed by Fletcher, Drysdale, Dudgeon, Reith and others to explain the action of homœopathic remedies. Dr. Jousset thus states the doctrine in relation to dose: (†)

"1. Every medicine produces on the healthy body two successive actions, primary and secondary. These two actions are always opposite one to another.

"2. The stronger the dose of the medicine the less marked is the primary action. If the dose is excessive, the secondary action only is developed.

"3. The weaker the dose the more manifest the primary action."

As Dr. Sharp now teaches that between the large and the

---

* See *Brit. Journ. of Hom.*, xxxi., 756.
† *L'Art Médical*, xlv., 182.

small dose, with their opposite actions, there is an intermediate point at which the medicine produces the two effects in succession, his doctrine becomes harmonious with that of his predecessors and colleagues.

I entirely subscribe to it, and teach it you from this chair, as a feature of the action of *certain* drugs. But I cannot go with Dr. Sharp, or indeed with Dr. Jousset, in affirming it of the action of *all* drugs. Hahnemann admitted two qualifications of his general statement as to the opposite primary and secondary action of medicines. The first was, that there were some (of which he specifies the metals, as arsenic, mercury, and lead) which " continue their primary action uninterruptedly, of the same kind, though always diminishing in degree, until after some time no trace of their action can be detected, and the natural condition of the organism supervenes." The second is expressed in a phrase he uses in the *Organon*—" the exact opposite condition to the primary effect, *if there be an opposite condition.*" Truly, there is much virtue in this " if." It is obvious that opposition can only be predicated of functional states which admit of a *plus* and *minus*, as excretions and secretions, sleep, muscular and nervous tone, and the like. These are the conditions which vegetable drugs—being mostly neurotics and eliminants—influence, and hence Hahnemann's description of primary and secondary actions applies chiefly to medicines of this order ; while the metals, which rather produce inflammation and other organic changes, do not manifest such phenomena. " The possibility, then," writes Dr. Carroll Dunham, " of classifying symptoms into primary and secondary on the basis of the relative nature of the symptoms, is not co-extensive with symptomatology ; it is partial, confined to a moderate number of conceivable morbid phenomena." I quote from a paper published by this physician in the *Hahnemannian Monthly* for May, 1876, and reprinted in his *Homœopathy the Science of Therapeutics* (1877), to which I would direct the attention of all who desire to have clear thought upon the subject.

Regarding then, as I do, the whole group of actions at present under discussion as limited in their sphere, I cannot go with those who explain by means of them the action of homœopathically-selected remedies. I am under the misfortune of disagreeing herein with my much-esteemed colleague in this School, Dr. Dyce Brown. Maintaining as he does (with Dr. Sharp) the opposite action of all drugs in health according to the quantity in which ·they are given, he would argue that when we give in disease small doses of a substance which in

large doses has caused a similar condition to that before us, we are administering an agent whose influence is in direct opposition to the morbid state. The curative process is thus antipathic, though the principle of selection is homœopathic. Now here I must recall the distinctions we have already established. In those functional exaltations and depressions which many a drug causes, common to it with others, and producible at will if a certain quantity is administered—in such a region we may have primary and secondary actions, we may have opposite effects from different doses ; and our cures may be wrought by counteracting secondary states in disease with primary states caused by the drug, or by opposing the action of one dose to morbid conditions similar to those producible by another.*
Such antipathic medication, whether practised under homœopathic appearances or without them, may accomplish all we require. But I think that *plus* or *minus* functional states like these, though frequent enough in pathogenesy, are far from being common occurrences in the actual disorders we have to treat. When existing at all, they are often indications of some nutritive disturbance at their root, or single features of a complex state similarly induced. How rarely is paralysis, for example, a purely " functional " disorder ! Nearly every form of it is traceable to inflammation or softening of the nervous substance ; even the diphtheritic variety, which did seem to have no lesion associated with it, has been found on deeper investigation to be connected with definite central alterations. So that, although the antipathic cure of functional excess or defect is easier or conception, and perhaps more in accordance with fact than the homœopathic, I do not think that we are therefore justified in inferring that all or even the greater part of apparent homœopathy is real antipathy. When we come to nutritive disturbances—to those alterations which in their full development are inflammation and fever, we have entered a different region. There is no *plus* and *minus* of opposition possible here, no conceivable reverse action of large and small doses in health. We have got beyond dose as an important element in the result : if the contingent susceptibility be present, the drug will cause disorder in almost any quantity, and cure it in almost any. You have only to read a few detailed provings, and a chapter or two of Rückert or Beauvais, to see that this is so. Such a law as that propounded by Dr. Yeldham about the curative dose being as little below the physiological as possible fails here, however it may hold good in the absolute region ; for there is no physiological dose for

* See Camphor.

contingent effects. It is very significant that Dr. Sharp admits that he has not yet touched the subject of infinitesimals ; all his statements about " large " and " small " apply to differences between grains and hundredths of grains. In like manner I think he will find that he has not yet touched the subject of nutritive as distinct from functional disorder. While in the latter the curative operation of apparently homœopathic remedies may be antipathic, in the former I can see no room for such working and no evidence but against it. *Aut simile, aut nihil ;* there is no trace of anything but homœopathy from the surface to the deepest root.

And there is yet one caution more to be observed. All these theories of primary and secondary action, and of the opposite effect of large and small doses, impose a limitation on the class of pathogenetic effects which we can employ in homœopathic practice. If homœopathy means opposing morbid conditions answering to the secondary effects of drugs by inducing the primary action of the latter, we must use such secondary phenomena only in selecting the *simile*. If we are, by giving a small dose, producing an opposite action to that of a large one, we must only take the effect of large doses into account. But facts are entirely against such limitation, and it would be disastrous to work by it. Hahnemann held just the contrary view, and believed that only the primary effects of drugs could be used in homœopathising. He therefore took special care to obtain such primary effects in his provings, and used small doses accordingly, as he himself tells us. Consequently, the pathogeneses he has furnished us, and which constitute the very core of our Materia Medica, are quite unsuited for the purposes of those whose views I am now considering. Upon Dr. Sharp's principles, he ought to give large doses instead of small to patients presenting groups of symptoms analogous to those found in Hahnemann's provings. That he does not do so, but gets excellent results from following an opposite course, shows (I submit) that his theory fails, at least in being conterminous with homœopathic action. Moreover, upon Dr. Sharp's showing, all those opposite effects of the same drug—constipation and diarrhœa, sopor and insomnia, excitement and depression, and so forth—which we find in nearly every pathogenesis, must be either primary and secondary actions of a single dose, or the effects of large and small doses respectively. Hahnemann, however, clearly perceived that this was not so. He would use none but primary actions for homœopathic application, as Dr. Sharp would use none but secondary ; but he soon found that the primary action of many drugs included two opposite states, either or both of which might be induced by it in the small doses used in his provings, and either or both removed by it in the still smaller quantities he administered to the sick. Such oppositions (antinomies, we might call them) he styled "alternating effects," and distinguished them sharply from the mere "secondary effects" of functional exhaustion, which last he considered unavailable for homœopathic purposes. I think that his discernment was entirely sound, and that Dr. Sharp is unduly limiting the range of the treatment by similars in fixing it to one set of oppositions in the action of each drug. Veratrum album, for instance, causes diarrhœa in large doses, and checks it in small, because (he thinks) in the latter it constipates. But he would find it—in smaller doses still—an excellent remedy for the kind of constipation itself causes; and this cannot be because these smaller doses purge. It is wiser, therefore, to say with Hahnemann that constipation and diarrhœa are alternating effects of the primary action of Veratrum,—that action probably being a depression of the functional activity of the intestinal nerves; and that either, if the other symptoms coincide, may be used in prescribing homœopathically. The same thing is true when opposite effects occur in succession as part of the primary action of a drug. They are then to be reckoned as part of the order and sequence of such action, and are to be fitted to corresponding successions occurring in disease. Thus, Aconite causes both the chill and the heat of fever; it is, therefore, homœopathic to fevers consisting of chill and heat, and in either stage. Here, too, the explanation is probably the same, that it sets up in the healthy that essential change of which the febrile heat and chill are the complementary expression, and neutralises the same change when present in disease.

In two lectures "On the Rationale of Homœopathic Cure," delivered at our Hospital in February, 1877, and printed in the *Monthly Homœopathic Review* for the March and April of that year, I have gone more fully into these questions of the primary and secondary actions of drugs, and of the opposite effects of large and small doses. I have examined the views propounded on these subjects, and the endeavours to explain by them the action of similar remedies, of Hahnemann and Fletcher in the past, and of my living colleagues, Drs. Drysdale, Dudgeon, Bayes, Sharp, Pope, and Dyce Brown. To those lectures I must refer you for my reasons in detail for being unable to agree *in toto* with the doctrine of any of them. The only further contribution which has been made to the subject

since their appearance is the paper " On the Double and Opposite Action of Drugs," which was read by Dr. Drysdale at
the British Homœopathic Congress of 1877.* I fully agree
with the criticisms he there makes upon Dr. Sharp's arguments, and am pleased to find him stating that he and I agree
in our present views more nearly than I had supposed. I may
quote the following passage in evidence thereof. " At the
same time," Dr. Drysdale writes, " I admit that the bare principle of a primary excitation, followed by a secondary collapse
or exhaustion, is insufficient, *per se*, to explain numerous and
important *qualitative* changes in the living matter produced
by the exciting causes of disease, and by drugs, and which are
met by the homœopathic law of cure. Here, I think, we had
better still rest the homœopathic law on an inductive basis,
viz. : that it simply expresses a general fact established by a
sufficient number of experiments. . . . . In diseases of mere
plus and *minus* of vital action, on the other hand, the Brunonian
theory of excitement and exhaustion gives an *à priori* explanation of the double and opposite action of drugs, and of the
homœopathic law of cure." This is in complete accordance
with the distinction between functional and nutritive disorders
which I was drawing a few minutes ago.†

I must now say a few words upon another part which dose
has been made to play in drug-action. I shall be here on
common ground with those whose views I discuss as to either
of two opposite effects of a drug being available for therapeutic comparison. But I must inquire how far they are
warranted in maintaining that the opposite phenomena displayed by certain medicines are dependent upon difference
of dosage, and that corresponding variations must be made
in the quantity administered when we come to apply them to
the treatment of disease.

The advocates of this doctrine are three of our American
colleagues—Drs. Hering, Hempel, and Hale, who, however,
differ considerably in their way of putting the matter.

1. Dr. Hering distinguishes primary and secondary symptoms only as those occurring earlier or later in the provings,
and states that observation will show the effects of the more
attenuated doses to correspond, not to the primary, but to the
secondary action of larger quantities. He would, accordingly,
advise the administration of the higher potencies when the
symptoms of the case before us have more resemblance to the
later symptoms of the drug, of the lower when the similarity is
between them and its earlier working.

* See *Monthly Hom. Review*, xxi., 656. † See p. 69.

2. Dr. Hempel takes a somewhat similar view, though going further in the interpretation of the phenomena. Let me cite a short passage from one of his lectures.

" I shall have frequent occasion to show you that drugs seem to affect the organism in two opposite ways, and may therefore be homœopathic to two pathological conditions, holding towards each other relations of antagonism. We may illustrate this point by the well-known condition of fever. The first stage of an inflammatory fever is not a full and bounding pulse, a hot and dry skin, flushed face, and so forth; an opposite group of symptoms occur. The patient experiences a chill or cold creepings along the back; he looks pale, hollow-eyed, the hands and feet are cold, the pulse is thin, feeble, rather slower than naturally; or, at any rate, not much accelerated. This condition is soon superseded by the opposite group of phenomena generally designated as fever. The chill is the primary effect of the disease; the fever constitutes a secondary effect, or the re-action of the organism. In selecting a remedial agent for this derangement, it should be homœopathic, not only to the primary chill, but also to the secondary group, fever. Aconite is such a remedy. Aconite is homœopathic to the chill, which marks the first invasion of the disease, and to the fever which marks the beginning of the organic re-action. We are seldom called to a patient during the primary invasion of the disease; the organic re-action is generally fully established when we first see the patient. Nevertheless we prescribe Aconite, knowing full well that the inflammatory stage must have been preceded by a chill.

" We say that Aconite is homœopathic to the chill, and we prove this experimentally by taking a large dose of this drug, of course within conservative limits, which will uniformly cause a more or less perceptible chill, coldness of the skin, depression of the pulse, all which symptoms disappear after a certain interval of time, and are followed by the opposite condition, fever. A small dose of Aconite will not produce the primary chill, but will at once excite the organic re-action characterised by the usual phenomena of heat, flushed face, dryness of the mouth, &c. This shows the importance of proving drugs in massive doses. It is massive doses that develop the primary drug-symptoms; small doses do not develop these primary symptoms, because the organic re-action very speedily supersedes them.

" In practice it is of the utmost importance that we should discriminate between the primary and secondary action. If we are called upon to prescribe for a group of symptoms corresponding with the primary action of a drug, we give a larger dose than we should do, if we had to prescribe for a group corresponding with the secondary action, or organic re-action."

Dr. Hempel adds as illustrations of the possibility of a medicine being homœopathic to two opposite conditions, that " Aconite and Nux may be used as true homœopathic remedies in paralysis as well as tetanus; Ipecacuanha may remove perfect atony as well as spasmodic irritability of the stomach; Opium cures diarrhœa as well as constipation, excessive wakefulness as well as drowsiness and stupor; Mercurius will check as well as promote the secretory action of the pancreas;

Secale answers in uterine hæmorrhage from atony of this organ as well as in spasmodic uterine contractions."

3. And now of Dr. E. M. Hale. In consulting the work of this author entitled *New Remedies,* which I have already brought before you, you will find frequent references to what he calls his law of dose. This law he states as follows :

"In any case of disease we must select a remedy whose primary and secondary symptoms correspond with those of the malady to be treated.

" If the primary symptoms of a disease are present, and we are combating them with a remedy whose primary symptoms correspond, we must make the dose the smallest compatible with reason ; and if we are treating the secondary symptoms of a malady with a remedy whose secondary symptoms correspond, we must use as large a dose as we can with safety." Under the latter circumstances he speaks of drugs as " secondarily homœopathic " to the morbid condition present ; and by means of this qualification maintains that we are still practising the method of Hahnemann though we should treat relaxed states with the ordinary doses of astringents, and states of excitement with those of narcotics.

Proceeding now to an examination of these views, it will be seen, in the first place, that we must be agreed as to what are primary symptoms. We have hitherto understood them— with Hahnemann and all who have followed him—to be the least possible effect of a drug, the expression of the direction in which the function affected by it deviates from the right line. It is obvious that an increase of the disturbing influence would but push it farther and farther still on the same side of the normal path, and that in proportion as it did so a pendulum-like swing to the opposite side would (when its action was over) become more and more apparent. Thus the re-active and secondary phenomena of the drug—when it exhibited any —would be opposite to its least possible effect, while Drs. Hering and Hempel would make them parallel thereto.

I think, nevertheless, that there can be no doubt of the reality of the facts to which they have directed attention ; and that Dr. Hempel's explanation of them is the true account of their meaning. This organism of ours into which we introduce drugs to prove them is a living one : it does not merely passively suffer under what is done to it, but re-acts thereupon. If the impression made by a foreign agent is sufficiently potent, it bends before it, with such subsequent recoil as the case demands. But it is readily conceivable that the impression may be so slight that the only notice taken of it by the organism is, so to speak, a resenting push in the opposite direction ; and this also may be the earliest response to the influence of a drug, while, as its action gathers force, it bends the function it modifies in its own way. I think that in this way are explained those temporary phenomena of excitation under paralysing agents—such as curare—which led Claude Bernard to the generalisation that " every substance which in large doses abolishes the property of an organic element stimulates it if given in small ones," and again, that " all those causes which exhaust the vital properties of a tissue or of an organic element commence by exciting them." I cannot, indeed, think him warranted in further maintaining that " they are paralysers because they are first excitants that exhaust ;" for the period of excitation is so short and its symptoms so slight that it cannot be conceived of as causing a collapse which should account for the long-lasting paralysis which ensues. Dr. Hempel's view that it is a re-action of the organism seems to me exactly to explain it ; and it puts it accordingly with all phenomena of the same kind in a separate class by themselves, standing on the hither side of the true primary action of drugs, in which the organism does not act but only suffers.

I therefore accept Dr. Hale's view as to what is primary and what secondary in the action of drugs, following here in the track of all the older observers. I agree with him also that " in any case of disease we must select a remedy whose primary and secondary symptoms correspond with those of the malady to be treated," always adding the proviso that there be such a succession of opposite states in either or both, which does not by any means hold good in all cases. But when I am told I must make a difference in dose according as the primary or secondary stage of the disease is present, I pause, and ask why ? The only answer it seems possible to give is that in the one case I shall be administering a remedy whose action is the same direction with that of the disease, and which therefore might aggravate if the doses were too large ; while in the other I should be as it were pushing the morbid process the opposite way, and must increase my force accordingly to the utmost point consistent with the safety of the organism at large. That is, in plain words, in one I shall be practising homœopathy, in the other antipathy.

It is well to perceive the true position to which we are led by this proposed rule of Dr. Hale's. It has more than one aspect in relation to our present subject. It suggests that even in the functional states of *plus* and *minus* of which I have spoken—and to which alone I conceive it to apply—there may be a real and not merely an apparent homœopathy practised. Our attention has been already called to this point by one among ourselves, of the same name phonetically though not literally as our Chicago colleague : I mean Dr. Hayle, of Rochdale. In his Presidential Address at the Congress of 1876, he pointed out* that Dr. Sharp's explanation of apparent similars as being real opposites could not hold good if both the double actions of medicines are to be used for homœopathic application. Nux vomica might cure paralysed conditions by its power of stimulating ; but if it be also useful in spasm and irritation we cannot invoke any such opposite influence, especially as we have to give it in smaller doses. Thus the practitioners who habitually employ attenuated medicines are in all probability homœopathising really and not apparently only ; while the remedies Dr. Sharp would give—he having, as we have seen, hardly entered the field of infinitesimals— may be such as are actually antipathic to the condition present, though on the surface seeming to be similars.

So far I think we can fully accept Dr. Hale's canon. But it is another thing to affirm that we should use all the secondary reactions which are observed in drug-effects as homœopathic indications, even though remedies so chosen should have to be given in the most substantial doses. It is obvious that such a mode of proceeding would lead us into the whole sphere of antipathic treatment, without even the appearance of homœopathicity about it. It would be impossible to convince others, difficult, I should think, even to satisfy ourselves, that we were practising the method of Hahnemann in giving (say) twenty grains of ergot to contract a flabby uterus after parturition. Dr. Hale would argue—The primary action of ergot is indeed to induce contraction of the womb ; but after a time, by the law of action and re-action, this over-rigid condition must be succeeded by one of relaxation. Ergot is therefore primarily homœopathic to the former, secondarily homœopathic to the latter ; and we are quite within the sphere of the law of similarity in giving it to induce contraction, while the dosage must be such as is sufficient to effect the purpose.

I shall certainly not teach you to apply the idea of homœopathy to such practices as these, but shall frankly acknowledge them to be what they are. At the same time I entirely assent to Dr. Hempel's statement that a medicine may be homœopathic to two apparently opposite conditions. It may be (as I have already suggested in the instances of Aconite and

* See *Monthly Hom. Review*, xx., 668.

Veratrum album) a similar to the underlying vital disturbance, of which these two states are the successive or the alternative expressions. It may produce one class of effects by acting on one element of the part, and the opposite of these by acting on another; and so it may homœopathically cure either. It may begin its action by increasing the secretion of an organ, but its prolonged influence may cause so much congestion that secretion is diminished or arrested. In these and in many other ways, of all which we have had or shall have examples, a medicine may be a true similar to two apparently opposite states. Nux vomica, as well as Veratrum, is applicable to both constipation and diarrhœa: Secale will check some forms of menorrhagia and counteract a certain form of uterine exhaustion : Scilla will arrest diuresis and restore the diminished secretion of acute renal dropsy. But in all these cases no difference of dose is necessary in the two spheres of action, or at least no such difference as that contemplated by Dr. Hale. We are really practising homœopathy, not inducing the physiological action of our remedy under its guise ; and our posology can be determined by the considerations which guide us in all other cases.

There are, indeed, only two ways of employing in disease the power which a drug has of disordering the healthy body. You may use it either to induce this physiological action in the patient, or to neutralise such action if it be already present. The former is (to use Hahnemann's nomenclature) antipathy or allœopathy, according as you are acting on the disordered part or not: the latter, and this alone, is homœopathy. For the former purpose some such dosage is required as is sufficient to develope the change in question in the healthy : for the latter no such quantitative administration is necessary. When, therefore,—to take an instance from another writer—Dr. Jousset tells us that for cardiac dropsy Digitalis has to be given in spoonfuls of a decoction representing not less than two grains of the powdered leaves, but maintains that such practice is homœopathic, because the drug causes an " asystolia " similar to that which is present in such cases, we must pause before assenting. And a very little inquiry, I apprehend, is needed to show that such asystolia in the case of Digitalis is but the functional exhaustion consequent upon the precisely opposite effect of the drug, and that to administer it for a similar condition in full doses is merely to induce such a contrary state in your patient as by the same means you could set up in the healthy. If this is homœopathy, I know not what is antipathy.

Of Dr. Hering's and Dr. Hempel's rules of dose, I can say little. They seem based upon the view that the larger the dose which produced the pathogenetic effect, the lower should be the attenuation given to counteract its *simile* in disease. Of this, however, we have no certain evidence.

I have now, I think, said sufficient to acquaint you with the principles as to drug-action which will regulate the teaching on the subject I shall give in this place. Very often, indeed, I shall have simply to present the phenomena of pathogenesy to you, and to state their therapeutic applications. But wherever analysis and interpretation are possible, they will proceed upon the physiological and pathological bases now laid down. How far they are absolutely true, I cannot say; they are the best at which I can arrive at present, and that is all I can do. Our comfort is, that however they may shift in the progress of time and knowledge, homœopathy, as a mode of the art of healing, is not dependent on them. The relation it establishes is between the observed facts of drug-action on the one hand, and of disease on the other; and no alteration in our view of the meaning of either can affect it one whit.

LECTURE VII.

HOMŒOPATHY—WHAT IT IS.

I must yet detain you a little longer on the threshold of our subject. I have spoken of several things pertaining to homœopathy ; but I have said nothing as yet about homœopathy itself. It seems desirable that, befo e I begin to tell you how to study and use medicines in the h omœopathic manner, I should explain to you what that manne: is, as I myself understand it. It is the more necessary that I should do so, as you will soon discover (if you have not already done so) that there are two distinct ways of conceiving and applying the method of Hahnemann prevalent among those who adopt it. You ought to know from me what is the position I take up in the controversy between the advocates of these two views, and on what principles I propose to conduct the present course of instruction.

Now both the homœopathies which exist at the present day find their origin in Hahnemann himself, though both are departures from his stand-point—the one diverging under the attraction of modern science, the other prolonging his own line of advance into regions unknown and undreamt-of by him. I can best present them to you, therefore, by tracing the history of the master's own mind, from his first conception of the new method to his final elaboration of it. Let us dwell, then, upon the history of homœopathy.

In the year of our Lord 1790, when the eyes of all Europe were fixed upon the rapidly evolving drama of which France was the theatre, there was a man in Germany intent upon far different matters. This man was a physician, in the prime of his life ; his name was Samuel Hahnemann. An accomplished scholar, both in medical and general letters ; a profound chemist ; the friend of the illustrious Hufeland,—he was utterly dissatisfied with the state of therapeutics in his day. One of its few bright spots seemed to him to be the treatment of ague by bark. He pondered much over the rationale of this curative action—so simple, so direct, so effectual. How

could other medicines be so used ?   How could other diseases
be so treated ?   It occurred to him to try the effect of this
bark in health : he experimented on his own person. He
found that it set up a fever very like that which it cured : the
relation between its disease-producing and disease-curing properties was that of similarity.   Its operation, therefore, was
an instance of that "similia similibus" which Hippocrates
had recognised as occasionally holding good, and whose
claims to notice and possibilities of fruitfulness as a therapeutic principle had been noticed by more than one writer.   If it
obtained in the present notable instance, the inference was
obvious.   Was it not possible that other cure-work like that
of bark in ague might rest upon such relationship between
drug and disease—might have been got from it occasionally
in the past, might be got from it continuously in the future?
The question was a reasonable one; but it was only a
question.   It had to be answered by observation and experiment—by reviewing the cures on record, and endeavouring to
obtain new ones.   Both were fully carried out.   Hahnemann's
Organon (the systematic exposition of his method, first published in 1810) contains a copious list, drawn up from medical
literature, of cures of disease effected by drugs which on no
less satisfactory testimony were declared capable of causing
similar conditions in the healthy.   And his own experience,
which was published from time to time, showed him that the
power of similarly acting medicines was most undoubted, and
their manner of curing greatly preferable.   He now considered
that the question had been answered affirmatively, the induction deductively verified ; and, after suggesting it as a new
method in 1796,* in 1806† he confidently put forth *similia
similibus*, ὁμοιοπαθεία, as the cardinal principle of therapeutics.

He had not gone far, however, in working out the method,
when he found that to do so properly required a much fuller
knowledge of pathogenetics than that possessed at the time.
Records of poisoning and over-dosing were not scanty ; but
they referred only to a small number of very active substances,
and to the large and crude effects of these.   A few typical
and severe diseases were here pictured, and served for the
early application of the method.   But if it was to be carried
out systematically, if the great variety of morbid conditions

* In his "Essay on a new principle for ascertaining the curative
power of drugs" (*Hufeland's Journal*, vol. ii.   See Dudgeons's
translation of his Lesser Writings, p. 295).

† "The Medicine of Experience" (*Hufeland's Journal* for 1806.
See translation, p. 497).

which come before the physicians were to be "covered" by corresponding drug effects, his knowledge of the latter must be indefinitely increased. With Hahnemann, to perceive this need was to feel the obligation of supplying it; and to feel the obligation was to fulfil it. He at once set to work to "prove" medicines on his own body and that of other healthy persons. In 1805 he had collected sufficient material of the kind for publication; and it appeared in his treatise *Fragmenta de viribus medicamentorum positivis*, of which I have already spoken to you, and which contains (as you will remember) pathogenetic effects of twenty-seven drugs, obtained from the ingestion of single full doses.

But yet another step had been taken before this time. In prescribing medicines according to the rule *similia similibus*, Hahnemann of course gave them singly, and without the complex admixtures so common in his day. He administered them, however, in the usual doses. It is not surprising that his patient's symptoms, even though ultimately removed, were often in the first instance severely aggravated. It needs no argument to show that the ordinary doses of Arsenic, against which even a healthy stomach needs to be shielded, would increase the irritation of one already inflamed—for which, nevertheless, the homœopathic principle would direct its being given. So Hahnemann found, and he reduced his doses accordingly. He did so by mixing his solutions or tinctures with definite proportions of some menstruum, as water or alcohol. The now well-known advantages of dilution came out in this process; and he found that attenuation could be carried to an extent hitherto undreamt of without the remedial power of the drug being lost. Accordingly, in his treatise on the *Cure and Prevention of Scarlet Fever*, published in 1801, we find him recommending Belladonna, Opium, and Chamomilla in fractional quantities about equivalent to our third centesimal dilution, and defending his practice in *Hufeland's Journal* of the same year.

His complete method, constituted as now described, is set forth in the luminous essay entitled "The Medicine of Experience," published by him in the same journal for 1806. He there expresses his conviction that "as the wise and beneficent Creator has permitted those innumerable states of the human body differing from health, which we call diseases, He must at the same time have revealed to us a *distinct* mode whereby we may obtain a knowledge of diseases that shall enable us to employ the remedies capable of subduing them; He must also have shown to us an equally distinct mode, whereby we may

discover in medicines those properties that render them suitable for the cure of diseases." To obtain this practically
useful knowledge of disease, he maintains, we must abandon
all speculation as to its essence, and content ourselves with a
faithful and detailed picture of its manifestations, with their
predisposing and exciting causes when these can be discovered. To ascertain the properties of medicines we must
experiment with them on the healthy human body, noting the
symptoms which result in their order and connection. We
must, then, if we wish a permanent and curative effect,
administer in disease that drug whose effect most nearly
resembles the morbid condition before us. To give, as is
ordinarily done, remedies whose primary action is opposed to
the diseased state we have to treat (as opium for sleeplessness), is mere palliation, and useful and necessary in but
few cases. Finally, curative—because similarly acting—remedies must be given in comparatively small doses, lest excessive
aggravation or undue reaction should occur ; and so sensitive
is the diseased body to their influence, and so purely dynamic
their mode of operation, that doses of extreme minuteness—
even to a millionth part of those ordinarily given—will often
suffice for the end proposed. Such medicines, also, should be
given singly ; and the doses should not be needlessly repeated
—each being left to work within its ascertained term of action.
"If," he sums up, "as is not unfrequently the case when there
is a sufficient supply of well known medicines, a positive
remedy perfectly appropriate to the accurately investigated
case of disease be selected, administered in a suitably small
dose, and repeated after the expiry of its special duration of
action, should no great obstacles come in the way (such as
unavoidable evolutions of nature, violent passions, or enormous
violations of regiminal rules), and should there be no serious
disorganisation of important viscera, the cure of acute and
chronic diseases, be they ever so threatening, ever so serious,
and of ever so long continuance, takes place so rapidly, so
perfectly, and so imperceptibly, that the patient seems to be
transformed almost immediately into the state of true health,
as if by a new creation."

The facts, dates, and quotations I have thus brought before
you present several aspects for consideration.

I. It would, I think, be impossible for any unprejudiced
person at the present day, standing in the light of the medical
knowledge now enjoyed, and having some acquaintance with
the doctrine and practice current in Hahnemann's time, to
doubt that the reform thus proposed by him was a real and

most beneficent one. Pathology, at the end of the eighteenth and the beginning of the nineteenth century, was a tissue of the most baseless hypotheses : the therapeutics associated with it were a mixture of violence and confusion. Men were treating, as Hahnemann says, "unknown morbid states with unknown medicines," opposing fancies about the one to fancies about the other. In the stead of this most unsatisfactory system he proposed a method alike simple, intelligible, and innocuous. It consisted, as we have seen, in the following elements :—

1. The apprehension of disease by its symptoms, *i.e.*, as we say at the present day, by its clinical characters and history.

2. The ascertainment of the powers of drugs by experimentation on the healthy human body.

3. The application of drugs to disease by a principle which at least insured directness of aim.

4. The administration of remedies singly, instead of in complex admixture.

5. Their prescription in doses too small to aggravate existing troubles or cause extraneous ones.

Who can doubt the blessing it would have been to mankind had such a method been adopted when Hahnemann promulgated it ? Who can reckon the thousands that would have been saved from the murderous and poisonous doings universally prevalent in the days when bleeding and mercurialisation reigned supreme in therapeutics ? If the profession can go no farther with Hahnemann ; if even they feel his system imperfect for fully dealing with disease in all its forms, let them at least admit the vast advance it made upon the practice of its day, and its anticipation of much that is now regarded of unquestionable importance.

But the point to which I wish especially to direct your attention is the relation of Hahnemann's first conception of his method, as now described, to the homœopathy practised in the present day.

The great majority of those known as homœopathists, at least in the old world, have been converts from the recognised modes of practice. The expositions of the system which have satisfied their reason, the cures which have established their faith, have been of the kind we have seen in the earlier writings and practice of its founder. They have accepted his method as he himself then conceived it—with its law of similarity, its provings of medicines on the healthy, its single medicine, and its small dose. But they do not think they need follow him in the rejection of the pathology of their day, as he in that of his. They find him allowing the existence of certain specific diseases, always essentially identical, for which fixed remedies can be ascertained ; and they think that the advance of knowledge has identified many more of the same kind. They prefer to work the rule *similia similibus* with pathological similarities where these are attainable ; though in their default, and to fill in the outline they present, they thankfully use the comparison of symptoms. Accepting his statement that attenuation within the millionth degree hardly weakens the power of a drug for good, while it robs it of power to harm, they freely use such fractional quantities ; but they rarely go beyond this limit, and as a rule steer closer to the other end of the scale. They do not mix medicines, but they often alternate them ; and (besides the occasional use of antipathic palliatives, which Hahnemann at this epoch recognised as sometimes allowable) they supplement them more or less freely with such agents as—lying outside the range of pure homœopathic medication—are commonly called auxiliaries.

On the other hand, there are many—especially in America —whose views of homœopathy have been formed upon the later teachings of the master, of which I shall subsequently speak ; and some of these have become more Hahnemannian than was Hahnemann himself. Among these colleagues of ours there has often displayed itself an intolerant spirit towards such as occupy the more independent position I have described above. Hard words are used of them, of which "mongrel " seems the favourite ; and they are bidden to depart from the associations of the true followers of Hahnemann, and to profane the name of homœopathy no more. Homœopathists of this kind are also exposed to considerable animadversion from their brethren of the old school. They are accused of sailing under false colours, because their practice is not exclusively of the kind denoted by their name, and are called upon—if they would vindicate their honesty—to withdraw from all fellowship from the societies, hospitals, journals, and other institutions which are consecrated to homœopathic therapeutics.

Now I maintain that great injustice is done to such men (who indeed form the great bulk of the homœopathists of the present day) by the attack of either side. It is not their fault that they, and the associations to which they belong, are known by a distinctive name. It is the fault of those who have refused to allow the views denoted by that name to be advocated, tested, and freely practised within the bounds of ordinary professional fellowship. Grant to homœopathy the same

liberty which is accorded to all other ways of thinking, however novel and unlike those ordinarily received, and the *raison
d'être* of homœopathic institutions will have disappeared.
But, till then, it must not be supposed that men who do believe
in homœopathy, however little they make it the exclusive rule
of their practice, will consent to put themselves in positions
where all employment of and reference to it is tabooed.   They
join themselves to homœopathic societies and journals because
there alone do they find the liberty of opinion and action they
require.   And why should their stricter colleagues be impatient
of their fellowship ?   Their practice is surely good practice as
far as it goes—far superior to that of one who rejects the
master's teachings altogether.   Pathological similarity must be
better than no similarity at all.   It may be a pity to alternate,
but it is less injurious than to mix.   Auxiliaries may be used
more freely than is needful ; but that is better than using nothing else.   Of course, there may be so frequent an employment of extraneous measures, and so little cultivation of the
method of similarity, that homœopathy ceases to be the predominant feature in a man's practice ; and in that case the less
he is connected with the name the better.   But this is a rare
occurrence ; as a rule, the adoption of homœopathy leads, by its
own intrinsic value, to a subordination of all other methods of
treatment, which is as evident to the observation of others as to
the consciousness of the practitioner.

Hitherto I have been vindicating the legitimacy of the
homœopathy taught by Hahnemann up to 1806 to be called by
that name, and to be practised by professed acceptors of the
system.   But it is another question whether it is wise to pause
there ; and whether, in declining to follow him further in the
elaboration of his method, there may not be involved the
neglect of a more excellent way.
It will be remembered that, when he wrote the *Medicine of
Experience*, Hahnemann was only fifty-two years of age.   In
the ordinary course of things, supposing health and strength
to be spared, there were at least twenty years of work
remaining to him ere age should begin to dim his perceptions
and enfeeble his faculties.   Such work, moreover, if less
original than that of earlier life, ought to be more matured ;
it should naturally contain the ripest fruits of a man's thought
and observation.   Now the twenty-two years which followed
1806 were those of Hahnemann's greatest activity as a practitioner and a writer.   To this period belong the first four
editions of the *Organon*, the first and second of the *Reine*

Arzneimittellehre, and the first of the *Chronischen Krankheiten*. He is at Torgau from 1806 to 1810, and at Leipsic from 1810 up to 1821, in both enjoying large opportunities of practice ; while from 1821 to 1828, at Cœthen, he has leisure to weigh the results of his experience, and to consider the problems of chronic disease presented by the sufferers of this kind who resorted to him there for treatment. It can hardly be doubted that whatever practical developments his method received during such a series of years are entitled to the most respectful consideration of those who accept that method in its essence.

There are four points, it seems to me, at which we discern a distinct advance and elaboration on Hahnemann's part at this time.

1. The first has regard to the principle on which selection by similarity should be carried out. Of course, wherever all the symptoms of a disease are reproduced in the pathogenesis of a drug, there is no difficulty ; and where no drug has them all, *cæteris paribus* the one which possesses the greater number would have the preference. But Hahnemann found after a time that this *cæteris paribus* involved a good deal. A mere quantitative dealing with symptoms proved insufficient : they must, he saw, be weighed as well as counted ; they must be treated qualitatively. And now, in seeking to appreciate the relative value of symptoms, he was led to two important conclusions : viz., that peculiar and unusual features, both of drugs and diseases, should count for more than common ones ; and that subjective symptoms—and especially those of the mind and disposition—should preponderate over such as were objective and physical. These views led him to attach less importance than he had formerly done to the disease—as nosologically or pathologically defined—which was before him, and to think more of the special sufferings of each patient. The result was the doctrine expressed in the phrase " individualisation," with the provisoes I have mentioned as regards the relative value of the symptoms present.

2. Up to 1806 Hahnemann had affirmed nothing more about the minute doses he had been led to employ, than that they hardly lost any of the efficacy of the medicines, while they robbed them of power to injure. But as he went on attenuating the more potent drugs employed, and as he applied the same process to substances comparatively or absolutely inert, he seemed to find a real development of power to be brought about. While all physical and · chemical qualities disappeared, such as odour and colour, alkalescence or acidity ; while all actively poisonous properties were lost,—

the medicines gained a penetrating energy as curative agents hitherto unknown to him, and a much wider range of action. Some of them retained this even up to the 30th or decillionth dilution ; some seemed to act best in other potencies of the scale, as from the 2nd to the 24th ; very few were the better for no attenuation at all.* Hahnemann's second point, as made at this period, was the positive efficacy of infinitesimal doses, as prepared according to his manner ; and their general superiority for the homœopathic treatment of disease.

3. Hahnemann had already warned against the needless repetition of doses. In the *Medicine of Experience* he had advised the duration of each drug's action to be ascertained, and the dose to be repeated accordingly. In the first edition of the *Organon* (1810) he substitutes for this rule, as based on an uncertain quantity, one which directed that the effects of a first dose should be allowed to subside ere another (if necessary) was given. But, whether by one plan or the other, treatment by single doses became increasingly Hahnemann's ideal throughout this period. It shows itself in every piece of practice he mentions, and in every case he records.

4. It may be thought strange that I should name, as a fourth step of advance on Hahnemann's part, his doctrine of chronic diseases. It would be so, did I mean by so doing to endorse the psora-theory, in its definite dependence on the entity itch. Hahnemann was indubitably in error about the pathological significance of this disease, as was Autenrieth and many another before him and after him. But, stripping his doctrine of all reference to this particular disease, it remains, in its essential substance, a most valuable induction from observation and guide to practice.† It is the affirmation that when disease becomes chronic it is because of some morbid diathesis, some constitutional taint; that the manifestations of this condition must not be treated as if they were mere local affections ; that even the ordinary internal specifics of homœopathy are mostly insufficient for their cure, and must be supplemented by new medicines, of a profound reach and long duration of action. It was this thought which led Hahnemann to introduce the so-called " anti-psorics " into medicine—which enriched the Materia Medica with Alumina, Baryta, Calcarea, Graphites, Kali carbonicum, Lycopodium, Natrum muriaticum, Sepia, and Silica.

What I have said about the distinction between the speculative theory and the practical doctrine of chronic diseases applies to much else in Hahnemann's work at this time. His

* See Appendix, " Hahnemann's Dosage." † See Sulphur.

discovery of the efficacy and sufficiency of infinitesimals, for example, was mixed up with hypotheses of all disease being a derangement of the " vital force," and of a " dynamisation " effected in medicines by the processes of trituration and succussion to which he subjected them. All this may be rejected, as it generally has been rejected ; but the discovery remains. It is thus with the various explanations he suggested of likes being cured by likes. Few receive these, but that *similia similibus curantur* is acknowledged by all his disciples.

Dismissing, therefore, the theories of the master as of doubtful value and only speculative interest, let us fix our attention upon him in the sphere of his true greatness, and consider his practical rules. I can but very briefly indicate the facts and arguments by which they have been substantiated. In so doing, I shall draw chiefly on the writings of Dr. Carroll Dunham. I feel that I am indebted to him for the conviction of the reasonableness of Hahnemann's fuller doctrine, as I was to Dr. Madden many years ago in respect of homœopathy generally.

1. And first, as regards individualisation. It is pointed out that while a few leading symptoms are sufficient to enable us to diagnose the nature of a case, and for this purpose we may ignore the rest, it cannot be so when we are to treat it by the method of similarity. Every appearance the patient presents, every sensation he experiences, every circumstance of amelioration or aggravation of his sufferings, must have some pathological basis, and must be taken into account in the choice of a remedy. Just in proportion as a drug has been found capable of causing all these concomitants and characteristics, will it be the rapid and certain cure for the case in which they occur. If it is otherwise, then, although the drug may have produced the actual disease, nosologically speaking, by which our patient is attacked, yet it may not be essentially homœopathic to the form of the disease now before us. It may be fever we are treating, and our medicine may be truly pyretogenetic. But suppose that the pyrexia it causes is accompanied with great restlessness and anxiety, while the febrile sufferer under our care lies dull and listless, there is a lack of true homœopathicity between disease and drug. Adherence to the " totality of symptoms " would set us right, though we could not define or explain the difference between the two cases. Again, our patient may have rheumatic joints ; but their painfulness may be either increased by continued motion or the reverse. It is obvious that this distinction may depend on the presence or absence of an inflammatory condition of the

parts, and may modify accordingly our whole management of
the case.   But, even though we knew not its significance, it
would symptomatically guide us to the choice between Bryonia
and Rhus as the medicinal remédy.

The individualisation of each case, therefore, by the totality
of its symptoms, is the only certain method of arriving at the
true *similimum* for it among medicines.   The more we gene-
ralise, and refer it to a class, the less happy we shall be in our
drug-selection for it.   And, should there be no drugs which
correspond to it as whole to whole, we should select that one
which has caused any peculiar features it may have, if we have
good reason to believe such remedy suited to the essential
malady present.   Correspondence at such special points indicates a very close relationship between disease and drug—far
more so than if common characters only were in question.
Subjective symptoms outweigh objective ones in such differentiation, for they present less of the common than of the
peculiar features of a case.   They are, moreover, of great value,
as being the earliest signs of disorder, before organic change
has begun; they constitute the main phenomena of a malady
at a stage in which it is still curable.   I should have liked, had
time permitted, to have read you an extract from the Address
on Medicine, delivered by Dr. Russell Reynolds before the
British Medical Association in 1874, enforcing the importance
of subjective and mental symptoms.   "We are bound to remember," he concludes, "that there are many affections of
which they furnish the earliest indication, and there are not a
few of which they are throughout the only signs."*

2. And now as to the infinitesimal doses of this period, by
which I mean the dilutions from the 2nd to the 30th.   Evidence as to their positive efficacy, and as to the comparative
inertness of many medicines unless thus attenuated, is abundant.   The best proof of the latter point is that in the practice
of those who confine themselves to the lowest potencies such
remedies find little estimation or use.   But a good deal of
consideration is also due, I think, to the position of those who
affirm the relative superiority of infinitesimal over more substantial doses.   Besides Hahnemann himself, this class includes
Dunham, Hoppe, von Grauvogl, and Chargé; and—to some
extent at least, as evidenced by their practice—Tessier and
his foremost disciple Jousset.   The first-named has shown,
from the comparative statistics of Wurmb and Caspar's

* See also Dr. Madden, " On Subjective Symptoms," in *Brit. Journ.
of Hom.*, xxvii., 458; and Dr. C. Dunham, in *Homœopathy the
Science of Therapeutics*, p. 89—92.

Hospital, that in pneumonia the action of the 30th decimal dilution was more certain and more rapid than that of the 15th and the 6th, while of the two last the 15th bore away the palm.*   There is, moreover, in the general tone of those who employ highly attenuated medicines, a confidence in their remedies, an habitual sense of power and success, which cannot be disregarded.

3. Regarding the use of single doses, instead of a series of them, allowing the medicine thus given to act undisturbed for a reasonable length of time, I can say little at present.   When we find so scientific a physician as Professor Hoppe maintaining the reasonableness of this practice,† and a veteran like Jahr saying that his best cures have been achieved in this way, which—he truly says—was that of Hahnemann and all his disciples for the first twenty years of homœopathy, it merits our best consideration.

4. And, lastly, as to the doctrine of chronic diseases. I think there can be no doubt of the immense benefit which has resulted therefrom in the past, in the tendency it has given us to look to the possible constitutional origin of local and superficial affections, and to treat them accordingly. This view, and our possession of the " anti-psoric " medicines, has placed us on the same vantage-ground towards all such affections, as, e.g., the knowledge of the syphilitic origin of many examples of nervous disease has afforded in general medicine.   There is a tendency in a certain school of homœopathists to think of all disease as local, and to neglect medicines which have not an absolute physiological action dependent on dose. Such, for instance, would be the result of Dr. Sharp's system, if it were allowed to embrace the whole sphere of therapeutics. We need, I think, to be recalled to Hahnemann's sounder standpoint if we are not to lose many of the triumphs over chronic disease which have hitherto waited on the steps of those who have adopted his method.

The second of our two homœopathies is now before us. It is that which Hahnemann taught and practised between 1806 and 1828. With the further modifications which took place subsequent to the latter date I have nothing at present to do. The new points which a man makes after seventy-four have no à priori recommendation in their favour ; and that the first of them here was the fixing the 30th attenuation as the uniform

* See Op. cit., p. 240.
† See his article in Hirschel's Neue Zeitschrift, ii., 3, transl. in Brit. Journ. of Hom., xx., 369.

dose of all medicines, whether for provings or for curative purposes, does not invite us to welcome the rest. To make the
Hahnemann of 1830-43 our guide is, I think, to commit ourselves to his senility. But the second homœopathy which I
have just been expounding is the fruit of his ripest manhood,
and I think it ought to be more cultivated than it is in
England at this time. I doubt whether it is, at least in all
hands, applicable to the exigencies of every-day practice and
the treatment on a large scale of acute disease. For this purpose I commend to you rather the earlier and simpler method
I have previously exhibited. But when there is more leisure,
and especially when chronic disease comes before you, I think
that your best hope of making certain and speedy cures,
whose brilliancy shall recall the earlier days of our history, will
lie in your adherence to that (shall I call it?) higher homœopathy which the genius and toil of its discoverer have
elaborated for us.

It is under these convictions that I shall set about teaching
you Materia Medica and Therapeutics from the homœopathic
point of view. I must avow at once that my ordinary stand-
point is that taken up by the followers of Hahnemann's earlier
method. It must almost necessarily be so. Lectures on
Materia Medica, like those on the Practice of Medicine, must
contemplate *diseases* as their objects, while the purer homœopathic therapeutics regard rather the sick person in his individuality. The similarities, moreover, which I shall seek to
establish between drug-action and disease will be in the main
pathological. When, again, I see reason to conclude that any
recognised use of a drug—as that of Amyl nitrite in angina
pectoris, and of Belladonna in nocturnal enuresis—is antipathic and palliative only, I shall not therefore advise you to
reject it from your practice. I shall also tell you of many
applications of remedies which, though truly homœopathic, are
(in my judgment and according to experience) best carried out
with appreciable doses. On the other hand, I shall be far from
ignoring such subjective and peculiar symptoms of drugs as
may aid in the task of individualisation : I shall frankly accept
the efficacy of infinitesimal doses, both in pathogenetic and in
therapeutic action ; and I shall assume the soundness of
Hahnemann's psora-doctrine, as I have now explained it, and
devote much attention to the new and recondite remedies
which it has led him to introduce to our notice.

The homœopathy you will learn from me will thus be no
narrow or imperfect thing, but will embrace the whole range
of Hahnemann's progress as a thinker and discoverer, while

content to receive some modification of its form from the
advances of modern investigation. It will be such as he (I
apprehend) would not fail to recognise as his offspring, while in
no disciple of the scientific medicine of to-day will it be likely
to excite repugnance or contempt.

LECTURE VII.

HOMŒOPATHIC POSOLOGY.

There is one more topic on which I must enlarge ere we begin our detailed study of the Materia Medica. I have spoken of the modifications imposed upon this course of instruction by the fact of its being delivered in a School of *Homœopathy*. But I find that I have omitted any special notice of what to many minds would seem the most peculiar feature of that which I shall say. I refer to the minute dosage with which I shall so often have to deal. The pharmaceutic processes I have described as characteristic of homœopathy have for their main objects the reduction of the drug to fractional proportions, of which the third degree already represents the millionth part of a grain or a drop, while I shall have to speak familiarly of the sixth, the twelfth, and even the thirtieth. You will be warranted in demanding of me some explanation and vindication of such unwonted dosage; and it will be my pleasure as well as my duty to give it you.

Now the first and chief reason of my dealing with these minute quantities of drugs is that their use is a fact in the history of homœopathy. I have already told you how Hahnemann early followed up the enunciation of his new principle by a reduction of the dose of medicines given in accordance with it, and how in later times he pushed the attenuation of his remedies to the elevated degrees I have just mentioned. If any of you desire to follow him step by step in his progress, from 1796 to 1839, you will find the means of doing so in the article on the subject contained in the *British Journal of Homœopathy* for April, 1878.* As it was not till after 1811 that he began to make professional converts to his system, it came to them all with the infinitesimal dose as a part of it, and was by them all carried out therewith. Most of them, moreover, went on with their master in his further development of attenuation, and some have since pushed far beyond him in the process. The result is that the great bulk of the

* Reprinted in the Appendix to this volume.

homœopathic experience on record has been obtained by means of minute dosage, and no little of its pathogenesy owns a similar origin. I, as a teacher in a School of Homœopathy, have to deal with it historically—as it actually is and has been ; and, whether I myself approved of them or not, infinitesimals must necessarily play a large part in the lessons it is my duty to give.

But I am fully prepared to maintain the tenableness in itself of the homœopathic posology, and to advocate it as a most important and beneficent part of Hahnemann's therapeutic reform.

In the first place, comparative smallness of dosage is the logical and obvious corollary of *similia similibus curantur*. It needs no argument, as I have said, to show that the ordinary doses of Arsenic, against which even a healthy stomach needs to be shielded, would increase the irritation of one already inflamed, for which, nevertheless, the homœopathic principle would direct its being given. The quantity administered must be reduced accordingly. Nor are Hahnemann and his avowed followers the only witnesses to the practical necessity of this proceeding. Whenever a piece of homœopathic practice has been borrowed by the practitioners of the old school, the small dose has always gone hand in hand with the similar remedy. Drops of Ipecacuanha wine were unknown to the ordinary posology until the drug began to be used to check vomiting instead of to cause it ; and similar novelties in the way of dosage abound in the *Therapeutics* of Dr. Ringer, and in the like-minded communications of Dr. Dessau to his New York colleagues.* I may appeal to such facts as the best answer to the argument lately advanced by Dr. Decaisne in France, and Dr. Barr Meadows in this country, that the aggravation caused by similarly-acting remedies in the ordinary quantities proves their unsuitableness, and that the diminution of dose merely evades the difficulty by reducing their action to nullity.

But this argument, valid as it is, establishes only the relative smallness of the homœopathic dose. We must go farther to ascertain what its positive littleness may be, and to warrant any measure of the astonishing exiguity it has actually attained.

Now I would here suggest that dose is, to begin with, a mere arbitrary matter. There is nothing in nature corresponding to drachms and scruples and grains, and there is no reason why that particular number of molecules which go to make up the

* *New York Medical Record*, July 28, 1877.

last-named quantity should be designated by a whole number, while all below it must be expressed by fractions. Yet the result of its being so is that in the grain we seem to have got to the *ultima Thule* of ordinary smallness, and any further division strikes us as strange. Again, it is evident that all our notions of dosage are derived from the quantities of drugs it has been found necessary to give to produce their physiological effects on the system—to set up purgation or emesis, the sedation of an aching nerve or the relaxation of muscular spasm. If the so-called "alterative" medication had attained a larger place in therapeutics, these notions might have been modified. It has always been recognised that a different posology holds good with regard to remedies of this kind; that, as no physiological effect was sought, but only a gradual extinguishment of the morbid state, the dose necessary to be given was purely a matter of experience. Now it cannot be too clearly recognised that all homœopathic remedies are "alteratives" in this sense; and hence that any standard of dosage taken from such medication as aims to produce physiological effects is inapplicable to them.

Further, it is obvious that, even without taking such distinctions into account, dose is a shifting quantity. It varies, as every one admits, within certain limits, according to age and sex, the strength or weakness of the patient, and the amount of medicinal susceptibility he possesses. It varies through a still wider range with the different drugs we administer. Take, for instance, two remedies renowned of old in the treatment of cutaneous disease—Dulcamara and Arsenic. Carrére, the introducer of the former, administered it in tablespoonfuls of a decoction made in the proportion of an ounce to a pint; while the latter is given in small doses of a solution (Fowler's) which contains only 1 part in 120, sometimes requiring (as in a case of Mr. Hunt's) that even minims of this shall be broken up into fractions, which yet prove curative. So, when another potent substance—Phosphorus—is introduced (as lately by Mr. Ashburton Thompson) into the ordinary practice, no one is surprised at his recommending its employment in hundredths of a grain. With the alkaloids we get further still in the realm of minuteness, even as regards physiological action. Take the influence of atropia in dilating the pupil. The "atropised gelatin" prepared by Savory and Moore under the direction of Mr. Ernest Hart purports to contain but $\frac{1}{100000}$th of a grain in each disk; yet it answers its purpose excellently well. Professor Donders (cited in the fourth edition of Pereira's *Materia Medica*) finds that in dogs the attenuation of atropia may be carried up to $\frac{1}{700000}$th before the effect becomes doubtful ; and it is possible, from the experiments of Rossbach and Frölich, that the doubtfulness arose from contraction being produced by the drug when reduced below the dilating point. Professor Donders, moreover, adds :—" The sensitiveness of the eye to atropia, indeed, excites astonishment, when we consider that of the single drop of attenuated solution which suffices to produce dilatation probably not a fiftieth part is absorbed." Nor is it the pupil only that these dilute applications to the eye can affect. Dr. Harley records an observation of " congestion of the entire conjunctiva, with dryness of the membrane and dull aching pain in the eyeball, lasting for several hours," occurring after the instillation of twelve drops of a solution of one part in 400,000 of water. We have only to go somewhat lower in the scale of fractional minuteness to see the drug affecting the whole organism from within. Dr. Ringer finds the 200th of a grain of Atropia, subcutaneously injected, sufficient to dry up the whole surface of the body, even when freely perspiring in the Turkish bath ; and Dr. Harley writes of this substance—" An infinitesimal quantity— a mere atom—as soon as it enters the blood originates an action which is closely allied to, if it be not identical with, that which induces the circulatory and nervous phenomena accompanying meningitis, enteric, or typhus fever." Aconitine carries us a step farther. The 300th of a grain of this alkaloid was found by Dr. Milner Fothergill sufficient actually to kill a rabbit of three lbs. weight ; while guinea pigs are so extraordinarily sensitive to its lethal influence that one weighing a pound died in three hours and a half after the administration of $\frac{1}{1130}$th of a grain. After these experiences you will not be surprised to hear that Professor Arnold, of Heidelberg, found tetanus readily produced in frogs by $\frac{1}{10000}$th of a grain of strychnia. Even the $\frac{1}{1000000}$th caused increased reflex excitability ; and in one of these creatures, which the day before had been tetanic for some hours, after $\frac{1}{10000}$th had been administered to it, but had quite recovered, a slight attack came on in half an hour after receiving the $\frac{1}{1000000}$th, which ended, after some hours, in its death.

With these poisons and alkaloids, then, we have clearly got far on the road to another standard of dosage. The French *milligramme*—*i.e.* (about) $\frac{1}{64}$th of a grain—is found the most convenient unit for them, and even this (as M. Gubler has announced in regard to aconitine) has to be further divided. We have got a long way towards infinitesimals, even for the production of physiological effects: and it would be very unwise if we refused to look ahead, and see what further reduction may be necessary when we seek for pure therapeutic results on the principle of similarity. If drop doses of Ipecacuanha wine are sufficient to check vomiting, while drachms are needed to cause it, then, if " an infinitesimal quantity—a mere atom " of atropia will originate the pyrexial process in the blood, how minute must be the quantity which, on the same principle, will be appropriate to extinguish it !

Yet again. There are many substances which are inert in their crude state, but which, when rubbed up with some indifferent vehicle so as to insure a fine division of their particles, become active enough. We have a familiar instance in Mercury, which as pure quicksilver may be swallowed by the pound, but which, when intimately mixed with confection of roses or with chalk, becomes a potent drug. It is now recognised that the amount of oxidation which takes place in the preparation of blue-pill and grey powder is very small, and that minute subdivision is the essence of the process. Now Hahnemann, as you are aware, has largely developed this mode of preparing drugs, introducing the improved method of a graduated trituration with sugar of milk. The metals— gold, silver, platinum, zinc, together with such neutral substances as charcoal, flint, and lycopodium, are awakened to energy by this potent process, and show themselves capable of no little influence upon the organism. It is obvious that since in this way a real development of power is effected, there must be a certain stage in the process at which the drug, inert in its crude state, begins to be active, and another at which this newly-awakened energy is at its height, after which all further attenuation must have a contrary effect. At this second stage the triturated substance stands on the same level with a medicine of similar character which is active from the first; so that a grain of Silica 2 may be equal to one of Hepar sulphuris ϕ, though in actual quantity of the drug the latter is to the former as 10,000 to 1. Thus, with the medicines made such by trituration a very minute fraction may be the unit of their strength and the standard of their physiological activity ; while a still more infinitesimal quantity will be appropriate when they are used as remedies upon the homœopathic principle. I have mentioned the second trituration here because it was in those from the first (as Aurum and Argentum) to the third (as Carbo) that Hahnemann proved medicines of this kind.

We have arrived, then, at the conclusion that, when administered in conditions similar to those which they cause, medicines must be given in smaller doses than would be necessary for such causation ; and that the exiguity thus required may, from the natural activity of the substance, or from the degree of attenuation at which its energies begin to appear, be very considerable, reaching sometimes to such fractions as the thousandth, the ten-thousandth, and even the millionth of a grain. It may have to go thus far, but it need hardly go farther. To attenuations of this degree Hahnemann was led when first (in 1799) he began to use infinitesimals ; and for some years after he seems to have remained at the same point, more often descending below it than rising above it. To such potencies, moreover, a number of his followers—and these not of least eminence—have confined themselves, when they have found it necessary to ascend above the mother tincture or the crude drug. Drysdale and Kidd, Yeldham and Black in this country ; Trinks and Arnold in Germany ; Cretin in France ; Gray in America—these are homœopathists of no small note, who tell us that in the first six decimal potencies they find all the attenuation they need, *when they need any at all.* On the other hand, the reasonableness of so far diluting potent drugs, when homœopathically employed, is denied by none. Dr. Ringer may recommend his hundredth-of-a-grain doses of corrosive sublimate in dysentery, and Mr. Hunt may come down to the 480th of a grain of Arsenic in psoriasis, and no one will gainsay them. One of the latest critics of Homœopathy—Dr. Rogers, in his *Present State of Therapeutics*, says : —" I can well imagine that certain energetic remedies may act more or less in doses of the 1st, 2nd, or 3rd dilutions of the decimal scale," *i.e.*, in the tenth, hundredth, or thousandth of a grain.

So far you have, I imagine, followed me without difficulty. There is nothing in reason, nothing in the nature of things to render doubtful the apparent testimony of experience, when it speaks of the efficacy of similarly-acting medicines in the attenuations from the 3rd or 2nd downwards. If homœopathic posology had only taken this range, I should have had nothing further to urge, and could now have left the subject in your hands, confident of your acceptance of my position. I wish indeed that I could have done so, and that the method of Hahnemann had not been weighted with anything in the way of dosage less defensible than the thousandths and millionths with which I have been dealing. But here again I must remind you that my duty is not to express my own preferences, but to teach you homœopathy as actually existing and historically developed. I must, therefore, take into account that, from 1808 onwards, Hahnemann is found raising the potencies of several of his medicines far above the 3rd, dealing with billionths, trillionths, quadrillionths, octillionths, at length reaching the decillionth, and in 1829 fixing this last proportion as most suitable for all drugs. I must recognise the fact that the majority of his disciples have followed him in the employment of these higher fractions, and are using them more or less largely in their practice at the present day. Nor can I shut my eyes to the later development of attenuation up to the 200th dilution ; and to the knowledge that potencies of this strength, of undoubted pharmaceutic reality, have been warranted as active by such men as Bönninghausen, Dunham, Tessier, and von Grauvogl, and by the first two at least esteemed of more efficacy—both in acute and chronic disease —than any lower dilutions. I cannot ignore these facts ; and more, I do not feel justified in presenting them to you as a mere recorder, with such unsympathetic reluctance as to influence you against their acceptance. Much as I regret the necessity of employing the higher infinitesimals, I cannot but acknowledge it. The testimony in their favour is overwhelming; the evidence of their efficacy undeniable. My own experience of such dilutions as the 6th and 12th, and (with some remedies) of the 30th, is such as to make me join with unquestioning acclamation in their praise. I have no practical knowledge of the 200ths ; but if I had no other fact before me than their constant use by so scientific and successful a physician as Carroll Dunham, I should be content to acknowledge their legitimacy.

But here, too, we must inquire how far the apparent testimony of experience is supported by reason, by science, by observation.

1. I fear that reason has nothing to say in our favour. We have good logical ground for reducing our dose below the point at which it can aggravate the existing malady, or injure healthy parts ; but we have none for carrying our attenuation further than this. We seem, therefore, to have effected all reasonable ends, even with the most potent poisons, when we have reached the thousandths and millionths of which I have hitherto spoken ; and the same may be said of the inert substances whose properties are first elicited by trituration and dilution. Unless some evidence should be brought before us to prove that we actually develope power, as we go on attenuating after the Hahnemannian method, reason must certainly frown upon the higher potencies. I shall examine presently the theories of " dynamisation " which have been put forward

to support this conclusion, and I fear I shall not be able to endorse them. I must, then, for myself at least, give up any countenance from the side of reason for this part of my position.

2. The relation of science to us, however, is at first sight very encouraging. No one can have followed the researches of the last thirty years, and considered the sizes dealt with in thermal and luminous undulations, and in the molecules and atoms of matter, without feeling that infinitesimals of a most minute character are acquiring undoubted place and reality in the world of being. All the work of the universe, all the actions of life, are seen to be carried on by these tiny existences; in their little microcosm forces of all kinds play, and in them begin all changes whether normal or morbid. It seems at first sight, I say, that we are only following in the same track when we present our drugs in a state of the finest molecular subdivision, when we seek to counteract abnormal motions of the ultimate particles of matter by vibrations as minute as their own.

And to a great extent we are, I think, quite justified in claiming the support of science for our proceedings. The existence and the energy of the infinitely little have been substantiated thereby, and no one is now warranted in rejecting effects because their supposed causes are inappreciable by coarse sensation. But I fear that if we make too much of the analogies of the minute quantities with which scientific speculation deals, we shall find we have enlisted a dangerous ally, one who will leave us when most we need assistance. It must be remembered that the conception of the atomic constitution of matter, while suggesting how infinitesimally small are its ultimate particles, implies also that it is not infinitely (in the strict sense of the word) divisible. You must come at last to atoms ($\dot{a}$, $\tau\acute{\epsilon}\mu\nu\omega$)—particles which can be divided no farther; and then any subsequent attenuation can but reduce their number until all trace of them disappears from the vehicle. Now molecular science has so far advanced that it has seemed practicable to estimate approximately the size of the ultimate atoms of matter. Sir W. Thompson, Clerk-Maxwell and others have attacked this problem, and, though their solutions of it differ pretty widely, none have gone further than the affirmation that a trillion of such atoms may be contained in a space of $\frac{1}{1000}$th of an inch cube.* Now, making all allowance for the molecular contraction which, as Jolly has shown,

* See *Monthly Microscopical Journal*, March 1876, p. 113.

attends upon all attenuation of chemical solutions,* this will hardly carry us beyond our 12th potency. At higher degrees than this the presence of any atoms of matter whatever must become increasingly doubtful.

This is the latest word of theoretical science on the subject, and its practical observations point in the same direction. Chemical tests, applied to those substances which are readily recognised thereby, follow them up with decreasing clearness to the third attenuation, and there—or thereabouts—lose them. The spectroscope carries our vision further still ; but the 9th dilution is the highest point from which any response has been forthcoming to this potent detector. The microscope, used upon the triturations, has yielded similar results.† Under a power of 300 diameters, Dr. Mayrhofer has traced metallic particles up to the 10th, 11th, and (in the case of precipitated tin) even the 13th and 14th attenuations, but no further. "Moreover, the visible particles of the substances," he says, "become gradually smaller and fewer as the triturations advance, and at last cease altogether." Up to a certain point, then, we gain by this process. "A patient who takes a grain of the 3rd trituration of tin or arsenic, swallows no less than 576,000,000 particles, each of which possesses all the properties of the metal, and from their minute size can freely penetrate to all parts of the organism, and develope their peculiar effects on every part." But, if trituration is carried on, "the atoms, becoming always smaller and more mobile, at length come to be so much so that they elude the triturating force." If, on the other hand, they are (according to our usual plan) mixed from this point with a fluid menstruum, either they are suspended therein, when it is obvious that their number must decrease a hundredfold with each successive dilution, or they undergo a true solution, when they are as divisible as matter itself, but no farther.

When now we turn to observations on the animal body, corresponding conclusions have to be drawn. M. Davaine, in experimenting with septicæmic blood, was led to try in what fractional proportion it still retains its virulence. He found that by employing the graduated Hahnemannian method of dilution, he could reproduce the disorder by inoculating other animals (rabbits) with the millionth, the billionth, the trillionth, and at last the ten-trillionth of a drop of blood. Above this

* See v. Grauvogl's *Text-book of Hom.*, pt. ii., § 221.

† Dr. Conrad Wesselhœft's recent examination of our triturations has yielded results still less favourable ; but his work is regarded as still *sub judice.*

point, however, no effects were produced. Again, therefore, science goes a long way with us. It shows that matter can be carried by the homœopathic process of attenuation above the 9th centesimal degree without ceasing to be present or losing the activity proper to it. But at this point it leaves us in the lurch, and—without denying it—gives no warrant to the supposition that the same thing will hold good at further stages of the process.

From science as such, then—science unconnected with Medicine—we receive countenance for our infinitesimals so far, that up to about the 12th centesimal dilution we can depend upon the presence of some particles, however few or small, of the original drug. But the very support which it gives us up to this point turns into opposition when we go beyond it ; for, if every test finds less and less response as we mount higher in the scale of dilution, it implies that there is a progressive diminution in the quantity and energy of the matter present, and that we must at last get to an end of it. And, again, if when we have reached the ultimately visible particles of matter, we see them diminishing in number as we attenuate farther, must it not be so with those still smaller particles into which matter is ultimately divisible? At the 12th dilution we are a good way off from the 30th, and there is a great gulf between us and the 200th. How are we to bridge it over ? how fill up the yawning void ? Now at this point come in the theories of " dynamisation " which have attracted so much attention in the homœopathic controversy—much more, indeed, than their intrinsic importance deserves. They imply that the processes of trituration and succussion with which our attenuations are made more than compensate for the reduction of the mass of the medicinal substance, that they actually develope power, and this to an indefinite extent, so that the higher dilutions are more potent as medicines than the lower, the 30th than the 3rd, the 200th than the 30th, and so on *ad infinitum*. By some of Hahnemann's followers, who are more imaginative than philosophical, this dynamisation has been supposed to result from a transference of the whole thing from the realm of matter to that of spirit.* I can only say that

---

* I must admit that his own language in later days favours the same idea, but I think that he used the term " spiritualisation " metaphorically. He supposed matter to be infinitely divisible, saying in the last edition of the *Organon* (1833) : " A substance divided into ever so many parts must still always contain in its smallest conceivable parts *somewhat* of this substance, and the smallest conceivable part does not cease to be *some* of this substance, and cannot possibly become nothing."

I know nothing of such conceptions as applied to natural things : they are to me alike uncongenial and unintelligible. Others, with a more just idea of the matter in hand, have endeavoured to apply to it the doctrine of the correlation of force, and have argued that the energy put forth by the triturator or succusser must be converted into increased force on the part of the drug so treated. But they have not shown, on the one hand, that it may not be accounted for by the heat and electricity developed in the process, and on the other, that the power of drugs to affect the organism is a " force," in the sense that heat and light and such like are forces, so that it has equivalence and correlation with other modes of motion. It seems rather to be a fixed and inalienable property, peculiar to each substance possessing it. The same objection holds good to the hypothesis advanced by my friend Dr. Allen,* that the energy of the drug is transferred to the vehicle, so that although no particles of the original substance remain therein the medicinal force is not lost. If, moreover, it were so, it is obvious that no further potentisation would be possible when once the drug had attained its ultimate subdivision, and, parting with its force to the surrounding menstruum, disappeared from the scene. From about the 12th to the 18th dilution, then (if the calculations I have specified are correct), all capacity of change must cease, and we have in hand nothing but a medicated water or spirit, incapable of further dynamisation. Dr. Allen refers to the French observations with septic blood as illustrating this transference of energy to a vehicle. But he forgets that after the ten-trillionth (*i.e.*, 19th decimal) dilution had been reached, which is about the estimated extent of the divisibility of matter, no further effect was manifested.

I may refer you to a short but able paper by Mr. Proctor in the thirty-first volume of the *British Journal of Homœopathy*, on " The Theory of Dynamisation," as a complete examination and, I think, refutation of these ideas.

You will observe that I have said nothing about the potencies lately employed in America, in which the 1000th becomes a new unit, and the scale is run rapidly up until now the millionth and ten-millionth are supposed to have been reached. I must reject these, not upon the grounds of science and reason, but upon those of pharmacy. They are simple impossibilities. It is easy to calculate that, if Hahnemann's directions are followed, upwards of 2,000 gallons of spirits of wine would be required for making the millionth potency of a single medicine, to say nothing of a million clean bottles ; and, as not more

* See *New York Journ. of Hom.*, ii., 1.

than four potencies could be made in a minute, each receiving
its due number of shakes, that incessant labour at the rate of
twelve hours a day, and six days a week, would yet occupy
more than a year in the process ! Even if machinery be employed, the time taken could not be reduced much more than
one half, and as power of some kind must be supplied, considerable expenditure would be incurred. Whenever, accordingly, we are able to learn the process by which these potencies
are prepared (and the tendency is to keep it a secret), we
always find it other than that recognised among us, and
illegitimate in itself. Jenichen's preparations, which first
broke ground in the new field, are now believed to be simply
succussions of an ordinary attenuation without further dilution
—ten of such shakes being reckoned as producing a potency
one step higher in the scale. The preparations which go
under the names of Fincke and Swan are manufactured by
what is called "fluxion," *i.e.*, by allowing a stream of water to
be propelled with some force into a phial containing a hundredth part of a drug, each emptying of which is reckoned as
diluting it one step farther in the centesimal scale. Even in
this way an immense time must be taken to produce such
potencies as are named ; * and how utterly untrustworthy is the
result ! † My advice to you, therefore, is to keep altogether
clear of these obscure and objectionable practices, and to set
down any results which seem to have been obtained by medicines so prepared to their being other than what they assume
to be.

Putting these, then, out of sight, and limiting ourselves
to such attenuations as have been, and can be, prepared in a
proper way, our conclusion must be that while we are fully
warranted in expecting action from those below the 3rd, and
are not without countenance in similar hopes from those up to
the 12th, beyond this range we have nothing to depend upon

---

* Jenichen purported to produce the 60,000th potency. Dr. Dudgeon
has shown that, working five hours a day, and allowing a second for
each shake, it would take him five weeks to raise—according to his
method—a single drug to this height.

† Dr. Burdick, of New York, who has eminent scientific qualifications,
has lately shown, by calculation and microscopical investigation, that
the potency which Dr. Swan represents as m.m. (*i.e.*, thousand thousandth, or millionth), "cannot exceed the tenth centesimal of Hahnemann, and is liable to be much lower" (*Hahn. Monthly*, Nov., 1877).
It has been cruelly suggested (and not without warrant) that the
reason why these preparations have been found so efficacious is that
they are really much *lower* attenuations than their adopters have been
accustomed to employ.

but observation and experience. While we are not, therefore to ignore curative results obtained from 30ths and 200ths, we must be wary about admitting them, requiring the warrant either of the capacity of the observer, or of a full statement of the facts of each case. Upon these principles I shall act in dealing with the materials of my present course. They are applicable also, and with even greater force, to provings which purport to have been made with infinitesimal doses, many of which will come before us as we proceed. The altered sensibility to stimuli of diseased organs, and the similarity of the action of the drug to the morbid cause, combine to suggest that homœopathic remedies may cause aggravation, and that their doses should be small and may be minute. Upon the healthy there is no such *à priori* probability of the action of infinitesimals : it is a pure question of fact. Well : I can here also affirm that, in my judgment, the facts bear out the doctrine that such quantities *may* produce effects. Let me mention three crucial instances :—

1. Dr. Imbert-Gourbeyre, whose bibliographical and personal collections of the effects of Arsenic will connect his name indissolubly with this drug, has recorded several instances of its physiological action in infinitesimal doses.[*] Among these are,—from the fourth trituration (gr. $\frac{1}{10000000}$), pruritus, erythema, papules, and burning of the eyes with lachrymation ; from the eighth (gr. $\frac{1}{100000000000000}$) a confluent miliary rash with great malaise (this was in a healthy prover, a medical student).

2. Dr. von Grauvogl, to whose transcendent ability his *Lehrbuch der Homöopathie* bears unquestioned witness, proved the same drug on himself. The 3rd and 10th decimal attenuations made him ill : the 30th decimal did not do this, but it brought on the insatiable thirst which he subsequently experienced when suffering from the stronger doses, and which he therefore knew to be arsenical.[†] The 30th decimal = the 15th centesimal attenuation ; *i.e.,* a drop of it represents the quintillionth of a grain.

3. Arsenic is a virulent poison in its crude state. But of the drugs which, inert thus, develope energy in the process of trituration we have a typical example in Natrum muriaticum. This substance was re-proved in Vienna, under the superintendence of Dr. Watzke, a most competent observer, and with all his prejudices the other way. But he writes—" I am,

* See especially his " Etudes sur quelques symptômes de l'arsenic " in the *Gazette Médicale* for 1862.
† *Text-book of Hom.* (trans. by Shipman), ii., 59.

alas! (I say, alas! for I would much rather have upheld the larger doses which accord with current views) I am compelled to declare myself for the higher dilutions. *The physiological experiments made with Natrum muriaticum,* as well as the great majority of the clinical results obtained therewith, speak decisively and distinctly for these preparations."

In the face of such facts (which might easily be multiplied, both from the Austrian* and the later American provings) we are not justified, I think, in rejecting symptoms purporting to be obtained by infinitesimal doses of drugs, as such. They possess, however, in enhanced degree the uncertainty which hangs about all provings on the healthy subject. Dr. Hamilton showed us some years ago[+] how many slight deviations from the norm will occur in a man presumably healthy, who notes his own feelings and doings for a few days. Dr. Conrad Wesselhœft, of Boston, has recently shown[‡] the same thing on a larger scale by a crucial experiment. Having to conduct a re-proving of Carbo vegetabilis, he began by furnishing his fellow-workers with a number of blank powders of sugar of milk. No inconsiderable array of symptoms were reported to him as the result of the ingestion of these placebos, before a single particle of the drug had been absorbed. Except, therefore, where care has been taken to eliminate this source of error, we must accept with considerable reservation the results purporting to be obtained from infinitesimal doses, especially when they are of the subjective and fleeting character which mostly belongs to them. When, as in Dr. Imbert-Gourbeyre's cases, they are objective, or when, as with Dr. von Grauvogl's, they are marked and recurring, there need be no doubt of their reality.

I believe these to be reasonable grounds on which to proceed in dealing with the difficult subject of Homœopathic Posology

* See *Brit. Journ. of Hom.,* vi., 10.
+ See *Ibid.,* xxix., 565.
‡ See Transactions of the American Institute of Homœopathy for 1877.

LECTURE VIII.

ACIDUM BENZOICUM, CARBOLICUM, FLUORICUM, HYDRO-CYANICUM, MURIATICUM.

We now proceed to the consideration of the several substances constituting the Homœopathic Materia Medica. Various classifications of drugs have been adopted by teachers and writers of the old school, as the order in which they should be discussed. I venture to think that all these, whether based on natural history, on physiological action, or on therapeutic properties, assume more relation between drugs than really exists. In homœopathy we are led to regard each drug as an individual, and it will be more in accordance with the genius of this system to adopt an order which assumes nothing as to the action of its constituents. This is, obviously, the *alphabetical*.

Most homœopathic authors, in adopting this plan, begin with Aconite, and at once plunge therewith into the very thickest of the fight. I shall ask your previous attention to the *acids* used in our practice. By Hahnemann and Jahr these were named after the substance which yields them, as Nitri acidum, Sulphuris acidum ; and took place in their alphabetical catalogues accordingly. Dr. Allen has them similarly scattered throughout his volumes, through their being called Benzoicum acidum, Fluoricum acidum, and so forth. I much prefer grouping them all together, with their *adjectiva* in the second place : their names will then stand first on our list. We shall gain this advantage thereby, that several minor yet not unimportant medicines will have come under our notice, and will have initiated us in the study of Materia Medica on homœopathic principles, ere we grapple with one of the most eminent of the series.

The first medicine we shall consider, therefore, is—

Acidum benzoicum.

This acid is obtained by sublimation from benzoin, a balsamic resin which exudes from the incised bark of the

Styrax Benzoin.　It is dissolved in rectified spirit, or tritu-rated.

Nothing was known of the physiological effects of Benzoic acid (save the alteration of the urine which it causes) till it was proved by the American Institute of Homœopathy.　The report of these experiments, by Dr. Jeanes, is contained in the *Materia Medica of American Provings*.　Another pathogenesis of the drug was then published by Dr. Petroz, and may be found in his colleeted writings.　An " arrangement " of our knowledge concerning the drug forms one of Hering's *Ameri-kanische Arzneiprufungen*, and may be read in English in Dr. Shipman's translation of v. Grauvogl's *Text-Book of Homœopathy*.　It contains many additional observations.　Dr. Allen's article includes all these materials, but is somewhat spoiled by a commingling of clinical with pathogenetic symp-toms, the former being not always distinguished by their proper mark.

The pathogenesis of Benzoic acid does not lend itself readily to interpretation or analytic statement.　It is one of those which are utilised therapeutically rather by the *à posteriori* than by the *à priori* method of homœopathising.　The account to be given of it is therefore the statement of what application has been made of it to practice.

After taking Benzoic acid in quantity, hippuric acid appears in the urine.　This seems merely a chemical change, as hippuric acid under the influence of acids is converted into Benzoic acid and gelatine sugar, and the opposite transforma-tion has every opportunity and material for its occurrence.　It was supposed, however, by Mr. Alexander Ure that in this process the lithic acid of the urine disappeared ; and hence he proposed to use Benzoic acid in gouty subjects to prevent concretions and calculi.　Later investigations have not con-firmed this observation as to lithic acid, nor Dr. Garrod's statement that under these circumstances the urea is dimi-nished.　But Lehmann has demonstrated that the Benzoic is one of the few acids which manifestly increase the acidity of the urine.　It has accordingly been used, with decided tem-porary benefit, in cases of irritable bladder with alkaline urine and muco-purulent or phosphatic deposits.

The dynamic properties of the drug seem to centre at the same spot.　Dr. Jeanes has found a deep red (almost brown) colour of the urine, and a great intensification of its natural odour, an almost unfailing characteristic for the drug.　A minute dose even will change these features of the secretion, and therewith ameliorate the morbid conditions associated with them. Among these he mentions especially syphilitic and gonorrhœal affections occurring after suppression of the primary symptoms, but also recurring quinsy and nephritic colic, infantile diarrhœa (the stools being pale and fœtid), ulcerations of the mouth and tongue, and rheumatic and gouty arthritis. In all these, Benzoic acid, prescribed mainly because of the presence of the characteristic urine, relieved greatly or cured. Subsequent experience and testimonies are in the same direction. In the enuresis of children* and old persons where this condition is present; in dysuria similarly accompanied;† and in acute articular rheumatism having the same feature,‡ the drug has been found of the utmost value. Dr. Guernsey states that the odour of the urine is more characteristic than the colour, and that it must be present when the urine is freshly voided.

These are the main uses of Benzoic acid; but a few miscellaneous observations must be added.

1. Benzoin and other balsams—as those of Peru and Tolu—are regarded as having a specific influence upon the mucous membranes, especially that of the respiratory tract, which (say Trousseau and Pidoux) they affect as the turpentines that of the urinary organs. They are used to check excessive expectoration. Now although, when swallowed in substance, their resinous constituents might have much to do with this action, yet the more common mode of applying them to the bronchial membrane is by fumigation, and here it is the acid they contain which becomes the active agent. In the case of benzoin this acid is, as we have seen, our present drug; which thus appears to exert a special action on the respiratory mucous tract. Accordingly, we find that when Schreiber had taken in two days about half an ounce of the acid, he noted—among other effects—an increase of the pulse-rate amounting to thirty beats per minute, *with increased secretion and excretion of phlegm;* while Pereira states that he has repeatedly tried the acid in bronchial affections, but has more frequently seen it augment than relieve the cough. Perhaps in the smaller doses we should use it would prove more beneficial.

2. Dr. Hering says that "the more Benzoic acid is used in

* *North Am. Journ. of Hom.*, iii., 334. Marcy and Peters, p. 14. Stillé says that incontinence of urine, without an altered condition of the secretion, has been treated successfully by means of benzoic acid; but Bartholow thinks that in such cases the urine was too alkaline.

† See *Brit. Journ. of Hom.* xxvi, 489.

‡ Von Grauvogl's *Text Book* (Engl. transl.), ii., 127. It is much used in this disease in the Leopoldstadt Hospital at Vienna (*Annals,* iv., 514).

gout the more it will be prized." The swelling of the fingers noted by Nusser, one of his provers, who took eighty grains of the second trituration in one dose, points in this direction; and the facts we have just mentioned suggest the drug in gouty bronchitis.

3. Dr. Bayes states that he found it rapidly curative in a case of tendinous swelling at the back of the wrist of long standing; he does not say in what dose. I have myself frequently obtained much reduction in size of ganglia situated in this region by its external application in an ointment containing five grains to the drachm. But Dr. Turrel has communicated to the eighth volume of the *Bibliothèque Homœopathique* (p. 354) five cases in which such tumours were dispersed by the medicine given internally in the dilutions from the 12th to the 30th. He mentions that horses are liable to an analogous affection (" wind-galls "), and suggests that it may be owing to the considerable proportion of Benzoic acid which exists in their forage. This latter fact may account for the uric acid in their renal secretion undergoing that modification which has given it the name " hippuric," and which accounts for the strong odour of horse-urine. In one of Dr. Turrel's cases the urine had a remarkable fœtor.

There is no homœopathic medicine I can compare with Benzoic acid.

Its chemical action on the urine seems attainable with about ten-grain doses. Its homœopathic uses have been carried out with quantities varying from gr. $\frac{1}{20}$th to the 3rd and (as we have seen) higher dilutions.

I have next to speak of the product of the distillation of coal-tar known as

Acidum carbolicum.

The Pharmacopœial preparation is a solution in rectified spirit.

Some excellent provings of this substance (mainly with the medium dilutions), in which upwards of thirty persons took part, have been made in America. Their results, together with a good many effects of poisoning, are given by Dr. Allen. Some of the provings are related at length, together with some clinical experience obtained with the drug, in the fourth volume of the *Pathogénésies Nouvelles* appended to the *Bibliothèque Homœopathique*, which you will find in the library of this School. There is a good account of its crude physiological effects in Dr. H. Wood's treatise.

It is needless to speak here of the action of Carbolic acid as an antiseptic and as a local anæsthetic. These are properties of the substance which medical men of all schools can and do utilise. Our present interest is with its dynamic influences and specific remedial powers.

The most marked symptoms of poisoning by this acid are those of the nervous centres, which are congested and prostrated by it, so that coma (with contracted pupils) and paralysis result. In animals clonic convulsions are not uncommon, which seem to be epileptiform in seat and character. In the provers these effects take the milder form of languor of mind and body, with headache and vertigo, and sometimes spinal pain and tenderness. The headache implies great fulness of the cerebral vessels, being generally compared to a sensation as if a tight band were stretched around the forehead and temples. Sometimes it becomes neuralgic in character, and is then especially felt over the right eye. We next have marked effects upon the *stomach*. Vomiting is often produced, even when the acid has been absorbed from a wound; and flatulent distension, causing frequent sighing or belching, is a constant symptom with the provers. One of these speaks of himself as suffering throughout his experiments from a veritable acute dyspepsia, though the doses he took were too small to produce any local caustic effect. These are the main seats of its action in the provers; but experiments on animals give us also fatty degeneration of the liver and kidneys, with epithelium and albumen in the urine; keratitis and conjunctivitis; and—post-mortem—pseudo-membranous and purulent inflammation of the bronchial tubes, with disseminated lobular pneumonia or else congestion of the lungs. It is not certain how far the human body is susceptible of these actions.

Of the therapeutic powers of Carbolic acid we know little as yet; but, so far as they go, they correspond with its pathogenetic action. It is especially in gastric affections that it has been found useful,—in vomiting (H. C. Wood) and flatulent distension (Ringer) in the old school, and in some complicated dyspepsias in homœopathic practice. Migraine, moreover, when the pain is seated above the right eye, has yielded to its use. Its physiological influence on the skin is uncertain, though itching and vesiculo-pustular eruptions occasionally appeared among the provers. But it has been found very useful, not only in such forms of cutaneous disorder, but also (by my friend Dr. Guerin Ménéville, of Paris) in psoriasis.

It can hardly be doubted that more has yet to be made of this potent agent. What it can do against purulent formations and malignant febrile and inflammatory conditions is probably due to its antiseptic influence, and needs material doses of the acid itself or of the sulpho-carbolates. My colleague Dr. Cooper has communicated to me an excellent cure of hepatic abscess and dysentery thus effected. A female prover experienced great relief from a lumbo-sacral pain which had long troubled her. The head symptoms, moreover, are so strikingly apoplectic that some use ought to be made of the analogy. It seems once at least to have cured acute hydrocephalus, and might be useful in uræmic coma. Davidson and Bähr esteem it highly in diphtheria.*

Carbolic acid compares with *Gelsemium* in its action on the nervous centres, with *Carbo vegetablis* and (naturally) *Kreosote* in the gastric sphere.

Its homœopathic cures have been effected with the dilutions from the first to the third.

The next in order is—

Acidum fluoricum.

This acid—more strictly hydrofluoric—is peculiar to homœopathic practice. The primary dilutions of it are, of course, prepared with water ; and, owing to the solvent action of the acid upon glass, must be kept in gutta-percha bottles.

The homœopathic school possesses an exhaustive proving of the dilute acid. It was conducted by Dr. Hering, assisted by thirteen others, and its results may be read in the *Materia Medica of American Provings*, or in Allen's *Encyclopædia*.

This is another pathogenesis of which no general account can give an adequate idea. But the main curative sphere of Fluoric acid has been ascertained by applying certain of its indications to practice. It may be defined as consisting in chronic irritations of mucous membrane, and in morbid conditions of the more lowly organized tissues. Cases are on record in which the acid, in dilutions from the 5th decimal upward, has proved curative of chronic diarrhœa, of secondary syphilis of the throat and tongue,† and of osseous caries.‡ These are from the late Dr. Laurie's pen ; but in Hering's article we read

---

* See Oehme's *Therapeutics of Diphtheritis*, p. 24.
† See *Brit. Journ. of Hom.*, xxiv., 154.
‡ Laurie's *Elements of Hom. Practice of Physic*, p. 609.

how under the use of the drug whitlows have been blighted, fistulæ—lachrymal and dental—have closed, varicose veins have shrunk to half their size, fresh hair has grown on a bald head, and moist palms have regained their healthy dryness. Chronic rhinitis also has been cured, and rectal troubles alleviated. Other directions in which it may profitably be applied will probably appear. My own experience with it in old cases of varicosis of the leg, such as we see at the hospital, is very favourable.

The following seem to be prominent among its physiological effects :

1. Disagreeable and inimical mood.

2. Sense in the brain as if on the verge of being struck by apoplexy. (After smelling the strong acid. The first effect was to irritate the throat : then an influence seemed to pass to the brain.)

3. Retinal excitement, with red photopsia.

4. Urine of strong odour (once with purple sediment).

5. Great excitement of the sexual instinct in men, and in a woman premature appearance of the catamenia.

6. Pains in the bones generally.

7. Numbness and lameness of the hands.

8. Itching and redness of old cicatrices of the skin.

9. Perspiration, glutinous or sour.

M. Maumené has been led from his observations and experiments to believe that the cause of goitre is the presence of fluorides in drinking water. He asserts that they are peculiarly abundant in the water of goitrous districts. In corroboration of his views he cites an experiment in which a true and permanent bronchocele was established in a dog by a five months' course of fluoride of potassium. This is a hint not to be neglected.

I have already mentioned the doses in which this acid has been given in homœopathic practice. It is a close analogue of *Silica*, of which we shall have hereafter to speak.

I have now a more familiar drug to introduce to you,— prussic acid, or

Acidum hydrocyanicum.

"Equal measures of the officinal acid" (which contains 2 per cent. of anhydrous prussic acid) "and rectified spirit will make the first centesimal dilution :" so writes the British Homœo pathic Pharmacopœia.

I

Hydrocyanic acid has not been experimented with in the school of Hahnemann. But an excellent proving of it has been furnished by Professor Jörg, in which five persons tested the acid itself, and sixteen the distilled waters of the two natural substances which contain it most largely—the bitter almond and the cherry laurel. Some of the numerous cases of poisoning by this agent have been collated, and their physiological and therapeutical significance analysed, in a paper on the acid by Dr. Madden and myself in the twentieth volume of the *British Journal of Homœopathy*, to which reference may be made for more details than can find place here. Dr. Allen's pathogenesis embraces the above materials and many other symptoms from poisonings.

This potent poison, reputed in many disorders since its discovery in 1782, appears in Ringer's *Handbook* as sometimes relieving pain and vomiting in chronic gastric diseases; and that is all. Stillé allows also some power on its part over nervous coughs, including pertussis. In homœopathic practice it is very rarely mentioned. I venture to think that this is undeserved neglect; and that we have in Hydrocyanic acid, given according to the law of similars, a very useful medicine.

It should be so, indeed, according to its physiological action, which pictures several severe diseases.

1. The first of these is *epilepsy*. There is a large *consensus* of authority as to the essential similarity between the phenomena of poisoning with this acid and the epileptic paroxysm. Pereira, Christison and Taylor all affirm it, and it need not be argued afresh here. The first case of poisoning we have cited in our paper was taken by the medical attendant for an epileptic fit; and there is nothing surprising in the mistake. The sudden falling and loss of consciousness, the subsequent laryngismus, empurpled face, foam at the mouth and convulsions together form a perfect picture of the attack of this disease. Excitation of the cervical sympathetic, which is now regarded as (through the contraction of the cerebral arteries it produces) the proximate cause of epilepsy, was undoubtedly present in this case, as indicated by the dilated pupils, with prominent, glistening eyeballs. Pereira's statement seems to be correct, that " whatever be the precise pathological condition of the brain in poisoning by this drug, it is probably identical with that which occurs during an epileptic paroxysm, and with that produced by loss of blood."* The sensations in

---

* This argument will be found more fully drawn out in a paper contributed by me to the World's Convention of 1876, and published in its Transactions.

the head described by provers are in entire harmony with this view, and forcibly suggest the epileptic vertigo.

The homœopathic inference from these facts must be that Hydrocyanic acid ought to find a very prominent place among anti-epileptic remedies. Its use in this affection hitherto has been only limited. It was hardly to be expected that it should play any large part in the old-school therapeutics of epilepsy : nevertheless, some experience of the kind is on record. Hartlaub and Trinks, in the preface to their proving of Laurocerasus, mention that Gremmler found the acid diminish the frequency and severity of the paroxysms, though he could not effect a radical cure with it ; and that Remer praises it in the epileptic convulsions of pregnant women. They also refer to a cure of epilepsy by cherry-laurel water, communicated by one Müller to *Hufeland's Journal.* I find that the patient here was a woman of twenty-two, who had had the fits for seven years, often twice a day. Aqua laurocerasi was prescribed, in doses increasing from twenty to eighty drops daily. By the time that four ounces had been taken, the patient was quite cured. Frank, in the first volume of his *Magazin* (p. 320), relates three of Gremmler's cases, which seem to warrant a more favourable account than that given of them by Hartlaub and Trinks ; and also one from Koehler, in which a complete cure was effected. In his fourth volume he cites a narrative from the *Bulletin* of the French Academy of Medicine, which tells how an epileptic dog, being delivered over to be poisoned, instead of being destroyed by the prussic acid given him with this intent, lost his fits and became quite healthy.

In homœopathic literature I know of no record of the treatment of epilepsy by this drug. Baertl, in the exhaustive collection of cases of the disease which he communicated to the *Vierteljahrschrift* in 1863 (translated in the twenty-second volume of the *British Journal of Homœopathy*), finds no place for Hydrocyanic acid. He mentions, indeed, some favourable results from Ferrum hydrocyanatum ; but this compound seems to have none of the active properties of the acid. I can only, therefore, speak from my own experience with the medicine.

Dr. Madden and myself were so struck with that homœopathicity to epilepsy which I have now claimed for it that we proceeded to use it largely in the treatment of the disease. Our results at first were encouraging, and we hoped to be able to communicate many instances of cure from its administration. But in all save recent cases the fits soon returned.

We thought that Dr. Russell had noted a fatal weakness in the medicine when he pointed out the evanescent character of its action, and we supposed that thus our fleeting successes were explained.

Save, then, in recent epilepsies—as from fright—I made little use of Hydrocyanic acid until 1875. Having then to lecture on the drug at the London Homœopathic Hospital, the fresh and more extended survey of the facts which I made led me to think that I had been hasty in abandoning it as an anti-epileptic. I thought it likely that some part of our failure had arisen from not giving the medicine strong enough or long enough, and that thus the evanescence of its effects might obtain compensation. I altered my plan accordingly, and am much better pleased with my results. It is my practice now to give from five drops of the 3rd decimal attenuation to three drops of the first centesimal three times a day.

Drs. Croucher and Holland have recently reported cases of epilepsy cured by the acid where the sudden cry so characteristic of poisoning by it has ushered in the paroxysms.

2. Secondly, Hydrocyanic acid causes undoubted *tetanus*. There is not, as with Strychnia, evidence of increased reflex excitability ; but, as with Aconite and Cicuta, persistent tonic spasm. This it produces by direct action upon the spinal cord ; for, when the cord was divided (by Wedemeyer) between the last dorsal and the first lumbar vertebræ, and prussic acid introduced into one of the hind legs, these, as well as the forelegs, were immediately convulsed.

We have thus in our medicine another anti-tetanic. The only instance of its use of which I am aware is a case of the traumatic form of the disease successfully treated by Dr. George Moore with drop doses of Scheele's acid.* The curative action here seems undoubted.

3. The tonic spasm excited by Hydrocyanic acid is nowhere more marked than in the organs of respiration. This also is the general testimony of toxicologists. " Spasmodic respiration " is noted by all observers of acute poisoning, Boehm† pointing out that it is to the expiratory stage that this character especially belongs; and Wood mentions among the chronic effects of the vapour "difficult respiration, constriction of throat, feelings of suffocation." " The only marked post-mortem phenomenon," he writes, " is a universal venous congestion, proving that the circulation had been arrested in the lungs."

* *Brit. Journ. of Hom.*, xxiv., 506.
† Ziemssen's *Cyclopædia*, xvii., 509.

Now it is in spasmodic disorders of the respiratory organs that, next to gastric affections, Hydrocyanic acid has obtained its chief reputation. In whooping-cough Dr. West says that " it sometimes exerts an almost magical influence, diminishing the frequency and severity of the paroxysms almost immediately." In recent and uncomplicated asthma I have a high opinion of it : it is to this disease as to epilepsy. Dr. Russell, in his work on *Epidemic Cholera*, relates a case in which it gave great and speedy relief to an intense spasmodic oppression of the chest, which came on in a cholera patient; and Dr. Sircar, from his Indian experience, speaks highly of it in such conditions.

4. Any poison which through the nervous centres can affect the respiration is capable through the same channels (pneumogastric and others) of disturbing the action of the heart. Hence the palpitations, anxiety, diminished pulse, and tendency to syncope, noted alike in poisonings and provings by this acid.

The value of prussic acid in cardiac affections is fairly stated in this sentence of Dr. George Wood's. " In palpitation and other irregularities in the function of the organ, of no very energetic character, whether purely nervous or associated with organic disease, I know no medicine better calculated to alleviate the disturbance of the function, and afford ease and comfort to the patient." It has been recommended in angina pectoris, which is indeed of a piece with the gastrodynia and enterodynia in which it has proved so useful. There are testimonies extant to its efficacy.* I had an interesting case some time ago, in which epilepsy and angina pectoris coincided in the same patient. Hydrocyanic acid was of very great benefit for both disorders.

5. The curative power of Hydrocyanic acid in pain at the stomach and vomiting must also, I think, be traced to its homœopathicity thereto. "An overdose," writes the late Dr. Elliotson, one of its warmest advocates, " will in every person occasion nausea, vomiting, and pain and tightness at the præcordia. Even applied externally, it has caused nausea, vomiting, vertigo, and syncope. It appears therefore," he concludes, " to act specifically upon the stomach." It is evident that here, as often elsewhere, "specifically" means homœopathically. And, indeed, some such action seems required to account for the brilliant and permanent cures of gastrodynia and enterodynia recorded by this physician, and

* " New Materia Medica," by Drs. Marcy and Peters, appended to *North American Journ. of Hom.*, p. 25.

also by Pereira and Granville. Here also, as in whooping-cough, is displayed that *contingent* character which belongs to all the best homœopathic medication. Its beneficent effects are sometimes astonishing, while at others there is utter failure. When benefit does result, it is exceedingly rapid, so that there is no need to persist in the use of the drug for many days ; and, as its action is of very short duration, it may be repeated pretty frequently. Whether in the instances of success the pains are from spasm, and therefore the acid homœopathic, while in those of disappointment they are neuralgic, I cannot say : if it were so, I should apply the same principle to the treatment of angina pectoris. The gastralgia which indicates this medicine I find always worse when the stomach is empty, and relieved by food.

There is good evidence of the action of Hydrocyanic acid on the solar plexus. Sir B. Brodie applied one drop of the essential oil of bitter almonds to his tongue. He immediately felt a remarkable and unpleasant sensation at the epigastrium, with such weakness in the limbs and loss of power in the muscles, that he thought he should have fallen. I have frequently removed by it the distressing feeling known as " sinking at the stomach," when this has been unconnected with the climacteric age.

The outline of the sphere of Hydrocyanic acid is now very clearly before us. It affects the whole cranio-spinal axis and associated sympathetic ganglia, setting up that disturbance which induces tonic spasm in the muscles. Hence the phenomena of head, heart, lungs, stomach, and trunk in general ; and hence its therapeutic value in similar idiopathic conditions. It will be a profitable task if any one will undertake from study of the provings and from clinical observation to fill in this outline, and define for us the precise place of the medicine in specific therapeutics.

You may ask—is this description of prussic acid warranted by toxicology ? It is commonly supposed to be a paralysing rather than a tetanising agent; and is set down in ordinary classifications of the Materia Medica as a pure sedative. But a few cases of poisoning will dissipate the first notion,* and will show you that the second arises from observation of its curative action only.

* See also Stillé (ii., 252, 254-5):—" the immediate consequences of a fatal dose of the acid are general spasm of the muscular system, and death from an arrest of the action of the heart and lungs ; " and Boehm (*loc. cit.*, p. 505)—" we consider the convulsions of prussic acid poisoning the result of a transient but energetic irritation of the central apparatus of the brain and spinal cord."

For its action on the spinal cord Hydrocyanic acid may be compared with *Aconite* and *Cicuta*. As an epileptifacient, its only analogue is *Œnanthe crocata.*

I have generally used Hydrocyanic acid in the dilutions from the third to the sixth decimal. The experience of the ordinary practice would seem to show that in whooping-cough and gastrodynia the first attenuation may be used with advantage.

As the salts of Hydrocyanic acid and the plants containing it owe their active properties to its presence, it will be well to consider here any that demand our notice. I shall speak only of the cyanide of potassium among the former, and of the cherry-laurel among the latter : others are probably conformable to these types.

Kali cyanatum.—As a poison this salt seems identical with Hydrocyanic acid. It has been proved, in the first, second, and third attenuations, by two members of the Massachusetts Homœopathic Society (1861-2) : the record of their experiments may be read in the twenty-second volume of the *British Journal of Homœopathy* (p. 496). Lembke also has experimented with it. The results obtained by these provings, with effects of poisoning, enable Dr. Allen to present a pathogenesis of 228 symptoms. It presents little that is noteworthy, save as it covers the same ground as the acid. My only reason for mentioning the drug is that in the hands of the late Dr. Petroz it effected a remarkable cure of disease of the tongue, which may be cited here :—

"In 1829 a woman living in the Rue St. Nicolas, whose family was known to me, came to ask my advice about a disease of the tongue, for which she had been under the care of Dr. L'Herminier. The organ was profoundly altered by an ulcer, which appeared to me cancerous, and which occupied its right side ; the edges, especially posteriorly, were indurated, raised, and knotty ; speech was difficult, indistinct, and accompanied with much pain. The patient could only take liquid nourishment. Distrusting my own diagnosis, I sent her to Professor Marjolin. She brought me back the following judgment : ' Cancerous ulcer ; no chance of cure but from operation ; and this impossible, for the base of the tongue is involved.'

" In the presence of so grave a disease, I turned my thoughts to diminish her sufferings. I prescribed the $\frac{1}{100}$th of a grain cf hydrocyanate of potassa, to be repeated every fourth day. After fifteen days I again saw the patient. She suffered less ; the tongue appeared to me not so thick, the edges less hard, the speech easier. The medicine was continued in the same way. Fifteen days later the patient, whose countenance had lost its grey hue and drawn features, said to me with joy, ' I begin to be able to eat a crumb of bread.' The hydrocyanate was continued for a month longer, when the cure was complete. It is now eighteen years ago, and there has been no relapse."

Laurocerasus.—The cherry-laurel has found a place of its own in homœopathic medicine, from having been proved in an elaborate manner by Professor Jörg and eleven of his pupils, and subsequently by Drs. Hartlaub and Trinks. The article on the drug in the first volume of the latter's *Arznei-mittellehre* contains Jörg's symptoms and their own, with many observations of poisoning and overdosing ; Dr. Allen's pathogenesis is a reproduction of this, Jörg's provings being transcribed from the original. A tincture is prepared for homœopathic practice ; but the distilled water (Aqua laurocerasi) is generally the favourite preparation.

I am myself unable to see in either the pathogenetic or the curative effects of Laurocerasus anything specifically distinct from those of Hydrocyanic acid. It has, moreover, the disadvantage of very uncertain strength. Nevertheless, Dr. Phillips seems to have used it with good effect in the gastric, cardiac, and respiratory affections for which the acid itself is recommended. His doses are from five to thirty minims of the distilled water. It has been very little used in homœopathic practice. Dr. Guernsey considers the sense of tightness about the heart and chest which prussic acid causes a characteristic indication for Laurocerasus ; and mentions that it has been very beneficial in his hands for the cyanosis of childhood, when a little exercise produces gasping for breath and increased blueness. A gurgling sound in the œsophagus when swallowing is regarded as indicating this medicine in gastro-intestinal disorders.

Last, on the present occasion, we come to

Acidum muriaticum.

This is of course the acid now called hydrochloric. The attenuations are necessarily aqueous,—10 minims of the acid of the British Pharmacopœia with twenty-one minims of distilled water making the 1^x dilution.

Nothing is known in extra-homœopathic literature of the physiological action (save the local poisonous effects) of Muriatic acid. Hahnemann's first proving of it appears in the fifth volume of the *Reine Arzneimittellehre,* containing (in the second edition) 61 symptoms of his own, 196 from six fellow observers, and 22 from authors. A later pathogenesis in the fourth volume of the *Chronic Diseases* adds 295 symptoms more, contributed by Hahnemann himself and two others (Rummel and Nenning). Dr. Allen reproduces this last, adding a few symptoms from poisonings.

I have already explained why I can make no use of the symptoms of the *Chronic Diseases*. Moreover, since the attenuations of the acid are directed to be made with diluted alcohol for the first, and undiluted subsequently—a process which would go far to change it into ether, even the symptoms of Hahnemann and his fellow provers in the *Materia Medica Pura* are somewhat vitiated as indications for the use of true Muriatic acid. Again, the twenty-two symptoms (made into twenty-four in the later pathogenesis) from authors are strangely irrelevant for their purpose and incongruous with their surroundings. Hahnemann himself tells us of some as the effect of "aqua oxymuriatica," *i.e.*, solution of chlorine (Schmidtmuller, Crawford, Sachse, Humboldt), of others as the troubles of workmen in salt-mines (Ramazzini); while sneezing and cough with hæmoptysis are the local effects of inhaling the acid in gaseous form (Theiner, &c.).

Happily, our clinical experience is sufficient to define pretty closely its sphere of action. This may be said to be *a low febrile condition of the blood, with ulceration of mucous membranes and eczema of neighbouring cutaneous surfaces.* Its use in low fever is common to both schools of medicine. Of old, its action in these cases was ascribed to a power of modifying a supposed putrescence of the fluids ; and the medicine was given also in malignant scarlatina and putrid sore throat. Now-a-days its use seems pretty well confined to true "fever," and it is considered to act by neutralizing superabundant alkali (Richardson) or by supplying deficient acid (Chambers). I am disposed to believe that its (undoubted) action in this malady is, after all, dynamic ; for it is certain that Muriatic acid, in doses too small to exert any chemical action, has a very high reputation in homœopathic practice as a remedy for low fever. Dr. Trinks* warmly commends it (in the first dilution) in the type known of old as "nervosa versatilis," where it does great things in calming and cooling. Its homœopathicity to the erethism of the circulation and nervous centres present in this stage is evident from Stillé's description of its physiological effects. "In small doses," he writes, "medicinal muriatic acid occasions . . . generally some quickening of the pulse, . . . flushing of the face, and an increased flow of urine. In larger doses it excites the brain in a peculiar manner, causing giddiness, confusion of the senses, a sort of intoxication, in fine." Teste extols it later on, to modify the

* *Brit. Journ. of Hom.*, xxix., 293.

intestinal ulceration, over which he thinks it has as much power as when the same morbid condition exists in the mouth or throat. He says that "the almost constant and frequently immediate effect of this drug is to modify the character of the intestinal secretions, and to take away their foul smell; and, after this result is accomplished, almost all the other symptoms improve, and the course of the malady is considerably shortened." With this coincides, from another point of view, the testimony of Dr. George Johnson.* He thinks that the diarrhœa of typhoid may well be increased by the mineral acids (usually the hydrochloric) commonly given; and ascribes its diminution at King's College Hospital to their discontinuance.

Bähr, Guernsey, Bayes and Espanet concur in commending Muriatic acid in typhoid; and add to the above as indications for it slipping down to the foot of the bed, tendency to involuntary evacuations, utter aversion to food, and copious urination, with putrescent phenomena.

A similar condition of blood and mucous membrane exists in malignant scarlatina and perhaps in diphtheria. In the former disease Muriatic acid is of great value for the affections of the nose and ears, especially when they occur as *sequelæ;* and it vies with Mercury in the ulcerations of mouth and throat. About its action in true diphtheria I cannot speak with any confidence, though I think (and herein Dr. Kidd confirms me†) that it has some efficacy when symptoms of blood-poisoning are prominent. The following case by the late Dr. Russell will show what it can sometimes do here; and we should not forget the value set upon it by Bretonneau as a local application.

"The case was that of a lady about sixty years of age, who had been ill for two days. He found the pulse very small and quick, as high as 130. There was great prostration; the expression of the countenance almost like that of cholera, from the sunken, exhausted look—very remarkable, considering the shortness of the illness, and indicating the action of some poison. There was great fœtor of the breath, and on examining the fauces the whole surface was of a dark red, approaching violet hue, and spotted over with white membranous deposit. He gave a drop of the 1st dilution of Muriatic acid every hour, and next day found great improvement. From the first dose the patient was sensible of benefit, which continued till she got well. The disease had been increasing up to the time of the administration of the medicine, and from that time declined." ‡

Muriatic acid also plays an important part in ulcerations of

* *Practitioner*, Jan., 1875.
† *Brit. Journ. of Hom.*, xxviii., 742.
‡ *Annals*, i., 231.

the mouth and throat independent of these acute diseases, though probably connected with similar constitutional conditions, as indicated by the " low " character of the local mischief. Mercurial sores and aphthæ often come under this category. It seems to have a special affinity for the tongue. To this attention has been called by Dr. Cooper.* The symptoms of Letocha in Hahnemann's pathogenesis, which he cites, are not to be found at the place referred to ; and, until verified, can hardly be relied on as dynamic effects of the acid. But his cases of cure are quite valid ; and, embracing as they do induration, fungous swelling, ulceration, and that so-called psoriasis linguæ which so often proves incipient cancer, encourage us to confident use of the acid in affections of this organ. In a letter of Hahnemann's, which is on record, we find him prescribing Muriatic acid for cancer of the tongue ;† and I have myself employed it in recurring ulcers of the organ with the best effect.

Several other uses of the drug, but all falling within the general description I have given, are mentioned by Dr. Marcy in the *New Materia Medica*. His, too, are the fullest statements of its usefulness in cutaneous affections, where itching papules or vesicles seem to indicate it both internally and externally. Its employment in dyspepsia, so well defined by Dr. Ringer, seems beyond the sphere of its specific operation. It acts here either by locally checking excess of formation of gastric juice, or by supplying deficient acid to the digestive process. It is esteemed by some in piles and other troubles at the anus, when a great sensitiveness of the parts is present. There may also be much itching, and a paretic condition of the sphincter, in which case it is doubly indicated.

Nitric acid is the only medicine with which, as it seems to me, Muriatic acid can be advantageously compared ; though it has some points of contact with *Baptisia*, and perhaps with *Rhus*.

There seems no advantage in raising Muriatic acid above the 3rd attenuation, and the 1st and 2nd are those most commonly used.

* *United States Med. and Surg. Journal,* ix., 268.
† See *Brit Journ. of Hom,* xiii., 149.

ACIDUM NITRICUM, OXALICUM, PHOSPHORICUM, PICRICUM, SALICYLICUM, SULPHURICUM.

The acid with which we begin to-day is one of the most important members of our group—

Acidum nitricum.

Ten minims of the acid of the British Pharmacopœia with sixty minims of water make our 1^x attenuation, which is thus of about the same strength as the ordinary dilute acid. The subsequent attenuations must, of course, be aqueous.

Our only pathogenesis of Nitric acid was first published in the second edition of the *Chronic Diseases*. It contains 1426 symptoms, of which about 130 were supplied by fellow provers, and 30 taken from authors, the remaining 1260 being Hahnemann's own. Dr. Allen's additions are chiefly toxicological.

The reasons I have alleged for ignoring the pathogeneses of the *Chronic Diseases* press with double force in the case of Nitric acid. Hahnemann's age and practice at the time make it certain that his symptoms—six sevenths of the whole—were observed on patients ; and his globules of the 30th have but a doubtful relation to Nitric *acid*, as alcohol was used to make the dilutions from the 2nd upwards. His cited symptoms, moreover, are rarely pure ; being too often observed upon syphilitic subjects. An exception to this statement is formed by the symptoms ascribed to Scott, which—as they constitute almost our only genuine proving of the medicine—I will give in some detail from the original.*

Mr. Scott, an Indian army surgeon, suffering from chronic hepatitis, was led to think that Nitric acid might be an effective substitute for the usual mercurials in his case. He took accordingly a drachm daily of the strong acid, in divided doses.

* Duncan's *Annals of Medicine*, 1796, i., 375.

On the third day the gums began to be somewhat red and enlarged. He slept ill; but could lie for a length of time on his left side, which the disease of the liver prevented him from doing for many months previous to this period. He also felt a pain in the back of his head,* resembling what he had commonly experienced when taking mercury. On the fourth day his gums were a little tender; headache and pain about his jaws still troubled him; but the symptoms of his liver complaint had already left him. The acid was continued on the fourth, fifth, and sixth days, the soreness of the mouth increasing, and salivation taking place. On the seventh day he felt his mouth so troublesome that he took no more.

Other observers have confirmed this effect of Nitric acid upon the mouth, adding looseness of the teeth and bleeding from the gums to the symptoms mentioned by Scott. The action is not a local one, as Richter has found it produced by baths containing the acid. It is ordinarily unaccompanied by the fœtor of the breath or the tendency to ulceration of the gums which characterises the mercurial sore mouth; but Prioleau has seen these symptoms also, with swelling of the sub-maxillary glands, occur under its use, when given for syphilis. All these observers, moreover, find it somewhat diuretic.

Save these effects on the mouth, then, we know little about the dynamic pathogenetic action of Nitric acid. Clinical experience with it, however, is large and definite; and allows its sphere to be assigned with much precision.

1. I would first speak of its action on the *muco-cutaneous outlets*—those parts where mucous membrane is exposed to the external air, and where skin is so shielded and moistened that it approximates in character to mucous membrane. Its ptyalism and gingivitis suggest its Mercury-like affinity for the mouth, which is very strong: it antidotes its analogue here, and cures ulceration of the buccal mucous membrane. Dr. Ringer recognises this " further action " (*i.e.*, beyond the chemical) " on the mucous membrane of the mouth," and recommends it where this is reddened, inflamed, and glazed, in connexion with irritation of the digestive organs. The same thing may be said of it as regards the throat. Then, leaping over the intermediate digestive tract, it exhibits a singular power over the rectum and anus: it is reported to have cured prolapsus, fistula, and especially fissure. The evidence of its

---

* A case of chronic headache seated in the occipital protuberance, cured by Nitric acid, may be read in the *New York State Hom. Society's Transactions*, iv., 365.

power over this last-named trouble is quite satisfactory : the
sharpness of the pain excited by stool is most felt at the time
of passing.   In the respiratory tract it controls the ocular,
nasal, and laryngeal mucous membranes.   Dr. Goullon, in his
treatise on Scrofula, assigns it a high place in the treatment of
obstinate strumous ophthalmia, and considers it useful in superficial ulcers of the conjunctiva corneæ, and indispensable in
ophthalmia neonatorum.   Jahr praises it in gonorrhœal
ophthalmia.   It has been commended for the affection of the
nose which obtains in malignant scarlatina, for ozæna, and for
chronic laryngeal affections.   Acting on the genito-urinary
membrane, it is a valuable remedy (according to Dr. Marcy)
for chronic vaginal leucorrhœa, which may be tenacious, and
flesh-coloured or green, in cachectic subjects ; and has cured a
long-lasting itching of the urethra left behind after gonorrhœa.*
Dr. Guernsey recommends it for pruritus vulvæ.

Dr. Hempel truly says that "Nitric acid is principally
adapted to disease depending upon the presence of some
virulent miasm, especially the scrofulous, syphilitic, and mercurial."   But it is chiefly when these muco-cutaneous outlets
are the seat of the mischief that it proves an antidote : it hardly
penetrates deeper.   As regards syphilis, it supplements Mercury in soft chancres occurring in weakly or scrofulous subjects,
and often supplants it in secondary ulcerations of the mucous
membranes (Jahr extolling it also for inflamed bubo). It becomes
the prime remedy when even a hard chancre begins to sprout
into vegetations, and for the "mucous patches" which occur
at this stage of the malady, and which always haunt its favourite
seats of action.   We are thus led to that curious offset or ally
of syphilis which Hahnemann distinguishes as "sycosis," whose
local manifestations are condylomata.   Whether he was right
or wrong (and he is not alone) in thinking this a separate
disease, at least we do well in following him as to its remedies ;
and these are Thuja and Nitric acid.†   I shall have more to
say on the subject when we come to the former medicine.

2. Next in importance to the foregoing is the action of
Nitric acid on the *liver*.   The experiments of Scott, which
first brought it into notice, related to its power over hepatic
disease : it was only later that they suggested its use in
syphilis.   He cured with it chronic hepatitis and the "liver-

---

* *New Mat. Med.*,p. 54.
† "Small syphilitic warts and condylomata, kept constantly moist
with a wash of diluted nitric acid, are removed certainly and painlessly.
A drachm or two of the dilute acid to a pint of water is sufficient "
(Ringer.)

cake" of ague; and it has always continued a favourite
medicine in Indian practice. Of late, the combination with
Muriatic acid has been preferred for this purpose. Dr. Horatio
Wood praises this Nitro-muriatic acid for hepatic congestion,
" biliousness," non-obstructive jaundice, and commencing
cirrhosis; he says it should always be freshly prepared. It is
also used in baths and compresses. Considering its virtues
in oxaluria also—in which, since Golding Bird's time, it has
been considered almost specific—it deserves a good proving.
Dr. Allen gives a short pathogenesis of it, obtained by three
provers, using small doses; and in his supplement cites an
observation by Scott of its effect when used as a bath. It produced on him the same beneficial influence on the liver, and
the same irritation of the mouth and salivary glands which he
experienced from Nitric acid; but the sensations of the
stomatitis extended down the gullet, and in the buccal
cavity and on the tongue small superficial ulcerations appeared. Sometimes, he says, the compound acid "very
suddenly increases the secretion of bile." It also (in him)
increased the perspiration.

3. Of late years, Nitric acid has come to the front as a
remedy for *cough*. The late Sir Duncan Gibb wrote a book
on pertussis expressly to extol its virtues. Dr. Bayes says—
"Another affection in which Nitric acid has proved serviceable is a chronic laryngeal cough, without expectoration, which
is characterised by a stinging or smarting sensation, as if a
small ulcer were there, and is generally felt on one side. The
3rd dilution of the medicine often speedily arrests and cures
this cough." I have myself long used it with benefit in
laryngeal coughs, dry and violent. But Dr. Dyce Brown has
led us to extend the sphere of this acid in coughs. He commends it in several forms of disease in which this symptom is
the prominent feature, and especially when there is much
general physical depression. He even extends its use to
pneumonic phthisis after the more active symptoms have been
removed by other means. A good many typical cases are
related in his communication, which you will find in the
eighteenth volume of the *Monthly Homœopathic Review*.
I myself have certainly been led by it to prescribe Nitric acid
more largely in chronic coughs; and have found it very
beneficial, both to these and to the gastric irritation and
general cachexia which often accompany them.

Dr. Brown mentions constipation as a marked indication for
the acid in cough cases; and adds that he has found this symptom so often to disappear under its use that he has been led to

use it as a remedy for the trouble itself, and with such success
that he now places it in the front rank of available means in its
treatment. Dr. Wilde has communicated some confirmatory
evidence. Hahnemann (as Dr. Brown notices) expresses himself
to just the contrary effect, saying that " it is more suitable to
those chronic patients who are disposed to looseness : it is very
seldom useful to those who suffer from constipation." It is
possible that infinitesimal doses of the acid, prepared according to his method, may have an action of their own. But
there is another intestinal affection in which Nitric acid may
prove useful, and this is dysentery. " The dysenteric process,"
says Rokitansky, " offers the greatest analogy to the corrosion
of the mucous membrane produced by a caustic acid ;" and
in the present instance we have evidence that the action is
not local only. Wunderlich observed a case fatal on the
eighth day after the ingestion of a teaspoonful of the strong acid,
in which the usual lesions were found in the mouth, fauces,
œsophagus, and stomach, but the small intestine was sound.
The colon, nevertheless, was " intensely and deeply ulcerated."*

Dr. Ludlam, speaking of Nitric acid as indicated generally
" in those hæmorrhages from the mucous surfaces which
depend upon the destruction and desquamation of the investing epithelium," commends it highly in menorrhagia following
upon abortion or continued dysmenorrhœa ; and says that
a similar condition sometimes exists at the climacteric age,
and is to be treated in the same manner.†

Dr. Guernsey's indications for Nitric acid are chiefly offensive urine, smelling like that of horses, restlessness after
midnight, and (in women) violent downward pressure in the
pelvis, with pain in back and thighs. Amelioration from
riding in a carriage is also mentioned by him, and of this Dr.
Hoyne‡ gives a curious illustration.

Nitric acid compares with *Muriatic acid,* with *Mercury,* and
with *Thuja.*

Dr. Brown advises two or three drop doses of the first
decimal dilution ; and with this or the potencies near to it all
the successes of Nitric acid have been obtained, save those in
the rectal and anal troubles. Here the 30th Hahnemannian
attenuation is reputed to have effected the cures.

---

* Stillé.—Boehm, who also mentions this case, adds that the symp
toms of acute morbus Brightii were present.
† *Diseases of Women,* 2nd ed., p. 565.
‡ *Clinical Therapeutics,* i., 455.

For our next acid we have once more the advantage of a good pathogenesis; it is

Acidum oxalicum.

This well-known acid is almost unused in ordinary practice. For homœopathic use it is triturated or dissolved in rectified spirit.

Our toxicological knowledge of Oxalic acid is both extensive, from its frequent use in suicide and ingestion by mistake for Epsom salts, and precise, from the full experimentation to which it has been subjected, chiefly by Drs. Christison and Coindet.* It has received a full proving (by six persons taking the 1st and 2nd triturations) under the auspices of the American Institute, and Koch and Reil also have experimented with it. Arrangements of these materials exist, from Dr. Neidhard in the *Materia Medica of American Provings*, from Dr. Hering in his *Amerikanische Arzneiprufungen*, and from Dr. Allen, who adds numerous symptoms from poisonings.

Oxalic acid is an irritant poison; and the great body of the symptoms induced by its ingestion in bulk are due to inflammation of the alimentary mucous membrane. There is, however, no evidence of intestinal irritation when the poison is otherwise introduced into the system; so that we have here a local rather than a specific effect. Oxalic acid would thus be truly homœopathic to irritation of this tract only where it was of local origin, and would need to be given in semi-material doses. A Dr. Nardo, of Turin, is reported by Marcy and Peters to have used it (in grain doses) with uniform success for many years in gastritis; and it has been useful in glossitis and chronic angina.

When absorbed into the system, its elective affinities manifest themselves in the sphere of the lungs and of the nervous centres. The former present—*post mortem*—either scarlet patches or a uniform scarlet redness over their anterior surface, but without effusion; and the provers had lancinating pains through them, especially on the base of the left side. The trachea also has been found reddened after death; and the provers experienced some irritation in it. Marcy and Peters mention some experience suggestive of its value in chronic inflammations of the respiratory mucous membrane, and even in phthisis pulmonalis.

But the most important action of the poison is that

* *Edinb. Med. and Surg. Journ.*, xix.

K

which it exerts upon the nervous centres. The facts are as
follows :—

When administered to animals in such a manner as that it
can be absorbed, "the first unequivocal sign of its action is
generally a slight permanent stiffness of the hind legs and
increased frequency of the pulse. About the same time there
appears a slight sudden check in inspiration, from the respiratory muscles contracting before the chest is fully expanded.
Gradually several of these come together, so as to constitute
paroxysms of short, hurried breathing, with intervals of ease.
Meanwhile the stiffness of the hind legs increases ; they become likewise insensible, and often the spasm gives place to
paralysis ; he jerks the head occasionally backwards, walks
with a peculiar stiff gait, and assumes very odd postures, from
inability to regulate the motions of the limbs. As the poisoning advances, the motions of the chest during the paroxysms
become more and more confined by spasms of the muscles ;
and at last there is a period towards the close of each
paroxysm, when the spasm is so great as completely to suspend the respiration. This is commonly accompanied with
more or less extension of the head, tail, and extremities,
sometimes amounting to violent opisthotonos. . . . The
insensibility, hitherto limited to the hind legs, now extends to
the trunk and fore-legs, and lastly to the head. As the insensibility increases, the breathing diminishes in frequency, the
spasmodic paroxysms become more and more obscure, and
then cease altogether. For some time, however, they may be
slightly renewed, by striking the back and limbs ; but at last
the animal falls into a state of deep pure coma, with complete
relaxation of the whole body. The heart can now scarcely be
felt ; the breathing is low, regular, and short, and becomes
gradually more obscure, till finally life is extinguished without
a struggle." If the dose be larger, "the fits of spasm come on
early and with great violence, the intervals are marked by
remissions only, and the animal expires in a paroxysm, before
the stage of insensibility begins. . . . Death may be produced in this manner in three, five, or ten minutes. If on the
other hand the dose be much diminished, there may be stiffness of the hind legs, much dulness, drooping of the whole
body, and a sort of somnolency, without insensibility, or even
without spasmodic paroxysms, and then the animal will commonly recover."

This summary is taken from the original paper in the
Edinburgh Medical and Surgical Journal by Drs. Christison
and Coindet. The former, in his *Treatise on Poisons*, adds the

following as regards the effects of the acid on the human subject. "The best instance yet related of the development of nervous symptoms in man is a case described by Dr. Scott of Cupar, of a girl who swallowed by mistake a solution kept for cleaning brass, and containing about two drachms. She did not vomit until emetics were given, but complained much of pain, which was succeeded by great lassitude and weakness of the limbs, and next morning by numbness and weakness there as well as in the back. This affection was at first so severe that she could hardly walk upstairs; but in a few days she recovered entirely. There is also evidence to the same effect both in Mr. Hebb's patient and in Dr. Arrowsmith's case. The first thing that the former complained of was acute pain in the back, gradually extending down the thighs, occasioning ere long great torture, and continuing almost till the moment of his death. Dr. Arrowsmith's patient had the same symptoms, complained more of the pain shooting down from the loins to the limbs than of the pain in the belly, and was constantly seeking relief in a fresh change of posture. Mr. Fraser's patient had from an early period a peculiar general numbness, approaching to palsy." Boehm adds "formication both on the trunk and on the extremities," and "numbness and anæsthesia of the finger tips."

I think there can be no doubt that the phenomena thus described are those of inflammation of the membranes and substance of the cord. In no post-mortem has the spinal column been opened for examination; and we thus want ocular evidence. But the stiffness of the limbs and paroxysms of spasmodic dyspnœa point plainly to irritation of the spinal meninges; and the anæsthesia, neuralgia and loss of power indicate a similar affection of the spinal marrow itself. I once had the painful duty of watching a chronic case of this disease until its termination in death; and the symptoms I then observed come vividly back to my mind as I cite these descriptions of poisoning by Oxalic acid. I hope that some use may be made of the analogy. I am myself learning to depend with great confidence on the drug as a means of checking the tendency to spasmodic constriction of the chest which manifests itself in several forms of spinal disease.

Dr. Burnett has recently given us* an excellent study of Oxalic acid. As regards its physiological action, he shows that later German experiment has brought out in greater relief the paralysing action on the heart which Christison noted. He also mentions three cases in which it caused loss

* See *Brit. Journ. of Hom.*, xxxv., 309.

of voice, and suggests its use in aphonia. But the most interesting thing in his paper is a series of cases treated by him in
which anomalous pains in the head and spine, like those it
causes, have disappeared under its use, and in which its elective
affinity for the left lung near its base was utilised by treating
congestion and inflammation with it when localised there.
In these last instances it manifested remarkable powers,
obviously touching the mischief when the ordinary remedies
had failed. Dr. Burnett takes exception to my view that
the lungs are specifically irritated by Oxalic acid, suggesting
that the hyperæmia found in them *post mortem* may have been
secondary to disorder of the nervous centres or the heart.
His own clinical observations are, I think, the best facts I can
adduce in support of my statement. Unless the poison can
directly inflame the lungs in health, it could not have cured
pneumonia and pulmonary congestion in the way it did in his
hands.

Christison says that in minimum doses the effect is mainly
on the brain; and most of the provers seem to have felt it
acting there, especially on the vertex and forehead, where it
causes (and has removed) a dull headache. The following
symptom was produced by it, and has been verified in practice: " immediately after lying down in bed at night, palpitation of the heart for half an hour, three nights consecutively."
Colic about the navel, with difficult emission of flatulence, and
irritation of the genito-urinary tract, with diuresis, are other
marked symptoms of the proving; to which may be added
great exhilaration of spirits.

Oxalic acid has more analogies with *Arsenicum* than with
any other drug in the Pharmacopœia.

The 2nd and 3rd triturations seem to have been those
mainly used, though Dr. Marcy speaks well of the 12th. Dr.
Burnett gave the 3rd in his cases.

The acid I am now coming upon is a special favourite of
my own. It is

Acidum phosphoricum.

The " dilute phosphoric acid " of the British Pharmacopœia
forms our 1^x attenuation, and water is used for subsequent
dilutions up to the 2nd centesimal.

The original proving of Phosphoric acid is in the fifth
volume of the *Materia Medica Pura*. It contains (in the
second edition) 268 symptoms from Hahnemann himself, and

411 from twelve fellow observers. A later pathogenesis appears in the fifth part of the *Chronic Diseases.* It is increased by 139 symptoms, most of which are credited to Hering, and were probably observed on the patients mentioned in the preface as cured by him with the acid. Five persons have proved it since, one in the pure substance, four in the dilutions : their symptoms are incorporated with Hahnemann's by Allen.

Hahnemann's directions in the *Materia Medica Pura* for the attenuation of Phosphoric acid are not so destructive as those for the other acids, as the dilute alcohol of the 1st potency is to contain nine parts of water to one of spirit. Perhaps the provings were made with this preparation. At any rate, they impress one with a greater sense of reality than those of the others; and Hahnemann characterises them as "remarkable, pure symptoms of artificial disease elicited by Phosphoric acid in the healthy body." They will well repay study and analysis. I shall best help this here by sketching and characterising the therapeutic action of the drug.

The chief sphere of this is the *nervous system ;* and the condition it influences here is one of debility without erethism (in this contrasted with China). When we find brain* or cord,† sight or hearing thus affected—as from continued grief, overexertion of mind or body, sexual excess, or drain on the system, or remaining after typhus or typhoid‡—Phosphoric acid is an invaluable remedy, well deserving the name of "tonic." Failure in memory is reputed a special indication for it in cerebral depression : the emotional condition is one of apathy and indifference. It is to " nervous debility " what iron is to anæmia. In virtue of this action (as I believe) is its curative power in its two chief local spheres, the *renal* and the *male sexual organs.*

1. Phosphoric acid has no known action on the kidneys themselves ; but it exerts a remarkable control over those changes in the composition of the urine which arise farther back than the secreting organs. Dr. Sutherland has directed attention to its usefulness in phosphatic deposits ;§ it is obviously indicated for these when, as commonly, depending on waste of nervous tissue or on alkalinity of urine from nervous depression. It cures, as Hering‖ and Chapman¶ have pointed

* *Brit. Journ. of Hom.,* vii., 391. *Hahn. Monthly,* Aug., 1876.
† Bayes, *Appl. Hom.,* 138.
‡ *Monthly Hom. Review,* x.
§ *Brit. Journ. of Hom.,* vi., 410.
‖ Preface to pathogenesis in *Chron. Diseases.*
¶ *Brit. Journ. of Hom.,* vii., 391.

out, those derangements in children connected with a milky state of the renal secretion; and would probably help (unless the affection be a mere mechanical leaking) in the West Indian "chylous urine," whose constitutional symptoms are very characteristic of the drug. But it is in *diabetes* that Phosphoric acid has won its greenest laurels. Not only in the "insipid" form—"chronic diuresis" or "polyuria" as we should now call it—but in true glycosuria cure has repeatedly resulted from the administration of this acid.* It is possibly a similar to the essential symptom of the disease; for Dr. Pavy† found saccharine urine to result from its injection into the general venous system, or introduction into the intestinal canal, and Griesinger, who gave it in diabetes to the extent of an ounce a day, found the sugar rather increased thereby. But the frequent origin of diabetes in the nervous centres (as suggested by Claude Bernard's well-known experiment) commends it still more forcibly; and in the only case out of those I have myself recorded in which I have needed it to re-inforce the nitrate of Uranium the disease obviously began in this way.‡ It will therefore be in diabetes of nervous origin that we shall expect to get the best results from Phosphoric acid; and this continues to be my own experience with it. Moreover, since Bernard found albuminuria to result from a central nervous lesion hard by that which occasions glycosuria, there may well be cases of this malady in which Phosphoric acid is indicated. Two cures by it are on record,—in one of which the albuminuria was associated with chorea,§ and in the other followed upon typhoid.‖ The presence of simple diuresis—especially when quantities of colourless urine are passed at night—is an indication in favour of the choice of the medicine in morbid conditions in general.

2. It is the nervous apparatus of the male sexual organs which is influenced by Phosphoric acid. It has no relation to

* *Brit. Journ. of Hom.*, xxiv., 260; xxxvii., 371.—The last reference is to Dr. Black's elaborate and interesting essay on diabetes. He there shows that we must not lay much stress upon the evidence I have cited above as to the causation of glycosuria by the acid: he also demonstrates that the remedy was known in the old school twenty years or more before it was employed in homœopathic practice. I do not think, however, that his criticism, judiciously sceptical as it is, has robbed Phosphoric acid of the laurels with which I have ventured to crown it in respect to this disease. The cases collected by himself suffice to show its power; and for my own part I rarely prescribe it without satisfaction.

† *On Diabetes*, p. 82.

‡ *Brit. Journ. of Hom.*, xxxi., 369.

§ Hempel, ii., 46.

‖ *Monthly Hom. Rev.*, x., 527.

their inflammatory states ; but in simple debility and relaxation—even to impotence—of these organs, resulting from excess or unnatural use, it is the most important of remedies. Frequent weak emissions and dragging aching in the testes may also be removed by it..

This action on the nervous system, peculiar to the Phosphoric among the mineral acids, is probably due to the nature of its base. From the same source may come its action on the *blood* and on the *bones*. In low fevers, indeed, it is indicated when the nervous system rather than the blood is affected by the poison, and only in milder cases here,—standing on the same level as Muriatic acid in their respective spheres ;* but it has more than once proved curative in purpura and passive hæmorrhages. As regards the bones, it is spoken highly of by German writers of the old school as a remedy for caries, and our own Hartmann recommends it strongly in rachitis. Its physical relation to osseous tissue is obviously an intimate one ; and there is good reason to believe that such facts may be used as suggestive of medicinal affinities.

In all these affections, the Phosphoric acid patient is characterised by tendency to passive flux from skin and mucous membrane. The medicine (which herein may be compared with China and Iodine) often first displays its power by checking these, as the perspiration of phthisis and the diarrhœa of rachitic or otherwise weakly children : the diarrhœa, I should say, is painless, and the stools are grayish-white. It has even cured ague when this condition, in the shape of profuse sweat, was the prominent feature of the case.† I know not whether the ozæna, and the thin and acrid leucorrhœa, in which Dr. Marcy has found it curative, come under this head ; or the falling of the hair, as from debility after fevers, in which I have often seen it successful. Dr. Hoyne says it is equally good when the loss of hair results from depressing emotions. This writer also praises it for the pressive headache on the vertex which so often accompanies cerebral anæmia, and for which we shall see Cactus and China recommended. Dr. Guernsey commends it for physometra, and mentions pain in the hepatic region during the menses as a noteworthy indication for it in women.

Phosphoric acid works side by side with *Phosphorus* throughout its action. Besides this, it touches at some points *Fluoric acid* and *Silica ; China ; Anacardium ; Ignatia ;* and the mineral acids in general.

* See *Brit. Journ. of Hom.*, xii.,23.—Jousset also commends it here, and thinks that I hardly sufficiently value it.

† *Annals* i., 457 ; *Monthly Hom. Review*, xiv., 544.

In nervous affections, in milky urine, in nutritive derangement, in fever, and in passive fluxes, Phosphoric acid seems to
act well in the attenuations from the 3rd to the 12th.   But as
a sexual tonic, in purpura, the phosphatic diathesis, diabetes
and caries, it does best in doses of several drops of the 1st
decimal dilution.

I have now to introduce you to two new members of our
group of acids—the picric and the salicylic.

Acidum picricum

(or, as it used to be called, carbazoticum) is the product of
the action of nitric acid upon several substances, among which
I may mention (as suggesting one of its relationships) carbolic
acid and salicin.   It forms in whitish-yellow prisms ; and is
soluble in alcohol, which will accordingly be its pharmaceutical
vehicle, unless triturations are preferred.

Dr. Allen is able to give us a pathogenesis of Picric acid
containing 469 symptoms, obtained by 18 provers.   Three of
the observations laid under contribution are from an old-
school source (Parisel), seven are from the provings instituted
by Dr. L. B. Couch in 1874,* and five from some very thorough
experiments made at the Michigan University by Professor
S. A. Jones.   The latter has furnished from time to time†
some elaborate analyses of the drug's effects, more especially
of those which it causes in the blood and the urine.   Drs. Couch
and Jones have unhappily fallen out of late over their offspring ;‡ but their controversy, though personally lamentable,
has elicited still farther the action of the new remedy.

Our fullest information as to the toxic influence of Picric
acid is contained in an essay by Erb, of Würzburg, entitled
*Die Pikrinsaüre, ihre physiologischen und therapeutischen Wirk-
ungen* (1865).   The conclusions arrived at bv this experimenter
are stated by him as follows :—

" 1. Picric acid, in combination with potash or soda, is
absorbed into the blood, enters nearly all the tissues of the
animal organism, and is in most part excreted with the urine.

" 2. The entrance of large doses of an alkaline picrate into
the blood brings about the destruction of a great part of the
red blood-corpuscles, and a consequent increase of the colourless (artificial leucocythæmia).

* See *New York Journ. of Hom.*, ii., 145.
† See *North Amer. Journ. of Hom.*, xxiii., 443.   Transactions of
World's Convention, vol. ii.   *Amer. Hom. Observer*, xiv., 395.
‡ See *Hom. Times*, April—July, 1878.

" 3. Under the same circumstances, a transitory icterus is produced.

" 4. Small quantities of the alkaline picrates are borne quite well for a long time : larger doses, after long use, cause death with the phenomena of inanition : very large doses produce (probably through destruction of the blood) a collapse which after a short time ends in death."

Dr. Jones, in some experiments made upon two students, found Picric acid to cause increase of the uric and phosphoric acids in the urine, and diminution of the sulphates and chlorides; *i.e.*, it diminished oxidation. He connected this action with Erb's observations of the destructive influence of the alkaline picrates upon the red corpuscles (the oxygen-carriers) of the blood ; and when lecturing on former occasions I have followed him in so doing. Dr. Couch, however, has objected that Erb's results were obtained equally when the picrates were mingled with blood outside the body; and no alteration was found in the blood in dogs poisoned by himself with the pure Picric acid crystals. He justly infers, therefore, that the action is a chemical one only, and is probably due to the action of the alkaline bases rather than to the acid with which they were united. But I cannot follow him when he goes on to impeach Dr. Jones' own experiments as failing to evidence any real power on the part of the drug to cause sub-oxidation. He argues that the deviations from the normal standard discovered in the provers' urine were not greater than occur in health. But if you will look at the tabular views given of these, in the case of the principal prover, in Allen's *Encyclopædia*, I think you will come to a different conclusion. They display the proportion of the constituents of the urine, first, in health ; secondly, whilst taking the acid ; and, thirdly, for some time afterwards. It is quite apparent that although the increase of uric and phosphoric acid, and the diminution of the chlorides,* which occurred during the medication, might not exceed the oscillations of average health, they greatly exceeded those of the health of the prover in question. Moreover, Dr. Jones has verified his experiments by therapeutic results. He joined his earlier provers in testing the acid, being at the time out of health ; " markedly indisposed to either mental or physical exertion ; easily fatigued ; readily blown by walking up hill ; inclined to day-sleepiness," with poor appetite and a general sense of tor-

---

* In the table at p. 528, the decimal point of the mean chlorides during medication is put in the wrong place. Instead of 76·911, the figures should stand as 7·6911.

pidity. The effect of the drug on his urine was the precise opposite of that experienced by his two fellow-provers, who were in good health. Uric acid and phosphoric acid were diminished : urea increased to the extent of two grammes per diem : the sulphates and chlorides were in excess. Therewith was experienced "an improved appetite, a general feeling of well-being, a renewed vigour in the morning, and an ability to rise much earlier than usual." In a later communication* he relates a still more striking case. It was one of profound anæmia, with prostration and vomiting : uro-hæmatin was discovered in the urine, which showed also the evidences of sub-oxidation mentioned above. Under the third trituration of Picric acid improvement speedily set in; and in a few weeks strength and colour had returned, and the same changes had occurred in the urine as those experienced by Dr. Jones himself, though in a greater degree.

Dr. Couch, indeed, states that his experiments on animals show, from small doses of the acid, a primary increase of all the constituents of the urine, with secondary diminution,—from large doses, the converse sequence of phenomena. Whatever be the value of these observations, they cannot outweigh Dr. Jones' provings on the human subject, confirmed as they are by the therapeutic results obtained from the drug when given as a remedy in accordance therewith. They give us *sub-oxidation* as its essential and fundamental action upon nutrition, which can be used upon the principle *similia similibus* for curative purposes; and they thereby add another potent weapon to our armoury.

Dr. Couch's earlier experiments on dogs, however, brought to light another action of the acid, viz.: that which it exerts on the nervous centres. These were found *post mortem* soft, pulpy, and apparently completely disorganised,—the focus of the mischief being from the mesocephale to the upper cord, but extending more or less forwards and backwards. The symptoms during life were of the paralytic character which might have been expected. In later investigations† of the same kind, entire anæsthesia and analgesia of the posterior extremities was noted. The poison was also found to produce "spasms, both tonic and clonic, which had a striking resemblance to those produced by strychnia." This may seem curious, when it is added that "under the influence of the drug the animals betray great weakness and lassitude ; especially is this noticeable of the hind legs, they being

* See *Hom. Times*, June, 1878.
† See *Ibid*, April, 1878.

scarcely able to support the already attenuated body, which sways constantly from side to side; the tail, too, is as limp as a wet rag, and cannot be made to either wag or curl." But Drs. Ringer and Murrell have recently adduced considerations which tend to account for this apparent anomaly.* They maintain that tetaniform phenomena are due to a diminution or destruction of the *resistance* of the cord, "so that an impression conveyed through an afferent nerve can spread throughout the reflex portion of the central nervous system, and produce tetanus." Such diminished resistance may coincide with unimpaired functional activity of the cord, as with strychnia; or with more or less paralysis of it, as they have ascertained in relation to Gelsemium and the buxus sempervirens, and as Dr. Couch seems now to have shown with Picric acid.

The symptoms of the provers show a very similar condition, though of course of lower grade. Their legs were cold, weak, and heavy like lead; and they experienced a feeling of great lassitude and debility, which with one was accompanied by cold clammy sweats. Nor does the marked excitement of the sexual organs, shown by priapism and profuse emissions, and finding its parallel in Dr. Couch's dogs, contradict these indications, when we remember how often such a condition exists in the early stages of chronic disease of the craniospinal axis, or as the result of injury to it.† Everything points —as Dr. Jones argues—to a profound depression and anæmia set up in the nervous centres, going on to softening.

Little use has yet been made of this action of Picric acid. It has served me very well to complete the cure of a case of spinal exhaustion following acute disease, which Phosphorus had begun. I gave it in the twelfth dilution. It should be helpful in white softening of the cord. Dr. Jones mentions a cure of satyriasis of three years standing effected by it, given in the third trituration; and Dr. Couch relates a case of masturbation, in which the 30th dilution, given to "cool the blood," proved (according to the patient) "altogether too cooling" It will probably play an important part ere long in the treatment of central nervous disease. In this connexion, the severe headaches it causes must be taken into account. They all begin in the occipital region, and thence extend forwards and downwards. Dr. Hale has found it very useful in headaches so localised, when the slightest excitement or

* See *Medico-Chirurgical Transactions* for 1876, and *Journal of Anatomy and Physiology*, vol. xi.
† As in a case recorded by Harley, *Old Vegetable Neurotics*, p. 50.

even use of the brain would bring on the attacks ; and I have in one instance verified his experience. Here, too, I should mention its effects upon the visual organs. In two of the provers the sight was much obscured ; and in the dogs poisoned with it the veins of the retina were found (ophthalmoscopically) much enlarged. In one, examined by Dr. Norton, "immense white patches of exudation were observed, with some hæmorrhagic spots." On post-mortem examination, the lesions thus manifested were found to be seated in the nervous elements of the eyeball, both nerve-entrance and retina showing infiltration and extravasation. Such phenomena suggest the possible usefulness of the drug in albuminuric and syphilitic retinitis, while the optic neuritis displayed completes the evidence of its homœopathicity to organic brain-mischief.

In two provers Picric acid caused "small, painful, reddish elevations, like furuncles " on the face, going on to suppuration ; and Dr. Houghton, writing of that troublesome affection, boils in the auditory neatus, says :—"during the last year I have used Picric acid here with the greatest satisfaction, and find it nearer to a specific for the disease than any other medicine."

Dr. Jones very justly compares Picric acid with *Phosphorus* and *Argentum nitricum.*

I have mentioned the doses in which it has hitherto been successfully used. The provings seem to show it as active in the 30th as in the 1st attenuation, and to produce effects of a similar kind.

My other new acid is

Acidum salicylicum,

which, as its name imports, is obtained from salicin, an active principle contained in the bark of the willow (Salix). It is not yet officinal in our Pharmacopœia ; but will form either dilutions with alcohol (in which it is quite soluble), or triturations. The latter form would be most suitable for salicin itself ; and the salicylate of soda, which has been much used as a substitute for the acid, and exerts similar properties, is best prepared in aqueous solution.

Salicin has been proved to some extent on the healthy subject by Ringer and a few others in the old school, and by Mr. Nankivell in our own ranks. The physiological effects of the acid, and of its compound with soda, we know mainly from observations of overdosing. These, with the results of such

provings as we have, may be found collated in Dr. Allen's
Encyclopœdia and its supplement under the heads of Salicinum,
Salicylicum acidum, and Natrum salicylicum.

Salicylic acid was first introduced as a rival of the carbolic
in point of antizymotic power, and for internal administration
with this view—as in cases of fermentation of the food in the
stomach—is preferable to that substance, having no offensive
odour or actively toxic properties. The popular repute of
willow-bark, and the proved efficacy of salicin in malarious
fevers, then led to the employment of salicylic acid therein.
It was found to exert an undoubted, though not extensive, influence upon cases of this kind ; and the interesting fact came
out that (as we shall see presently) it resembled quinine in
pathogenetic as well as curative action. It thus came to be
tried, like that drug, as an anti-pyretic in general, and especially in febrile states presumably depending on a zymotic
process, or on the development of disease-germs. It exerted a
certain amount of influence over these also, but hardly sufficient to give it any recognised place in their treatment, unless
it be in septicæmia. Its most striking effects were manifested
in a non-contagious fever, which had hitherto been classed
separately from the zymoses : I speak of acute rheumatism.
As a remedy for this malady it has received the warmest commendation from all quarters. It seems to find its opportunity
when the temperature is high, and joint after joint is being
involved, with severe pain : its administration at this time
rarely fails to bring down the fever and relieve the pains in the
space of 36 or 48 hours. Salicin, in Dr. Maclagan's hands,
has yielded results as good as those obtained with the acid,
without the occasional unpleasant effects of the latter ;* and
the combination with an alkali—as in the form of the salicylate of soda—seems in no way to weaken its properties, while
it gives a more soluble preparation.

In the face of these facts, we disciples of Hahnemann had to
consider what we ought to do. The results of our treatment
of acute rheumatism, though satisfactory enough, were certainly
not so good as those claimed for this remedy ; so that, even
could we not recognise its action as an instance of the law of
similars, we should have felt bound—as being physicians, and
not mere homœopathists—to have entertained the question of
its employment. At first this seemed to be the position of
affairs. The acid was found by Fürbringer to cause no elevation of the temperature in healthy animals, and Dr. Ringer
found the same negative results from salicin in the human

* See *Practitioner*, Nov., 1877, and *Lancet*, June 21, 1879.

subject. Of late, however, some observations on the other side have appeared. Dr. Wheeier, in a paper communicated to the British Homœopathic Society,* relates a proving of Mr. Nankivell's on himself, in which ten grains of salicin on two occasions brought on a feverish attack of twenty-four hours duration, in the first of which the temperature rose to 101°. He also cites a case of acute rheumatism, treated with this substance in such large and frequent doses that in the four or five days the patient was under its influence he must have taken at least 1,400 grains. Under this medication the temperature steadily rose until death occurred, when the thermometer registered 111°. Two Neapolitan physicians, moreover, have lately ascertained on dogs and rabbits that Salicylic acid, both free and in the state of salicylate, lowers the temperature, but within restricted limits. In a somewhat larger dose, it not only does not lower the temperature, but sometimes considerably increases it.†

Now as it is in febrile rheumatism that the drug displays its great powers, there is some suggestion in these facts of its possible homœopathicity thereto. A similar conclusion follows from the small dosage which sometimes proves sufficient. Those of our own school who have used it, and have reported successes surprisingly good in comparison with those to which they had been accustomed—among whom I may name Drs. Hale and Lilienthal in America, besides Dr. Wheeler among ourselves—have all found doses of from two to five grains of the soda salt sufficient for their purpose. On the other hand, I apprehend that such results are exceptional, and that it is only occasionally that the drug is truly homœopathic to the disorder. Its employment in the old school seems to me to rest upon an altogether different basis. There are three ways in which acute rheumatism has been and can be treated, and the medicines which have been in repute for it fall into three classes accordingly. You may endeavour to neutralise chemically the presumably acid *materies morbi*, as by alkalies, neutral salts, or lemon juice. You may seek to check the formation of this peccant matter : such, I apprehend, must be the action of such medicines as the colchicum and propylamine of old-school practice, and of our homœopathic remedies (as Bryonia). Or, thirdly, you may forcibly (as it were) repress fever and deaden pain, while leaving untouched the specific morbid process present. I suppose that a good deal of the success obtained from Aconite by Lombard and Fleming is to be thus explained ; and I am sure that in this way Briquet and his

* *Annals*, viii., 363.
† See *Lond. Med. Record*, April 15, 1878.

imitators gained their results with full doses of quinine. Salicin and its derivatives, I consider, act in acute rheumatism like the last-named drug; and the necessary dosage has similar inconveniences. It has been said that " cerebral rheumatism " was almost unknown in France until the quinine treatment of the original malady became fashionable. Accidents of this kind have been common enough under the free use of salicylic acid and its compounds, and have more than once ended fatally. The great defect of such remedies, moreover, is that, leaving the essential malady untouched, and only hushing up its expressions, they favour the tendency to relapse—strong enough already in rheumatic fever, and so unduly protract the illness. That it is so with the salicylates was the conclusion reached at the discussion of the subject at this year's meeting of the British Medical Association,* and has since been shown by the statistics of the Middlesex Hospital.†

While, then, I cannot give to our present drug any important place in the homœopathic therapeutics of acute rheumatism, indications for uses of it of this kind are sure to result from the symptoms of overdosing with it now so often reported. Dr. Ringer's experiments on the human subject with salicin show that it affects the head like quinine. " The aspect," he writes, " of a patient under full medicinal doses is very characteristic, being in many respects similar to that of a patient suffering from cinchonism." Amongst other symptoms of this state he mentions—" The patient, made more or less deaf, often complains of noises in the ears." This effect, noted by Dr. Tuckwell from salicylic acid, has been most definitely described by Dr. Gowers, of University College Hospital, as occurring during the administration of salicylate of soda; and he, besides the deafness and tinnitus, found vertigo to exist.‡ We have thus, as Dr. Gowers perceived, the essential features of Meniére's disease (" auditory nerve vertigo "). He himself curiously enough made some tentative prescriptions of the drug in this very affection. Dr. McClatchey, of Philadelphia, initiated the systematic application of drug to disease in the homœopathic school by reporting§ a striking cure with it,— the salicylate being given in two-grain doses. Dr. Dyce Brown has since followed up with others, in which the dilutions from the 1st to the 3rd decimal seem to have done

* See *Brit. Med. Journ.*, Aug., 25, 1879, p. 283.
† See *Lancet*, Sept. 20, 1879.
‡ See *Brit. Med. Journ.*, April 21, 1877.
§ *Hahn. Monthly.* Aug. 1877.

everything that was required ;* and Dr. Claude reports from
Paris that the third trituration of salicylic acid is becoming
quite a favourite medicine with him for simple deafness with
tinnitus. My own experience has been quite as favourable
with it in this class of cases.

The power of the drug to disorganise osseous tissue has
also been utilised by Mr. S. H. Blake in a case of scrofulous
caries.†

I have already mentioned *Quinine* as the analogue of our
present drug, and suggested the dosage in which it will
probably have to be given.

The last of my group is

Acidum sulphuricum.

"Ten grains by weight of the officinal acid of the British
Pharmacopœia, mixed with sufficient distilled water to measure
eighty minims, will constitute our 1^x preparation." I quote
the British Homœopathic Pharmacopœia.

The only pathogenesis of Sulphuric acid we have is that
contained in the second edition of the *Chronic Diseases*. It
contains 513 symptoms from Hahnemann and five fellow-
observers, and 8 from authors.

The first dilution of this acid is here directed to be made
with distilled water, and the subsequent ones with alcohol.
If we could suppose the former to have been used for the
proving, we might attach some importance to the symptoms
recorded ; but the epoch of their appearance compels us to
refer them to the category of those supposed to result from
globules of the 30th. Of the eight symptoms from authors
five are those of a typhoid from which the patients taking it
were suffering. The only valid ones are S. 148 ("salivation"),
151 ("aphthæ in the mouth") and 198 ("hiccough"—this
repeatedly recurred after the administration of clysters containing the acid).

We thus know next to nothing about the dynamic physiological effects of Sulphuric acid ; and, judging from its therapeutic position in homœopathic practice, these are probably of
more limited range than in the case of the other mineral acids.
It has been mainly used in disorders of the alimentary canal.
Hahnemann‡ speaks of "a very small dose of a high dilution"

* *Monthly Hom. Review*, Sept. and Oct., 1878.
† *Ibid*, xxii., 415.
‡ *Organon*, note on p. 10 of Dudgeon's translation.

as curative of acidity of stomach.   Dr. Bayes mentions a form
of gastralgia in which he found it very useful; and Dr.
Schneider commends it in obstinate hiccough, to which it is
certainly homœopathic.   Its undoubted power, now so generally recognised, over diarrhœa is also a homœopathic action;
for it is admitted by all therapeutists that its continued use
tends to loosen the bowels.*   The same may be said of its
influence over cutaneous disorder: "occasionally" writes
Christison of acute poisoning by it "eruptions break out over
the body."   Pereira says that "no remedy is so successful in
relieving the distressing itching, tingling, and formication of the
skin of lichen, prurigo, and chronic urticaria, as sulphuric acid
taken internally."   Teste has cured syphilitic maculæ with it.

But there are those who would have it that our use of
Sulphuric acid has been too limited hitherto.   Among these
are Drs. Espanet and Cooper.   The former thinks that it is
the antiphlogistic of cachectic subjects, as Aconite is that of
the robust.   The latter† considers that Sulphuric, like Phosphoric, acid shares the virtues of its base, and is an anti-
neuralgic and a possible anti-periodic.   He gives a good case
of chronic gastralgia cured by it.   The special relation of this
acid to cutaneous affections seems to support his position:
it was, indeed, on this ground that it was first used in them.‡

It must also be mentioned that later observation shows that,
in poisoning by Sulphuric acid, some absorption into the blood
does take place, leading to a great increase in the elimination
of sulphates in the urine, and the setting up of an acute parenchymatous nephritis thereby, manifested during life by albuminuria and fibrinous casts.   In several cases, moreover, there
have been observed during convalescence from the immediate
local effects "neuralgic affections of the intercostal and
abdominal nerves; also, in isolated cases, extended and severe
hyperæsthesia over the whole trunk." §

Dr. Guernsey considers Sulphuric acid indicated by a
general sense of tremulousness, without actual tremor; and by
a hurried feeling on the patient's part.   The former symptom
seems connected with general debility ("the weaker the patient

* Dr. Ringer moreover says, "A small dose often benefits diarrhœa,
whilst a full one, by increasing the acidity of the canal, may even
aggravate it;" and Stillé—"A caution should be observed in treating
bowel affections with sulphuric acid, which is, not to persevere in it if
the first few doses fail to mitigate the symptoms, for in that case it is
almost certain to aggravate them."

† *Brit. Journ. of Hom.*, xxix. 699.
‡ See *Med. and Phys. Journ.*, iv., 484.
§ *Ziemssen's Cyclopædia*, vol. xvii., *sub voce.*

is, the more tremulous she becomes ") ; otherwise its association with hurriedness would suggest an incipient stage of the tremor and festination of multiple cerebral sclerosis.

The Sulphuric may be compared with the other mineral acids, and with Sulphur. The 2nd and 3rd decimal have been its usual attenuations.*

* A comparative view of the action of some of these acids, by Dr. H. V. Miller, may be read in the *Hahn. Monthly*, Nov., 1877, and *Mon. Hom. Review*, xxii., 30.

LECTURE X.

ACONITE.

The survey we have now completed of the acids used in our practice has exhibited the weakness as well as the strength of Homœopathy as it at present exists. But in the medicine we have now to study its strength aione is seen, and that at its full. If Homœopathy had done nothing for therapeutics but reveal the virtues of

Aconitum,

it might even die content.

The Homœopathic tincture is prepared from the Aconitum napellus. By Hahnemann the whole plant was used. The British Homœopathic Pharmacopœia directs the employment of the leaves and flowering tops, freshly collected, with the fresh or dry root. This is the tincture ordinarily dispensed ; but an alternative (and of course much stronger) one made with rectified spirit from the dry root alone can be had if ordered.

Hahnemann's proving of Aconite is contained in the first volume of his *Materia Medica Pura*. It contains (in the latest edition) 541 symptoms, of which 431 are from himself and seven fellow-observers, and 110 from authors. Aconite was, moreover, one of the medicines selected for re-proving by the Austrian Provers' Society. Their work was carried out in the most thorough manner, sixteen persons co-operating in it, two of whom were women : the record of the experiments is contained in the first volume of the *Oesterreichische Zeitschrift für Homöopathie*. These two provings, with all additional matter available, are collated by Dr. Dudgeon in the first part of the *Hahnemann Materia Medica*, and by Dr. Allen in his *Encyclopædia*. There are also (besides the well-known treatise* of Fleming from the other school) studies of Aconite by

* *An Enquiry into the Physiological and Medicinal Properties of the Aconitum Napellus.* 1845.

Hartmann ;* by Reil (in the form of the first prize essay of the German Central Verein),† and by Carroll Dunham in his Lectures. Hempel and the *New Materia Medica* give numerous cases of poisoning ; and all the systematic writers devote large space to the discussion of the action of the drug.

It is impossible to begin to speak of Aconite without a thrill of gratification and pride. The inestimable benefits which are daily being obtained from this remedy as an anti-pyretic and antiphlogistic, and which are now—at least in this country and America—obtaining general recognition, are the direct result of homœopathy. Fleming indeed, in 1845, was led by his experiments to infer that Aconite was an arterial sedative, and to recommend and employ it accord-ingly in fever and inflammation. But, as might have been expected, so indiscriminate a use of the drug made little way ; and the place it occupies in Pereira's great work as a mere benumber of pain, and its rejection as dangerous and useless by Trousseau and Pidoux, sufficiently characterise its recep-tion in the old school twenty years ago. When, ever and anon, our brethren without have caught a glimpse of its precious virtues, it has been from its use by homœopathists that they have done so ; though they have generally (Liston being a noble exception ‡) proclaimed them in the medical journals with a sneer at the source of their information. The present English use of the drug is not handed down from Fleming, but is the result especially of the persistent teaching of Dr. Ringer, whose inspiration is not dubious. But this writer had to say, as late as 1874, first, indeed, that " perhaps no drug is more valuable than Aconite," but then, that "its virtues are only beginning to be appreciated."§

On the other hand, the therapeutics of homœopathy exhibit a continuous use of Aconite as an antipyretic and antiphlo-gistic from the earliest years of the present century down to this day. The knowledge of this property of the drug it owes to Hahnemann himself; and the history of his discovery is of importance, alike as vindicatory of his own fame and as illus-trative of the working of his method.

On his first mention of the plant—in his " Essay on a new

* *Practical Observations on some of the chief Homœopathic Remedies*, trans. by Okie. First Series, 1841.
† Translated into English by Millard. 1860.
‡ See *Lancet*, April 13, 1836.
§ *Handbook of Therapeutics*, 4th ed.—Dr. Ringer's first memoir on Aconite appeared in the *Lancet* for Jan. 9th, 1869, and closely follows the article on it in the first edition of this Manual, which was published in 1867.

principle for ascertaining the curative power of drugs," published in *Hufeland's Journal* in 1796—he evidently knew no
more of it than was known by the toxicologists and therapeutists of his day. He describes its familiar poisonous effects,
and suggests that, upon the "new principle" of similarity
which he was now advocating, it might be given in rheumatic,
paralytic, convulsive and eruptive affections, in some of
which he states that it had already displayed no trifling efficacy.

When, however, in the first edition of his *Materia Medica
Pura* (1811) he publishes a pathogenesis of Aconite, he prefixes thereto the following remarks :—

"There is hardly any vegetable medicine but Opium whose
primary action is characterised by the production of heat ;
and so those medicines serve just as effectively in acute
diseases, whose primary action is compounded of several
alternate states of chill (or coldness) and heat. To plants of
this class belong Aconite, Ignatia, and some others. Since,
moreover, the action of Aconite is of very short duration, and
nearly always over in twenty-four hours, it thus becomes intelligible, that for the most part it is in acute diseases only that
this plant can be permanently helpful ; and that it but seldom
suffices in chronic disorders, which are subject to far fewer
of those alternations of condition which constitute the main
essence of the action of this substance.

"Where Aconite is suitable as regards the rest of its symptoms, it becomes nevertheless so much the more helpful as the
state of the patient's disposition presents at the same time a
predominant resemblance to that which is expressed in its
symptoms."

This is entirely a new thought about the drug, and is the
germ of our present knowledge regarding it. When we
enquire how Hahnemann came to this thought, the answer is
plain. In the year 1805, he had issued his *Fragmenta de
viribus medicamentorum positivis*, which contained pathogenetic
effects of a number of substances obtained by provings on the
healthy human body. Among them was Aconite, and in a
note to his article upon it Hahnemann had written : "through
the whole course of action of this plant, its effects of the first
and second order were repeated in short paroxysms two, three
or four times before the whole effect ceased, which it did in
from eight to sixteen hours." And these effects he describes
thus :—"coldness of the whole body, and dry internal heat ;
chilliness. Sense of heat first in the hands, then in the whole
body, especially in the thorax, without sensible external heat.
Alternating paroxysms (during the third, fourth, and fifth

hours); general sense of heat, with red cheeks and headache, worse on moving the eyeballs upwards and laterally, then shuddering of the whole body with red cheeks and hot head ; then shuddering and lachrymation with pressing headache and red cheeks."

It was from his provings, then, and upon the the principle of similarity, that Hahnemann inferred the usefulness of Aconite in acute diseases, in which it had hitherto found no employment. In what forms of these disorders it would be serviceable he does not indicate at present, save that he points to the mental and moral symptoms of the drug as those especially to be looked for in the patient. When, however, we next hear from him on the subject, he is able to be much more explicit. I quote from the preface to the pathogenesis of Aconite in the first volume of the second edition of the *Materia Medica Pura*, published in 1822.

"Although the following symptoms do not yet express the whole significance of this most valuable plant, they nevertheless disclose to reflecting homœopathic physicians a prospect of help in morbid conditions, in which the ordinary practice employs its most dangerous means, viz., copious venesections and the whole antiphlogistic apparatus,—measures very often injurious, and nearly always followed by disastrous after-effects. I mean the so-called pure inflammatory fevers, in which the smallest dose of Aconite renders unnecessary all the antipathic measures hitherto in use, and cures rapidly and without *sequelæ*. In measles, in purple-rash, and in the most intense pleuritic fevers its remedial power is something miraculous, when—the patient observing a somewhat cooling regimen, and avoiding everything else of a medicinal kind, especially vegetable acids—a dose of a small part of a drop of the octillionth" (*i.e.*, the 24th) "attenuation is administered. Seldom is a second dose, thirty-six or forty-eight hours after the first, required.

"But to remove from our conscientious method all influence of the ordinary practice, which is too ready to be regulated by (often imaginary) names of disease, it is necessary also that in all morbid conditions in which Aconite is indicated, the principal symptoms of the patient, as well as those of the (acute) disease, should suitably correspond as likes to likes with those of the remedy.

"The result is then surprising.

"It is just in the cases where Allopathy most prides itself, in the great inflammatory fevers where they look to bold and free blood-letting as the only means of salvation, and consider that herein they have a huge advantage over homœopathic modes of help, that they are most utterly mistaken. Just here appears the infinite superiority of homœopathy, that—without the need of spilling a drop of that precious life-juice, so irreparable, which Allopathy relentlessly sheds in streams—it not seldom transforms those frightful fevers to health in as many hours as the life-reducing proceedings of Allopathy require months for the full restoration of the patient, if perchance he has escaped actual death, and has only had to struggle with the chronic *sequelæ* which have been artificially produced.

"It is sometimes necessary, in these acute attacks of disease, to have recourse to an intermediate homœopathic remedy for the symptoms which remain after Aconite has acted for twelve or sixteen hours, and still seldomer (as I have said) to a second dose of Aconite after this intermediate remedy.

"When the careful employment of Aconite is practised in the morbid conditions mentioned, four hours will not have passed ere all fear for life has been removed, and the excited circulation then returns from hour to hour to its habitual tranquil course."

He goes on to say that it is occasionally a useful auxiliary even in chronic diseases where tension of the fibre is present ; and that most of the symptoms in the appended list which seem contrary one to the other are really alternating states, either of which can be used as curative indications, although those of a "tonic" character are of most value. Lastly, he repeats his admonition as to the importance of securing similarity in the symptoms of the mind and disposition.

Eight years more gave him little to add upon the subject. The preface to Aconite in the third edition of the first volume of the *Materia Medica Pura* (1830) is almost identical with that of the second, save that for the 24th he substitutes the 30th dilution, and mentions the value of the remedy in preventing the injurious effects of fright or vexation when occurring in women during the catamenial flow, which these emotions are very apt to suppress. He also inserts one other new paragraph which must be transcribed. "So also," he writes, "is Aconite the first and chief remedy (in the attenuated doses mentioned) in inflammation of the windpipe (croup, angina membranacea), in several kinds of inflammation of the throat and gullet, and in like manner in acute local inflammations elsewhere, especially when, with thirst and rapid pulse, an anxious impatience, an unappeasable restlessness, and an agonised tossing about are conjoined." These last are evidently the "symptoms of the disposition" (Gemüths-symptomen) on which Hahnemann had always laid so much stress as indications for its choice.

And when again we enquire how Hahnemann came to these applications of Aconite—how from a general fitness for acute diseases he was led to see its especial appropriateness to active states of fever and inflammation, we find that it was (in all probability) from these very mental conditions that the discovery was made. Dr. Quin—the honoured pioneer of Homœopathy in this country—was well acquainted with Hahnemann, and has related how "in 1826 he asked him how he had discovered the great antiphlogistic power of Aconite, as that was not evident from the proving. Hahnemann replied, that he had not directly discovered this property from the proving, but that whilst treating some inflammatory disorders he was led to the employment of Aconite from the similarity of some of the concomitant symptoms with some in the pathogenesis of Aconite, and he had found its administration followed by a great diminution in frequency of the pulse, and a cessation of the febrile state."*

From the facts and dates now brought forward the following conclusions seem to result :—

1st. The antipyretic and antiphlogistic properties of Aconite were an original discovery of Hahnemann's, made by him many years before any thought of the kind occurred (if it ever did occur at first instance) to a practitioner of the old school.

2nd. The discovery was made by pure induction from the symptoms produced by the drug when proved upon the healthy human body, applying these to disease according to the relation of likes to likes.

3rd. The application which led to the discovery was regulated primarily by the similarity of the mental symptoms of the drug to those of the morbid condition present.

4th. The antiphlogistic and antipyretic virtues of Aconite were first ascertained and obtained by means of infinitesimal doses.

But although the actual discovery of the power of Aconite over fever was made by means of the associated mental symptoms rather than by the febrile phenomena themselves, yet there can be no doubt of the real homœopathicity of the drug to the latter also. It is true that a hasty glance at the symptoms of poisoning by this plant has led to its being set down as a mere cardiac depressant. But a closer look reveals that the condition set up is one answering to the chill of fever and ague and the collapse of cholera. The pale face, the quick and contracted pulse, the general coldness within and without; the signs (should death result) of extreme venous congestion—these speak of a corresponding excitation of the vaso-motor nerves throughout the body. Had the thermometer been applied, it is probable that here as there[*] the temperature would have been found already on the rise. That this is the true explanation of the symptoms appears from what follows. For mark, that, should reaction take place, the condition of febrile heat succeeds that of chill: as Dr. Geo. Wood states, "the circulation, respiration, and general temperature are somewhat increased." The same statement is made and illustrated by Fleming (pp. 34, 148). This is well seen in such a case as the tenth of Hempel's series. The pulse, at first collapsed, became fuller, and rose to 100; the skin being hot and dry and the tongue coated, with headache and sleeplessness. His twelfth case exhibits a similar succession of phenomena. But the power of Aconite to induce fever is still more evident in the provings, and especially those of the Austrian Society.[†] One of the latter experimenters was so distressed by the febrile heat induced, that, not knowing what drug he had been proving, he commenced taking Aconite to obtain relief. The fever in these subjects was generally accompanied by signs of arterial congestion of the head and chest. If further confirmation of the pyreto-genetic power of Aconite had been needed, it would have been supplied by the experiments of Professor Schroff.[‡] Their main interest to us lies in the evidence they afford of the influence of Aconite upon the trigeminal nerve. But repeatedly in their record we meet with expressions like these —" much febrile movement," "general internal and external heat, with quick pulse," " the whole body was burning," " he passes from the midst of cold to the midst of heat," "alternately hot or cold." Dr. Mackenzie, also, as the result of his recent experiments on animals, states that Aconite increases the temperature until asphyxia sets in,—the thermometer in the ear of a rabbit rising from two to four degrees Fahrenheit under its influence.

---

[*] That the temperature is rising during the collapse of cholera is proved by Erman's observations (see *London Medical Record*, i., 580). I need not argue the point with reference to fever and ague.

[†] See Symptoms 777-782 in Dr. Dudgeon's arrangement.

[‡] Translated from the *Präger Vierteljahrschrift* and *Journal für Pharmakodynamik*, in *L'Union Médicale* for June and July, 1854. Reil also gives the earlier set of experiments *in extenso*.

I maintain, then, that it is in virtue of its power of setting up the essential phenomena of fever, of its action upon the same parts and in a similar manner, that it controls this condition when already present. It is febrifuge because it is febrigenic. But it is not every kind of fever which Aconite can remove. Like every other specifically acting drug, it has its proper sphere, beyond which it is less useful. The sphere of Aconite may be defined by two negations.

First, it has little control over the fevers resulting from morbid poisons. Its use in typhus and typhoid is mere waste of precious time. In variola it will not lower the circulation until the eruption comes out; nor will it touch the high temperature of pyæmia. It is more frequently useful in measles and scarlatina, though in the latter only when of a sthenic type, i.e., when the blood-poisoning is but slight. I need hardly say that it will do nothing to prevent the recurrence of the paroxysms of hectic or of the malarial fevers.

Secondly, Aconite will do little for a fever which is symptomatic of an acute local inflammation. The excellent cases of pneumonia which Tessier has put on record* well illustrate this: it is most interesting to notice how the pulse defied Aconite, but went down rapidly when Bryonia or Phosphorus touched the local mischief. There are, indeed, a few inflammations in which Aconite may alone effect a cure, as being a specific irritant of the part affected. These are especially, as we shall see, the rheumatic inflammations. But even in non-rheumatic pleurisy, in its plastic form, and also in some kinds of croup and angina tonsillaris, Aconite is, as Hahnemann has said, a potent remedy. With these exceptions, it may be laid down that in proportion as true inflammatory changes in a part have actually begun, it ceases to exert remedial influence; and a medicine homœopathic to the local mischief must take its place.†

These negatives suggest the positive we desiderate. The fever in which Aconite is specific is neurotic, not toxæmic or sympathetic in nature. It is the "synocha" of the old authors,

---

* *Récherches cliniques sur le traitement de la Pneumonie et du Choléra, suivant la methode de Hahnemann.* Paris, 1850.

† Dr. Ringer supplies another contra-indication to the use of Aconite in inflammation, viz., the absence of increased temperature, as shown by the thermometer. When this obtains—as in some forms of angina—the remedy will be ineffectual. Dr. Imbert-Gourbeyre, in pre-thermometric days, had shown the same thing symptomatically (*Brit. Journ. of Hom.*, xiv).

the " pure inflammatory fever " indicated by Hahnemann, the fever in which the fibrin of the blood is in excess (so that its clot would be buffed and cupped), while the corpuscles are unpoisoned and the tissues are yet intact. It is the kind of fever which follows in some sensitive persons upon the passing of a catheter, or which any one may experience from exposure to (especially dry) cold. Let the morbid impression known as a "chill" be made upon the vascular nerves; let the arterioles under their influence first contract to produce the cold stage, and then dilate for the hot stage of simple fever; and we have the everyday occurrence for which Aconite is the unfailing remedy. Whether the chill or the heat be present the medicine is no less indicated ; and let the storm of arterial excitement be ever so high, a few doses will quiet its fury. " In as short a time as four hours after the administration of Aconite in the morbid states in question, all danger to life is past, and the excited circulation returns from hour to hour to its more tranquil course." So (as I have reminded you) wrote Hahnemann in 1822, pointing out to us this most important use of our medicine. Indeed, it may be laid down, that unless a fever (not being rheumatic, of which more anon) has greatly abated within twenty-four hours of commencing Aconite, it is one for which the remedy is unsuited.

The relation of Aconite to inflammation and inflammatory fever is well stated by Teste ;* and still more fully by Dr. Dunham. He (the latter) well points out its accordance with the symptomatic indications given for the drug by Hahnemann himself, i.e. (as you will remember) when " in conjunction with thirst and a rapid pulse there are present an anxious impatience, a restlessness not to be quieted, distress, and an agonised tossing about." These are the symptoms of inflammatory fever before it has well localised itself. When exudation has set in at the affected part, the tension of the circulation and nervous system diminishes ; and such fever as continues is sympathetic, and of like character with the local changes. He illustrates the phenomena by the passing of a tempest over a village, which may subside to perfect calm ; but which may leave behind it a cottage on fire, that shall be in its turn the centre of agitation and mischief. Aconite will subdue the storm ; but it will not put out the conflagration. The same symptomatic indications admirably harmonize with the relation of our drug to the essential fevers. The condition of the patient in typhoid and other toxæmic pyrexiæ is one of

* It is, he says, " in phlegmasiæ primarily general, and only secondarily localised " that Aconite is curative.

heaviness and oppression, rather than of the *anxietas* characteristic of Aconite.

It is right to add that all these observers—Hahnemann himself, Tessier, Teste, Dunham (and I may add Dr. Guernsey in
the same strain)—speak of the action of the higher dilutions
of the medicine, which alone they were accustomed to employ.
Those who have used stronger preparations seem inclined to
give it a wider range. " The power of this drug over inflammation," writes Dr. Ringer, " is little less than marvellous ; "*
and Hempel seems to know no limit to its action here.   Dr.
Bayes speaks highly of it, in the first decimal dilution, in acute
otitis, to which it has no proved homœopathic relation.
Wurmb, who gave it high, allows it no place in typhoid ; but
Trinks, who used the lowest dilutions, thinks it of real service
in the incipience of the less asthenic forms.   It is here as
elsewhere.   Infinitesimals, at least in the higher grades, act
only when the homœopathicity is perfect ; though they then
display such brilliant powers that one may well become
enamoured of them.   A nearer approach to the crude drug
widens the range of action, and enables us to be content with
a *simile* instead of searching for an often unattainable and
still more often illusory *similimum*.   But on the other hand,
the farther you get from the *punctum saliens* of minute symptomatic resemblance, and increase your doses accordingly,
you are in peril of coming to employ the drug in quantities
large enough to induce its physiological action as an " arterial
sedative," in which it ranks with Digitalis, Tartar emetic, and
other drugs, like them retarding the heart's action through the
vagi, and relaxing the system through the induction of nausea.
It is such an application of the drug which was advised by
Fleming (in 1845) on the strength of his experiments with it ;
and it is this, mainly, which, through Ringer and Phillips, has
come into vogue again now.   It is not without its merits ; but
I am anxious to impress upon you that it is not homœopathy,
and that you must not claim it as such.   It is not that antipyretic and antiphlogistic use of Aconite which was discovered by Hahnemann before 1822, and which has ever
since constituted (as you may see by Reil's and Dudgeon's
quotations) one of the most cherished practices of his school.

The condition, then, to which Aconite is homœopathic, and
which makes it our great febrifuge, is one of *tension* of the
nervous and arterial systems, manifesting itself by restless

---

* This was his language in 1874. In his seventh edition (1879) he
employs more qualified language, and inclines to the views expressed
above.

anxiety in the one, and chill and heat, with thirst, in the other. It is easy to see that a large class of acute affections beyond those hitherto specified may thus come within its range. In active hæmorrhage, especially hæmoptysis ; in acute congestion of almost any part ; and in recent febrile dropsy, Aconite will always commence and often complete a cure. The same thing may be said of acute sthenic erysipelas and puerperal fever, and (as I have said) of the " urethral fever " which in some subjects ensues upon catheterism. In cholera infantum Dr. Madden found it indispensable in Australia ;* and Dr. Guernsey writes of it—" if a child is suffering from a watery diarrhœa, is crying and complaining very much, biting his fists, and is sleepless, Aconite will usually settle this trouble in a short time." In the collapse of Asiatic cholera itself, where the chill is so deadly that were it not for the consecutive fever its true nature would be hardly recognisable, but where (as in ague) the temperature is already rising, Aconite will assert its power. It is due to Dr. Hempel to say that from early times he has maintained the homœopathicity and potency of the medicine here. In the epidemic of 1865, a French physician (Dr. Cramoisy) reported twelve severe cases recovering under this remedy alone, given in drop doses of the mother tincture.† It is especially when collapse comes on very rapidly, with little or no premonitory illness, and unattended by copious evacuations, that Aconite is indicated. Arsenic is the medicine generally prescribed in such cases ; but its sphere and that of Aconite intersect and overlap each other at this point, and the greater rapidity of the action of the latter would seem to turn the scale in its favour.

The power of rectifying the disordered balance of the circulation shown in these instances gives Aconite an important place in the treatment of many morbid conditions not strictly febrile. In apoplexy and in puerperal convulsions, where there is much arterial excitement, Aconite will do everything for which the lancet used to be thought indispensable. In suppression of the menses from a chill, with its accompanying congestive phenomena, there is no more valuable medicine. Again, where the tension is in the nervous system alone, Aconite (especially in the higher dilutions) is of signal service. Dr. Bayes speaks well of it in the insomnia of aged persons, and Dr. Guernsey in erethistic states occurring during dentition and parturition ; while Hahnemann writes—" It produces

* *Annals*, v. 57.
† *Bull. de la Soc. Méd. de France*, 1865, pp. 604 and 652. See also Dr. Cramoisy's further experience in *L'Art Médical*, xlviii., 414.

all the morbid states which are manifested in persons whose
minds have been excited by fear, joined with vexation ; and it
is also the surest means of curing them rapidly." Fear itself
(especially the fear of death), when urgently present, has been
found an unerring indication for it.

This leads me to say a few words upon the action of Aconite
in the musculo-motor sphere of the nervous system. We find
here a similar tension induced to that already seen in the vaso-
motor division. Not paralysis, but spasm, is excited, and that
nearly always of a tonic character. Trismus is a common
symptom in cases of poisoning ; the sufferers frequently complain of constriction at the throat, of local cramps and spasms,
and of stiffness and difficulty of moving the limbs ; and there
are several cases on record in which complete opisthotonos
existed, and the pseudo-tetanic state was induced as completely
as by Strychnia. There is, however, none of the reflex excitability present which characterises that medicine.

These statements as to the musculo-motor action of Aconite
(which I have always made) are of course in direct opposition
to the common notions about the poison, which assume it to
be a pure paralyser. They are fully borne out, however, by
the most recent experiments with it on animals—those of Drs.
Harley* and Mackenzie.† The former infers from his observations that Aconite affects the cranio-spinal axis from the
centres of the third nerves to the origin of the phrenics, as
Strychnia does the whole ; and exhibits well the spasmodic
dysphagia and dyspnœa which result from its administration.
Dr. Mackenzie extends the statement to the whole sphere
under consideration. " In the earlier stage of aconitism," he
writes, " the irritability of the muscles and motor nerves is
augmented ; their excessive functional activity induces a period
of exhaustion, which disappears, however, if they be allowed
time for recuperation."

Correspondingly, Aconite has considerable power over some
spasmodic affections. Its usefulness—generally in alternation
with other more locally acting medicines—in the incipience of
the neuro-phlogoses we call croup and whooping-cough is
probably to some extent of this kind. In the asthmatic
paroxysm, and in that of the so-called "spasmodic croup"
(not real laryngismus stridulus), when excited by cold dry air,
it will often give relief. In simple trismus and many other local
cramps and spasms, especially when owning a similar origin,
it should always be thought of : Teste relates a striking case

* St. Thomas' Hospital Reports, vol. v.
† Practitioner for 1878-79.

of the kind in which the pectoralis muscle was at fault, and simulated cardiac disease. But, above all, it bids fair to be a valuable medicine in tetanus. There are seven cases of the traumatic form of the disease now on record, in which Aconite, in ordinary doses, was the main remedy used; and in six recovery was the result. It would be still more suitable to the idiopathic form of the disease, from exposure to cold and wet; and to the "tetany" described by Trousseau. The numbness and tingling with which the spasms of the latter begin, their probable rheumatic origin, the occasional presence of febrile symptoms, and the benefit observed from blood-letting—all point to Aconite.

We come next to the action of Aconite in the sensory sphere of the nervous system. To the mind of a physician of the old school, this is a very simple matter. In poisoning by the drug, he would say, and in experiments with it upon animals, loss of sensibility is one of the most obvious phenomena. Aconite, accordingly, is a paralyser of the sensory nerves; and may often prove useful in neuralgia and other simple pains, to which—when the affected parts can be reached—it is best applied locally.

But a little further enquiry will show that such a conception is simple only because of its poverty, and that it fails to embrace the whole series of facts under notice. In experiments on animals, indeed, loss of sensibility of the skin is always noted. But no better instance can be given of the inadequacy of this mode of pathogenetic research than the present. You have only to read a few cases of poisoning by the drug to find that, while the surface of the patient's body is insensible to external impressions, it is not so to his own consciousness. He will complain of at least an uneasy sense of numbness and tingling, or of pricking and burning; and not seldom of actual pain. The condition set up is evidently a dysæsthesia, and not a mere impairment of sensation. Still more evident is this when we come to deliberate provings on the human subject. Those of Professor Schroff have most bearing on the point. "Aconitine," he says, "produces a peculiar feeling of drawing and pressure in the cheeks, the upper jaw, the forehead—in a word, in the parts supplied by the trigeminal nerve. This feeling increases little by little in intensity, and is transformed at first into a remittent pain which shifts its place, later into a continued pain of considerable severity." In one of his provers the extract of Aconitum neomontanum caused "drawing and tension in the range of the fifth nerve, which soon gave place to a lancinating pain," and Rothansel, in the Austrian experiments, experienced a similar effect.[*]

The action of Aconite upon the sensory nerves is thus to develope in them that morbid condition which shows itself in neuralgic pain. Nor need its production of anæsthesia be regarded as in any way inconsistent with this statement. It has often been shown (and by none better than the late Dr. Anstie) that pain is not hyperæsthesia, but something entirely different if not opposite ; and that neuralgic pain especially is nearly always associated with diminution of healthy function, and may even exist in the presence of almost entire destruction of the nervous substance which is its seat. That Aconite causes anæsthesia, therefore, is in favour of rather than against its development of neuralgia ; and, therapeutically, it suggests its appropriate place to be in those instances where the two conditions most obviously coincide.

And now again,—if Aconite showed itself useful in neuralgia only when applied to the painful nerve, its operation might be conceived of as a mere local benumbing. But its chief reputation in this disease has been obtained by its internal use. In an article in the *Gazette Médicale de Paris* for 1854, Dr. Imbert Gourbeyre has collected numerous testimonies to its efficacy ; and at the present day Professor Gubler[†] declares it " almost specific " in facial neuralgia, especially of congestive form, saying that he has yet to see a case in which it fails to be of at least some benefit, even if it does not cure. Dr. Ringer concurs with him that it is where the fifth nerve is affected that it proves most useful; and this exactly corresponds with Schroff's statement, that " Aconite, as also aconitine, given internally, appears to have an elective and special action upon the trigeminal nerve, producing in all parts animated by the sensitive branches of this nerve peculiar sensations, most frequently painful." But the general pains experienced by many subjects of its influence show that it has in some degree the same action everywhere ; and Dr. Imbert Gourbeyre's collection of evidence proves that its efficacy is not limited to prosopalgia. It has proved very useful, for instance, in sciatica.

The kind of neuralgia to which Aconite is homœopathically appropriate has been sufficiently exhibited. It is most suitable to recent cases, occurring in comparatively young subjects, and especially when traceable to cold draughts. Dr. Gubler's experience, however, may lead us to trust to it—especially in the form of aconitine—in more chronic and deeply-rooted cases.

---

[*] See Allen, s. 419.　　† *Bulletin de Thérapeutique*, Feb. 25, 1877.

The numbness and tingling of Aconite may have another significance : they may suggest that which, felt in the extremities, is so frequent and grave a warning of impending apoplexy or paralysis. Dr. Hempel has laid much stress upon this ; but I confess that I rather thought of the anæsthetic influence of the drug as being exerted upon the extremities of the sensory nerves, reaching them through the blood which bathes them. Liegois and Hottot,* however, seem of late to have demonstrated that it produces the effect by acting upon a supra-spinal sensory centre—possibly the optic thalamus. If this be so, we have in aconitism a condition precisely similar to that which obtains in threatened hemiplegia, into which in two of the older records of poisoning cited by Hahnemann—those of Matthiolus and of Richard—it seems to have actually developed ; and Dr. Hempel is quite justified in urging us to use it as a homœopathic remedy in corresponding morbid states. He relates several cases of cerebral paralysis, imminent or present, in which its use was of the utmost advantage.

You will also think of Aconite whenever you meet with anæsthesia as such, general or local, at any rate when it is complained of. It would hardly be suitable to the form of it met with in hysteria, which has of late excited so much interest in connection with the "metallo-thérapie" of Burq ; for here the patient is unaware of the loss of sensibility till it is ascertained from without. But whenever an "anæsthesia dolorosa" is present, give its subject the benefit of Aconite.†

Yet another application of the elective action of Aconite on the trigeminus has been made by Dr. Dekeersmaecker, of Brussels, when he reports its efficacy in incipient glaucoma. It is when the ocular affection is associated with anæsthesia or neuralgic pain in the parts supplied by the fifth that he finds it so useful ; and these symptoms obviously suggest its dependence on disorder at the origin of that nerve.‡

I cannot pass from this part of my subject without pointing out to you how beautifully the facts which have just come before us illustrate the method of Hahnemann. By the proving on the healthy human body which medicine owes to him the *modus operandi* of a valuable piece of practice is ascertained, and hence rendered more sure and definite for the future ; while, by applying the results obtained according to

---

* The later experiments of Drs. Ringer and Murrell lead them to a similar conclusion.

† See a case of my own in vol. viii. of the *Annals*, p. 491. This patient has since continued almost entirely free from her ailment.

‡ See *L' Hom. Militante*, i., 271.

the rule of similarity he has enunciated, other uses of the medicine are gained which give us a remedy for morbid conditions, one of which is of the utmost importance.

We pass now to another great sphere of the action of Aconite,—its anti-rheumatic virtues. It cannot be said that these also were proclaimed by Hahnemann, or are discoveries of the law of similars. The names of Störck,* Lombard† and Fleming are most prominent as advocates of Aconite in this connection. The first found it curative in many old rheumatisms, improvement generally setting in with critical sweats or eruptions. The second ascribed to it a specific action against acute articular rheumatism. And the third says of its use in the same affection that the average time required for cure is from five to six days; that the drug seems to protect the patient from cardiac complications ; that the convalescence is very short ; and that much less stiffness of the joints is left than under the ordinary treatment.

Nevertheless, though otherwise arrived at, the anti-rheumatic virtues of Aconite are truly homœopathic. Aconite is an irritant as well as a neurotic poison ; and the tissues its irritation affects (when introduced into the circulation) and the kind of trouble it causes are distinctly those of rheumatism. Pains in the joints, muscles, and fibrous tissues generally, of a cutting, tearing, and shooting character, are very frequent in the provers ; and they are attested by Ringer and Schroff. Schneller, in the experiments of the Vienna Proving Society, developed genuine muscular rheumatism in his own back and loins.‡ One of the Austrian provers had, alternating with his articular sufferings, painful palpitation of the heart and præcordial anxiety; and Dr. Jousset says that he has introduced into the circulation of rabbits increasing doses of the extract, with the invariable result of producing lesions of the mitral valve. Very painful hyperæmia of the eyes has been more than once observed,§ and looks like rheumatic ophthalmia. Lastly, in post-mortem examinations decided evidences of inflammation of the pleura and peritoneum have been found ; and the symptoms elicited by some of the provers are in full harmony therewith.

All this is in closest analogy with the action of the rheumatic materies morbi ; and in the hands of those who avail

* *Exp. et Obs. circa usum internum Stram., Hyosc., et Aconiti.* 1762.

† *Gazette Médicale de Paris*, 1835.

‡ *Brit. Journ. of Hom.*, vi., 271.

§ See case 7 in the *New Materia Medica*, and Cases XV. and XVI. in the Appendix to Fleming's monograph.

themselves of the lower potencies, Aconite is reckoned the prime homœopathic remedy for acute rheumatism. In higher attenuations it seems to have less power, and is thus little favoured by Wurmb : there is indeed none of the nervous tension here which seems indispensable if it is to act well in infinitesimal doses. But there is fever, with which is increase of the fibrin of the blood ; it is (ordinarily) of synochal type, and would by itself demand the remedy. It is as yet unknown whether Aconite can subdue the dangerous hyper-pyrexia sometimes observed in this disease ; but I should think it likely to impede its supervention by moderating the ordinary rise of temperature, which it unquestionably does. The rheumatic being a toxæmic fever, and not departing in its characteristic perspiration, cannot be expected to disappear under the Aconite in a few hours ; but it will yield in good time. It is obvious, moreover, that the supervention of any of the common complications of acute rheumatism would not render this medicine less truly indicated ; for we have seen it acting similarly on the heart and the serous membranes. It may, however, be sometimes aided by medicines acting more powerfully upon the tissues affected, as Bryonia in pleurisy, Colchicum in pericarditis, Spigelia in endocarditis.

In acute local rheumatisms, moreover, Aconite is often most effectual, as in stiff-neck or lumbago resulting from a draught, and in sciatica where the sheath of the nerve is affected. It is also of great value in the primary stage of rheumatic ophthalmia. It is not so effective in iritis as in what we used to call sclerotitis. We are now taught that the sclerotic is rarely inflamed, and that the redness of its hyperæmia appears in patches. But clinically I mean by sclerotitis a *painful* inflammation of the eyes, brought on by exposure to cold, and presenting a crimson and straight-lined injection of the ball instead of the scarlet network of catarrhal ophthalmia. Here Aconite—*meipso teste*—is most effective. It is also highly praised by oculists of both schools* for its power of checking incipient inflammation of the eye after mechanical injury, whether accidental or operative. Look out, says Dr. Vilas, for the ciliary zone, and directly it appears put in your Aconite. Homœopathy has hardly put it to the proof in those chronic rheumatic conditions for which Störck and his followers have so lauded it ; and what are the nature and conditions of its action here remains to be seen.

I have only yet to speak of the action of Aconite on the

---

* See the experience of Dr. Cade in *Journ. des conn. med.-chir.*, 1856, Nos. 9 and 10.

heart. It has hitherto been generally assumed that it depresses and ultimately paralyses this organ. But such conclusions have been arrived at from cases of poisoning, and from experiments on animals with large quantities. Schroen, Arnold and Sharp* in the homœopathic school concur to testify that in small doses it quickens the cardiac action in man, at any rate at first; and Rudolph Boehm has lately obtained similar results from fractions of a milligramme of aconitine in frogs.† The acceleration cannot be, he says, from removal of inhibition through paralysis of the vagi; as atropine, which effects this, leaves the number of beats unaltered in the frog. It can only be, therefore, from excitation of the motor nervous supply of the heart. This is further confirmed by the second stage of the phenomena resulting from these minute quantities. Spasms of the heart set in, and these " far more decided and outspoken than with larger doses." The ultimate stage is, indeed, diastolic absence of motion; but this, he says, is clearly a cessation from weariness,—the heart showing all the characters of an organ semi-paralysed and tired out by excess of activity and irritation. He calls attention, moreover, to the remarkable consonance between the action of higher degrees of *heat* (as observed by Cyon) and that of aconitine upon the heart. The " palpitation " so constantly noted by the provers of Aconite points in the same direction; and the whole phenomena are precisely analogous to those observed by Dr. Mackenzie in the muscles generally.

Aconite is thus perfectly homœopathic to the condition of the heart which obtains in the sthenic fevers; but it also has an important place in primary disorder of that organ. Of its value in the cardiac inflammations of acute rheumatism I have already spoken. It is very useful in all diseases of the heart characterised by increased action, especially where the left side is chiefly involved. Its continued use gives much relief to the distress of hypertrophy. In one case of the rare spasm of the heart I saw almost instantaneous relief follow its administration; and in palpitation, where the heart retains its vigour, it is the best soother.

The therapeutic powers of Aconite have now been passed in review. The conclusion is that—beyond many other applications—it is the precious remedy which fills that important

---

* Dudgeon, p. 27, note. *Monthly Hom. Rev.*, xvii., 603.
† *Brit. Journ of Hom.*, xxxi., 194. The full account of these experiments gives a very different impression from that conveyed by Dr. H. C. Wood's *résumé* of them.

place so long occupied by venesection.   It was Aconite which, in days when the lancet was in universal use, enabled Hahnemann and his disciples to dispense with it ; and it is Aconite only which will prevent its revivification now.   Ten years ago I should have said that the revival of venesection was far from improbable ; for, save our present drug, no such potent antipyretic exists.   Wilks and Ringer had merely repeated what Fleming and Routh in their time had proclaimed ; and with these as with those it seemed likely that, from want of knowledge how to use the remedy, they would let it go again.   But a deeper and wider impression seems now to have been made ; and it may be trusted that throughout the prefession the conviction is growing that in Aconite we possess a remedy which has all the energy without the inconveniences of bleeding, so that by it the place of the lancet is irrevocably taken.

As regards allied medicines, it seems to me that Aconite is perfectly unique in its action in the sphere of the circulation, and the same thing may be said as to its action upon the sensory nerves.   In the musculo-motor sphere, it may be compared with *Cicuta* and *Hydrocyanic acid.*   Its relation to rheumatism classes it with *Bryonia* and *Actœa racemosa ;* and in its influence upon the heart it resembles somewhat *Cactus grandiflorus*, *Naja*, and *Spigelia*—which last acts like it upon the fibrous tissue of the eye-balls.

And now as to dose.   I cannot deny that Hahnemann and his immediate successors seem to have found success from the plan recommended by him, of administering in fever a single dose of a high dilution of Aconite (18th to 30th), and allowing it to act.   But it is no less certain that the homœopathic practice of the present day in all countries is to give frequently repeated doses of (generally) a low dilution until the fever departs in perspiration.   I have myself never adopted any other practice than this ; so that I have no other to recommend to you.   The dilutions I use are the 1st, 3rd, and 6th of the decimal scale.   The first I prefer in high fever, in acute rheumatism and rheumatic or other inflammations, in cholera, croup, cardiac spasm, and tetanus : also in neuralgia, where I often give Aconitine (3rd decimal) with advantage.   The 3rd is sufficient in less violent febrile conditions, or when the anxietas of Aconite is very marked, in whooping-cough and asthma, and when the symptoms requiring the drug occur in young children.   The 6th I think best in the febrile chill, in sub-acute circulatory disturbance connected with menstruation, in chronic heart disease, and generally where the medicine has to be taken continuously for some time.   I have also, like Dr.

Bayes, used with advantage in nervous excitement the 12th and even the 30th; and Dr. Hempel has shown that in such dilutions it should be used even as an antipyretic when the patient's strength has been much reduced by depleting measures.

LECTURE XI.

ACTÆA, ÆSCULUS, ÆTHUSA, AGARICUS, AGNUS CASTUS, AILANTHUS.

We begin to-day the consideration of a series of minor medicines which, in our alphabetical order, follow upon Aconite.

The first is the

Actæa racemosa.

By this, its Linnæan name, I venture still to designate the plant; though it is now more commonly called—less beautifully, and with no pleasing suggestiveness—Cimicifuga.

A tincture is made from the root. The "concentrated" preparation, cimicifugin or macrotin (which is a resin obtained by evaporation of or precipitation from the tincture), seems to contain most, if not all, of the virtues of the plant: it is triturated, or dissolved in alcohol.

Actæa has been fairly proved, and by many persons. Some of the original experiments may be read in the third volume of the *North American Journal of Homœopathy*, and in Dr. Hempel's *Materia Medica*. Dr. Allen gives a full pathogenesis of it, containing 447 symptoms derived from twenty distinct sources; and Dr. Hale, in the second volume of the fourth edition of his *New Remedies*, supplies a complete account of its therapeutic virtues. Both call it Cimicifuga.

Drs. Phillips and Horatio Wood concur in saying that we have little or no knowledge of the physiological action of Actæa. This is an ignoring of the labours of homœopathists, because such, which is hardly creditable to either, and which ignorance cannot palliate in the former, as he refers to Dr. Hale's book. Perhaps it would not be welcome to either to admit that restlessness is so markedly caused by it; for it was first introduced into ordinary practice as a remedy for chorea, and upon the prevailing theory of medicinal action it ought to exercise a sedative rather than a disturbing influence upon the nervous centres. There is, however, abundant evidence from provings and overdosings to show that the latter is its real action. Agitation and pain are the signs of its influence everywhere. The head aches severely, with especial involvement of the eyeballs ; the mind is irritable and distressed, and even a condition resembling delirium tremens has been induced. There is great bodily restlessness, which is next door to jactitation, with pains in the spine, the muscles (including the heart), and the joints. One prover had sharp pleurodynia more than once during his experiments ; and another, examining his urine, found urea and uric acid in considerable excess.

Now, if the principle of homœopathy be sound, Actæa ought to prove a remedy for some forms of *rheumatism*, and especially when the nervous centres and the muscles are the seat of the disorder. On the other hand, since it causes no febrile symptoms, it cannot vie with Aconite in rheumatic fever. Well, this is just what experience has established. In the acute and local muscular rheumatisms, as pleurodynia, lumbago, and torticollis, Actæa has gained commendation from all. The only exception is Dr. Ringer ; but he extols it highly in some of the sub-acute articular forms of the disease. He specifies rheumatoid arthritis, especially when of uterine origin, and when the pains are worse at night and in wet or windy weather. It relieves these, and the cramps which often accompany them, to a very considerable extent. Another form simulates gonorrhœal rheumatism, but without any history of gonorrhœa. Here not only may the pains be almost immediately relieved, but the joints may become supple and useful again. This by the way ; but I am persuaded that it is in muscular rheumatisms that Actæa will best sustain its reputation. Among these must be included the sufferings which the heart and the uterus often undergo from the influence of the rheumatic poison. The provings recorded by Dr. Hempel—the experimenter was a pupil of his—make it evident that Actæa affects the heart very powerfully. When rheumatism attacks this organ, not setting up inflammation, but as it does other muscles, we have a valuable remedy in our present drug. In a case of the kind cured by Dr. Hale the symptoms resembled angina pectoris, the attacks of pain recurring several times a day. Last, it is here (I think) that we must place the undoubted power of Actæa over chorea. The frequency of the rheumatic origin of this disorder is well known ; and Dr. Ringer actually states that it is only when chorea owns this causation that he finds the medicine curative.

He might, however, have extended its efficacy to cases having the *uterus* for their starting-point. Actæa has an undoubted action upon this organ; though in the absence of female provers we can say only that it is abortifacient and ecbolic, producing miscarriage without the inflammatory irritation of Sabina, and exciting in labour less unremitting contractions than Secale. But its therapeutic virtues in this region are numerous and well established. It is especially when the uterus is presumedly rheumatic that it influences it for good, relieving dysmenorrhœa and after-pains, checking the tendency to abortion, and facilitating parturition. When the " irritable uterus " is traceable to this origin, Actæa helps it greatly. But beyond this, when morb d uterine conditions show themselves elsewhere than in the organ itself by the pains and agitations characteristic of the drug, it comes potently to their relief. It cures uterine epilepsy and hysteria; puerperal melancholia (the case published by the late Sir James Simpson is a brilliant instance); the nervousness of pregnancy; and the restless and unhappy state of mind so often seen in uterine patients.* The co-existence of sleeplessness is said by Dr. Hale to be a special indication for it in these mental states. It dissipates the infra-mammary pain in unmarried females, which is to the uterus what pain in the shoulder is to the liver; and also pains in the mammæ themselves so arising. It is above all useful in the sufferings of the climacteric age, relieving the sinking at the stomach (which is one of its marked pathogenetic symptoms), the pain at the vertex and the irritability of disposition better than any other medicine.

While connecting the influence of Actæa on muscular tissue with that of rheumatism, I have no idea of limiting its remedial power to rheumatic myoses. It has removed simple myalgia when not traceable (as with Arnica) to fatigue. Of this Dr. Madden has recorded some instances; and one of very striking character in which the diaphragm was the seat of the affection, and where he was not only physician but patient. The malady had lasted nine years; and the narrative of its diagnosis and cure is one of the most interesting things in medical literature. It is to be read in the twenty-fifth volume of the *British Journal of Homœopathy* (p. 493).

The same remark applies to the nervous centres. It may be only rheumatic chorea in which Actæa is curative, but there

* See cases in *Brit. Journ. of Hom.*, xxvi., 168, 662; xxviii., 159, 248.

are certainly other nervous affections in which no such origin can be traced, and in which nevertheless the medicine acts perfectly well. We have seen this in the uterine neuroses; but it holds good no less elsewhere. Thus Dr. Hale has seen it useful in what he calls "chorea of the heart," in the sleeplessness of children from dentition, and in melancholia of all kinds, and Dr. Phillips in the hypochondriasis of spermatorrhœa: it has also more than once removed the spasms of cerebro-spinal meningitis.

Last, as to the eyes. I have mentioned before the severe aching pain in the forehead and eyeballs caused by the drug; this is, indeed, the characteristic symptom of actæism. Dr. Hale commends it in headaches resulting from loss of sleep or mental strain and worry. It would seem to be the muscles of the eyes in which its pains are situated, and it would be indicated when these were aching from undue exercise or from rheumatic influences. Dr. Angell has been led to use it largely, in the form of macrotin, in accommodative and muscular asthenopia, to remove the evil consequences of prolonged exertion of eyes thus affected, as hyperæmia and photophobia. It should be useful (as Dr. Hale suggests, and as its influence on nervous system plainly indicates) in the ocular hyperæsthesia which Mr. Hutchinson has lately described so well, when it is use of the eyes which brings on the aching. I know not if "muscular rheumatism" ever affects its appropriate parts in the optical apparatus: if it did, Actæa would be quite in place in its treatment.

Actæa may be compared with *Caulophyllum* and *Secale* in its uterine relations, and with *Aconite* in its influence over rheumatic disorders. Its effects on the nervous system somewhat resemble those of the last medicine, and of *Ignatia*, but they are *sui generis*. Physiologically, Dr. Bartholow considers that it acts on the circulation and the unstriped muscular fibre much like Digitalis and Secale respectively, but less actively than either; and Dr. Stillé compares it to Colchicum.

It is used in homœopathic practice mainly in the dilutions from the first decimal to the third centesimal.

We have next to speak of the

Æsculus Hippocastanum.

This medicine—the horse-chesnut—is known only in homœopathic practice. A tincture is prepared from the nut, and is certainly efficacious. Pharmaceutically, however, it would seem better to make triturations; which indeed were mainly used in the provings.

Æsculus was first proved—on seven persons—by Dr. Buchmann; an account of his experiments is translated from the *Hom. Vierteljahrschrift* in the eighteenth volume of the *British Journal of Homœopathy.* In the second edition of Dr. Hale's *New Remedies* six more provings are detailed, and the many reports of its clinical use which have appeared in Homœopathic journals are brought together. Æsculus also forms the first of a very instructive series of "Studies in the Materia Medica" which Dr. Dyce Brown has contributed to the *Monthly Homœopathic Review* for 1876 and the subsequent years.

The region most constantly and strongly affected by the horse-chestnut is that of the *rectum* and *anus.* No prover escaped its influence there; and beyond the many forms of distress experienced by others—dryness, fulness, constriction, sense as if a foreign body were there, heat, itching, in two, one of whom had never had piles before, these morbid growths were produced. Correspondingly, Æsculus has acquired a high reputation in the homœopathic school as an anti-hæmorrhoidal medicine. I have several times affirmed and illustrated its value;* and Dr. Hale cites numerous testimonies of like import. The form of the disease in which I have found it specially efficient is that in which the only connected symptom or appreciable cause is constipation, and where there is much uneasiness and pain but little bleeding. Dr. Hale, who agrees with me in the latter qualification, disputes the former, maintaining that the hæmorrhoids of Æsculus belong to congestion of the liver and portal system, in which he is supported by Dr. Hart, of Wyoming.† Dr. Minor, of New York, too, gives "absence of constipation" as an indication for Æsculus, distinguishing it thereby from Collinsonia.‡ Putting all these things together, it would seem that our medicine has a very wide range of anti-hæmorrhoidal activity. I think, too, that we may carry it a point farther. The older authors used to describe an hæmorrhoidal diathesis, of which the local occurrence of these excrescences was but the main feature. Dr. Jousset, in his *Eléments de Médêcine Pratique*, maintains that we have suffered loss by losing sight of this conception, and

* *Brit. Journ. of Hom.*, xxiii., 294, 485; xxv., 428. *Manual of Therapeutics*, (1st ed.), p. 280.
† *Amer. Hom. Observer*, xi., 208.
‡ *Brit. Journ. of Hom.*, xxxv., 141.

draws a picture of the "hæmorrhoidaire." Now if side by side therewith you will read Dr. Brown's description of the "person under the influence of Æsculus," you will observe a close correspondence to one aspect of the hæmorrhoidal diathesis, viz.: that which in its depression, irritability, portal congestion and catarrh of mucous membrane approaches to the gouty. The other elements of the picture—the varicosis and hæmorrhages—are supplied by Hamamelis, which takes the place of Æsculus in bleeding piles. We may then add these two medicines to Nux vomica and Sulphur as remedies for the hæmorrhoidal diathesis.

Aching in the lumbo-sacral region is very marked in the provers of Æsculus, and is a well-known concomitant of hæmorrhoids. Dr. Guernsey attaches great importance to this pain as a "key-note" for the remedy. He considers it situated in the sacro-iliac symphysis. "The pain," he writes "in this region is not severe, more a sensation of painful weakness, and is brought on by exercise and relieved by rest. When attempting to walk about or attend to usual occupations the back 'gives out,' and the patient is obliged to rest." When this symptom occurs in connection with disorder of the rectum or the sexual organs, we are (he says) to think of Æsculus.

When first writing about Æsculus I called attention to its action on the throat, where it has caused a dark-red congestion of the fauces, with dryness and soreness, similar to that which is set up in the rectum. I mentioned then a case in which it had removed such a condition when occurring idiopathically; and Dr. Meyhoffer has since put another on record, in which constipation and hæmorrhoids co-existed, and all yielded to the remedy.* The case was one of follicular pharyngo-laryngitis; and Dr. Meyhoffer mentions that other means were required to remove the granulations. In the *Monthly Homœopathic Review* for September, 1877, Dr. Brown highly commends Æsculus in this affection of the pharynx; and, with an interesting consilience of thought, Mr. Clifton contributes to the same number a series of eleven cases of the disease, occurring as a recent affection and within a short space of time, where he was led by the similarity of the symptoms to give the horse-chestnut, and with rapid success. "Angine granuleuse," I may mention, is one of the local manifestations, according to Dr. Jousset, of the hæmorrhoidal diathesis.

The paper to which I have referred, by Dr. Hart, of

* *Brit. Journ. of Hom.*, xxvii., 549.

Wyoming, has some interesting remarks on Æsculus. He extends its sphere to all active abdominal and pelvic congestions, especially when characterised by a sense of throbbing; and speaks warmly of its value herein.

Æsculus seems to act the better for dilution to some extent. The second and third potencies have been those I have used, and Dr. Hart gets his results with the sixth.

I have next to speak of the

Æthusa cynapium.

This is the "garden hemlock," the "fools' parsley" of popular nomenclature. The tincture is prepared from the whole fresh plant for homœopathic practice, in which alone it is used.

A pathogenesis of Æthusa was published by Hartlaub and Trinks in the fourth volume of their *Annalen* (1833). An analysis of this, with the sources of the cited symptoms in full, is given by Dr. Roth in the second volume of the *Revue de la Matière Médicale Spécifique*. In 1847 Dr. Petroz published another pathogenesis, consisting of symptoms observed by himself.* Dr. Roth has combined the two collections, with revision and additions, in his Materia Medica (I. 169). His article is translated by Metcalf. The cases of poisoning on record are pretty fully given by Hempel; and Allen, in his supplement, adds some new provings.

The result of Dr. Roth's examination of the pathogenesis of Hartlaub and Trinks was to discredit it sadly; as nearly all the symptoms were supplied by Nenning, whose contributions to the Materia Medica are in his eyes of very dubious value. But Dr. John Harley would leave us still more destitute. In an article in the fourth volume of the *St. Thomas's Hospital Reports* he examines the recorded cases of poisoning by Æthusa, and records sixteen experiments of his own in which large doses of the juice were entirely inoperative; coming to the conclusion that toxicologists have hitherto been under a delusion, and that the fools' parsley is a harmless plant. I must confess that his experiments have much negative force, and they have been repeated with similar results by Dr. Allen.† I do not, however, feel satisfied with the principles on which he determines the validity of the poisoning cases, and must think the question still *sub judice*. However it be settled, the

* See his *Etudes de la Thérapeutique*, and also Teste's *Materia Medica*.
† *Encyclopædia*, x., 262.

therapeutic virtues of the drug may yet be believed ; and you
must allow me for the present to connect them with its
physiological effects as hitherto accepted.

Supposing this acceptation to be well-founded, Æthusa is a
poison of no mean intensity. One of the narcotico-acrids of
toxicology, its irritant influence is manifested not so much by
inflammation as by pain, which is generally very severe. The
nervous symptoms are convulsive, somewhat epileptiform in
character ; in one case (in a child) it is noted that the thumbs
were bent inwards, and the eyes turned downwards. The
lower jaw is tetanically fixed. In less severe cases there
is much complaint of headache ; the face is usually red, and
in one instance the eyes were painfully inflamed and the
cheeks œdematous. As regards the provings, I have
nothing to say of those of Hartlaub and Trinks. No information is given as to the manner in which Petroz'
observations were made ; nor is there anything very specific
about them, except pain and swelling in the axillary and
other glands. Dr. Allen's provers experienced little but
gastric disturbance. Æthusa has been seldom used in practice.
From Petroz' experience it would seem most useful in sub-
acute inflammations of the ocular and palpebral conjunctiva,
associated with swelling of the glands and cutaneous eruptions,
—in a word, in mild cases of strumous ophthalmia. Dr. Roth
also reports a cure of this malady. The action of Æthusa on
the eyes deserves further investigation. Kallenbach speaks
very highly of its value in intolerance of milk in children.*
I agree with Mr. Clifton† that the inference as to this from the
pathogenetic symptoms is a misunderstanding ; but it may be
a true action nevertheless. Dr. Guernsey entirely confirms it,
and esteems Æthusa highly in cholera infantum. He says
that " this remedy is one of the most important in the Materia
Medica, and is not so well known as it should be." He gives
as indications for it, great anguish and crying ; disposition to
jump out of bed or escape from the room ; great anxiety
expressed by the face, often accompanied with the linea
nasalis ; regurgitation of food an hour after it has been taken ;
swelling of external glands with lancinating pains ; startings
preventing sleep ; heat without thirst. It should be of service
in the convulsive affections of childhood : Mr. Clifton reports
it useful in these, when gastro-enteric irritation is present.

Hahnemann mentions facts about Æthusa which suggest
that it has some action upon the brain. After saying that it

* *Gazette Hom. de Paris,* 1850, No. IX.
† *Monthly Hom. Review,* xii., 399.

specifically produces imbecility, and should be of use in this condition, he goes on to state that once when he found himself, from much mental work of various kinds coming upon him in rapid succession, distracted and incapable of reading any more, he took a grain of a good extract of it, prepared by himself. The effect was an uncommon disposition for mental labour, which lasted for several hours, until bed time ; but had passed off by next day.*

Æthusa is comparable with *Cicuta virosa* and *Œnanthe crocata* in its toxic effects ; with *Cistus, Bovista, Clematis,* and *Sulphur* in its finer actions and curative powers.

The 6th dilution seems to have been that mainly used.

And now, of

Agaricus muscarius.

This is the mushroom popularly known as fly or bug agaric ; it is the *fausse orange* of the French, the *amanita* of the Italians. For homœopathic practice (in which alone it is now used) a tincture is made of the fresh, or triturations of the dried fungus.

The pathogenesis of Agaricus appears first in the second edition of Hahnemann's treatise on *Chronic Diseases.* He acknowledges ten fellow-observers ; and the 715 symptoms recorded belong almost exclusively to these. They are indeed, as Dr. Hering shows,† a selection from several provings of various kinds, previously published. There are but twenty-one symptoms from authors ; so that little use has been made of observations of poisoning by the fungus. In the tenth volume of the *Vierteljahrschrift*‡ Dr. Roth has analysed the pathogenesis with condemnatory results, and has given a schema of what he considers the genuine effects of the drug. Since then, it has been re-proved by the Austrian Society in their usual exhaustive manner, under the auspices of Prof. Zlatarowich. Nineteen persons took part in these experiments, the record of which appeared in the *Zeitschrift d. Ver. d. Hom. Ærzte Œst.* for 1863. An account of them is given by Hempel (in his second edition) ; and in Allen's *Encyclopædia*

---

* *Lesser Writings,* (trans. by Dudgeon), p. 318.

† *Guiding Symptoms,* i., 144.

‡ Trans. in *Brit. Journ. of Hom.,* xviii., 268.—Dr. Roth shows that five of the symptoms were supposed to have resulted from holding a solution of *Agaricus* 9 or 30 in a full glass before the opened right eye of the patient !

the symptoms obtained are incorporated with Hahnemann's and those of poisonings (the last fully given by Marcy and Peters), making a grand total of 2495. Upon this important pathogenesis Dr. Brown has given us another of his valuable studies.*

Agaricus appears, from the poisonings and Austrian provings (which alone I feel able to use as materials), to exert its chief influence upon the nervous centres. Upon the brain it acts as an intoxicating agent, like alcohol, opium, and haschisch : it is used for the purpose by the Kamschatkans. The drunkenness is more vertiginous at the outset, and more delirious afterwards than that induced by alcohol : it is often accompanied by increased muscular force. The disordered exaggeration of function ending in suspension, which intoxication implies in the cerebral centres, is also manifested in the other divisions of the nervous system. Neuralgic pains are experienced as though sharp ice touched the parts, or cold needles ran through the nerves—in this contrasted with the Arsenic neuralgia, in which the imaginary needles are redhot : or again, the sensory nerves lose their elasticity and power of resistance, so that when even feeble pressure is applied to a spot, it pains a long while after. The motor centres suffer quite as severely. Tremors and choreiform twitchings are produced by it; convulsions of epileptiform type are not uncommon in poisonings; and in several of the provers were developed symptoms of a profound affection of the spinal cord. Here are the symptoms obtained by Baumgartner :—while taking some of the lower decimal attenuations he had pain between the eighth and ninth dorsal vertebræ, heaviness and langour in the lower extremities, and a sensation of coldness in the glutei muscles. Under large doses of the mother tincture the latter symptoms increased, the gait became unsteady, and formication was felt in the feet. The pain was then felt also in the region of the first and second lumbar vertebræ, and in the sacrum. Next followed paralytic weakness of the sphincter ani and involuntary dribbling of the urine. Three hundred drops caused, among other symptoms, " lassitude and trembling of the lower extremities ; coldness and insensibility of the glutei muscles ; continual twitching in the small of the back and the lower extremities ; sensation as if a cool current of air were passing from the spine over the whole body." The prover experienced a fulness and a sensation of weight, with pressure, in the small of the back, a creaking in the fingers and toes when moving

* *Monthly Hom. Rev.*, xx., 334.

them, with stinging pains in the same, and in the integuments generally. Another prover, after taking ten drops of the mother tincture, was suddenly attacked with a violent stitch in the small of the back, attended with vertigo and nausea, so that he had to vomit; the pain gradually extending along the whole spine, as far as the medulla oblongata. On touching the vertebral column, it was painful in several places. Prof. Zlatarovich himself had "crawling and pricking sensation in the nerves, a feeling of painful tension in the fascia of the thigh, painful sensitiveness of the spinal column, drawing and tensive pain in the spinal cord, and occasional fugitive pains in the track of the spinal nerves."

There are many other characteristic symptoms induced by Agaricus, which as yet defy classification. Thus the mucous membranes are found coated with a yellow mucus; on the skin a lichenous eruption (lichen pilaris urticatus) has been developed, with crawling, stinging, and burning; the liver is seen in autopsies greatly enlarged; pains, as though innumerable splinters were in them, are felt in the muscles, especially in the deltoid, where a small abscess even developed itself; and great constriction was complained of in the chest. The testicles were much retracted in several provers; and the urine often had a whitish sediment, which one tested and found to be phosphate of magnesia.

The employment of Agaricus has been hardly commensurate with its physiological importance. It is quite disused in ordinary practice, though formerly reputed in epilepsy, to which it is homœopathic enough. In our practice it has often cured chorea, to the idiopathic form of which it is a precise simile: it is said to be especially indicated when the twitchings cease during sleep, but this they almost always do. Drs. Allen and Norton commend it highly in spasmodic affections of the eyelids and muscles of the eye-ball, especially of the internal recti. Dr. Roth, from his study of its toxicological effects, recommended it in ataxic typhus; and Dr. Drysdale has recorded two cases of this form of the fever in which it proved effective in his hands.* Dr. Simmons has communicated a still larger experience of the same kind; and an American writer has followed suit. All agree that tremor, restlessness and constant desire to get out of bed are the indications for it; and that the mother-tincture must be used for the purpose. Some of its spinal symptoms point to congestion of the cord; but most of them, I think, belong to that ill-understood condition which we call spinal irritation. I am glad to find that in this

* *Brit. Journ. of Hom.*, xxi., 401.

opinion I have the concurrence of Dr. Brown. Mr. Clifton, in
some interesting observations on Agaricus,* speaks of having
gained much advantage from its use in this complaint. He
also commends it from experience in delirium tremens and its
non-alcoholic analogue, in enlargement of liver and spleen,
and in chilblains. It is thoroughly homœopathic to the last-
named trouble, judging from S. 492, 1947, and 2250 of Allen's
pathogenesis, which show such a condition of skin in ears,
hands and feet ; and Dr. Guernsey considers chilblains a key-
note for the remedy. Hahnemann says—" Apelt has found
this drug serviceable in pains of the upper jaw-bone and the
teeth ; also in pains of the bones of the lower extremities (as
if in the marrow), in confluent eruptions of itching papules of
the size of a millet-seed, and in lassitude after coition."

Dr. Brown's article is very suggestive in respect of further
uses of Agaricus. Amongst other things, he thinks it likely
to be useful in spasmodic conditions of the respiratory organs,
with some irritation of the mucous surface, herein resembling
Ipecacuanha. I cannot quite follow him in expecting good
from it in the " douleurs fulgurantes " of locomotor ataxy ;
the inflammatory induration which is at the basis of these
pains lies, I think, beyond the range of the action of the
drug. The pains of Agaricus radiating from the cord seem
rather those of " spinal irritation."

The medicines most allied to Agaricus seem to be *Actæa*,
Cannabis Indica, *Hyoscyamus*, and *Opium*.

The lower medium dilutions (3-6), and not uncommonly the
mother tincture, have been employed.

Before leaving Agaricus, I must say a few words about the
alkaloid which has been recently obtained from it and called
Muscaria. It had been noted of old† that in some cases of
poisoning by fungi the power of the vascular system was
remarkably depressed. The provers, also, invariably report
reduction of the frequency of the pulse. Physiological experimentation has now proved that this property resides in
the muscaria of the fungus, and that its rationale is excitation
of the inhibitory nervous apparatus, slowing the heart's action,
and ultimately arresting it in diastole. The irritability of the
organ itself is unimpaired ; and a dose of atropine, which
depresses the inhibition, sets it going again. M. Prevost, of

---

* *Monthly Hom. Review*, xii., 400.—In a later communication (vol.
xxiii., p. 255), he speaks of obtaining continued success with it in
splenic congestions and enlargements.

† See Pereira, ii., 59.

Geneva, has lately instituted experiments on animals which, confirming these results, show that muscaria has much power over the secretions, increasing the lachrymal, salivary, hepatic, and pancreatic, but diminishing the renal to entire suppression. Atropine is antidotal to it on all sides in this sphere also ; so that the whole action is neurotic, and probably connected with variations in the blood-pressure, which atropine increases, and muscaria lowers.

Still more recently,* Drs. Ringer and Morehead have experimented with muscaria, and on the human subject, injecting fractions of a grain subcutaneously. They confirm M. Prevost's results as regards lachrymation and salivation, but find that it also acts as a sudorific, producing perspiration almost as constantly and as profusely as Jaborandi. Not much influence was noted on the pulse. The pupils were contracted ; but, when a ten per cent. solution was locally applied, they became widely dilated. In this respect muscaria corresponds with Gelsemium, and differs from pilocarpia—the alkaloid of Jaborandi—which contracts the pupil whether internally or externally exhibited. Its internal administration, however, has not so potent an effect of this kind as has that of muscaria. The pupillary changes of the latter drug are unaccompanied with disturbance of vision, so that it probably has little action on the accommodative apparatus. In animals great dyspnœa has been observed from muscaria, and Dr. Brunton has found the pulmonary blood-vessels strongly contracted, the lungs blanched, and the right heart much distended ; but no disorder of respiration was noted in the four men on whom Drs. Ringer and Morehead experimented. On the whole, muscaria possesses properties closely analogous to those of pilocarpin and eserin—the alkaloid of Physostigma, and antagonistic to those of atropine.

No application has yet, to my knowledge, been made of these properties of muscaria. The drug ought to be a useful antipathic palliative for palpitation.

My next medicine is

Agnus castus.

This plant is only used in homœopathic practice. A tincture is made from the berries in the usual way.

The pathogenesis of Agnus castus is in Stapf's *Beiträge ;* and it is prefaced by a summary of all that is known concerning the drug. The provers were Hahnemann and six others.

* *Lancet*, Aug. 11, 1877.

The name of this plant hints at its special action ; and its history points the same way.   It was used by Athenian women during religious solemnities, and by mediæval monks, to repress carnal desire.   Its provings show that it really has this property, depressing sexual instinct and energy without previous excitation.   It is even reported to have caused in one case permanent extinction of virility.   Its therapeutic use has accordingly been directed against atonic conditions of the sexual organs.   In the hands of Drs. Stapf and Marcy it has cured simple impotence in males ; and Dioscorides states that it promotes menstruation and the secretion of milk.   Its elective affinity for the sexual organs seems even to render it effectual against their local diseases; for it is said to have been occasionally curative of gonorrhœa, gleet, induration of the testes, and leucorrhœa.   Dr. Guernsey considers as characteristic of Agnus castus a mental state in which the patient thinks that it is of no use to do anything, as death is sure to come soon (this is different from what obtains with Aconite, where there is fear of immediate death).   It might thus be useful in some cases of sexual melancholia.

Camphor, Conium, Kali bromatum, Nuphar luteum and *Phosphoric acid* are the medicines which in the sexual sphere invite comparison with Agnus castus.

Drs. Marcy and Stapf both report the 6th dilution as that with which their success was obtained.

I have last to introduce you to the

Ailanthus glandulosa.

A tincture is prepared from the flowers of this " tree of heaven," as it is popularly called.

Some few provings of Ailanthus have been made, and are collected in the article on it in Allen's *Encyclopœdia*.   But its real history as a medicine is to be found in the three papers to which I shall presently refer.

The story of Ailanthus is a very interesting one.   One of our most accomplished American physicians, Dr. Wells of Brooklyn, supplies its first chapter.*   A child of his own was seized with all the symptoms of the invasion of malignant scarlet fever.   There was " violent vomiting ; severe headache ; intolerance of light ; dizziness ; hot, red face ; inability to sit up ; rapid, small pulse ; drowsiness, and at the same time great restlessness ; much anxiety ; two hours later, the drowsiness

* *Amer. Hom. Review*, iv., 385.

had become insensibility, with constant muttering delirium ; and she did not recognise the members of her family. She was now covered, in patches, with an eruption of miliary rash, with efflorescence between its points, all of a dark, almost a livid colour ; the eruption was more profuse upon the forehead and face than elsewhere." Dr. Wells gave up his child for lost. But in a few hours a change came about which gave a new aspect to the case ; and inquiry ascertained that she had largely sucked the juice of the stalks of the Ailanthus. Dr. Wells ends his tale by suggesting that we have here a possible aid in those frightful cases of scarlatina which prove fatal in the first stage, with the symptoms of cerebral toxication.

This was written in 1864. But, published in a journal little known, it seemed to have made no impression. In 1867, however, Dr. Pope, discerning the significance and value of these facts, called the attention of English readers to them.* His remarks soon bore fruit. In 1868, Dr. Chalmers found himself in the midst of an epidemic of malignant scarlatina. New at that time to the use of homœopathic remedies, he was disappointed (as we all have probably been) at their action here ; though the traditional practice had nothing better to offer him. His attention was then called to Dr. Pope's paper. He procured the Ailanthus, and at once found that he had the agent he needed. The fever was characterised by a dark-coloured and partial eruption ; and the effects of the medicine were constantly shown in the change of this to a rash more bright-hued and general. With this there was a marked diminution in the frequency, with more regularity and firmness, of the pulse, along with restoration to consciousness. " The result of the treatment by this drug was, and is, to me " he writes " a source of sincere gratification and thankfulness."†

I have seen no records of the use of Ailanthus since ; but from private information I have reason to know that it fully answers expectation. Dr. Madden used to tell me—and there was (alas ! that it should be " was ") no better observer —that from what he had seen of its action in London, he had no doubt of its direct specificity and eminent value. Dr. Fischer, of Sydney, who was present the last time but one that I lectured on this drug, informed me afterwards that he had had large experience with it in scarlatina, and could entirely corroborate the favourable reports of its use which I had mentioned. He said, however, that he found it necessary to discontinue it when once the eruption had began to decline,

* *Monthly Hom. Review*, xi., 286.
† *Ibid*, xii., 713.

under the penalty of causing a pemphigoid rash to annoy the patient during or after desquamation.

I should have let this main use of Ailanthus stand by itself, illustrating so vividly as it does the fruitfulness of the law of similars. But Dr. Dyce Brown, who has made the drug the subject of one of his " Studies,"* has directed our attention to the symptoms it produced in several of the provers, as forcibly suggesting its probable usefulness in some forms of cerebral and spinal congestion. Its effect on the head and mental faculties is very like the dull heavy headache, with confusion and incapacity for labour, which arises from brain—fag or over-worry ; while the pains in the back, all up the spinal column, the contractive feeling in the chest and abdomen, and the numbness and tingling in the upper and lower extremities are the symptoms of spinal congestion, and give us another remedy for it in addition to Gelsemium. Dr. Brown also suggests it in bad cases of measles, where the eruption fails to come out, or retrocedes suddenly, or is livid ; in diphtheritic and other low forms of sore throat ; and in epidemic cerebro-spinal meningitis. Such an action as that which it displays in malignant scarlatina certainly ought not to stand alone.

In Dr. Chalmers' cases, and by Dr. Madden, the first decimal dilution was used.

* *Monthly Hom. Review*, xxi., 288.

LECTURE XII.

ALLIUM CEPA AND SATIVUM, ALOES, ALUMEN, ALUMINA, AMBRA, AMMONIUM CARBONICUM AND MURIATICUM, AMYL NITRITE, ANACARDIUM, ANGUSTURA.

You may be amused when, as my first medicine to-day, I mention the common onion. You will find, however, if you read Dr. Hering's preface to its proving, that this vegetable was highly esteemed as a remedy by the ancients, and was credited with considerable pathogenetic activity. We prepare the

Allium Cepa

by making a tincture from the mature bulb of the red onion.

Dr. Hering proved the onion, chiefly in the mother tincture, on some dozen persons in 1847. His results, with the statements of old authors about it, form one of the pathogeneses of his *Amerikanische Arzneiprufungen*, and are translated therefrom in the fifth volume of the *American Homœopathic Review*, and in Allen's *Encyclopædia*.

It is evident from this proving that the well-known irritation of the eyes and nose produced by the emanations from the onion are specific effects, as they also result from the internal use of the tincture. It is hence recommended for fluent coryza and other nasal defluxions,—Dr. Guernsey says, with acrid secretions. Whether it is needed to occupy a place in the treatment of these conditions which Euphrasia, Arsenicum and Kali iodatum do not already fill, experience only can decide. Dr. Dunham describes clearly* a catarrhal condition which he considers suitable for it,—a dry cough causing splitting sensation in the larynx being its most noteworthy feature.

The medicines I have named are the analogues of Cepa in its relation to the conjunctival and nasal mucous membranes. Dr. Hering thinks it occupies a middle place between Aconite and Ipecacuanha.

* *Lectures*, ii., 105.

The transition from onions to garlic is as natural as it is alphabetical. We will speak of

Allium sativum.

A tincture prepared like that of Allium Cepa is used in homœopathic practice.

A pathogenesis of garlic, with clinical remarks, was presented by the late Dr. Petroz to the Société Gallicane in 1852, and published in the third volume of its journal.   It is translated, with additional symptoms and therapeutic notes, by Teste in his *Materia Medica;* and some further additions are made by Allen.

Eructations with salivation ; profuse whitish urine, which becomes cloudy on the addition of nitric acid ; much cough, with glutinous mucus and pains beneath the ribs ; swelling and tenderness of the mammæ, and severe pain in the conjoined psoas and iliacus muscles when put in action—these seem the most characteristic symptoms of Allium sativum.   It has cured chronic cough, with profuse mucous expectoration ; and morbid sensibility to the influence of cold air.   Petroz wrote of it—" Allium sativum has been of remarkable service in cases where the herpetic diathesis has manifested itself in the respiratory or digestive mucous membrane."   He considered a pale red appearance of the tongue, with effaced papillæ, pathognomonic of this affection.   The old authors esteemed garlic an excellent remedy for " phlegm."

The 6th dilution was most probably that used by Petroz and Teste.

My next medicine is one familiar to you as a purgative, though new as a specific remedy.   I speak of

Aloes.

Of the best Socotrine Aloes we make a solution in proof spirit for our tincture.

A copious pathogenesis of Aloes, obtained from twenty-four provers, mainly with material doses, is contained in Hering's *Amerikanische Arzneiprufungen.* Some fresh provings are incorporated in Allen's *Encyclopœdia,* where the medicine has 1180 symptoms

Although, as I say, you have hardly thought of Aloes as a specific remedy, you yet know a good deal about its specific action. You know that it is no mere aperient, but has peculiar properties. That it purges, however introduced into the system ; that it affects the large intestine only, especially the rectum; that here also it excites the action of the muscular coat rather than the secretions of the mucous membrane, being thus (as Dr. Druitt calls it) " eccoprotic ;" that it not unfrequently irritates the rectum and anus, causing heat, tenesmus, and even hæmorrhoids ; and that the determination of blood it induces towards the lower bowel extends itself also to the other pelvic viscera, so that the bladder becomes irritated, and menstruation excited,—these are the teachings of every work on Materia Medica. Our provings confirm them in every particular. They add evidence that the sexual instinct also is excited : that the whole abdomen shares though to a less degree in the congestion of the pelvis, becoming distended and tender; and that, probably in sympathy with the latter affection, a heavy headache is caused by the drug.

They also support what Wedekind and Giacomini have maintained, but which is much forgotten at the present day, that Aloes has a decided action upon the liver. Uneasiness, heat, pressure and tension are occasioned there; and the stools betray evidence of increased secretion of bile, which indeed Dr. Rutherford has lately ascertained to be the effect of Aloes on animals. They enlarge, moreover, our knowledge of the action of the drug upon the rectum, showing its tendency to produce such weakness of the sphincter ani as leads to involuntary stools. " The diarrhœa of Aloes," writes Dr. Dunham, " occurs especially in the morning, say from 2 A.M. to 10 A.M. : the desire for stool is sudden and extremely urgent, being felt in the hypogastrium and in the rectum, and being so urgent that the patient can scarcely retain the fæces long enough to effect the necessary strategic ' change of base ' : during this brief interval, he fears to evacuate wind by the anus, or to make any physical exertion, or even to strain to pass water, lest he should have an involuntary evacuation of the bowels. . . . There is also a similar frequency or urgency of the desire to pass urine, with a similar uncertainty in the tenure of that excretion."*

The use of Aloes in the homœopathic school has been mainly carried on in the treatment of hæmorrhoids, of diarrhœa of the kind above described, and of dysentery. Heat, rawness and soreness of the parts, with loose motions, indicate it in piles ; and in dysentery it is preferable to other medicines where the rectum is much affected, the tenesmus severe, and

* *Lectures*, sub voce.

where there is faintness after each stool. Dr. Holcombe writes—" Aloes 3rd, a single pellet, once cured for me almost instantaneously a tenesmus which had endured for a week or ten days after recovery from dysentery." The want of confidence in the sphincter ani of which I have spoken is a characteristic symptom for it, if present, in all these affections; and a similar condition is a sense of insecurity in the bowels, as if diarrhœa might occur at any minute, for which Dr. Wells recommends it, and which he says is especially prevalent during an epidemic of Asiatic cholera. The same physician has found it useful in the kind of headache it causes—a peculiar, heavy, dull, pressing pain in the forehead, of no great severity, but which indisposes to or even incapacitates for all exertion, especially for intellectual labour. Dr. Dunham had a case in which such a headache, prevailing in winter time, alternated in summer with the characteristic Aloes diarrhœa ; and the remedy cured both. He mentions also a feeling as if it were necessary to contract the eyes and make them very small in order to see as characteristic for it here.

Aloes should, I think, be more used in hepatic, abdominal, and pelvic congestions than it has been. I have recorded a case in the twenty-seventh volume of the *British Journal of Homœopathy* in which the last-named yielded very satisfactorily to its use. It is a sub-acute condition which it sets up, and *heat* is its chief subjective symptom. Dr. Guernsey commends it in what might be called rectal catarrh, *i.e.*, where masses of mucus come frequently away by stool.

Teste promulgates some curious experience relative to the power of Aloes in causing and curing falling of the hair, but it does not seem to have been confirmed by others.

Æsculus, Collinsonia, Nux vomica and *Sulphur* compare with Aloes.

In dysentery, the potencies from the 1st to the 3rd have been used; but Drs. Dunham and Wells have obtained their successes from the 200th.

We have next the well-known sulphate of aluminium and potassium,

Alumen,

or, as commonly called, alum. It was prepared by trituration in the provings, but the British Homœopathic Pharmacopœia directs aqueous solutions to be made.

Alum has been proved by ten persons in the third and

higher attenuations. The symptoms obtained were published by Dr. Hering in his *Materia Medica*, and are also to be found in Allen's *Encyclopædia*.

Of this proving I cannot say much as yet; and little use has been made of the medicine in homœopathic practice. I should not have thought that it had any action beyond that which it exerts as an astringent, were it not for the high commendation it receives from many quarters in lead colic and constipation, where it must surely act as a *simile*. It is not as a chemical antidote to lead that it operates, for it is praised by others as a remedy for simple constipation and for enteralgia in general. It should be tried for the disorder in small doses, should Opium ever fail in our hands. The rectal symptoms of the drug also seem worthy of attention.

I can, of course, say nothing at present of allied medicines or dose.

And now for

Alumina,

the oxide of aluminium. It is prepared by trituration.

Alumina was proved by Hahnemann for the second edition of the *Chronic Diseases*, where it has 1161 symptoms from himself and five fellow-observers. I think you will learn most of the drug's sphere of action by reading the clinical remarks of Teste, of Marcy and Peters, and of Hoyne, in their articles upon it.

Alumina seems to affect chiefly the sexual system and the mucous membranes. Teste says, "I have often derived the greatest advantages from the use of this drug in the case of aged females, against diseases that had been apparently seated in the sexual system, but whose primary symptoms had disappeared with the complete cessation of the menstrual periods." It has cured in his hands chronic gonorrhœa and leucorrhœa, chronic post-gonorrhœal induration of the testicles, and "raised itching spots" in the vulva and vagina. In the mucous membranes, the characteristic feature indicating Alumina seems to be *dryness* with more or less irritation. Thus it has proved curative in morbid sensitiveness of the nasal mucous membrane to cold; in chronic dry catarrh of the conjunctiva, even when it is granular; in chronic pharyngitis where the membrane looks dry, glazed, and red; in dry hacking coughs from pharyngeal or laryngeal irritation; in dyspepsia from deficiency of gastric juice; and in constipation from lack of intestinal secretion. It has also cured a frequent desire to urinate during the night, occurring in an old paralytic.—All the affections to which Alumina is suitable are of a chronic character, and occur in old people, or in dry and thin subjects. I have little experience of the drug myself : it is but rarely used. Dr. Guernsey says that great difficulty in the expulsion of stools, even when soft, is characteristic of it; also an inability to pass water except when straining at stool. It is commended by him when a similar condition to that of the rectum exists in the œsophagus, causing dysphagia. Dr. Hoyne has some good illustrations of its value in violent dry coughs,—Dr. Dunham recommending it for these when excited by an elongated uvula. He himself affirms that " for the sore-throat of clergymen and other public speakers who are thin in flesh there is no remedy equal to it," and says the same of ·the constipation of infants, whether naturally or artificially nourished.

Its analogues are *Baryta, Conium*, and *Plumbum*, and, as regards the rectum, *Veratrum album ;* and its dilutions those high in the scale.

We will now speak of ambergris,

Ambra grisea.

The substance, as met with in commerce, is triturated for homœopathic uses.

The proving of Ambra is in the sixth volume of the *Materia Medica Pura :* the symptoms (490 in number) were furnished by Hahnemann himself and von Gersdorff. Dr. Marcy, in the *New Materia Medica*, contributes some therapeutic information concerning the drug.

Ambergris is one of those strongly scented substances, like musk, castor, and valerian, which disturb sharply but superficially the functions of the nervous system. The symptoms of its pathogenesis all answer to this description. " Choking and vomiting can hardly be avoided when hawking up phlegm from the fauces ; " frequent tenesmus, whatever be the character of the stool ; frequent micturition of pale and copious urine ; some sexual excitement (it was esteemed of old as an aphrodisiac) and irritation of the female genitals—are symptoms of this kind. Ambra is obviously what the therapeutists of the old school call a " nervine : " it finds its place in the treatment of nervous and hysterical affections. Depression, with anxiety, sleeplessness, diminished sight and hearing from mental trouble, spasmodic choking and convulsive cough in hysterical subjects,—are some maladies of this kind which Ambra is reported to have cured. Dr. Lawrence Newton has communicated a case in which Ambra relieved retention of fæces, from nervous causes, after parturition.* Ambra is also much commended for nervous vertigo, especially in old people.

Dr. Guérin-Méneville has recently given us, in the fortieth volume of *L' Art Médical*, an interesting study of Ambra. But he has made a mistake in directing our attention to an article in the *Gazette des Hôpitaux* for 1871, by Dr. Révillout, in which "ambre" is much praised as a subduer of excited reflex action. The author is speaking there of amber (succinum), not of ambergris. We are indebted to Dr. Ozanam for pointing out this error, into which I confess myself to have fallen, though I consulted the original article in the *Gazette*. He is to the point, however, when he calls attention to the irritation of the skin caused by Ambra, and refers to a case of Croserio's, where an obstinate prurigo was cured by it. The pudenda seem especially affected in this way by the drug, and Dr. Guernsey commends it in pruritus vulvæ. I am also indebted to this writer for another indication for Ambra, viz., tendency to sanguineous flow on the least provocation during the menstrual intervals, which led me to it with great advantage in a troublesome case.

As I have already suggested, Ambra is closely allied with such medicines as *Asafœtida*, *Moschus*, and *Valerian*.

Hahnemann recommends the third potency, and Marcy the sixth and twelfth.

I have now to give you some account of the homœopathic uses of ammonia and its salts. The specific properties of these substances are few compared with those of a chemical nature : hence they play a far less important part in homœopathic therapeutics than in those of the old school. Nevertheless, they exert some dynamic action, of which we must take cognizance.

There are two salts of ammonia which have been proved, and of which we have some slight clinical knowledge. The first is the carbonate,

Ammonium carbonicum,

of which we make at first watery and subsequently spirituous dilutions.

* *Brit. Journ. of Hom.*, xxvii., 364. See Hahnemann's S. 185.

A pathogenesis of Ammonium carbonicum appeared in the first edition of the *Chronic Diseases*, containing 159 symptoms. It was subsequently proved by Nenning on several persons; and 479 symptoms from him, including a few from the editors, appear in Hartlaub and Trinks' *Arzneimittellehre*. In the second edition of the *Chronic Diseases* the foregoing observations are united with some fresh ones from Hahnemann himself and three others to make a total of 789. The drug has since been proved by Professor Martin of Jena on himself and eleven pupils. The results may be read translated from the *Vierteljahrschrift* in the eighteenth volume of the *British Journal of Homœopathy*. The symptoms from all these sources are incorporated in Allen's article, making a total of 1010.

Very little result followed the doses of a few grains of the salt taken by the last-named provers. The elective affinities of Ammonium carbonicum appear to be with the mucous membranes of the respiratory tubes and of the small intestines. Wibmer found it to cause, on himself, an irritative cough and increased secretion of bronchial mucus; and bronchitis is a frequent occurrence in poisonings by ammonia, even where there has been no inhalation of the fumes. In both schools of medicine it is in repute for bronchitic conditions : its cough is an incessant one, excited by a sensation as of down in the larynx. A specific action on the small intestine has been ascertained by Mitscherlich in his experiments with it on animals; but has not been utilised in practice. It converts, he says, its epithelium into reddish mucus.

The power of this salt in moderate doses over scarlatina is vouched for by so many practitioners that there can be no doubt of its reality; and homœopathists have not unfrequently used it with advantage in this disease, especially where throat symptoms of a malignant character were prominent.

Dr. Hoyne commends it in the coryza of children, when the nares are seriously obstructed.

Carbonate of ammonia in full doses causes headache;* and in small ones relieves nervous forms of the malady, particularly when (Dr. Guernsey says) increased by closing the teeth. This well corresponds with the fact that the tension and throbbing of the headache ammonia causes is chiefly felt in the temples.

The lowest dilutions have been generally employed.

The other ammonia salt whose proving has given it a place

* See Allen, x. 286.

in the Materia Medica of Homœopathy is the chloride, sal-ammoniac, or, as we call it,

Ammonium muriaticum.

A trituration of the crystals or a solution in rectified spirit is used in our practice.

The pathogenesis of Ammonium muriaticum is in the second edition of the *Chronic Diseases*, and consists of 397 symptoms from Hahnemann and three fellow-observers. Some other experiments with it have been used by Dr. Allen, bringing the number in his *Encyclopœdia* to 600.

From the experiments of Gumpert it would appear that sal-ammoniac has the property, in large and long-continued doses, of causing a morbid increase in the secretions of all the mucous membranes in the body, a "status pituitosus," as the Germans call it. This is accompanied with chilliness; lassitude, sluggishness, and prostration; loss of appetite; and profuse sweating and urination. Later on, a true intermittent fever was induced, having the curious character of recurrence every seventh day. From Böcker's researches it would appear that Ammonium muriaticum greatly increases the elimination of urea.

Many of the uses of Ammonium muriaticum, though in large doses, are certainly dynamic. It exerts great power over the chronic catarrhs (the mucous flux of Chambers) which its pathogenetic effects so much resemble. As Dr. Ringer writes, "All the chlorides of the alkalies increase considerably the secretion of mucus from the digestive mucous membrane, and, indeed, do so from all the membranes of this class. They may even excite catarrh. This is notably the case with chloride of ammonium. . . . These substances, and especially sal-ammoniac, are not uncommonly used to remove catarrhal conditions of the intestines." It is in considerable repute for neuralgia of various kinds, particularly migraine, clavus, and prosopalgia; and, if the German physicians are not mistaken, it exerts an influence upon the liver which is doubtless of a specific character. Dr. Anstie found it very useful in the pain in the liver, with great depression of spirits but no other symptoms of functional disorder of the organ, which he calls hepatalgia. He also esteems it highly in myalgia. In these four spheres the action of the drug needs investigation, and its trial in small doses might be essayed. Dr. Dunham speaks of having had great success with it in sciatica, where the pain was worst in sitting, relieved somewhat by walking and entirely by lying down, Dr. Guernsey considers sense of contraction or actual contraction of the legs a prominent indication for its use. This physician also mentions loss of blood by stool during the catamenia as a special sympton calling for it.

Sal-ammoniac has some repute against intermittent fevers : it should be useful in those seven-day agues which are sometimes left after the suppression of quotidians by quinine.

In its action on the mucous membranes, Ammonium muriaticum closely resembles *Antimonium crudum* and *Pulsatilla*. Its dosage is undetermined.

The acetate of ammonia—*Ammonium aceticum*, as we should call it—has not been proved ; but I would suggest that its remarkable power of relieving dysmenorrhœa, as shown by the authorities cited by Marcy and Peters, is of a specific character. It may be given in the well-known " Spiritus Mindereri." The plain solution of ammonia—*Ammonium causticum*—is rarely used but in veterinary practice. Mr. Moore seems to esteem it highly in acute bronchial and pulmonary affections of a severe type occurring in animals.

I have next to speak of the nitrite of amyl—

Amyl nitrosum.

This now well-known substance—prepared by the action of nitric acid on fusel oil—is dissolved in rectified spirit for internal administration.

The history of Amyl nitrite as a remedy exhibits well the working of the two cardinal principles of therapeutics—the antipathic and the homœopathic method ; and for both is contained in the literature of the dominant school.

Amyl nitrite, when inhaled, was found to cause (after the fashion familiar to us in Glonoin) a rapid dilatation of the arteries in the head and also throughout the body, with quickened but weakened circulation. It was at once perceived that it might be useful in those morbid conditions in which the blood-vessels are spasmodically contracted. Such is the epileptic paroxysm and the cold stage of intermittents, and such are some forms of angina pectoris and of migraine. The inference was acted upon, and with most gratifying success. Angina is for most sufferers robbed of half its terrors by this means of relief. Migraine and other neuralgiæ accompanied with cold pallor of the surface are often arrested in their progress by it. When the epileptic aura precedes by an appreciable interval the actual paroxysms, and when the *petit mal* and even the *grand mal* are recurring frequently, a resort to this medicine does much to avert the mischief. The shivering aguish subject warms up under its influence, and his paroxysm is materially shortened. Its use has been occasionally beneficial in other spasms, as in asthma and spasmodic gastrodynia and dysmenorrhœa.

All this is pure antipathy, and affords an exquisite example of the method, both in its strength and in its weakness. In its strength—for the relief afforded is great and rapid ; in its weakness—for it is palliative and temporary only. The amyl arrests or mitigates the paroxysms ; but it does little to prevent their recurrence—to cure the disease. It has generally to be given in ever-increasing doses ; and though sometimes the reverse holds good, and the attacks gradually diminish in frequency, as a rule its influence is in time worn out, and it ceases to benefit. Nevertheless, such as it is, we thankfully avail ourselves of its aid. It is an utter mistake to suppose that we of the school of Hahnemann debar ourselves—it is an utterly false assumption to say that we are debarred—from using any remedy, whatever be its *modus operandi,* which promises good to our patients. We are as free as others to use antipathic palliatives : only we know them for what they are, and do not allow their fascination to lead us to abuse them, or to neglect to seek a more excellent way.*

This better way is the homœopathic and curative ; and in the case of nitrite of amyl it has been trodden for us by Dr. Ringer. There is a paroxysmal affection whose essence is not contraction, but dilatation, of arteries. It is the "flushing" so common in women at the change of life, but occasionally troubling them at other times also. This is just the condition which amyl nitrite causes ; and—administered in ordinary doses in the attack itself—it certainly would not benefit. But given every three hours, and in minute quantities, Dr. Ringer has found it of the utmost service in preventing the recurrence of the flushings. What he says about dose is very interesting. "The author began with a minim dose, but was obliged to reduce this quantity, and he ultimately found that, for the most part, these patients can bear one third of a minim without any disagreeable symptoms, but that a tenth, nay even a thirtieth, of a minim will in some patients produce the

---

* I am glad to see that the veteran Constantine Hering, generally reputed of the "straiter sect" of homœopathists, speaks out boldly in favour of the palliative use of amyl nitrite (*North Amer. Journ. of Hom.*, Feb., 1879).

desired effect on flushing." This is just the experience of Hahnemann and his school with medicines generally.

Among ourselves amyl nitrite has found the ground of flushings pre-occupied by the similarly-acting Glonoin, and by Lachesis. Nevertheless, it may have a shade of difference in its action peculiar to itself, and so help us in an occasional *non-plus*. Dr. Edward Blake, who was quick to perceive its suitableness to the affection in question,* has obtained very good results from it therein. He has also lately communicated to the *Practitioner* a case of exophthalmic goitre, in which great relief has been given to the patient's subjective sufferings by the remedy. Of a piece with this is Dr. Conrad Wesselhœft's testimony to its usefulness in tumultuous though feeble action of the heart, such as that which it causes.† This physician has given us several provings of the drug administered internally in diluted form.

In naming *Glonoin* I have mentioned a very close analogue of Amyl nitrite. I defer comparison between them till I come to speak of the former drug.

The drug I have next to introduce to you is one of the many of high repute of yore which had fallen into disuse, but which the Hahnemannian method has restored to its due place in medicine. It is the product of the marking-nut-tree,

Anacardium orientale.

This must not be confounded with the cashew nut (A. occidentale). The oily, dark substance which separates the husk from the kernel, and in which the active virtues of Anacardium seem to reside, is triturated with sugar of milk.

A pathogenesis of Anacardium appeared in the second volume of the *Archiv* (1823), containing 484 symptoms obtained from the powdered bean and tincture by Stapf and seven others, among whom was Hahnemann himself. The latter has reproduced these provings in the second edition of his *Chronic Diseases*, adding 138 fresh symptoms obtained in his later manner. Dr. Allen supplies some observations from three other sources as to the effects of Anacardium when applied to the skin, and some further information on this head is supplied in the *New Materia Medica* of Drs. Marcy and Peters.

The ancient reputation of Anacardium was as a remedy for

* *Monthly Hom. Review*, xv., 166.
† *New Engl. Med. Gaz.*, xi., 387.

weakness of the mind, memory, and senses : a preparation of it was known as the " confectio sapientium." Noack and Trinks mention that Caspar Hoffman called it rather " confectio stultorum," because many had lost their memory and become mad on account of using it too often and inconsiderately. They, therefore, fairly claim its remedial powers for homœopathy. Our provings arid therapeutic records confirm these observations of the old physicians. Anacardium appears from its pathogenesis to depress the cerebral centres (especially as regards memory) and the organs of special sense ; and it has frequently proved remedial in weakness of the brain caused by onanism, or remaining after acute diseases. Dr. Bayes writes—"When in Cambridge I found it very useful in steadying the nervous system in *funk* previous to examination, as also in removing nervous exhaustion induced by over-study. In sexual debility it is invaluable; also in cases of nervous prostration following seminal emissions (whether involuntary or not)." He gave the 12th dilution. It is an important remedy in dementia, and in too rapid loss of memory and mental vigour in old persons ; also in amblyopia and nervous deafness. It has removed an hallucination of a dyspeptic, which took the form of a belief that a demon was pursuing him ; and is said to have cured " paralysis of the tongue "—whatever that may be.

Later researches have shown that Anacardium has a remarkable influence on the skin. When taken internally, indeed, it has not been proved to do more than cause the burning itching noted by Hahnemann. But the effects of its external application, however slight or limited, are so extensive as to leave no doubt of its being a specific cutaneous irritant. Dr. Yeldham has recently recorded a case in point, which you may read in Dr. Allen's supplement ; and where, while the earlier part of the narrative exhibits well the dermatitis induced by the drug, the last paragraphs show the mental symptoms coming in. When painted locally on the skin, in its slightest degree of action it causes the appearance of wheals like those of urticaria tuberosa, with itching, burning, and swelling, terminating in desquamation. When operating more intensely it developes eczematous vesicles, and even bullæ.

I am not aware that Anacardium has been used much as yet as a cutaneous remedy* ; but it deserves attention in some forms of nettle-rash, eczema, and pemphigus,—perhaps also in

---

* A cure of eczema by it is mentioned in *Brit. Journ. of Hom.,* xxxiii., 546.

erythema nodosum and vesicular erysipelas. Dr. Sircar, after
relating some instances of dermatitis provoked by the juice,
mentions that in Hindoo medicine it has some repute against
leprosy ; while yet the native doctors are afraid of handling
the drug for fear of getting this very disease, which, he has
been told by his friends among them, has actually occurred in
some instances. He adds that he has been using the drug in
leprosy (in the 6th dilution), and can report remarkable benefit
from it.

Dr. Allen emphasises a sensation felt in several parts of the
body by Gross—" dull pressure, as of a plug being forced in "
—as characteristic of Anacardium. Dr. Dudgeon has communicated a cure of gastralgia by it,* and Dr. H. N. Martin
praises it highly in dyspepsia, when the symptoms disappear
during eating, and return again in two hours.

In the cerebral sphere Anacardium resembles *Phosphoric
acid* and *Zinc ;* in its action on the skin, *Apis, Croton, Mezereum,
Rhus*, and *Urtica.*

Both high and low dilutions seem to have been used with
advantage.

I have last to say a few words upon a medicine with which,
were it not one of Hahnemann's, I should not have burdened
your memory by introducing it here. It is

Angustura.

By this name I intend the Angustura vera, or cusparia, the
bark of the galipæa officinalis. The "vera" is necessitated
because of the occasional substitution of an Angustura spuria,
which is pretty certainly identified with the bark of the
strychnos nux vomica, or some allied species having the same
physiological action. Hahnemann, saying that the true Angustura likewise possesses great medicinal powers, cites in
illustration the symptoms of a case of poisoning by it, which
are evidently those of the spurious kind !

The true Angustura was proved by himself and eight associates : the 299 symptoms obtained are recorded in the sixth
volume of the *Reine Arzneimittellehre.* Dr. Allen adds some
from two other sources, but of equally unexplained origin.
There is little that is distinctive about any of them, nor has
Angustura any recognized therapeutical place. It is used in
its native marshes as a substitute for Cinchona in the treat-

* *Brit. Journ. of Hom.*, xxxvi., 159.

ment of remittent and intermittent fevers. Homœopathy has nothing to add to this, save one case of prosopalgia cured by it (in the first dilution) recorded by Dr. Marcy in the *New Materia Medica*. Indications for it in spinal affections—as those of Noack and Trinks—are untrustworthy, being based upon the effects of the spurious bark. Angustura vera has no spinal action.

It is prepared in tincture, but the Pharmacopœia recommends triturations as preferable.

ANTIMONIUM CRUDUM AND TARTARICUM, APOCYNUM.

Having now run rapidly through our minor medicines, we will address ourselves for the main portion of this lecture to the important remedies afforded by the preparations of Antimony.

Of these we have two in common use,—the ter-sulphide, *Antimonium crudum ;* and the potassio-tartrate, *Tartar emetic.* The former may be considered to represent the various preparations of the metal—"butter" and "glass of antimony," "crocus metallorum," "kermes mineral," and so forth—which gained its repute of old, and are still in use in France and Italy. The latter, while partaking of these properties, has a field of action all its own.

First, then, of

Antimonium crudum.

The purified ore is triturated for our use.

Antimonium crudum is the subject of one of the new pathogeneses of the second edition of the *Chronic Diseases.* But this is not therefore to be ignored ; for more than four-fifths of it are taken from an earlier pathogenesis, contained in the first volume of the *Arzneimittellehre* of Hartlaub and Trinks, and the symptoms therein are stated to have been observed on healthy persons taking fractional doses of the crude drug triturated with milk-sugar. These, therefore (appearing under the guarantee of Hartlaub and Caspari), may be accepted ; while the additions of Hahnemann and Langhammer may be passed by for the present. Hahnemann's pathogenesis also contains 71 symptoms from authors (of which 50 were collected by Hartlaub and Trinks). These are from various preparations,—most commonly from the so-called "glass of antimony," a sulphuretted ter-oxide, containing silica. They must be used with caution, as being too often the mere mechanical effects (as deafness and hernia) of the violent vomiting induced by the drug. With the pathogenesis of Antimonium crudum may be read a proving of the golden sulphide, in doses varying from gr. $\frac{1}{16}$ to gr. x, by Dr. Mayerhofer. It is translated from Hirschel's *Zeitschrift* (xix, 27) in Allen's *Encyclopædia*.

The condition set up by Antimonium crudum seems to be one of depressed vitality of the mucous membranes and the skin. The action hardly goes on to inflammation. The mucous membranes are loaded with mucus, giving rise to slow digestion with fermentation of the food, nausea, and occasional vomiting ; alternate constipation and diarrhœa, with mucous discharge from the anus ; much hawking and expectoration of phlegm ; and irritability of the bladder with mucous sediment. The secretions and the flatulence are of a foul odour ; and there is drowsiness. and loss of flesh and strength. This is the " mucous flux " I have already spoken of while upon Ammonium muriaticum ; but here there is no tendency to fever. The condition of mucous membrane described finds its parallel in the cutaneous disorder caused by Antimonium crudum. Parts readily become sore ; and pimples, tubercles, and pustular eruptions are developed. When these gastric and cutaneous affections appear in practice, Antimonium crudum will often prove an excellent remedy. I have the utmost confidence in it in chronic gastric catarrh, where the tongue is thickly coated with a milky or granular white fur. Eructations tasting of the ingesta are a symptomatic indication for it here. It is useful, says Dr. Hempel, in that " diseased condition of the intestinal lining in children which favours the development of worms ;" and Dr. Guernsey esteems it in diarrhœa when amidst the watery evacuations there is frequent passage of solid hard lumps. Among skin affections it has cured nettlerash when dependent on gastric disorder ; the sore eyelids, ears, and nose of scrofulous children ; and not unfrequently eczema.* Dr. Clotar Müller speaks of " its extraordinary efficacy in affections of the skin. I have reason to think," he writes, " that Antimonium crudum is an invaluable remedy in all cutaneous affections where pimples, pustules, pocks, or furuncular elevations arise primarily or secondarily, especially when at the same time there is severe continued pricking itching of the skin, and after rubbing tenderness and soreness."† It is particularly useful, he adds,

* See two cases of eczema impetiginodes cured by it in *Brit. Journ. of Hom.*, xxiv., 312.
† *Brit. Journ. of Hom.*, xxxii., 241.

when such phenomena occur on the face or the genitals, as in impetigo scroti. We shall see that these are the favourite habitat of the specif eruption of Tartar emetic.

A curious sympton recorded by Caspari is—"large horny places on the skin of the soles of the feet, close to where the toes commence, which pained like corns, and always returned after having been cut out." Hahnemann lays stress on a tendency to these callosities as indicative of Antimonium crudum ; and Hartlaub and Trinks mention several instances of their cure by it. A striking case of the kind is recorded by Dr. Alvarez Gonzales, where one of twenty years' standing, involving the entire sole, and very sensitive, was soon cured by the drug.*

Antimonium crudum may yet find a place in some of those syphilitic and other constitutional affections for which the antimonial preparations were of old reputed as alteratives, and which gave the metal its "currus triumphalis" in spite of the opposition of the profession.

Its analogues are *Ammonium muriaticum, Kali bichromicum, Petroleum,* and *Pulsatilla.*

The attenuations from the 3rd to the 12th have been most in use : I myself have generally employed the 6th.

And now of

Antimonium tartaricum.

Under this heading we will consider the "Tartar emetic," which is still the common name of the salt. As regards its preparation, " the 1^x, when required, must be a trituration, but its solubility in water admits of 1 being a solution. Dilute alcohol may be used after 2." So speaks the British Homœopathic Pharmacopœia. The "antimonial wine " of the old pharmacy is a convenient form : it contains two grains to the ounce, *i.e.,* about one part in 240.

Tartar emetic has no place in any of our classical collections of pathogenesy ; but provings of it have been made from time to time in our body, from Hahnemann downwards. These are collected, together with numerous poisonings, in the article on it in Allen's *Encyclopædia,* which has 970 symptoms. In addition to this, I would direct attention to the large collection of facts about its over-action contained in the *New Materia Medica ;* to a study of its influence on the skin, by Dr. Imbert-Gourbeyre, translated from the *Gazette Médicale de Paris* in

* *Amer. Journ. of Hom. Mat. Med.,* iii., 38.

the nineteenth volume of the *British Journal of Homœopathy ;*
and to a monograph on Antimony, by Dr. Madden and myself, in the twenty-fifth volume of the last-named periodical.

The best known action of Tartar emetic—that to which it
owes its name—is its power of producing nausea and vomiting.
The nausea which it causes is very intense and long lasting.
Dr. G. Wood thus describes the general condition, which, in
addition to the peculiar sensation referred to the epigastrium,
is known as " nausea." " The face," he writes, " is pale, the
skin cool, moist and relaxed,the pulse feeble, frequent, and often
irregular, the saliva flows copiously, and feelings are usually
experienced of gastric uneasiness, languor, and unusual weakness, which are sometimes in the highest degree distressing,
so much so as, if long continued, to render the patient utterly
prostrate in body and mind, and indifferent to all things
around him, even to life itself." To these symptoms should
be added universal muscular relaxation. The vomiting of
Tartar emetic comes on comparatively late, though sooner
than from Ipecacuanha. When it once begins it is energetic,
effectual, repeated, and prolonged. The vomited matters are
often bilious, from extension of the action to the duodenum.

The emetic influence of tartarized Antimony appears to be
purely neurotic in its *modus operandi.* The numerous muscular
movements whose harmonious play produces the complex act
called vomiting are under the control of the nervous centres
at the base of the brain and in the medulla oblongata. That
Tartar emetic acts directly on these centres is shown by the
fact that it causes vomiting when injected into the veins or
rectum, or rubbed into the skin, as well as when introduced
into the stomach, and in the latter mode of administration is
emetic in doses too small to irritate the mucous membrane ;
and, further, that (like Apomorphia, but unlike Ipecacuanha),
it produces the same effects when communication with the
stomach is severed by dividing both the vagi,* and even when
the stomach itself is replaced by a bladder. How the complex
act of vomiting is brought about, and how the general condition called nausea is connected with it, are problems which
physiology has not yet solved, and with which, therefore,
pharmacology may not trouble itself.

Entirely independent of the above phenomena, though
moving in the same sphere, and sometimes consentaneous with
them, are the remarkable effects of Tartar emetic upon the
circulation and respiration.

When this drug is administered in large doses, there is either

* See *Practitioner,* xiii., 281.

an entire absence of nausea, vomiting, and purging ; or, after a short time during which these symptoms continue, the system appears to become tolerant of the drug, and they subside. Then the pulse is found to have fallen one fifth or even one fourth of its normal number of beats, and the respiration to be lowered in even a greater ratio. Trousseau has known it fall from twenty and twenty-four times in a minute to six. It is rather curious that a corresponding effect on the respirations was observed by Dr. Sharp on his own person from a dose of the hundredth of a grain. Their number was reduced from 18 to 6 in fifty minutes, and they became " deep uncomfortable sighings." The pulse was hardly affected.* " It is singular," writes Dr. Wood, " that under these circumstances of great circulatory and respiratory depression the mind is wholly unaffected, the muscles retain their strength, and the organic functions, with the exception of the two referred to, appear not to suffer. Thus it is seen that this condition differs *toto cœlo* from that induced by nausea." It should be added that the force as well as the frequency of the heart's action is diminished by the drug, and that " sometimes, instead of being reduced regularly, the pulse becomes at first irregular and intermittent under its use," as is often noticed with Digitalis.

In seeking to explain these phenomena, we must obviously look for some source of influence common to the cardiac and respiratory movements, by means of which Antimony may consentaneously reduce the frequency of both ; and this we have in the pneumogastric nerves. It is well known that a moderately strong galvanic current passed through these nerves towards the heart will retard and ultimately stop the movements of the latter organ. It is not so well known that a strong current passed centripetally along these same nerves will stop the movements of respiration, the stimulus being reflected upon the diaphragm and the muscles of expiration, causing general tonic spasm. A less degree of the same excitation will simply retard the respiratory movements. We have only then to suppose that Tartar emetic excites centripetally the pulmonary and centrifugally the cardiac branches of the vagi, and we have its circulatory and respiratory depression explained. If it act upon the central origin of these nerves, it cannot but affect the pulmonary branches, which are centripetal, centripetally, and the cardiac branches, which are centrifugal, centrifugally ; and that it does act at this spot we have already shown when speaking of its power of producing vomiting.

* *Essays in Medicine*, p. 726.

The interest of these last phenomena is physiological rather than practical. The " contro-stimulant " method of Rasori, to which they belong, is rarely practised now ; and in the school of Hahnemann was excluded from the first. Nor does the emetic power of the drug play so important a part in homœopathic therapeutics as might be expected. We use it, of course, to check the kind of vomiting it causes; but this rarely comes before us in comparison with that of Ipecacuanha, of Kreosote, and of Apomorphia. Nevertheless, when it occurs—as in cases recorded by Drs. Bayes and Nankivell— Tartar emetic will do all that is required of it. The presence, moreover, of nausea and vomiting in diseases otherwise calling for it will always indicate it additionally ; and these will, as Dr. Ringer states in reference to bronchitis, be amongst the first symptoms to yield to its use. But its most important sphere of action for homœopathists lies in the mucous membranes and the skin (herein resembling Antimonium crudum, but acting much more sharply) ; and in the lungs.

1. There are two forms of morbid action set up by Tartar emetic in the mucous membranes. The first is that peculiar kind of inflammation we call catarrhal. In the second we have on the mucous membranes the same pustular eruption on an erythematous base which we shall see to be the specific effect of the drug upon the cutaneous tissues.

Thus, in the alimentary canal (in poisonings and experiments on animals) a catarrhal gastritis and enteritis are set up, which Dr. Richardson has found to occur however the drug is introduced into the system : the stomach and intestines are found after death lined with a whitish-yellow viscid secretion. In two cases of poisoning observed by Dr. Wood, the matters vomited and purged were white and liquid, without a trace of bile; resembling opaque rice-water. Post-mortem appearances show the stomach and small intestines to be most affected ;. the glands of the latter, especially those of the ileum, have not uncommonly been found enlarged. The subjective sensations accompanying these effects are best described by Dr. Mayerhofer, who took the drug in increasing doses, beginning with the hundredth of a grain. " When the quantity," I quote from Stillé, " was gradually augmented until an emetic dose was reached, the following effects were observed : the malaise and nausea, which had before existed, increased, with frequent eructation, and retching followed by vomiting ; the stools were frothy, and consisted of mucus and bile ; the abdomen was distended and painful ; the urine, which at first had been copious, became

scanty ; the region of the liver was tender upon pressure ;
rumbling and cooing sounds proceeded from the abdomen,
which was the seat of cutting, tearing, and griping pains ;
there were pains also in the lower limbs.   There was an
increased sense of warmth, alternating with chilliness, over the
whole body, and the skin itched. Anorexia was complete, and
if any food was taken, it renewed the nausea.   The throat felt
raw, and deglutition was somewhat difficult and painful.   The
tongue was covered with dirty mucus, and there was a pasty
and insipid taste in the mouth."   On the other hand, the
pustular eruption characteristic of Antimony has been seen in
the jejunum, the stomach, and the lower third of the œsophagus, but is most severe and constant about the mouth and
throat. In this latter region it begins with a feeling of tension,
and other disagreeable sensations, and a metallic taste ;
patches of erythematous inflammation then appear, upon
which come aphthæ, vesicles soon going on to pustules, and
even false membranes.   Upon the respiratory mucous membrane the influence of Tartar emetic is almost purely of the
catarrhal character, though pustules are said to have been
seen in the larynx.   The nares escape untouched ; but the
inflammation, beginning in the larynx, becomes intense in the
trachea and bronchi.   The production of this inflammation
under the influence of Tartar emetic has been established, not
only by post-mortem appearances in animals, but by the
symptoms of the living, as in the experiments of Dr. Molin of
which I shall immediately speak.   Irritation of the genito-
urinary mucous membrane is not marked among the effects of
Tartar emetic.

And now what of the lungs ?   Does the irritant influence
of Tartar emetic upon the respiratory mucous membrane
extend to the air-cells themselves, so as to set up pneumonia ?
The importance of the question is obvious, as its answer in
the affirmative would claim for homœopathy one of the most
cherished pieces of practice known.   You are probably aware
that Majendie so answered it.   In the dogs poisoned by him
he states that the lungs were always more or less affected ;
they were of an orange-red or violet colour (according to the
age of the animal) throughout, destitute of crepitation, gorged
with blood, and in some parts hepatized.   Before death the
respiration had been embarrassed and hurried.   Lepelletier
independently confirmed these observations ;   and naïvely
remarked—" One would imagine that, admitting its action in
man to be similar, far from being useful, its administration
would be particularly pernicious in pneumonia ; but it is

not so, for, instead of favouring engorgement of the lung, it promotes its resolution."

Such facts were too unpalatable for reception, although Majendie was an accredited observer, and his description of the phenomena unmistakeable. Counter experiments were performed by Rayer and Campbell, in which no pneumonia was set up by Tartar emetic; and Ackermann has more recently promulgated the same experience. But Dr. Molin of Paris, in an able thesis on the subject,* points out that the large doses used by Rayer produced death so rapidly that the inflammation of the lungs had no time to develope itself. His own experiments, in which the animals were slowly poisoned, corroborate those of Majendie : the post-mortem investigation showed pneumonia in its first or second stage, together with an intense tracheo-bronchitis characterised by abundant exudation. Still further to clear up the subject, Dr. Molin instituted some careful provings on his own person with small doses of the drug (gr. $\frac{1}{12}-\frac{1}{6}$). On two successive occasions he developed in himself all the signs, rational and physical, of the first stage of broncho-pneumonia, with marked inflammatory fever.† Some experiments on rabbits by Dr. Nevin, recorded by Marcy and Peters, corroborate those now stated. He says—" The lungs and trachea were frequently congested, sometimes highly inflamed, the two lungs seldom alike." I should mention that in Dr. Molin's experiments the inflammation of the bronchial tubes was observed, even where the animals died before the pneumonia had time to be developed.

The facts seem proved; and Ringer and Nothnagel in our own day accept them. Their moral is obvious. The well-known curative action of Tartar emetic in bronchitis and pneumonia is after all an instance of the law of similars. You have hitherto in all probability been taught that it acts in these cases by its general antiphlogistic power, in virtue of its depressing influence upon the circulation and liquefacient action on the blood. But were this its only or even chief *modus operandi*, it ought to be beneficial alike in all inflammations, wherever occurring. That it is not so, the therapeutists of the old school freely admit. In inflammations of the respiratory mucous membrane it is invaluable; when other parts, as

* *Des Spécifiques en Médécine.* 1847.
† An account of Dr. Molin's experiments is given in the sixth volume of the *Brit. Journ. of Hom.* Dr. Allen, who uses some subsequent provings by the same physician made with the dilutions, seems to have overlooked these.

the serous membranes, are affected, it does little or nothing. Even from this alone it would appear that the drug has some specific relation to this part of the organism. Nor will the theory that its influence here, though direct, is antipathic hold good. The " relaxed " condition we have seen it causing in skin and mucous membrane is part of the nausea it excites; while Dr. Bartholow expresses the general experience of the practitioners of the present day when he says that doses from the twentieth to the twelfth of a grain suffice here, " for it is not necessary that nausea should be excited." Now as we have, on the other hand, seen Tartar emetic acting as a specific irritant of the trachea, the bronchi, and the lungs, we seem warranted in concluding that it must be in virtue of its homœopathicity that it proves curative—whenever it does so —in tracheal, bronchial, and pulmonary inflammations. In actual homœopathic practice it has not played so prominent a part in the treatment of these maladies as in that of the old school,—mainly, in all probability, because we have better remedies for some of their forms and stages. But there is very general agreement as to its value in the second stage of bronchitis occurring in infants and aged persons, when the mucus is profuse and the expulsive power feeble, so that much rattling of phlegm is audible. As regards pneumonia, Bähr's statement well expresses the general view. " In un-complicated pneumonia Tartar emetic is scarcely ever indi-cated in the first stage, nor even at the beginning of the second. The time for this remedy commences with the resolution of the exudation. If this take place rapidly, and the reabsorption be slow, the dyspnœa generally becomes quite considerable, because the lungs are unable to remove the copious contents from their cells. If now great dyspnœa be present, and a spasmodic cough with expectoration that affords some relief, Tartar emetic will have a fine effect. This termination of pneumonia is generally characterised by a sinking of the temperature with an increased frequency of the pulse, great anxiety and restlessness, with a copious, cool perspiration, cerebral congestion with a livid or at least a strikingly pallid complexion. In contradistinction to Phos-phorus, the indications for Tartar emetic point to a deficient reaction; hence it is more suitable for old people than for vigorous and young persons." In broncho-pneumonia Tartar emetic is homœopathic enough, but in acute cases of this dangerous disease it yields in efficacy to Phosphorus. In pleuro-pneumonia I should not have thought it applicable at all, but Kafka seems to esteem it highly. The drug has also several times proved curative, in the hands of Drs. Wurmb and Caspar, of acute œdema of the lungs. I have myself much confidence in its power of removing this condition when occurring in the course of general dropsy. Tartar emetic is also very useful in chronic catarrhal coughs, when the expectoration is profuse and easy, and of a mucous nature. Dr. Ringer recommends it, in doses of $\frac{1}{80}$th of a grain or less, for children in whom bronchitic asthma occurs frequently ; and Dr. Bayes praises it in catarrhal croup.

We have little experience of Tartar emetic in affections of the alimentary canal. Dr. Dyce Brown has lately put on record a case of acute catarrhal gastro-enteritis, in which its curative action was manifest.* It should be serviceable in aphthous, pustular, and other eruptive diseases of the mucous membrane,—perhaps in the aphthous mouth and throat of those dying from exhausting diseases, as phthisis. The phenomena of over-dosing with it are—superficially—so like those of the collapse of cholera, that it has been natural for homœopathists to use the drug in choleraic affections. Save, however, as regards cholera nostras, I think the resemblance deceptive. The antimonial collapse is a result of extreme nausea, while no such condition is present in cholera ; and again, its diarrhœa is caused by the catarrhal enteritis it sets up, while cholera is non-inflammatory. Similar objections hold good to its employment in " cholera infantum," where it is (according to my experience) of little service.

2. I have yet to speak of the action of Tartar emetic upon the skin. You have been told of the peculiar pustular inflammation which is excited by the local application of the drug. If your memories need refreshing as to its characters, you will find them described at length in our article. But it may be a new idea to you, that this effect of Tartar emetic belongs to it, not as a mere local irritant, but as a dynamic agent. Nothing, however, can be more clearly demonstrated than is this thesis by Dr. Imbert-Gourbeyre, in the paper I have already referred to. He first quotes nineteen observations to show that, when Tartar emetic is used locally, pustular eruptions are apt to occur on other parts of the body, especially about the scrotum and labia, and the anus ; and this without the possibility of the mechanical transference of the ointment. He then cites five instances in which eruptions, closely resembling those produced by Tartar emetic ointment (and that also which characterises variola), have appeared during

* See *Monthly Hom. Review*, xxi., 153.

the internal administration of the drug.* Lastly, he adduces evidence to prove that the local effect of the drug is not produced till after a day or two, and sometimes does not appear at all at the spot of application, but on some other part of the body. Coupling these facts with the peculiar and specific character of the eruption, and with the frequent occurrence of similar pustules on the internal mucous surfaces under the use of the drug, he comes fairly to the conclusion that Antimony is a specific and dynamic "exanthematogenic,"—its characteristic eruption being pustular. I shall have to tell you, when I come to Arsenic, how these observations as to the specific action of Tartar emetic upon the skin have been supported by the results of experiments on animals and microscopical examination of the tissues as affected by it.

The precise form of cutaneous eruption to which Tartar emetic corresponds is *ecthyma*. "The pustules," says Erasmus Wilson, "following the irritation of tartarized antimony are ecthymatous." A case of this disease cured by Tartar emetic is given in the *New Materia Medica*. It is less suitable or serviceable in impetigo, save in one form of the disease, the impetigo erysipelatodes ; where I have found it as curative as it is homœopathic. Dr. Dudgeon, however, has (*Brit. Journ. of Hom.*, xxiv., 311, and xxix, 405) recorded two excellent cases of cure with it (given in the first and second triturations) of those disfiguring pustular eruptions which haunt the faces of young people. In the second case, the genitals also were involved. But the deepest interest of Tartar emetic in this sphere lies in its relation to *variola*. Not only does it cause a specific pustular eruption closely resembling that of smallpox, but its pathogenesis has also the vomiting, the pustules of mouth and throat, the viscid mucus clogging the air-passages, and the hypinosis of the blood, which no less characterise the disease. Still further, the inoculation of the lymph of Tartar emetic pustules appears to effect results analogous to those of vaccination. The pustules produced are precisely similar in appearance to those of cow-pock, and they in their turn can excite fresh pustules by inoculation ; though I cannot accept the statement that they further confer the same protection from smallpox. Correspondingly with this close homœopathicity, the power of Tartar emetic as a remedy for variola is very great. Testimonies to its value are collected by Drs. Marcy and Peters ; it is said to be especially useful in cases where the respiratory mucous membrane

* Two additional cases of this kind are cited in the *New Materia Medica*, and Tardieu recognises the fact.

is much affected. I myself have invariably used Tartar emetic (in the first trituration) as the medicine for smallpox, and have rarely had occasion to substitute any other. I cannot say that it cuts short the disease ; it is doubtful whether any medicine can. But it seems to me to conduct the cases through in a very satisfactory manner, decidedly mitigating all the incidental troubles, and leaving (even in non-vaccinated subjects) very little pitting behind.*

I have now described the three great spheres of the action of Tartar emetic,—the medulla oblongata, the respiratory mucous membrane, and the skin. There are other forms of disease in which it is often curative. One of these is delirium tremens, where much gastric disorder of saburral kind is present, as when beer has been the intoxicating drink employed. Another is lumbago, and similar so-called " muscular rheumatisms," in which Bähr and Lawrence Newton have praised it highly. It is also reckoned by Dr. Angell a prime remedy for photophobia ; I have recently had a good opportunity of verifying his recommendation. In connection with this it may be mentioned that Dr. Ringer recommends it, in doses of gr. $\frac{1}{30}$ to $\frac{1}{48}$, in strumous ophthalmia.

The correspondences and divergences of the application of Tartar emetic in the two schools respectively are surely very instructive. The drug is known as an emetic, a depressant of the circulation, and a specific remedy in acute pulmonary affections. Ours is the direct opposite of the first of these three uses ; for we cure vomiting with the drug instead of causing it. The second we reject utterly. The third we claim for homœopathy, and, in the light of the law of similars, define its range and precisionise its application.

Ipecacuanha is the medicine most closely allied to Tartar emetic. Then we have, as acting like it on the medulla, *Digitalis, Lobelia, Tabacum,* and *Veratrum viride ;* on the respiratory organs, *Phosphorus ;* on the skin, *Antimonium crudum* and *Clematis.*

The success of old-school practice with Tartar emetic in laryngitis, bronchitis and pneumonia shows that these diseases do not need very infinitesimal doses of the drug. In these, and in variola, the homœopathic school has generally used the second, rarely the third decimal potency. Higher dilutions (12—15) seem to answer well in œdema pulmonum.

My next medicine in alphabetical order would be Apis. But as I cannot begin so important a remedy at the fag end of a

* See case in *Manual of Therapeutics,* 2nd ed., i., 49.

P

lecture, I will skip it, and conclude our talk to-day with a few
words upon the

Apocynum cannabinum.

This plant is often called the " Indian hemp," but it must
not be confounded with the Cannabis Indica of Hindustan.
It is a Canadian herb, from whose root we make a tincture
with proof spirit.

Dr. Allen's *Encyclopædia* gives pathogenetic symptoms
obtained from Apocynum by four provers ; and Dr. Hale's
New Remedies relates all that is known regarding its clinical
use.

And (almost) all that is known is just this, that Apocynum
has virtues of a remarkable kind in the treatment of all
varieties of *dropsy*. Anasarca, hydrocephalus, hydrothorax,
and especially ascites, of all kinds and from all causes, occur
repeatedly among the cases cured by it which Dr. Hale has
collected in his second edition. I am unable at present to
distinguish the precise form of action of Apocynum in this
sphere ; and still less to suggest its rationale. It seems always
to require to be given in substantial doses, yet it is no diuretic,
that is, in healthy persons ; and, when proved by Drs. Peters
and Marcy, it actually diminished the urinary secretion in
both. I have not found it of any service in the hydrocephalus
of tubercular meningitis or the ascites of hepatic cirrhosis—
conditions for which we sadly want medicinal help ; but I
have seen simple hydrocephalus supervening upon typhoid
clear away very satisfactorily under its use. It is impossible
to read Dr. Hale's cases without feeling assured that Apocynum has a true place as a specific remedy for some forms of
dropsy. He himself thinks it permanently curative in renal
dropsy only ; and supposes that it temporarily relieves other
forms of the disease by its action on the kidneys.

Apocynum has also cured menorrhagia, to which it seems
homœopathic, and " stuffy " colds in the head. I have found
it of occasional service in dyspepsia where there is much
bloating after meals, and a frequent sensation of sinking at the
stomach—these two symptoms being very marked in the
provings of Drs. Peters and Marcy respectively.

Apis and *Helleborus* seem the most analogous medicines.
As regards dose,—the mother-tincture, from one to five drops
at a time, has sometimes proved effectual ; but more frequently
it has been found necessary to use the preparation known as

" Hunt's decoction," or to prepare an infusion from the fresh root (an ounce to a quart of water).

[The supplement to Dr. Allen's *Encyclopœdia* contains several fresh provings of Apocynum, the mother-tincture or an infusion being taken in every case. The most marked effect was great relaxation of the bowels,—the abdomen seeming to fill with wind and fluid, which must be hastily and explosively discharged. Great and lasting weakness of the sphincter ani was induced in connection therewith, somewhat resembling that we have seen under Aloes ; but the motions of Apocynum are much more copious, and they occur after food throughout the day, and not in the morning only. Apocynum ought to find place in the treatment of diarrhœa.]

LECTURE XIV.

APIS, ARGENTUM METALLICUM AND NITRICUM.

We will begin to-day's lecture with

Apis mellifica.

This is the poison of the honey bee, and is (it need hardly be said) peculiar to homœopathic practice. It is prepared for use in more than one way. A trituration of the whole bees, dried, and a tincture prepared by macerating their hinder parts, after killing them while in a state of excitement (which last is the preparation of our own Pharmacopœia), have been used, and seem to contain the virtues of the medicine. A better preparation still would be a solution of the virus itself in alcohol or glycerine. It can be obtained, as Dr. Hering suggests, by seizing the bee by its wings and causing it to eject its poison upon a piece of sugar, or by grasping the sting of a stupefied bee with a small pair of nippers, and gradually drawing out the sting and poison bags together.

Apis has been proved, both in trituration and in the solution of the virus above mentioned, by the Central New York State Homœopathic Society. The results, published in its *Transactions*, appear in schema form in Metcalf's collection. They are also published, incorporated with effects of beestings and with new symptoms obtained on the healthy or observed on patients taking the drug, in Hering's *Amerikanische Arzneiprufungen*, and again in Allen's *Encyclopœdia*. Numerous clinical cases are appended to Metcalf's arrangement; and others are to be read in Marcy and Peters, in the eleventh and twelfth volumes of the *British Journal of Homœopathy*, and in the *Bibliothèque Homœopathique* for 1874-75. We have, moreover, a special monograph on the therapeutic virtues of the honey-bee by Dr. C. W. Wolf, which has been translated into English.

The medicine now to be discussed differs in important respects from the substances we have been accustomed to regard as drugs. We have to believe that the symptoms known to result from the sting of a bee are also in some degree produced when the virus of the insect, in a diluted form, is taken into the stomach. In noting, moreover, the homœopathic indications for the remedial use of the virus, we shall depend much upon the phenomena of bee-stinging; and shall take it for granted that similar phenomena occurring in disease are properly treated by the internal administration of the poison. Such assumptions at one time raised considerable difficulty, on the ground of the supposed inertness of animal poisons when introduced through the digestive mucous membrane : and on former occasions I have had to discuss the subject. It is now needless to do so; for, as Drs. Brunton and Fayrer state,* it has been clearly shown that serpent-poison does act when introduced into the stomach, or when applied to a mucous or serous membrane. " The idea," say they, " that it is only effective when injected directly into the blood is erroneous; though it is, no doubt, more certainly and rapidly fatal when it enters the blood direct."

Let us consider the local effects of a bee-sting. The part rapidly swells up, becomes more or less hot and red, with a tense pain, and often considerable burning, tingling, and itching. This is the simplest and most characteristic form of the pathogenetic influence of Apis. It is an *acute œdema*, the cellular tissue being more affected than the skin. Whenever a similar condition occurs idiopathically, whether on cutaneous or mucous surfaces, Apis will be found curative. Acute œdema occurring on the skin is a form of *erysipelas;* and in this disease Apis is a prime remedy. It stands between Belladonna and Rhus, not controlling intense cutaneous inflammation like the former, or the tendency to form vesicles like the latter, but acting most efficiently in its own sphere of œdema. It is of course to traumatic erysipelas that Apis is especially suitable, and Dr. Bojanus—our eminent Russian confrére—highly eulogizes it here. " Since we have fully known the virtues of this remedy," he says, " we have undertaken plastic operations with much more confidence, all fear of bad results from erysipelas being removed." Dr. Kafka records a good case in which the disease followed upon circumcision, and was rapidly controlled by the remedy. Dr. Wolf—who esteems it specific against erysipelas of all kinds —suggests it in that fatal form of the malady which attacks new-born children, spreading from the umbilical wound.

* Trans. of Royal Society for Jan. 22, 1874, reported in *Lond. Med. Record*, ii., 109. See also *Monthly Hom. Review*, xvi., 673.

Then there is a species of sore throat in which Apis is specific.
There is no very great redness or pain as with Belladonna, nor
is the parenchyma of the tonsils inflamed as when Baryta
carbonica is the remedy; but there is general œdema of the
submucous cellular tissue covering the tonsils, uvula, soft
palate, and even the posterior portion of the hard palate.
When you look at the throat it seems as if a bee had flown in
and stung the patient there. If the numerous cases of angina
cured by Apis which have been put on record be studied they
will be found to have been of this character. Such a sore
throat is not uncommonly an extension of erysipelas, as the
late Dr. Todd describes it in his *Clinical Lectures*. It is often,
also, the beginning of œdema glottidis, in which Apis is the
great remedy. It has proved curative in more than one instance of this affection, where the cause was drinking boiling
water from a kettle.* Such cases are commonly fatal.

There are two specific diseases in which the throat is often
affected in the way of acute œdema, and to which Apis, thus
indicated, bears an important therapeutic relation. These are
diphtheria and *scarlatina*. Facts are accumulating which point
to Apis as a prime remedy in the former disease. Drs. Baumann and Veith Meyer in Germany, Kallenbach in Holland,
and Jahr in France, have concurred in esteeming it the best
anti-diphtheritic we have ;† and my own experience points in
the same direction .‡ In the last case I had I found it remove
everything but the coryza, which yielded to Kali bichromicum.
The great prostration, faintness, and even tendency to death
by syncope, noticed in those stung by bees, show that Apis
has more than local homœopathicity here. In scarlatina
Apis is obviously indicated for the anginose form, where there
is more œdema than ulceration. But it has also the action on
the kidneys and skin characteristic of this poison. Dr. Chepmell narrates a case of bee-sting causing scarlatinoid rash and
anasarca, which is so instructive as to the action of Apis, that
I will read it to you, as it is not given by Allen.

"Mr. D——, a middle-aged gentleman, of a bilious *sanguine* temperament, who rather prided himself upon his practical knowledge of
bee-keeping, had invited me to an inspection of his hives, warning me
at the same time that the bees were in a very excitable state, owing to
their having been disturbed some days before. Of this we soon had
experience ; for on approaching the hives we were immediately warned
off by a swarm of bees hovering angrily about us. Under the circum-

* *Monthly Hom. Rev.*, xiii., 364. *Hom. World*, xiv., 427.
† See *Brit. Journ. of Hom.*, xxviii., 613, 775.
‡ *Ibid*, p. 738.

stances we thought it best to beat a retreat, if haply we might escape the penalty of our rashness. After a time I was fortunate enough to get comfortably quit of some dozen bees, which were becoming more familiar with my physiognomy than I quite liked; and so was my friend, in respect of about an equal number similarly engaged upon his own face, with the exception of one eccentric *flaneur*, which persisted in a walking excursion behind his left ear. Annoyed by the obstinacy of this insect, he at last succeeded in brushing it off by a sudden dash with his hand. At the time he remarked to me that he was not quite sure whether he had or had not been stung; but he seemed to think no more about the matter when, shortly after, I took my leave. About half an hour later I was hastily summoned to attend him, as he had become seriously indisposed.

"I found my friend in bed, very anxious and alarmed about himself, although at times he was in a half unconscious state, and slightly delirious. He was *swollen all over*, but more especially about the face and neck, the abdomen, and the upper and lower extremities. The entire skin was covered with a *red rash, very much resembling scarlatina*, only, if anything, *of a less bright colour and somewhat rougher to the feel* than the common type of that exanthem (the smooth scarlatina of Sydenham). The skin was hot and dry, the breathing oppressed, and the pulse quick, but somewhat weak. He complained of fulness and confusion in the head; the face was flushed, and the eyes suffused. His wife informed me that, soon after I had left him, a sudden dizziness came over him, and his head began to feel so full, that he thought he was going to have a fit. These symptoms were succeeded by *rigors*, when he felt so ill and weak that he at once undressed and went to bed, not without considerable assistance. There was reason to believe that a suppression of the renal functions had also taken place; for he made a useless attempt to urinate, and the swelling and eruption almost immediately followed. I gave him, two or three times in succession, three drops of camphor tincture, at intervals of a few minutes; and then prescribed *Bell.* six drops, third solution, in doses of a sixth part, at first every ten or fifteen minutes; then every half-hour, hour, to two or three hours, according to circumstances. Under this treatment a speedy and salutary reaction took place; so that when I left him, at the end of an hour, he was quite comfortable and reassured about himself. In the meantime, all the discomfort about the head and the oppression of the breathing had ceased; and he had passed an unusually large amount of urine; after which (as I subsequently learnt) a gentle *diaphoresis* followed, and the swelling (*anasarcous* as it really was) seemed to subside as rapidly as it had arisen. He then fell into a refreshing sleep, which lasted some hours; and, when he awoke, all trace of his indisposition had vanished. I can only account for this extraordinarily severe effect of the sting of a single bee on the supposition that the poison must have been immediately carried, undiluted, into the cerebral circulation by the *internal carotid artery*. In whatever way this must have happened, the *pathogenetic* experiment is not the less interesting or instructive."

Mr. Nankivell noticed in a patient affected by it that a patch of skin on the arm remained white amid the surrounding redness, and was informed that this spot had been a short time previously the seat of the inflammation resulting from

the sting of a bee.   Both these gentlemen, as well as others,
have used it here with success.   It is especially indicated in
irregular and adynamic forms of the disease, as when the
eruption is repelled, or does not come out well : a typical case
of the kind is given by Dr. Chepmell in his *Hints*.   Dr.
Guernsey says that the alternation of perspiration and dryness
of the skin is characteristic of it here.   Dr. Wolf goes so far
as to say that "thanks to the curative powers of Apis, scarlatina has ceased to be a scourge to childhood."

Other forms of acute œdema are inflammations of the tongue
and of the labia pudendi, in both of which Apis has been
found curative (glossitis has frequently resulted from beestings in other parts of the body).   Indeed, if this pathological
condition be borne in mind as the keynote of the medicine, it
will rarely be used in vain.

We have still remaining the burning, itching, and tingling
of our bee-sting,—features by no means common in idiopathic
œdema.   They rather point to cutaneous dysæsthesiæ and
eruptions, into which, indeed, in the provers they are seen
developed.   The exanthem induced (both in these and in
persons stung by bees) generally resembles *urticaria*, in which
disorder Apis is our great remedy.   The following case is instructive in this connexion :—

"I was called to Mr. L. Stewart, banker, of this city, to see his little
son, who, the messenger stated, was suffering from ' a rash of some
kind.'   Knowing it to be the first time a homœopathic physician had
ever been called upon professionally by this family, I hastened to the
bedside of my patient, and found a little boy about ten years of age,
suffering from a severe attack of urticaria.   He was covered from head
to foot with elevated, circular, and oblong blotches, which soon ran
together, forming one entire blotch over the entire back, arms, and
legs.   The character of the eruption on its first appearance was white,
but on rubbing the parts the colour would change to a pinkish cast.   The
eruption was accompanied with intense itching, stinging, and burning,
which caused the little fellow to scratch and rub himself continually ;
the pulse was but slightly accelerated ; tongue clean.   The child appeared to feel well apart from the symptoms caused by the eruption.

"*Apis mel.* seemed to be so plainly indicated that further investigation appeared to be useless, and I was about to prescribe, when Mrs.
S—— inquired as to the cause of urticaria.   After making a satisfactory explanation, I inquired of my patient as to what he had been doing
through the day.   His reply was that he had done nothing except swim-
ming in the river, and that while dressing, a ' yellow jacket ' had stung
him on the right hand, and that immediately he commenced itching
and burning all over, and when he got home ' he was all broke out,'
and that was all he knew about it.   This bit of information changed
the programme.   Here was a part of the *pathogenesis* of almost the
very remedy I was about to prescribe.   Instead, therefore, of giving
Apis 4th, I prescribed *Ledum pal.*, 5th, gtt. x. in half-a-glass of water,

a teaspoonful every half-hour. I called again after two hours, and finding a decided improvement, I directed that a teaspoonful be given at
eight o'clock, and another at bed-time, and the medicine then discontinued. Early on the following morning I was notified by a messenger
that my patient was entirely well, and that it would not be necessary
for me to call."*

Apis has also cured cases of lichen and of erythema nodosum ; and is generally indicated in skin affections not going
on to destruction of tissue, but accompanied with excessive
itching, especially of a burning and stinging character.

Urticaria, like erysipelas, may manifest itself internally.
Here also we have acute œdema, but without the tendency to
suppuration belonging to the erysipelatous form. The distressing and sometimes even dangerous symptoms arising
from this cause have several times been successfully encountered by Apis.†

In acute œdema, erysipelatous and urticarious, we have the
pathological condition most characteristic of Apis ; and upon
this I am desirous of fixing your attention. But both provings and therapeutic records credit the medicine with a range
far wider than this, as will appear from what follows.

1. The mucous membranes are not influenced in their general extent by Apis ; but at certain spots it manifests great
power. It has frequently proved curative in catarrhal and
scrofulous ophthalmia. It is where the cornea is much involved
that its most striking curative results are seen. Dr. Casal,
of Mentone, has recorded a case where the sting of a wasp
(which seems pathogenetically identical with that of the bee),
inflicted near the right eye, caused—after a lapse of some
days—a sub-acute keratitis, first on that side and then on the
other. Dr. Jousset expresses great confidence in Apis as a
remedy for strumous ophthalmia affecting the cornea ; and finds
it important in these cases to use the solution of the virus, and
not the trituration of the whole bee. It causes hoarseness and
dry cough ; and is often useful in subacute and chronic laryngo-
tracheal irritation, of a mild type (it may be compared here
with Rumex crispus and Carbo vegetabilis). It irritates the
stomach, and somewhat the bowels : it is one of the best
remedies for diarrhœa *recurring every morning*, the motions
greenish-yellow and painless (here again corresponding with
Rumex crispus). Dr. Wolf commends it highly in acute
gastro-enteric catarrh, and in dysentery. It is very decidedly

* Dr. F. B. Smith, in *Hahn. Monthly* for Sept., 1875.
† See Erasmus Wilson, *Diseases of the Skin*, article "Urticaria,"
and cases 14, 16, 28 in Dr. Metcalf's paper.

irritant to the kidneys and neck of the bladder (like Cantharis). Dr. Marcy recommends it in incipient Bright's disease, in inflammation of the neck of the bladder, and in "irritable bladder."

2. Apis acts rather powerfully in the *ovario-uterine* sphere. Few medicines cause so many ovarian symptoms ; and it has more than once provoked miscarriage when given to pregnant women. It has proved curative in amenorrhœa, dysmenorrhœa, and menorrhagia, when resulting from active congestion of the ovaries ; and even in inflammations of the latter organs. The presence of a "stinging" pain is said to indicate it here.

3. I come now to the important question,—what power has Apis over *dropsy*, general and local ? It is credited with almost unbounded curative virtues in this disease ; but I think discrimination is needed. Its action on the kidneys is sufficient to make it a most useful, because homœopathic, remedy in acute febrile dropsy from a chill, in post-scarlatinal dropsy, in that of incipient Bright's disease, and in that which sometimes appears in the later months of pregnancy and lays the foundation of future puerperal convulsions. In all these forms of dropsy Apis has been used successfully, its curative action being generally announced by a great increase in the secretion of urine. Absence of thirst is regarded as a characteristic symptom for it in recent dropsies. Then there are the serous dropsies,—ascites, hydrothorax, hydrocephalus. These may be mechanical, from obstruction of the circulation ; as when ascites results from cirrhosis of the liver. In such cases, I cannot conceive of Apis dispersing the effusion ; nor do I see sufficient evidence that it has ever done so. It is otherwise when the dropsy is the unabsorbed effusion remaining after serous inflammation. There seems little doubt but that Apis acts specifically upon the serous membranes. I do not know that it has been much used in their acute inflammations ; but in ascites and hydrothorax remaining behind after peritonitis and pleurisy it has over and over again proved curative, and there is some reason to suppose that it has removed the effusion in cerebral meningitis (probably non-tubercular). Dr. Wolf speaks in the highest terms of it here. It must be remembered that in full doses Apis is diuretic, and in this way may remove—at any rate temporarily—dropsical effusions unconnected with the kidneys or the serous membranes, such as cardiac and ovarian dropsies, both of which are reported to have yielded to its use. Here, however, it must not be given in dilution ; and the Indian experience from which the remedy was first obtained suggests an infusion or trituration of the entire bee as the best preparation.

Apis seems to have the same action on the synovial as it has on the serous membranes. A lady who took two doses of 15 drops of the tincture found next morning her second right finger begin to swell, the middle joint especially being red and hot. Several cases of acute synovitis have been reported in which its curative powers were evident.* Whether, as Wolf thinks, it will meet the synovitis of morbus coxæ and white swelling of the knee, is a question.

Apis has some repute in intermittent fevers. Dr. Wolf declares it a universal specific for them. Dr. Nichol, of Montreal, considers that it is rarely suitable for malarial intermittents, but heads the column of the remedies with which we combat those of non-malarial origin. Its chief indications seem to be the commencement of the attack in the afternoon, absence of thirst, and a sensation during the chill as if the hands were dead. He relates a good case so characterised and speedily cured by it.†

We have once more in the case of Apis the advantage of one of Dr. Brown's "Studies." The only additional hint I can cull from it, however, is his suggestion of the drug as a remedy for dry catarrh of the nose and larynx, based on the view that the œdematous condition characteristic of the drug is present here.

I have indicated many of the medicines which in particular spheres of action correspond with that of Apis. Thus *Cantharis* and *Terebinthina* in the urinary organs, and *Rumex* in the morning diarrhœa and laryngeal symptoms, closely resemble the present medicine. For the cutaneous symptoms, *Anacardium, Belladonna, Croton, Rhus*, and *Urtica* may be compared ; and for the affections of the serous membranes, *Apocynum, Mercurius corrosivus*, and *Bryonia*. As a whole, the action of Apis more nearly resembles that of *Arsenic* than of any other drug.

The 3rd decimal dilution is that which I always employ in acute œdema in all its forms. In dropsies, Dr. Marcy prefers the lower dilutions, from the 3rd downwards; in cutaneous affections, from the 3rd upwards; in irritation of the bladder he says we ought never to go lower than the 6th. The most striking cures of ophthalmia have been made with the higher dilutions. Dr. Wolf uses the 3rd or the 30th according to the sensitiveness of the patient, and in most acute affections advises its alternation with Aconite to avoid excessive re-action.

* *N. Engl. Med. Gazette*, xii., 20 : Jousset, *Leçons*, p. 478.
† *Monthly Hom. Review*, xxi., 175.

Of the preparations of silver we use two, the pure metal itself, and the nitrate. First, of

Argentum metallicum.

The finest silver leaf was the form in which metallic silver was proved by Hahnemann. The precipitated metal is allowed as an alternative form by the British Homœopathic Pharmacopœia. Either is triturated for our use.

Metallic silver was proved, in the first trituration, by Hahnemann and seven others : the pathogenesis, containing 224 symptoms, appears in the fourth volume of the *Reine Arzneimittellehre.* Some later provings by Dr. Huber, in the potencies from 1 to 6, are recorded in the second volume of the *Œsterreichische Zeitschrift,* and amalgamated with Hahnemann's by Allen.

Dr. Huber sums up his proving by suggesting that the chief action of Argentum is on the articulations and their component elements,—bones, cartilages, ligaments, &c. It seems to produce arthralgia rather than arthritis ; and might be serviceable in hysterical joints. Dr. Sharp writes :—" a very long-lasting and severe case of coxalgia in a young woman, and another nearly similar affection of the knee, have been cured by it in my hands." It also causes some diuresis ; and—as Hahnemann suggested—is occasionally useful in diabetes (not *mellitus* indeed, but *insipidus*). Another sphere of its action is the larynx, where it has cured hoarseness and chronic laryngitis. Easy expectoration, looking like boiled starch, is said to indicate it.

We have yet to learn the influence of Argentum on the uterus, as there were no women among the provers. But Pereira's statement, that " in uterine diseases, especially when there are augmented discharges and great irritability, it has been beneficial," suggests a specific action here ; and Teste has related an interesting case of uterine cancer, in which the relief afforded by the drug was so great that for a time a cure seemed about to result.

Aurum, Platinum and *Selenium* are analogues of Argentum ; less so *Zincum.*

I know of no recorded experience from which to suggest the dose. Hahnemann recommends the 2nd trituration.

And now, of

Argentum nitricum.

This salt of silver is prepared in aqueous solution, and preserved with the usual precautions—yellow actinic bottles being recommended. It is sometimes triturated ; but the preparation must be uncertain.

Nitrate of silver only obtained a few symptoms in Hahnemann's hands, the 15th dilution being employed. But it has received an exhaustive proving from Dr. J. O. Müller, of Vienna, the record of which was published in the second volume of the *Œsterreichische Zeitschrift*, and may be read in Hempel's translation of Stapf's *Beiträge*. Four men and two women took part in it, using both the crude drug and the attenuations. Some physiological experiments with fractions of a grain ($\frac{1}{16}$—$\frac{3}{8}$) are related by Krahmer in his monograph on silver,* and may be read in Allen's supplement. The primary article in the latter's *Encyclopædia* adds to these numerous symptoms from poisonings.

I would first speak of the local application of nitrate of silver. Most of you would probably be loth to lose the advantages of the practice, and would wish to know if homœopathy forbids its continuance. She certainly does not ; but, on the contrary, claims it for herself. Let Trousseau be witness on the point. " Solutions of nitrate of silver," he says,† " at first applied to the pharynx and mucous lining of the mouth, passed into every-day use in the treatment of inflammations of the mucous membrane of the nose, eyes, urethra, vagina, and even of the intestines. . . . . It was soon perceived that the primary effect of this and similar agents was analogous to that produced by inflammation, and it was easy to understand that inflammation artificially induced in tissues already the seat of inflammation led to a cure of the original inflammatory attack. When this view was once acquired, there flowed from it the great therapeutical principle of *substitution*, which, at present, reigns supreme in medical practice." If we needed to know what Trousseau meant by " substitution," we should find it in what he says in his *Matière Médicale* :—" if now arsenic is employed " in inflammations " locally in very small proportions, *il agit homœopathiquement, c'est-a-dire, substitutivement.*"

Nevertheless, it is rarely that the disciple of Hahnemann has to avail himself of such medication. To direct his " substitutive " agents to the parts affected, he uses the elective affinities of drugs. He thus has a far wider range, and also a more radical kind of operation. Local cure of inflammation can be satisfactory only when the disease is of local origin. If, as so often happens, the inflammation is but an expression

* *Das Silber als Arzneimittel betrachtet*, von Dr. L. Krahmer. 1845.
† *Clinical Lectures* (New Syd. Soc.), ii., 19.

of blood-changes farther back, it is poor practice to blight the efflorescence while root and stem are untouched. A *simile* which acts from without can do this only. But one which acts from within will, if it be a true one, track the whole course of the disease, and " cover" it from its first origin to its ultimate manifestation ; for after a like manner itself is wont to behave. Hence, if it cures, it will do so thoroughly.

If, therefore, a beginner in homœopathy should ask me about the local use of nitrate of silver, I should reply, first of all, that homœopathy is affirmative, not negative. She forbids nothing—not even bleeding and blistering : she ousts them merely by curing without their aid. So, by all means, if you have an ulcer or a local inflammation which you cannot cure by specific internal medication, apply your lunar caustic. But try the internal treatment first. I venture to predict that, as that becomes perfected, the local treatment will cease to be required ; and the porte-caustique will take its place with the phlebotomy lancet among the disused instruments of torture.

We turn now to the internal use of our drug. What is generally known of it is that it inflames the gastro-intestinal canal, causing (in Pereira's words) " if the dose be too large, gastrodynia, sometimes nausea and vomiting, and occasionally purging ; " and that, when absorbed, it disorders the nervous centres, producing affections of a convulsive and paralytic character. Its uses are—according to the same authority— to allay chronic vomiting and relieve gastrodynia, while it occasionally displays curative powers in epilepsy and chorea. It is hardly necessary to argue that the virtues of the salt depend upon the operation of the law of similars.

But homœopathy requires more precision than this ; and we must look closer at both the irritant and the neurotic phenomena. As regards the former,—locally the nitrate may, of course, inflame and even ulcerate the whole alimentary canal. There is no evidence, however, of its elective affinity for any other parts of the tract than the mouth and throat, and the duodenum, which last was found inflamed in Orfila's dogs when the salt was injected into the veins. In provers the throat looks dark red, and feels dry, and as if a splinter or ulcer were there ; the tongue is sore, and the papillæ elevated. Tender and easily bleeding (but neither painful nor swollen) gums have been observed in patients under its influence, and in dogs treated by Krahmer like Orfila's. Other mucous membranes feel its influence, especially that of the eye. Dr. Müller himself had, from the second decimal trituration, a sharp attack of conjunctivitis, most severe in the canthi and carunculæ ; there was even an approach to chemosis. Symptoms of urethritis were experienced by the same prover : the canal was swollen, hard, and knotty to the touch, and the right testicle was enlarged and hard.

Then as to the nervous centres and nerves. " Both convulsions and paralysis are present," writes Dr. H. C. Wood, " in *argyria*, or silver-poisoning." The convulsions he describes as reflex, excited by the least peripheral irritation ; and as persisting after the complete abolition of voluntary movements. " Portal," says Stillé, " relates a case in which the exciting cause of epilepsy appeared to be a poisonous dose of lunar caustic." The paralysis is general, and is especially seen in the pulmonary branches of the vagi—death ensuing from asphyxia, with the same condition of the lungs as when their nerves are divided. In the provers the neurotic effect of the drug was manifest in headache deep in the substance of the brain, with low spirits ; vertigo ; want of mental power ; restless, dreamful sleep ; weakness of the spine, with pain at the small of the back ; and very marked debility of the lower extremities, almost approaching to paraplegia. In Dr. Müller this last was accompanied with emaciation of the legs. Krahmer developed in himself a long-lasting (left) infra-orbital neuralgia ; but as this succeeded to much gastric weakness and heartburn, it was probably sympathetic only.

But we have not yet exhausted the pathogenetic power of nitrate of silver. Dr. Bogolowsky, of Moscow, has recently experimented with it largely in rabbits, to ascertain its deeper and more chronic effects.* From these it appears that the salt has a direct and primary influence on the red corpuscles of the blood, causing their colouring matter to escape into the plasma, and so leading at first to ecchymosis and effusions, and later to interference with oxidation and ultimate chlorosis. As a result of the deficient nutrition (so he thinks) there occurs catarrh of the mucous membranes generally, and degeneration —rather of a granular than a fatty kind—of the renal and hepatic cells, and of the muscles, including the heart. There is also found a universal venous blood-stasis.

The therapeutic virtues of Argentum nitricum may be ranged in the same three categories.

1. Its previous repute in affections of the stomach seems well sustained in the present day, and some of it is echoed from the homœopathic ranks. In chronic inflammatory states of the organ its action must be local, and crude doses are

* See Virchow's *Archiv*, vi., 4, 1869 ; and *Practitioner*, iii., 65.

required. Its virtues in the round ulcer of the stomach are, as I shall show, no exception to this statement. But the marked gastric sufferings of the provers seem to show that the drug affects the nervous supply of the viscus, and may—in doses too small for local effect—modify its functional derangements. The same thing appears from the fact that many therapeutists ascribe no less virtue to the oxide of silver than to the nitrate. Dr. Bayes speaks highly of its power over what he calls "irritative flatulent cardialgia," where the wind comes away easily, rushing upwards through the mouth.* Dr. Holland communicates two excellent cases of cure by it of chronic dyspepsia disordering the heart's action.† This was a condition strikingly developed in Krahmer's provings. His chief trouble was heartburn; and the excess of acid on which this symptom usually depends was the prominent feature of two cases of gastrodynia recorded by Mr. Harmar Smith as cured by the nitrate.‡

The virtues ascribed by many writers to nitrate of silver as a remedy in chronic diarrhœa—as that of phthisis—must be referred to homœopathy, as all admit that in full doses the salt purges. But the action is probably, here as in the stomach, local only, and substantial though moderate doses are required. There is, however, a form of diarrhœa occurring in young children, in which the motions are green, like spinach in flakes; and in this Dr. Lippe finds the higher infinitesimals perfectly efficacious.

The specific irritant influence on the conjunctiva which Dr. Müller's experiments revealed led Dr. Dudgeon (in 1848) to argue that its local application, as practised in the old school, acted after a true specific manner, pointing out that, owing to the chemical and mechanical action of the lachrymal secretion upon it, the action of the caustic upon the eye is but momentary, and its quantity infinitesimal.§ I myself have been so satisfied with even its internal effects in ophthalmia neonatorum, that I have never had to resort to any external measures beyond those needed for cleanliness. The experience of our American oculists is quite confirmatory of its power over such purulent inflammations of the conjunctiva. Dr. Angell commends the remedy "in affections of the lining membrane of the lids, and of the lachrymal duct and sac, *when there is an abundant discharge of*

* *Brit. Journ. of Hom.*, xxx., 143.
† *Ibid*, xxxii., 85.
‡ *Ibid*, xxv., 504.
§ *Brit. Journ. of Hom.*, vi., 216.

pus ; " and Drs. Allen and Norton write :—" The greatest service that Argentum nitricum performs is in *purulent ophthalmia*. With large experience in both hospital and private practice, we have not lost a single eye from this disease, and every one has been treated with internal remedies, most of them with Argentum nitricum of a high potency, 30th or 200th. We have witnessed the most intense chemosis with strangulated vessels, most profuse purulent discharge, even the cornea beginning to get hazy and looking as though it would slough, subside rapidly under Argentum nitricum internally."

It is possible that there may be other mucous tracts to whose inflammations nitrate of silver is ordinarily applied locally, but where it acts by elective affinity. Such is certainly the throat, whose appearance and sensibilities in the provers are very like those of the follicular pharyngitis in which it is so much used, and probably the larynx, in whose chronic (even tubercular) affections Dr. Meyhoffer praises the drug given internally as well as by spray. Dr. Guernsey takes the same view of ulceration of the cervix uteri, in which he often gives the 200th dilution with marked results.

2. The anti-epileptic virtues of this salt have yet to be defined. They are undoubted, though only occasionally seen. Nor are large doses always required. A case of forty years' standing is cited by Hempel, in which the cure was effected by swallowing a silver coin which was ejected twenty months later but little diminished in size. The only contribution from the homœopathic school is that of Dr. Gray, of New York, who asserts that epilepsies originating in the brain may be promptly and durably cured by a few small doses, while those proceeding from abdominal irritation can be barely palliated by large quantities. In the paralytic sphere, considerable interest attaches to the medicine on account of its having been strongly recommended of late in locomotor ataxy. Some cases by Wunderlich and others have been published (you may read them in the twenty-first volume of the *British Journal of Homœopathy*), in which there appears no doubt of the nature of the disease, nor of its cure or great mitigation by the use of the nitrate of silver.* Trousseau, however, states that he has been disappointed in it. Dr. Bazire gave it in six cases : a very marked improvement took place in one, and a less marked one in another, but no appreciable result in other instances. Topinard, also, found an entire failure in twelve cases out of seventeen ; and in three only of the remaining five was the improvement decided.

* See also Ludlam's translation of Jousset's Clinical Lectures, p. 420.

Q

Friedreich's experience is still more negative. It is certain, therefore, that nitrate of silver is no specific remedy against locomotor ataxy as such; nor is it homœopathic thereto, as the proving points to a true paralysis of the legs as the effect of the drug, rather than a disorder of movements with retention of energy. In simple paraplegia from exhaustion I have more than once found it of signal service; and it has cured this condition when resulting from concussion or alcoholic excess, and also hysterical and diphtheritic paralysis. In dull chronic headaches of literary and business men Argentum nitricum is much commended. Dr. Guernsey indicates it in giddiness on the least mental or bodily exertion, and when time seems very long to the patient. Dr. Seip, of Alleghany, has recorded several interesting cures by the drug of hypochondriasis in men, traceable to alcoholism or venery;* and Dᵣ Woodyatt, of Chicago, speaks highly of it in paralytic weak ness of the ciliary muscle, causing imperfect accommodation of vision.†

3. But a no less interesting and important sphere of our medicine is that in which its influence on the blood and on nutrition is brought to bear. Not long before Dr. Bogolowsky published his results, Dr. von Grauvogl's *Lehrbuch der Homö-pathie* had appeared in Germany. This able work is, by the labours of Dr. Shipman, of Chicago, accessible to us in an English dress. The author—now (alas!) taken from us—considers that there are three principal " morbid constitutions;" that one of these is the carbo-nitrogenous, in which the oxidation of the blood is obstructed, giving rise to accumulation of carbon and nitrogen in excess; and that the chief remedy for this condition is nitrate of silver. Whatever may be thought of his pathological theory, the cases he gives amply bear out his commendation of the remedy; and the experiments of Dr. Bogolowsky supply the missing link by demonstrating its homœopathicity. We have thus another true *simile* for chlorosis and defective oxidation of the system; and from what I have myself seen I believe that the medicine will fully answer expectation in this direction. Shortness of breath (without lung or heart affection), as observed by Dr. Grauvogl, and sallowness rather than pallor of complexion, have proved my special indications for it. It is here that I will speak of the action of the drug in gastric ulcer, in which several of us think it almost specific. It is now well-known that this lesion is not of inflammatory nature, but a local

* See *Brit. Journ. of Hom.*, xxxiv., 347.
† *Ibid*, xxxii., 739; *Monthly Hom. Review*, xxii., 143.

innutrition; and that the patients most liable to it are young women who are the subjects of chlorosis. Upon this point I would refer you to some excellent remarks by Dr. Cooper, in connection with a case of the kind cured by our medicine reported in the thirty-fourth volume of the *British Journal of Homœopathy* (p. 485). He would, I think, quite concur with me that Argentum nitricum is appropriate to gastric ulcer just when it supervenes upon general chlorosis.

Argentum nitricum has obvious points of analogy with *Arsenic* and *Mercury ;* with *Phosphorus ;* and with *Hydrocyanic* and (as I have pointed out) *Picric acid.*

The potencies from the third decimal to the third centesimal have been those chiefly employed ; but von Grauvogl gave several drops of the first for a dose.

LECTURE XV.

ARNICA—ARSENIC.

Our attention is first to be directed to-day to the "leopard's bane,"

Arnica montana.

The tincture of the British Homœopathic Pharmacopœia is directed to be made either from the entire fresh plant, or from the dried flowers. Dr. Hering has recently shown good reason why the root, and this only, should be employed for the purpose. It seems that an insect is in the habit of depositing its eggs in the flowers, and that these have a peculiarly irritant effect on the skin; so that some at least of the disagreeable effects occasionally produced by its use are to be thus explained, and may be avoided by the exclusive selection of the root for pharmaceutic purposes.

Arnica has been well proved. Hahnemann supplies a pathogenesis of it in the first volume of the *Reine Arzneimittellehre*, to which nine persons besides himself have contributed. It contains (in the third edition) 638 symptoms, of which 47 are taken from authors, and are chiefly collateral or excessive effects of the drug when given to patients. Then we have the provings of Jörg and thirteen of his pupils, which were made sometimes with an infusion of the flowers, sometimes with the tincture of the root. Last come the experiments of Schneller and other members of the Vienna Proving Society, of which an account is given in the sixth volume of the *British Journal of Homœopathy*. Dr. Allen unites the symptoms from all these sources with many of its idiosyncratic effects upon patients in his Encyclopædia. A valuable study of Arnica, by Dr. Imbert-Gourbeyre, may be read in the forty-fourth volume of *L'Art Médical*.

Of the physiological effects elicited in these provings I shall best speak as I discuss the therapeutical powers of the drug. Of these let us take first the best known,—its remedial action in mechanical injuries.

1. This property of Arnica has come to be (in our own country at least) associated with homœopathy. But the method of Hahnemann cannot take credit for its discovery. He himself tells us, in the preface to his proving, that it had become known to the "common man," and the plant named "Fallkraut" accordingly; and that two hundred years before his time, a physician (Fehr) communicated this discovery of domestic practice to the profession, who then named the herb *panacea lapsorum*. The only credit homœopathy can claim in connection with Arnica is that she has kept the tradition alive. Satisfied with Hahnemann's inference from his provings, that " all the symptoms attending violent contusions and tearing of the fibres are analogically produced by Arnica in the healthy organism," and with the fact noticed by the older observers that the pains of such injuries were always at first aggravated by the full doses given, she has adopted the popular remedy into her list of similars. With her adherents to this day Arnica is to an injury what Aconite is to a chill ; and the most gratifying results are continually being obtained from it. In contrast, it may be mentioned that Ringer and Horatio Wood (in his first edition) omit Arnica altogether ; while Dr. Phillips " considers it a great pity that it has not (1874) come into more general use " in this direction.

I have said that Arnica is to an injury what Aconite is to a chill : that is, it will almost infallibly obviate the ill-effects, if given before organic mischief has been set up. It becomes thus the great remedy to be administered in all cases of concussion, sprain, or other suffering from violence. It removes, as Hahnemann says, " the pernicious consequences which often attend falls, contusions, blows, thrusts, straining, twisting or tearing the solid parts of our organism." But, unlike Aconite, it will follow up the cause to many of the changes it effects, even when of long standing and profound character. Such are those instanced by Dr. Bayes in his interesting article on the drug, viz. : the chronic muscular stiffness—called rheumatism—of old labourers,* and the cardiac hypertrophy of boating men. Mr. Nankivell has illustrated the same thing by some of the thoracic affections of the Cornish miners.†

The tissue affected in all these instances is the *muscular ;* and upon this Arnica specially acts. It is above all things a myotic. I learn, from Dr. Imbert-Gourbeyre, that the great organopathist, Rademacher, makes a similar observa-

* See also *New York State Hom. Society's Transactions*, viii., 473.
† *Brit. Journ. of Hom.*, xxiii., 177.

tion. It thus becomes the main remedy for those numerous
affections which Dr. Inman has so well described under the
term (*myalgia*) Over-exertion of healthy muscles, or the
normal use of weak muscles, will bring on these pains; and
Arnica will almost infallibly relieve them. As their occurrence is very common, it is a medicine in daily use. I need
only specify two of them. One is the form of pleurodynia
known as spurious pleurisy. This may readily be induced by
over-exertion, as in the following case reported by Dr. Inman.
" A party of gentlemen on a severe pedestrian excursion were
all tired on the first day, and that was all; on the second day
some began to have frequent stitches in the side, could not
sleep on the side, but only on the back; on the third day the
pains in the side were terribly increased, with so much tenderness that they could not bear the weight of the clothes." In
this not uncommon form of pleurodynia—the "rheumatic
pleurisy" of the old writers—Arnica gives rapid relief. It
must be distinguished from the muscular rheumatism so
called, which yields much more satisfactorily to Bryonia or
Actæa racemosa. Another myalgia which I would specify is
one of the forms of pain after food. The pain comes on immediately, even during the act of swallowing;* the patients
are weak and of lax fibre; and they often have or have had
myalgiæ elsewhere. Here too Arnica is an admirable remedy.

In this connexion I would recommend the perusal of an
excellent paper by Dr. Madden on " Myalgia," in the twenty-
fifth volume of the *British Journal of Homœopathy.* He, too,
places Arnica first among the anti-myalgics; and agrees with
Dr. Bayes in finding heart affections consequent on over
exertion amenable to its use. I may also mention that Dr.
von Grauvogl praised it highly for the " clergyman's sore
throat," or any other induced by loud speaking; and that
I myself have cured with it a chronic tenesmus of the bladder
produced by frequent long retentions necessitated by the
patient's business. Drs. Small and Hoyne have obtained
great relief from it in the passage of urinary calculi or
gravel. It is, moreover, serviceable against simple muscular
debility, such as shows itself in prolapsus and in involuntary
evacuations. It ought to be useful in asthenopia, from over-
exertion of the eyes.

But, though Arnica affects the muscles chiefly, we must not
limit its influence to these. It will check the hæmorrhages of
mechanical violence; quiet the nervous startings of a fractured
limb; and obviate the danger of re-action in concussion of

* See *Hoyne*, i., 200.

the brain and sudden apoplectic extravasation. It seems, moreover, to cover the whole remote effects of an injury. Give it to one whose frame cannot forget the shock of a far-back railway accident; and you and he will be alike delighted with the effect.

In external injuries Arnica may be used locally as well as inwardly; and will give speedy relief to pain, while promoting the restoration of the bruised part to its normal condition. Any one who has tried it when his finger has been jammed in a door will bear witness to the statement.* How it effects this is a difficult question. Dr. Garrod has shown that it has no "absorbent" power over mere sanguineous effusion, such as dry-cupping can produce. Violence seems always needed to call forth its remedial powers; but then they are indubitable.

In old times, the use of Arnica in injuries was extended to the suppurations and hectic therefrom resulting. Stoll declared it most effective in such conditions, and Dr. von Grauvogl—who was an army-surgeon—has revived its use and reputation. Let me read you what he says of it :—

"The results of Arnica provings on the healthy offer an array of symptoms so similar to traumatic fever and septicæmia by purulent infection, that hardly a better description of these states is to be found in works on surgery and obstetrics, and where there is traumatic fever there must have been previously, or still present, wounds; consequently Arnica is indicated according to the law of similars in wounds, and not only in their consequences, and in this respect it is an old renowned homœopathic remedy. Traumatic fever runs its course at first without any rise of temperature, which cannot therefore be accepted as the invariable sign of fever. It begins at once after every considerable mechanical inquiry, with which the whole habitus of the wounded person is shaken and often altered, so as to be unrecognisable. This condition improves manifestly under the use of Arnica, as also all signs of actual absorption of the decomposing elements of the secretions from the wound. Of all the ordinary mechanical injuries, compound fractures give the most profuse suppuration, and the attendant lacerations of the soft parts, that are often very extensive, like large operation wounds, predispose to the occurrence of pyæmic, or septicæmic fever. We do not always see these cases at the commencement, in the country generally not till after the lapse of several days, after the country doctor has done his best, and then we meet with most extensive suppurations. If here we give Arnica 30 x, four to five drops every hour, and apply compresses moistened with the same dilution, the patient feels a considerable alleviation of his pains in two, or at most four or five, hours, and the following day the suppuration is manifestly diminished. It decreases daily, and after a few days is reduced to a small quantity, during which time the wounds become cleaner. Things go on much more rapidly if we give every hour four to five drops of the 1 x dil., and

* See *Brit. Journ. of Hom.*, xviii., 132.

the same as a compress. On the following day, at latest in twenty-four hours, the suppuration is, as a rule, reduced almost to nothing, and the most favourable condition in every respect established.   In the military hospitals I directed the attention of the surgeons to the efficacy of this treatment, and showed them that this favourable effect would at once disappear, and a large quantity of pus be found on the bandages, on leaving off the Arnica. This happened constantly, so that the very next day the former quantity of pus was there, and the wounds of the soft parts gaped again, after they had nearly closed, so that I could not withhold any longer the employment of Arnica internally or externally.

" The renewed employment of this medicine had the same effect as before, and the cure took place in the shortest space of time, and to the astonishment of the allopathic lookers on, without further suppuration, granulation, or retraction of the edges of the wound , therefore quite differently to what they had hitherto been taught and had observed. I had ample opportunity of seeing the same thing done during the French war, but I found no imitators. The effect of Arnica in all sorts of wounds consists in this, that not only does the exudation of white corpuscles and the mortification of the injured parts, and consequently all suppuration, cease, but that the intercellular fluid dries up by continually parting with water to the blood-vessels and lymphatics ; that in consequence of this, the inflammatory swelling of the wound generally declines after a few hours ; therefore all the wounded part consolidates, and the edges, when they can be brought together, agglutinate very rapidly, or when that is not the case, spontaneously approach ever nearer to union, whilst the loss of substance is supplied without suppuration or rank granulations. For these reasons the primary inflammation cannot extend, and where there is no inflammation there is no fever; further, when there is no water there is no pus, no absorption of injurious substances ; thus diphtheria and septicæmia cannot occur. The relapse on leaving off the Arnica, especially externally, causes erythema, with formation of vesicles ; internally, in fractures of the bones, it causes a soft and scanty callus. It is doubtful if Lister's vaunted carbolic-acid method can show such favourable results as the Arnica treatment.''

2. The next most familiar action of Arnica is that which it exerts on the skin.   There is first an eruption, which in some susceptible persons results from its external application. The very scent of it is sometimes enough ; and I have known the eruption follow the internal use of the first dilution, while Dr. Dyce Brown has seen it result from still more attenuated doses.* It consists of a number of very fine vesicles on an erythematous base, with much heat, pricking, and itching. Dr. Phillips thinks that an aqueous infusion of the plant, by excluding the arnicine and etherial oil (which are insoluble in water), is preferable to a lotion made from the tincture for external application, as being non-irritating.

The precise Arnica-erysipelas is rarely met with as an idiopathic affection, and hence the drug is little used in this com-

* *Monthly Hom. Review*, xxii., 171.

plaint. Dr. Cooper thinks it unjustly neglected, and says that he gets more decisive results from it than from any other remedy. Hahnemann points out the resemblance of another of its cutaneous effects to a boil ; and recommends it as preventive and curative in that complaint. Dr. Müller found compresses of a drop of the tincture to an ounce of water very effectual to resolve these troubles. Teste cured with it an angina which seemed to result from the retrocession of boils, and von Grauvogl states that repeated doses will often abort a carbuncle.

3. Less known is the action of Arnica on the nervous tissue. It is reputed in Germany as a stimulant to the brain and spinal cord ; and seems to have cured in Collin's hands* many cases of amaurosis and paralysis. Improvement was generally preceded by peculiar sensations in the affected parts, as tingling and electric shocks. The provers suffered from congestive vertigo and headache ; and from pains down the spine. In one, the lower dorsal vertebræ became very sensitive, and pressure on the last caused radiating pains and sense of oppression of the chest. Van der Kolk (according to Phillips) found Arnica "invaluable in that condition of idiopathic mania where, the first excitement having diminished, the head nevertheless remains hot, and where a tendency to imbecility or to paralysis is shown." Hahnemann cured a chronic vertigo with it ; it was known of old by the name of "Schwindelkraut."

4. Arnica causes, according to both Jörg and Hahnemann, violent urging to stool, with scanty and natural fæces, as if the muscular coat only of the bowel was excited. This suggests the homœopathicity of its action in dysentery, for which it has long been in repute—Stoll calling it a specific antidysenteric. Hahnemann recommended it here himself ; but it had almost dropped out of use until it was revived in America by a curious accident, and has been highly esteemed there since.† Tormina and tenesmus would especially call for it.‡ It acts similarly on the stomach, causing contractive pain, flatulent distension, and hiccough.

Arnica has yet some minor actions, which may be briefly

---

* *Obs. circa morbos*, iv. and v.

† See *Philad. Journ. of Hom.*, ii., 94, 179.

‡ S. 261 of Hahnemann's pathogenesis (" purulent and bloody stool ") must not be regarded as proving the homœopathicity of Arnica to dysentery. It occurred in a child to whom Arnica was being given for a fall from a height. The reporter regarded it as a sign of internal contusion or extravasation.

mentioned. It causes two other marked gastric sensations,— a sense of repletion, and a feeling of canine hunger with (nevertheless) no appetite for food ; also eructations, smelling as of rotten eggs. It is recommended in whooping-cough, when children begin to cry as soon as they feel the cough coming on. It causes several kinds of hæmorrhage (especially epistaxis), and often finds place in the homœopathic treatment of this accident. It plays some part in the therapeutics of intermittents ; it was known of old as "le quinquina des pauvres," and is often useful when that drug has been abused.* It probably has some direct action upon the heart. Dr. H. N. Martin recommends it in angina pectoris, and Dr. Liedbeck confirmed in his own person Kafka's recommenda- tion of it for the dyspnœa accompanying fatty states of that organ.† Dr. Guernsey considers it as truly indicated when the patient feels " as if bruised," as when there has been actual mechanical violence. He also specifies heat of head with cool- ness of the rest of the body as a keynote for it, and recom- mends it when pregnant women feel pain from the movements of the child, in the varices which form in their vulvæ or vaginæ, and in simple cases of painful nipples. I need hardly say that he, in common with every homœopathic accoucheur, invariably gives it immediately after childbirth, and testifies to the good effects of so doing.

A sensitiveness of the body to pressure, so that everything on which the patient lies seems too hard, is another recognised symptomatic indication for Arnica. This feature is often met with in low fevers, and the medicine was not without repute in such disorders among the older homœopathists. A tendency to hæmorrhage is regarded as indicating it here.

Besides ordinary vertigo, Arnica has been suggested by Dr. Ravel as suitable for that associated with disorder in the semi- circular canals of the ear ; ‡ and Dr. Brown has recorded a case of the kind in which it was curative, being indicated by the apparent origin of the symptoms in a fall.§ I have myself had a similar case, in which I was led to try it by the circumstance of the patient having had several falls in the hunting-field.

In its antidotal power against mechanical violence Arnica is almost unique, finding only a point of contact here and there with *Rhus* and *Hypericum*. In its action on the muscles *Bryonia* and *Actæa* resemble it somewhat ; as a cutaneous irritant it is allied again to *Rhus*, and to *Croton*.

See *Brit. Journ. of Hom.*, xxxiv., 719. † *Ibid*, p. 738.
‡ *L'Art Médical*, xliv., 282.
§ *Monthly Hom. Review*, xxii., 595.

In all recent affections Arnica may be given in small or fractional doses of the mother tincture. But I must agree with Dr. Bayes, that if we desire to get good from it in the remote effects of injury, we must ascend to the region of infinitesimals.

We have now to gird up our loins, and summon all our strength, that we may master the greatest of medicines, because the greatest of poisons,

Arsenicum.

By this name a homœopathist means arsenious acid, the Arsenicum album of the old nomenclature. The British Homœopathic Pharmacopœia follows Hahnemann's original directions, and directs the primary (first centesimal) solution to be prepared by boiling. I incline, however, to think that its compilers would have done better to have gone on with him to his later practice, and to have ordered triturations to be made. Either form can be obtained of the homœopathic chemists.

The homœopathic literature of Arsenic is very extensive, and abounds in both original and collected material. Hahnemann published a proving of it in the second volume of the *Materia Medica Pura*, and subsequently another in the second edition of the *Chronic Diseases*. The former, in its latest shape (1833), consists of 1079 symptoms, of which 697 are from Hahnemann himself and seven fellow-observers, and 382 are cited from authors. Many of these last belong to records of poisoning with arsenious acid itself, or with other preparations of the drug—as orpiment, realgar, and cobalt. But a good many are vitiated by having been observed in sufferers from intermittents treated by the drug, where it is very difficult to decide how much is ague and how much Arsenic. The pathogenesis in the *Chronic Diseases* (1839) contains 202 additional symptoms, of which 79 are from a case of poisoning involving a whole family (Kaiser's), and the rest from observations made on patients taking globules of the 30th by Hahnemann himself and by Hering. Several studies and supplementings of Hahnemann's pathogenesis of Arsenic have been made. Dr. Wurmb has contributed one of the former, which may be read in English in the third and fourth volumes of the *British Journal of Homœopathy*. Dr. Black has given us a most valuable arrangement of the drug in the first part of the *Hahnemann Materia Medica*, where its symptomatology is revised and augmented, and illustrated by clinical comments. Dr. Roth has criticised Hahnemann's toxicological material, and has incorporated what he considers trustworthy in it with all that has since appeared in a schema of the drug which contains 1056 symptoms.* The matter from all these sources, with a more complete revision and illumination of Hahnemann's cited symptoms, is embodied in the article on Arsenic in Allen's *Encyclopædia*, where the list has swelled to 2872. Dr. Berridge has furnished a series of cases of poisoning by it as an appendix to the *British Journal* for 1875 and onwards to the present time. But,, next to Hahnemann himself, the most eminent and fruitful worker in the field of arsenical action has been Dr. Imbert-Gourbeyre, professor in the medical school of Clermont-Ferrand. His numerous writings on the subject—appearing during the last twenty years in the *Gazette Médicale de Paris*, the *Moniteur des Hôpitaux*, *L'Art Médical*, and other journals—I shall cite as I come to the several points of which they treat.

In considering how I should best present this abundant material to your notice, the history of Arsenic as a medicine seems to suggest the most instructive way. We find it to have been used of old, in China for ague, in India for chronic cutaneous diseases ; while at the present day it is chiefly esteemed as a "nerve-tonic" in such disorders as neuralgia and chorea. Now ague is a fever ; chronic skin affections are inflammations ; and neuralgia and chorea are neuroses. It has appeared best to me that I should discuss the action of Arsenic in reference to these three types of disease, bringing its pathogenetic effects before you in connection with its curative virtues. I think that from this clinical point of view we shall get a better idea of the great medicine before us than if we attempted to draw a detailed sketch of its physiological action, and then studied its therapeutic powers in corresponding categories.

But, before we pass to such considerations, I must bring before you certain general characters of the action of Arsenic which belong to it more or less in every sphere of its activity, and are of great importance as indications for its choice. I do not say that their presence is indispensable, nor that, when it obtains, it absolutely determines the prescription of the remedy. But I do claim for them a prerogative rank among the features which lead us to its use, and they may sometimes weigh so heavily as alone to turn the scale in its favour. They are seven in number.

* See *Brit. Journ. of Hom.*, xx.

1. The first is *periodicity*. Arsenic is—as we shall see—one of the few medicines capable of inducing a true recurrent fever; and remissions, intermissions, and more or less regular returns of the symptoms are noted by all observers of its poisonous action, and are manifest in its provings. Periodic recurrence is thus a true feature of its pathogenetic influence, and experience has shown the same character to belong to its therapeutic activity. It is not merely that such a phenomenon suggests the influence of malaria, and so guides to the drug as one of the antidotes for that poison. It is very true that it constitutes one element in the homœopathicity of Arsenic to malarious affections;* but even in the absence of all such influence it both manifests itself, and *cæteris paribus* calls for Arsenic. "In typical diseases of all kinds," wrote Hahnemann in 1796, "the type-exciting property of Arsenic in small doses becomes valuable."

2. The second is *adynamia*. Christison long ago pointed out that there were a set of cases of arsenical poisoning in which there was little sign of irritation in any part of the alimentary canal, but the patient was chiefly or solely affected with excessive prostration of strength and frequent fainting, death being seldom delayed beyond the fifth or sixth hour. This effect of the drug is doubtless traceable in part to the paralysing influence it has been found to exert upon the heart. But it seems something more than this; and it characterises (as Wurmb has shown) a great many of the symptoms observed by the provers. It has become a well-established indication for the remedy in practice, finding its analogue in the intense prostration characteristic of certain diseases—as influenza, diphtheria, &c.—which is in many cases quite out of proportion to the substantive disorder which accompanies it. "Great exhaustion after the slightest exertion" is the symptomatic way of describing it. We shall have numerous instances of its practical value.

3. The third is *malignity*. This is a feature of disease more easy to recognise than to describe. I do not mean by it so much that fatal onward march of a malady which Dr. Frédault denotes by the name, that " grave state in which there are no

* " Dr. A. T. Thomson states that the action of Arsenic is liable to exacerbations and remissions, and sometimes even intermissions. Thus we may suppose that there is a certain degree of analogy between its operation and that of the malarious poison, by virtue of which it may perhaps exert a corrective power over the working of the latter in the blood " (Headland *On the Action of Medicines in the System*, p. 224).

gleams of true amendment, no crises which give a respite, no signs of relief which encourage hope, and where there is an utter lack of amenability to treatment."* I mean rather that condition which may appear in any acute disease—as scarlatina or diphtheria—and which leads us to name them "malignant," a condition especially shown by darkened colour of the blood and fœtor of its excretions and exudates, with corresponding prostration and disorder of the nervous system. In all fevers, exanthemata, and inflammations where this tendency to putrescence and decomposition shows itself, Arsenic is one of the first remedies of which we think and on which we depend.

4. The next is *restlessness* and *anguish*—a feature constantly noted in the subjects of arsenical poisoning, and seldom absent from any acute morbid condition, not purely local, to which it is otherwise appropriate. It is something like that which I have described as the characteristic of Aconite, but more intense. I have advisedly used the term "anguish" to designate it, rather than "anxietas" as with the other medicine. Either, of course, is employed in its physical sense,—not in that of the emotional disturbance which by analogy has been similarly named ; and there is a difference, slight but real, between them. I can hardly put it into words, but you will feel what is anguish in a patient's condition, and what is anxietas.

5. The foregoing are characters belonging to the symptoms of Arsenic generally. I have now to speak of certain characteristics of its pains. The first of these is that they are most frequently *burning*. This has been accounted for by the circumstance that it is mucous membrane chiefly which is affected by the drug, and that the pain of inflammation of this tissue is always more or less of a burning kind, as that of serous membrane is cutting. But such an explanation is quite insufficient, for there are other pains indicating Arsenic— notably its neuralgia—which have this same feature, but which certainly do not belong to mucous membrane. Burning pain as such, accordingly, is characteristic of Arsenic. There is one caution, however, to be given, and that is that you do not class under this heading such disagreeable sensations of heat as are caused by acrid fluids, as the bile and the products of gastric fermentation. Patients annoyed by the presence of these irritants will complain of burning sensations, but you must not therefore think of Arsenic for them.

6. Another feature of the arsenical pains is that they are *worse at rest*, and therefore at night, and are *increased by cold*, being

* *L'Art Médical*, Dec., 1876.

of course, conversely, relieved by warmth, and diminishing during exercise. Teste considers these characters of pains to indicate that the drug to which they belong is of a depressing kind, and believes that the action of all such medicines is more marked on the left (as being the weaker) side of the body. How this may be with Arsenic, I cannot say; but I am sure that the aggravation of its pains—especially its neuralgia—during the rest of night and by cold air impinging on the surface is very distinctive of it.

7. The last characteristic of which I have to speak belongs to the *thirst* of Arsenic. This is an early and marked symptom of its action on the healthy body, and is always present in febrile states to which it is suitable. But it has been added that the Arsenic patient, unlike the one whose condition calls for Aconite, " drinks little but often." This statement is founded, pathogenetically, on observations obtained from Stapf and Wahle in Hahnemann's proving of Arsenic. It is also cited as from Richard ; but in this author's brief narrative of a case of poisoning to which reference is made I can find no trace of it. Nor does it appear in any of the numerous toxicological records on which Dr. Allen has drawn ; and in his *Encyclopœdia* the next symptom but two after the " drinks much, but little at a time " of Stapf and Wahle is—" thirst so violent that he drank eleven jugs of water in half a day." This is from a poisoning case. Therapeutically, I find that the symptom in question has been used as an indication for Arsenic in fevers, and with good results ; but there is no evidence that its absence, or the presence of thirst for large quantities, contra-indicates the remedy. Desire to drink, but inability from the irritable state of the stomach to take more than a small quantity at a time, is a frequent symptom of gastritis, and so might truly call for Arsenic when present ; while in inflammations occurring elsewhere, and in general fevers, the thirst may be as insatiable as possible without forbidding its employment.

I have now gone through the leading general indications for our medicine. Let me repeat my *caveat* that all such characters are to be taken as suggestive, not as decisive, of the choice of the remedy. Undoubtedly, the more of them that are present, and the sharper their definition (so to speak), the keener will be the action of the drug in removing the morbid state which they characterise, and the more minute may be its dosage. But there may be many a diseased condition in which they are entirely absent, and to which Arsenic is yet thoroughly homœopathic and curative. Never make such a misuse of

them as that which we shall see in the case of cholera, where
the want of minute symptomatic similarity (among other
points, in that very "drinking little but often" whose small
value I have shown above) was made a ground* for denying
to Arsenic a place in the therapeutics of this disease, which it
so truly causes, and which it has so often arrested.

I. We now pass to the special actions of Arsenic; and
shall begin, as I said, by considering it as an anti-pyretic.
In this capacity it appears as a leading remedy for the types
of fever known as malarious, hectic, and typhous, and also for
cholera.

The use of Arsenic as a remedy for the intermittent and
other fevers arising from malaria is of very ancient date in China
and India. In Europe its employment was for a long time
popular only, and it was not until the middle of the last
century that physicians (among whom our English Fowler
was prominent) took it up. Once again, however, as Stillé
says, "Arsenic fell into disuse, and was for a long time quite
neglected," until, in 1842, Boudin published a work which (in
the words of the same writer) "demonstrated its efficacy in
periodical fevers, and vigorously advocated its use, giving the
first impulse to those numerous researches into the action and
uses of the mineral which have since appeared."

Who was this Boudin, and how was he led to revive the forgotten employment of Arsenic in malarious fevers? The
answer supplies a curious and interesting chapter in medical
history. It is given by Dr. Chargé, of Marseilles, in a communication made by him to the World's Convention of 1876.†
Boudin was, in 1840, in chief medical charge of the great military hospital in that city. He one day lamented to Dr. Chargé,
with whom he was well acquainted, his want of success in the
intermittents of the soldiers returned from African service,
with whom at that time his wards were crowded. Our
colleague took him at his word, and begged him to try Arsenic
prepared according to the homœopathic manner. On his con-
senting to do so, he took from his pocket-case a tube
of globules of Arsenicum 30, and presented it to his friend.
Boudin took a few patients just as they came, put upon their
tongues a few globules of the medicine, and they were all
cured. It is to be regretted that this striking result did not
lead him to study and adopt the method of Hahnemann in its
entirety; but we know the obstacles which have prevented
many a man similarly situated from adventuring on such

---

* See *Monthly Hom. Review*, ix., 120.
† See *Bibliothèque Homœopathique*, March, 1877.

perilous investigations. However, he did follow up the special therapeutic point now made.   In his *Traité des fièvres inter-mittentes* he writes—" Arsenious acid, *suitably prepared,* pre-serves in the almost microscopic dose of a hundredth of a grain all its medicinal energy, not only in the treatment of marsh fevers, but also in that of a host of other maladies. Yet more, I have often obtained with a single dose of a hundredth of a grain of this drug the radical disappearance of fevers con-tracted in Algeria or Senegal, and which had till then resisted the most varied treatment, including sulphate of quinine and change of climate." And what was this " suitable prepara-tion " whereby the virtues of the drug were so preserved or rather developed ? Dr. Chargé gives the " formule de Boudin." " Take a centigramme of arsenious acid ; add by degrees, and in small portions at a time, a gramme of pulverised sugar of milk. Triturate in a glass mortar for a sufficiently long time (at least ten minutes), and divide into twenty packets, of which each represents a demi-milligramme of arsenious acid." He calls this a hundredth of a grain ; but, as the milligramme is about $\frac{1}{65}$ of a grain, it is rather a hundred and thirtieth. But it is obvious that the process is Hahnemann's, and hence the activity of the drug. Dr. Chargé well shows that the larger doses to which Boudin subsequently resorted are explained by the imperfect preparation the drug underwent at the hands of the ordinary chemists of Paris, where his later practice was carried on. While at Marseilles, his Arsenic was supplied him from a homœopathic pharmacy.

This by the way, to show that it was from the school of Hahnemann that Boudin received the impulse which made him the reviver of the use of Arsenic in malarious fevers. But let us now enquire what relation its physiological effects bear to the febrile condition, as such, and to the various forms it may assume.

Dr. Imbert-Gourbeyre has examined this point in an essay " On the febrigenic power of Arsenic,"* and demonstrates that fever is among the most constant and characteristic effects of the poison. It is obvious, however, that in the great majority of the observations he cites it was symptomatic of the gastro-enteric irritation set up, rather than a primary effect. When thus occurring, it is of the hectic type, often having marked evening exacerbations ; sometimes chill and heat, with thirst and headache, recur periodically, in somewhat irregular rota-tion. This is the condition set up in chronic arsenical poison-ing, as seen (for instance) in the victims of the *Aqua Toffana*

* *L'Art Médical,* 1865 ; and *Brit. Journ. of Hom.,* xxiv., 72.

R

of old.   Hahnemann describes the cachexia thus induced in
his usual graphic manner.   "It is" he says "a gradual sinking of the powers of life, without any violent symptoms ; a
nameless feeling of illness ; failure of the strength ; slight
feverishness ; want of sleep ; lividity of the countenance, and
an aversion to food and drink and all the other enjoyments of
life.   Dropsy closes the scene, often with colliquative vomiting and purging."*

But some of the evidence adduced by our author, and other
facts elsewhere obtainable, show that Arsenic can cause fever
without local irritation.   Of this kind is the observation of Dr.
v. Grauvogl, who, after some days' use of the 15th attenuation,
experienced nothing but an insatiable thirst.   From the 5th
potency he felt great languor and sleeplessness in addition to
the thirst ; and it was not until, some weeks after, he descended
to the 3rd decimal, that symptoms of the stomach and bowels
showed themselves.   Then Hahnemann remarked (1796)†—
" I have myself ascertained that Arsenic has a great tendency
to excite that spasm in the blood-vessels and shock in the
nervous system we call the febrile rigor.   If it be given in a
pretty large dose (one sixth or one fifth of a grain) to an
adult, this rigor becomes very evident."   It affects the vaso-
motor nerves as we have seen that Aconite does.   But the
subsequent phenomena are very different in the two drugs.
With Aconite a brief febrile reaction of synochal type occurs,
and then all ends with perspiration.   But from Arsenic we
have either a repetition of the chills at intervals, or a long-
lasting fever with typhoid symptoms.   Of the former Hahnemann speaks :—" It possesses," he says (*loc. cit.*), "the power,
observed by me, of exciting a daily recurring, though always
weaker paroyxsm, even although its use be discontinued."
Thus it may set up an affection undistinguishable from ague,
of which instances have been recorded by Boudin, Delaharpe,
Imbert-Gourbeyre, Clarus, and Dudgeon.‡   Of the typhoid
condition often induced in protracted arsenical poisoning an
exquisite example is afforded by one of Orfila's cases.   From
the eighteenth to the twenty-third day, it is said, " his appearance resembled that of a patient labouring under typhus."
By others, moreover (as Dr. Imbert-Gourbeyre shows), poisoning by Arsenic has been compared to the course of low fever ;
and once it has been mistaken for it.   Dr. Hausmann has

* Quoted from his *Arsenik-Vergiftung* by Christison (*Poisons,*
3rd ed., p. 296).
† *Lesser Writings* (tr. by Dudgeon), p. 336.
‡ See (for the two last) *Brit. Journ. of Hom.*, xi., 334, and xx., 204.

also shown, in an essay on the subject in the *Œsterreich. Zeitschrift* (1845), that the intestinal lesions of typhoid have often found their analogues in the autopsies of persons perishing from the effects of Arsenic.

It is thus evident that (as Hahnemann first argued and Boudin admits) Arsenic is homœopathic to the ague it undoubtedly cures ; and that, upon the principle of similarity, it ought to be useful in typhus and enteric fever. It is indeed so. My own experience would lead me to lay it down as a canon that what Aconite is to simple fever, that Arsenic is to its malignant form. Whenever the well-known " typhoid " symptoms occur —especially the dry tongue and the (often involuntary) diarrhœa—whether in continued fevers, in the exanthemata, as symptomatic of mortification, or as results of blood-poisoning, my advice is to put in your Arsenic, and use it freely and persistently. I have seen many an apparently desperate case cured by it. Dr. Imbert-Gourbeyre's paper will show that this canon obtains general acceptance in the homœopathic school, and is not without confirmation elsewhere. Fleischmann relied upon Arsenic almost exclusively in the treatment of typhoid at his hospital.

The irritative fever of Arsenic suggests (as Hahnemann perceived and pointed out) its use in hectic conditions, such as those which accompany tuberculosis and chronic mischief in the lungs or intestines. We have always made much use of it in the febrile marasmus of children (usually from mesenteric disease) and in phthisis. Recently it has been much commended in the latter disease, especially as diminishing the hectic. In our own school Dr. Herbert Nankivell has recorded much valuable experience with it, giving it usually in the form of the iodide.* Dr. Ringer confirms the statement that it reduces the temperature in tuberculosis ; and states that coincidently the symptoms. are relieved, and even—in some cases—apparent cure effected. Of a piece with this is von Grauvogl's commendation of it in pyæmia†. As regards ague, Arsenic has the highest repute as an anti-intermittent among homœopathists, and in quite infinitesimal doses. Wurmb and Caspar, from their experience in the Leopoldstadt Hospital at Vienna, place it first among the remedies for chronic agues (it is rarely indicated when they are recent). The special indications for it they epitomise thus :—" one stage absent ; heat burning; rapid prostration ; torpid weakness ; dropsical swellings ;

* *Brit. Journ. of Hom.*, xxx., 515 ; and *Monthly Hom. Review*, xvii., 621 ; xxiii.

† *Op. cit.*, i., 335.

cachexia ; abuse of quinine." But they add—" it will often cure when other remedies selected with the greatest care have failed." They were at this time using the 15th dilution exclusively in their wards.* Bähr praises the same potency as sovereign in malarial cachexia ; but in recent cases prefers the first three triturations. Of these, besides the ordinary symptomatic indications of the drug, he says—" Arsenicum is indicated the more specifically the cleaner the tongue remains, the more rapidly the strength is exhausted by a single paroxysm, and the sooner the characteristic sallow pallor makes its appearance." To the German authors now cited I may add the testimony of an American, whose residence in the Mississippi valley gives him large experience in marsh-fevers—Dr. Lucius Morse. "For the so-called dumb chills of malarious climates," he writes,† "Arsenic is a foremost remedy. In the outstart of acute attacks of intermittent fever, where the paroxysms are distinctly divided into stages, I have found it of little utility ; but as an intercurrent remedy, in the treatment of relapsing cases, I have found it to act admirably. It also deserves attention as a prophylactic of diseases resulting from malarious poisoning." Sensation of coldness of the body is regarded by him as especially significant for its choice. He gives the triturations from the second to the sixth decimal, and, preparing these himself, follows faithfully Hahnemann's injunction to triturate a good while, saying that the labour expended has been well repaid.

Dr. H. Wood praises it in the fever known in America as " typho-malarial."

Before leaving this part of our subject, I must speak of the action of Arsenic in cholera. I think I shall carry most pathologists with me at the present day, in maintaining (as I have long ago done)‡ that Asiatic cholera is essentially a pernicious malarial fever, in which the poison exhausts its influence in a single paroxysm. We have already seen Arsenic causing the primary chill and the consecutive fever of this malady ; and we shall hereafter find the cramps, the vomiting and purging, and the suppression of urine reproduced in its pathogenesis.§ So complete is the resemblance that Dr. H. C.

* *Brit. Journ. of Hom.*, vols. xii. xiii.
† *American Homœopathist*, ii., 6.
‡ *Brit. Journ. of Hom.*, xxiv., 485.
§ " Dr. Blachez describes another form of arsenical poisoning, characterised by choleraic symptoms of the intestinal canal, with suppression of urine, cramps, and progressive coldness of body " (Ringer, 7th ed., p. 281).

Wood can truly say that " arsenical poisoning has been mistaken for cholera, not only in life, but also after death, on the post-mortem table." He is probably referring in these last words to a case reported by Professor Virchow, in the forty-seventh volume of his *Archiv.** The very fungi described by Klob and others as peculiar to cholera were present in the rice-water fluid with which the intestines were filled ; and the condition of the mucous membranes was anatomically identical. The phenomena, moreover, which sometimes occur in arsenical poisoning, where the patient dies in a few hours in collapse, without symptoms of gastro-enteric irritation,— *sidération*, as the French call it, have been compared by many observers to the way in which cholera occasionally invades the system.

It is true that this is not always so ; and that the vomiting and purging of arsenical poisoning usually depend on gastro-enteritis, which is absent in cholera. Hence (as I have said) the minute symptomatology of the disease does not altogether correspond with that accepted as characteristic of the drug, though the internal burning of which cholera patients so often complain is a point in its favour. It was probably for this reason that Hahnemann, on first hearing an account of cholera when it invaded Europe in 1830, in naming the drugs most likely from their homœopathicity to be its antidotes, specified Camphor, Veratrum, and Cuprum, but omitted Arsenic. Further knowledge of the disease has shown that the features in which there is a true similarity are those of most importance; and Arsenic has accordingly been added to the three Hahnemannian medicines by those who care more for real lesions than for symptomatic minutiæ. With such it has become the sheet-anchor in the most desperate cases. In the epidemic of 1849, Dr. Russell at Edinburgh and Dr. Drysdale at Liverpool concurred in giving to Arsenic the chief place in the treatment of cholera, when the time for arresting it with Camphor had gone by ; and I believe this to be the general experience of homœopathists. I may add that with malarious fevers Boudin classes, not only cholera, but also yellow fever and plague, as being all "limnhæmic" affections; and accounts Arsenic the great remedy for them all.

We have now completed our consideration of Arsenic an an antipyretic. Before leaving the subject, let me say a few words by way of comparison between it and Aconite in this capacity. You will see at once that the contrast we observed between the pathogenetic effects of the two drugs shows itself

* See *Brit. Journ. of Hom.*, xxviii., 202.

as plainly, and as of the same kind, in their therapeutic virtues. Aconite is the remedy for acute and ephemeral fevers, Arsenic for those of some duration : the only point at which their spheres intersect is (as I have said) in the treatment of cholera. The fever of Aconite is neurotic : that of Arsenic commences in the blood or the tissues, and affects the nervous system secondarily. Aconite rapidly calms the violent but superficial storms to which the circulation is subject : Arsenic goes down with a slower but more penetrating movement into the inmost recesses of the pyrexial process, and there cools its ardour and steadies its agitation. They are both most precious febrifuges ; and we should be hard put to it to do without either.

LECTURE XVI.

ARSENIC *(continued)*.

At our last meeting we began the consideration of the great medicine supplied us by the metal Arsenic. We dwelt upon certain general characteristics of its action, both as a poison and as a remedy; and then studied its virtues as an anti-pyretic in connexion with its physiological effects in the same sphere.

II. We come now to the place of Arsenic in the treatment of inflammations. Here its general homœopathicity, at least, is evident; for no more characteristically irritant poison is known. It is only necessary on this score to enquire if the similarity extend to the seat and kind of the inflammatory action.

1. Let us first take the mucous membranes. To this tissue Arsenic may fairly be called a specific irritant; as it affects it in some measure wherever found, and however the poison is introduced into the system. The kind of inflammation produced is not (as with Tartar emetic) muco-purulent, but the membrane is dry, or exudes a thin ichorous discharge; and the further progress of the mischief is towards ulceration rather than suppuration. After this manner the alimentary canal is affected throughout, but more especially the mouth, throat, stomach, duodenum, and rectum. Of these the stomach may be called the central seat of the action of the drug, which has such affinity for it that Brodie found the gastritis more intense when the poison was applied to a wound than when it was swallowed; and yet, Boehm says, it is not eliminated by the gastric mucous membrane. Throughout the canal the inflammation is severe, and causes vomiting, diarrhœa, and dysentery; aphthæ in the mouth; ulceration of the stomach and intestine; and even gangrene at the anus. I should note what Hahnemann says of the arsenical vomiting, that it is more frequently a dry retching, with ineffectual efforts to vomit, than a true emesis. On the respiratory tract the influence of Arsenic is less virulent, save on the uppermost portion; but the whole

extent is affected, as shown by post-mortem redness, and cough and other symptoms of irritation during life. In the frontal sinus the irritation is shown by the dull, tight frontal headache so common in those exposed to its emanations. The arsenical conjunctivitis, which is as well known as the mercurial stomatitis, belongs to this category ; and there is also an arsenical coryza—not merely in those living in rooms papered with it (where it is constant, but might be a local effect merely), but also (as Dr. Imbert-Gourbeyre has shown) from its internal administration, even in infinitesimal doses. In cases of poisoning the conjunctivitis has been seen as purulent, and the coryza to consist of a profuse ichorous discharge, going on to ulceration. The genito-urinary mucous membrane is inflamed throughout, even—as in one case of Christison's—inside the uterus and Fallopian tubes ; in the penis, scrotum, and vulva (as in the anus) gangrene not unfrequently takes place. This last phenomenon is one of those specially studied by Dr. Imbert-Gourbeyre.*

These are the pathogenetic facts ; and now let us turn to those of therapeutics. If *similia similibus* were absurd ; if the presence of inflammation were, according to the old view, a contra-indication for an irritant, Arsenic ought to be utterly eschewed in gastritis and enteritis. Yet it is not so. Mr. Hunt tells us that when his patients with cutaneous disease had also chronic irritations of the alimentary canal, the Arsenic he gave them rather benefited these than otherwise. Dr. Thorowgood writes in the *Practitioner* to extol the medicine in "irritative dyspepsia" (v., 21) ; and Dr. Ringer, supporting this recommendation, adds the morning vomiting of drunkards, chronic ulcer of the stomach, and several other analogous affections, in all of which he says "it allays pain and checks vomiting." These gentlemen have but borrowed a remedy traditional in the homœopathic school. There are indeed few inflammatory diseases of the alimentary canal in which Arsenic is not of great service, though in some it is eclipsed by other remedies. Thus : in the mouth and throat Mercury, Nitric and Muriatic acids, Kali chloricum and Belladonna supersede it on ordinary occasions. But in cancrum oris,† in severe forms of aphthæ (especially such as appear at the close of exhausting diseases), and generally in malignant inflammations and phagedænic ulcerations (non-syphilitic) of these parts, Arsenic has no rival. In gastritis,

---

* See *Brit. Journ. of Hom.*, xxiii., 77.

† In an epidemic of this disease Dr. Arnold found it (in the 4th decimal trituration) of the utmost service (see *Brit. Journ. of Hom.*, xi., 149).

acute and chronic, and in duodenitis, it is the chief remedy ; and so in all dyspepsiæ resulting therefrom. In chronic gastric irritability, with such retching as that I described just now, it is often most efficacious. Dr. Guernsey praises it in the condition described by Dr. Chambers as " the indigestion of water." In ulcer of the stomach and intestines it might find a place, but generally yields the palm to Kali bichromicum, and also in the one to Uranium nitricum, and in the other to Mercurius corrosivus ; which last, moreover, is superior to it in dysentery, save where the rectum is most affected and where there is much prostration. As the purging caused by it depends upon intestinal inflammation, it is scarcely homœo-pathic to simple " functional " diarrhœa, however severe. But in most cases of chronic diarrhœa, where there is generally some disorganization, Arsenic is a glorious remedy ; and in " English cholera " it is esteemed by Dr. Black, of Chesterfield, a true specific.

Arsenic holds an important place in the treatment of the disorders of the upper portion of the respiratory mucous membrane. Here, too, we have the support of Dr. Ringer, who makes some interesting remarks on a variety of forms of paroxysmal coryza, sometimes running into bronchitis, in which he finds the medicine very useful. The sneezing and wheezing of these affections ally them to hay-fever and its asthma ; though here—probably because of the local presence of the specific irritant—remedies do not avail much. Nevertheless, Arsenic has often gained some credit in its treatment.* Dr. Ringer does not mention influenza. This, like cholera, is an epidemic disease characterised by vaso-motor disturbance, prostration, and copious flux. To the typical form of this malady Arsenic precisely corresponds ; and in my hands has always proved rapidly curative of it, unquestionably cutting short its progress. In sporadic coryzas approaching this type it is no less valuable. Here, too, I must speak of its use in ophthalmia. In simple chronic conjunctivitis I myself place great reliance upon it ; and in strumous ophthalmia my experience coincides with that of many others that it will often cure obstinate cases where every other medicine has failed. Dr. Angell commends it " in superficial and deep-seated ulcerations of the cornea.† especially in scrofulous subjects ; in catarrhal ophthalmia, wi

* See Watson's *Practice cf Physic* (4th ed.), ii., 55, and *Hahn. Monthly*, Aug., 1876.
† It has been found to affect the cornea in frogs similarly to the skin, —its influence upon which will come before us immediately.

thin secretion and irritation of the edges of the lids ; and in
ulceration of the tarsal edges, with thin secretion." Drs.
Allen and Norton make this same thinness of secretion a
prominent indication for Arsenic, adding excoriating quality
of the same, burning pains, and sense of dryness. In bronchitis it is rarely indicated, save when the constitutional
symptoms call for it, and there is much thin expectoration.
But Dr. Black and Dr. Bayes both think it should be used
oftener, especially in aged people. They are borne out here by
Hahnemann himself, who in a note to S. 584 of his pathogenesis of Arsenic in the third edition of the second volume of
the *Reine Arzneimittellehre*, writes—" Of a similar suffocative
catarrh, becoming much worse every evening after lying down,
and bringing me nigh to death, I cured myself rapidly with
Arsenic, and that with a dose of marvellous minuteness. The
other symptoms of my illness were obviously those of the
remedy."

In inflammation of the urinary tract Arsenic is more than
rivalled by other medicines, as Cantharis and its analogues.
In affections of the generative organs its chief use has been
in chronic menorrhagia, where it is praised by Sir Charles
Locock and Mr. Hunt ; and in endo-metritis. A thin, corrosive, burning leucorrhœa indicates it in uterine affections. It
will probably be found curative in noma pudendi, in cancer
scroti, and where the soft chancre runs into phagedæna or
sloughing.

2. The powerful irritant action of Arsenic upon the mucous
membranes makes it almost certain that it must exercise a
similar influence upon their external continuation, the skin.
That it does so, affirmed by Hahnemann,* is witnessed to also
by Hunt, Inman, Horatio Wood, and Christison ; and Ringer
and Warburton Begbie concur in stating that its first effect on
skin disease is to make it redder and more inflamed, worse in
fact than before the treatment was begun. But upon this
point we have one of Dr. Imbert-Gourbeyre's most valuable
contributions. In a monograph *de l'action de l'Arsenic sur la
peau* (Baillière, 1872) he has demonstrated from numerous
facts, collected and observed, that Arsenic has the power of
causing almost every form of cutaneous disorder. He gives
instances of its production of pruritus, erythema, erysipelas,
urticaria ; of papules, vesicles (including a true zona), pustules
and furuncles ; of discolorations ; and of falling of the hair
and nails. He does not mention squamæ in his list; but here
we have the testimony of Hunt and of Tilbury Fox, both of

---

* *Lesser Writings*, p. 337.

whom speak of pityriasis as a frequent effect of its use. Dr. Roberts gives a case of pityriasis rubra caused by it. Stillé enumerates among the effects of arsenical wall-papers—" the skin grows rough and scaly;" and says that its continued medicinal use " has in some few instances caused an eruption of urticaria, pityriasis, or psoriasis upon the skin. In one case," he writes," " of acute arsenical poisoning, and a fortnight after the patient had apparently recovered from its effects, the face, head, hands, and feet were swollen, and the whole surface of the body was of a bright red colour. After a few days the skin partially desquamated, and was tender to the touch; and this was followed by an attack of psoriasis which extended over the whole body. The hair of the head, the eyebrows and eyelashes fell off, as did also the nails." Of this last phenomenon he writes—" The continued use of Arsenic has in some cases caused the hair to fall out over the whole scalp, or in patches *(alopecia areata)*;" and Naunyn, in Ziemssen's *Cyclopædia*, enumerates among the symptoms of chronic arsenical poisoning, " falling out of the hair, and even of the nails, with or without the formation of ulcers at the edges of the nails."

Thus is convicted of unconscious homœopathicity one of the most generally accepted of all the virtues of Arsenic, viz., its power over cutaneous disease. To assume, as is ordinarily done, that it acts as a " nerve-tonic " in these disorders, is a mere evasion. And here also the small dose accompanies the law of similars. Mr. Hunt gives a case in which no more than the $\frac{1}{480}$th of a grain could be borne at a time; yet with such minute doses he cured a chronic psoriasis guttata. He recommends just enough to be given to keep the conjunctiva slightly affected throughout the course—a relic, probably, of the old mercurial practice; but Dr. Ringer finds it quite unnecessary "to induce these toxic symptoms to ensure the beneficial influence of the remedy."

At the present day the tendency among dermatologists seems rather to depreciate the unvarying prescription of Arsenic in skin disease which Mr. Hunt's success especially brought so into vogue. But it is still highly reputed for chronic pemphigus and the squamæ, and in general practice seems to be used pretty universally when the skin is affected. With us of the homœopathic school, having many other remedies for skin disease, it does not play so large a part or undergo so indiscriminate an employment. But in chronic cases of urticaria, eczema, pemphigus, lichen, prurigo, alopecia, pityriasis, psoriasis and lepra we esteem it as highly as our

brethren, and use it as the leading remedy. Where the constitution is coincidently affected in the arsenical manner, quite
high dilutions of the drug may suffice.* The innocuousness,
and even necessity, of more substantial doses in most chronic
dermatites corresponds with what Hahnemann says :—"in
cases where, along with a local affection, the general health
seems good, we must proceed from the at first small doses to
larger ones."

Further evidence as to the poisonous action of Arsenic on
the skin has been supplied by the recent observations of Drs.
Ringer and Murrell regarding its action on frogs. Experimenting with the view of studying its paralysing action, they
noticed " a curious action of arsenious acid on the skin of
these batrachia." Soon (5-8 hours) after the hypodermic
injection they found that they " could strip off the cuticle with
the greatest readiness over every part of the body." No such
phenomena appeared in frogs otherwise killed, save when
Tartar emetic was used, and then " the cuticle became softened
and reduced to a jelly-like condition, too soft to be stripped
off, though it could be easily scraped off every part of the
body."

Dr. Emily Nunn, of Boston, U.S., undertook, in the Physiological Laboratory of Cambridge, a microscopical examination
of the epidermis of frogs thus poisoned. Her conclusion with
regard to Arsenic is that " all the facts go to prove that the
changes are the result of the Arsenic acting directly on the
epidermic cells themselves," beginning with those lying
deepest. It is, she says, " obviously a specific effect," and
" not without interest in view of the remarkable therapeutic
value of Arsenic in skin diseases." Dr. Ringer also acknowledges this connexion ; and aptly points out that it is
diseases of the more superficial parts of the skin which are
most amenable to the influence of Arsenic. The action of
Antimony was, histologically, almost identical ; but was more
rapid and violent, and accompanied with a marked softening
of the ultimate elements of the tissue.

3. Arsenic affects the serous hardly less powerfully than
the mucous membranes. The inflammations here caused by
it are of a sub-acute character, with speedy and copious serous
(less often purulent) effusion. The pleuræ are most frequently
affected ; then the pericardium ; less often the peritoneum
and arachnoid. The post-mortem evidence of this is to be
read in every work on toxicology. And here too, as with
Apis, the synovial membranes are affected similarly with

* See *Brit. Journ. of Hom.*, iv., 349.

their serous analogues, though only during the convalescence from acute arsenical poisoning.

Correspondingly, Arsenic is highly esteemed in the school of Hahnemann in inflammations of the serous membranes, whenever very copious serous effusion is present. No remedy equals it here, especially when the pleura or pericardium is the part affected. It thus resembles Apis, and, like that medicine, is often very useful in chronic serous dropsies remaining after inflammation. Some capital cases in point are related by Dr. Yeldham in the third and fourth volumes of the *Annals* of the British Homœopathic Society. It is in some repute in the old school in the treatment of chronic articular rheumatism.

Besides these tissues, Arsenic has a potent influence upon three important organs of the body; and this is mainly of irritant nature, though not without other features. The organs I refer to are the lungs, the heart, and the kidneys.

4. As regards the lungs, Arsenic first of all congests and inflames them. This is evident from many symptoms during life, both in poisonings and provings; while autopsies frequently disclose great pulmonary engorgement and even pneumonia. But there is a dyspnœa manifest in most of these subjects which cannot always be thus accounted for; and it has long ago led homœopathists to use Arsenic largely in the curative treatment of asthma. Dr. Black writes— "There is no medicine which manifests so frequently and so closely the symptoms of asthma ; and in practice it proves an admirable remedy." Dr. Russell, who devotes two of his excellent *Clinical Lectures* to- asthma, recommends it where bronchitic asthma tends to become, or has become, chronic ; and furnishes several illustrative cases. But I find it very effective also in the more purely neurotic form of the malady, especially in weakly persons, and where the attacks recur periodically. This is another piece of homœopathic practice which has been appropriated by our brethren of the old school. The therapeutists of the stamp of Anstie and Ringer seem to rely much upon it : the latter praises it in the asthma of emphysema. In pneumonia Arsenic has found little employment as yet.

5. The action of Arsenic on the heart has been fully studied by the author I have so often cited, Dr. Imbert-Gourbeyre. In his treatise *de l' action de l' Arsenic sur le cœur* (Baillière, 1874) he adduces copious evidence of the elective affinity of the drug for this organ and of the profound changes it sets up. Of functional disorders he specifies palpitation and cardiac dyspnœa (to which he might have added præcordial

pain and anxiety, often severe); and as lesions produced in the heart he mentions endocarditis and hypertrophy. The heart sometimes also shares in the fatty-granular degeneration which occasionally results from arsenical poisoning.

This influence of Arsenic on the heart has been summed up by Trousseau and Pidoux in saying that it abolishes its contractility and often inflames its tissue. The feebleness of heart thus induced is probably an essential part of the prostration it causes, which is constantly accompanied with faintings ;* and we find in practice that the pulse grows stronger under its influence. Its combination with lime (Calcarea arsenica) is an excellent cardiac tonic. But the power of the poison to inflame the endocardium has led us to use it freely in chronic organic diseases of the organ. In these—especially in dilatation and valvular mischief—the testimony to its value is loud and unanimous. It relieves pain, palpitation, and dyspnœa, besides having (as we shall see directly) a marked influence over the anasarca always imminent in these cases.

Such use of Arsenic, long familiar to us homœopaths, seems now finding its way into the opposite school, especially among the French. That they employ the arseniate of antimony probably makes little difference beyond reducing the dose of the more potent element in the combination. But we are indebted to our brethren for the demonstration of the power of the drug over angina pectoris, to which nevertheless it is quite homœopathic, as no poison causes such severe præcordial pain and anxiety. An accidental cure by Alexander, in the last century, first called attention to it ; and the latest writer on the subject, Dr. Anstie, styles it "an invaluable remedy." He considers angina pectoris a cardiac neuralgia ; and I believe that it is when it is so that Arsenic will do it so much good. But I have strong reason to think that it is occasionally a muscular rather than a neurotic affection ; and here may come in other remedies, of which we have seen one in Hydrocyanic acid, and shall see another in Cuprum.

6. On the kidneys Arsenic exerts a very potent influence. In acute poisoning they share in the general irritation; so that their secretion is diminished or suppressed, and, if any urine is obtained, it is found to contain albumen. This presence of albumen is so constant a phenomenon that it has been assigned as a diagnostic mark between arsenical poison-

---

* " The poisonous or hurtful effects that we have to look out for, when arsenic has been prescribed, are a peculiar silvery whiteness of the tongue. . . . ; and, if the medicine be continued, *fainting* is often added " (Watson, *op. cit.*, ii., 785).

ing and antimonial. Of the more lasting renal effects of Arsenic we have full information from the experiments of Dr. Quaglio. He slowly poisoned six cats with the arsenite of potash, during periods of from one to ten months, and produced in all more or less completely developed Bright's disease. During life the urine was scanty, and contained albumen, fat-globules, renal epithelium, fibrin-casts, and blood-corpuscles ; it was neutral in reaction, and the proportion of solids was below the standard. The animals died comatose, and after death their kidneys were found enlarged and hyperæmic, and the epithelial cells charged with fat and granules.

Correspondingly, while the ischuria of acute arsenical poisoning forms one element of its homœopathicity to cholera, its deeper effects have led to its use in Bright's disease. It is apparently the large white kidney—the " tubal nephritis " of Dr. Dickinson—to which it is a simile ; and it is this form which seems to have been present in the cases of cure by it on record, which are numerous and brilliant.* Of the same nature is the post-scarlatinal nephritis, in which it is, perhaps, the favourite remedy in our school : it is certainly mine. It must be mentioned that in four out of the six cats experimented on by Dr. Quaglio there was found hypertrophy of the left ventricle. Dr. Buchner maintains that the renal mischief of Arsenic is always secondary to cardiac disease, and that the drug is only suitable to morbus Brightii thus arising. I cannot agree with him here, thinking both pathogenetic and clinical evidence to be against the theory. But a difficulty is created by the presence of hypertrophy of the ventricle under such circumstances, as it was supposed to belong only to granular degeneration. Dr. Dickinson now finds, however, that it may occur in tubular nephritis also, at any rate (as Baertels says) when secondary contraction has set in. The relation of Arsenic to inflammations of the serous membranes is an important element in its homœopathicity to Bright's disease, acute and chronic ; and indicates its employment, if not previously, at least when these occur.

It is in this place that we must speak of the power of Arsenic over dropsy. Its tendency to cause œdematous swellings, local or general, has been noticed by many observers, and among them by Fowler, whose name is indissolubly associated with the liquor potassæ arsenitis of the Pharmacopœia. Dr. Imbert-Gourbeyre has collected their

* See *Lancet*, Jan. 18, 1862 ; Black, p. 17, note ¹ ; and *Brit. Journ. of Hom.*, xii., 485 ; xiii., 556; xiv., 20 ; xvi., 219; xvii., 545, 573.

testimony in a chapter on the subject in his *l' action de l' Arsenic sur la peau*. One of the latest authors who has mentioned the arsenical anasarca is Dr. Weir Mitchell, of America.* In the cases which came under his notice he examined the urine, and generally found evidence, though slight, of renal disorder, either albuminuria or a few pale tube-casts. Stillé's description of the dropsy of Arsenic points plainly to its renal origin. " Under the influence of continued small doses," he writes, " a characteristic puffiness of the face arises, with œdema of the eyelids, which at first is most visible in the morning, but is afterwards more permanent and exten-sive, occupying the ankles, the limbs, and the abdomen with a dropsical effusion." It may also lead to dropsy by its depres-sing effect on the heart, and by the impoverishing influence which we shall see it exerting upon the blood. Whether from one or all of these causes, Arsenic is undoubtedly " hydro-pigenic ;" and among homœopathists it is always esteemed the most potent " hydropifuge." Thus Bähr writes—" Arsenicum is our most important diuretic. It is suitable in all forms of dropsy, more particularly in dropsy depending upon heart disease and œdema of the lungs. After giving Arsenicum, a copious diuresis will sometimes set in with astonishing rapidity, after which the dropsical swelling speedily disappears. The result is most doubtful if we have only ascites to contend against, and inasmuch as the medicine shows its good effects in a few days already, after a few doses have been taken, it is useless to continue it for a longer period, in the vain hope of eliciting good effects from it by persisting in its use." He recommends the low triturations ; but the higher dilutions have often been reported as doing great things, in cardiac dropsy especially.†

III. I come now to the neurotic influence of Arsenic, and the part played by it in the treatment of the neuroses.

It is universally recognised that Arsenic, like nitrate of silver, affects the nervous centres after its irritant influence has been more or less exhausted. The disorder induced sometimes takes the form of tremors and twitches, sometimes of epilepsy ; more rarely of tetanus. But the most frequent effect is paralysis. Dr. Imbert-Gourbeyre has given us some " Etudes sur la Paralysie Arsenicale " in the *Gazette Médicale de Paris* for 1858, in which he cites thirty-one observations of its occurrence. It is nearly always paraplegic ; though a case of arsenical hemiplegia is related, in which also the laryngo-

---

* *New York Medical Journal*, June, 1865.
† See *New York State Hom. Society's Transactions*, iv., 337.

scope detected paralysis of the vocal cord on the affected side.* The arms are involved nearly as often as the legs. Cramps and contractions in the paralysed limbs are common; but the most invariable concomitant is neuralgia. This generally coexists with loss of sensibility, at least to everything but cold, by which also the neuralgic pains are brought on or aggravated. The paralysis is most complete in the hands and feet, and spreads, if it do so, periphero-centrad. There is a sense of great restlessness in the limbs when the pains are present. The seat of the mischief seems to be the spinal cord. In a case observed by Huss the spine was found tender on pressure; and Wibmer says that in autopsies the cord is always seen to be affected, especially with congestion of the lumbar portion and cauda equina. Velpeau now announces that he has succeeded in developing an acute myelitis with it in a dog, and three undoubted cases of this inflammation in the human subject have been traced to its influence.†

Arsenic may thus occasionally find place in the treatment of myelitis and of epilepsy; but we have as yet little experience of it in these diseases. On the other hand, it is the prince of remedies in chorea and in neuralgia, to both of which the above facts show it to be homœopathic. " In simple, uncomplicated cases of chorea it is," Dr. Ringer says, " by far the best remedy ;" and Dr. Warburton Begbie says that in an experience of nearly thirty years, and in a large number of cases, he has never known it to fail. Neuralgia is a still more important, because more frequent, disorder ; and one cannot speak too highly of Arsenic in its treatment. In this estimate I have the concurrence of the late lamented Dr. Anstie, in his brilliant treatise on the disease. But I cannot at all concur in his view of the rationale of its action, which is that the drug has "a happy combination of powers as a blood-tonic and a special stimulant of the nervous system." The "blood-tonic" properties he ascribes to it are only seen in disease, as in malarial cachexia and the instance he cites in proof—of anæmic children suffering from chorea after rheumatism. Its influence in health is, as we shall see directly, of a very different kind. Its "special stimulation " of the nervous system is hardly shown by sensory paralysis, which he himself says is the chief chronic poisonous effect of Arsenic in this region ; nor would he at least argue that such an influence is antipathic to nerve-pain, for he has demonstrated the consistency and frequent coincidence of anæsthesia with neuralgia. When

* *Med. Times and Gazette*, Jan. 11th, 1862.
† See *L'Art Médical*, xliii., 48.

we consider, then, the undoubted production of neuralgic pains by Arsenic, and the excellent results obtained from it with the infinitesimal doses of homœopathy, I submit that we are shut up to the admission that its action is an instance of the operation of the law of similars.

Our experience certainly is that it far excels all other drugs in the treatment of the idiopathic disorder. The arsenical neuralgia is pure, *i.e.*, neither inflammatory, toxæmic, nor reflex. The pain is burning and agonising, accompanied with great restlessness and anguish ; it is often intermittent, with tendency to periodic return ; is generally made worse (even though at first relieved) by the application of cold ; is worse at rest, and diminished during exercise ; and usually affects (at least in the first instance) the left side. Such a neuralgia you often meet with as a consequence of malaria or influenza,— still more frequently as a symptom of pure debility. If you will read the cases published by Dr. Quin in the fourth volume, and myself in the twenty-second and thirty-first volumes of the *British Journal of Homœopathy*, you will see evidence that Arsenic exerts a magical influence over pure neuralgiæ, wherever occurring. Some of these were prosopalgiæ, some gastralgiæ, one sciatica ; and of the first more than one were instances of the terrible "tic-douloureux," or "epileptiform neuralgia," usually reckoned so intractable, but which Dr. Quin's skilful use of Arsenic entirely and permanently removed.

Here also the comparison of Arsenic with Aconite obviously suggests itself. In both there is the combination of anæsthesia with neuralgia ; but at this point the resemblance ceases. The neuralgia which Aconite induces is among its acute effects : it corresponds accordingly to the idiopathic affection when of recent origin and in fairly healthy subjects. The arsenical neuralgia is always associated with paralysis, and the drug becomes a remedy most appropriately in persons advanced in life or of exhausted constitution, where degenerative change may well be supposed to exist at the nerve-roots. Experience has fully confirmed these indications for the two drugs.

Before leaving the nervous system I must speak of the mental and moral symptoms which characterise the sufferings from Arsenic. These are so constant that I cannot but refer them to a direct action upon the ideational and emotional centres. As in the motor and sensory sphere, we have the mingling of depression and irritation. As there the paralysis is accompanied with cramps, and the anæsthesia with neuralgia, so here there is melancholy, but also restlessness, irritability, anxiety, and anguish. In some forms of melancholia and hypochondriasis we may take advantage of this action, as others have done with success.*

In the three great groups which have now passed before us —the fevers, the inflammations, and the neuroses—the part of Arsenic, as a poison and as a remedy, is mainly played. But there are other features of its action on which we must dwell, before we quit its consideration.

1. I must speak of the profound influence which Arsenic exerts upon the life of the blood. The researches of Schmidt, Sturzwage, and Harley have made it evident that it acts as a direct poison to the red corpuscles, either when formed or in the course of production. In small doses the only result of this influence of the drug is diminished metamorphosis of the food and tissues,—the excretion of carbonic acid and urea becoming notably less, and the change of the alimentary sugar into glycogen being impeded. Hence the *pseudo* "good condition" of the Styrian arsenicophagi, and of the Vienna horses, to whom the stable-keepers are accustomed to give the drug with the view of making them sleek and fat. These effects are reasonably traced to lowered functional power of the red corpuscles as oxygen-carriers, and a consequent suboxidation of the system,—the carbonaceous compounds, unconsumed, depositing themselves in the form of fat. A further degree of the same influence produces the "grayish cachectic appearance," and "all kinds of anæmic troubles," which Naunyn includes among the chronic effects of Arsenic; and, finally, the petechial effusions and hæmorrhages so often seen—the former of which have been studied by Dr. Imbert-Gourbeyre. In poisoning by arseniuretted hydrogen the red corpuscles suffer such rapid disintegration that abundant hæmoglobinuria is noted.

I may sum up this evidence in the words of Stillé. "The microscopical and chemical peculiarities of the blood under the action of Arsenic are of great importance in relation to the changes which the solids undergo, to the hæmorrhages from the nose, the digestive canal, the urinary passages, to the ecchymosis found in the lungs, pleura, pericardium, and heart, and to the occurrence of dropsy during the use of this medicine. The production of serous effusions as an ordinary effect, and of chronic anæmia as the consequence of prolonged exposure to arsenical influences, appear to furnish grounds for

* See Wurmb, §, 16; *Hom. Times*, vii., 2.

believing that, in sufficient doses, Arsenic, like Mercury, tends
to disintegrate the blood-corpuscles, to diminish the proportion of fibrin, and possibly, also, to attack still more directly
the vital principle upon which the normal qualities of the
blood depend." Since we have been able to count the blood-
corpuscles, this inference has been confirmed by actual inspection. "Drs. Cutler and Bradford, from their experiments
conducted according to Malassez' method, are led to conclude that Arsenic given in health causes a progressive
decrease of the number of the red and especially of the white
corpuscles" (Ringer).

It is now obvious in what fashion Arsenic is a "blood-
tonic." It is so upon the principle that likes are cured by
likes—that it enriches the blood in disease because it im-
poverishes it in health. But the likeness must be complete if
the medicine is to be entirely appropriate and strikingly
curative. Arsenic is, as Dr. Bartholow says, "one of the most
valuable agents which we possess in the treatment of chlorosis
and anæmia," but his only indication for its distinctive place
is that it is "especially adapted to those cases in which iron
does not agree or fails of effect." We, on the other hand,
should not think of giving Ferrum in those cases to which
Arsenic is suitable, and which we should recognise beforehand. "Excessive prostration, considerable œdema, violent
and irregular palpitations, with marked appetite for acids
and brandy, and, above all, extreme anxiety"—such are
Dr. Jousset's indications for it in chlorosis, in which he
recognises it as one of our best remedies, especially where
menorrhagia is present rather than the opposite state. "A
high degree of debility, with excessive irritability, œdematous
paleness, cardiac phenomena even during rest and complete
gastro-ataxia" are Bähr's signs for its choice in this affection:
in which, he says, "it is remarkable how soon after the administration of Arsenicum the normal appetite returns, and the
sickly complexion is replaced by a brighter hue." In anæmia
otherwise occurring, Arsenic is most suitable when the
poverty of blood has arisen from some miasmatic influence
or exhausting toxæmic disease. Such a condition is especially
seen in the malarial cachexia, where in both schools, and in
doses most wide apart in quantity, the drug is reckoned of
sovereign efficacy. Arsenic bids fair, moreover, to be our
great remedy in the malady now recognised as idiopathic, or
progressive pernicious, anæmia. The fever, the œdema and
the petechial effusion which characterise this form of the
disease all belong to our drug. Iron has been found quite

ineffective in it ; and a case has been published by an old-school physician, Dr. Bramwell, in which Arsenic proved completely curative.* More recently, our excellent colleague, Dr. C. H. Blackley, of Manchester, has communicated† to the British Homœopathic Society four cases which have come under his notice, in which a cure of this disease was effected by Arsenic, and in doses much smaller than those employed by Dr. Bramwell.

2. I would further direct your attention to the ulceration of the skin which is apt to follow upon acute, and to manifest itself in chronic, arsenical poisoning, and whose tendency is always to phagedæna and gangrene. I need not quote authorities on this point, but will use the fact as a peg on which to hang the evidence I shall bring before you of the remedial value of Arsenic in malignant ulcerations, including cancer. It has some reputation in rodent ulcer. In lupus exedens Mr. Hunt says that it is "not only our sheet-anchor but absolutely a specific," warning us that it must be per-severed with for a length of time—"half a life-time if neces-sary."‡ Of still greater importance is its use in carcinoma-tous affections. Here again I may quote Mr. Hunt, as one whose experience with this medicine is second to no man's. " Arsenic is always useful and necessary in cancer. Although I have rarely found a malignant tumour dissipated by Arsenic, I have as rarely known the mineral fail to check its onward course. It most assuredly exerts, when discreetly administered, a certain amount of specific influence over this disease." I think he might have spoken still more unreservedly, had he used his Arsenic exclusively or especially for carcinomatous *ulceration.* In the glandular tumours of this disease I prefer Hydrastis, and in its fungoid and bleeding growths Phos-phorus ; but in epithelial cancer—as of the lip, face, and tongue—Arsenic has unquestionably proved curative, and that not seldom. Dr. Bartholow recognises its power here, though doubting it as to other forms of cancer. Even in these, however, Arsenic may do much to relieve the lancinating

---

* *Med. Times and Gazette,* Oct. 20, 1877.

† See *Annals,* ix., 171.

‡ " In its operation, Arsenic is the slowest by far of all medicines. It never takes disease by storm, but gradually loosens its hold. . . . Month after month, and year after year, you watch for improvement under its use, and find none, until at length you utterly despair of making any impression ; and perhaps the very next week you examine the patient, and the crust has fallen off, the ulcer healed, and the disease of twenty years has gone, never to return." *Brit. Med. Journ.,* Jan., 4, 1862.)

pains, and promote a better sanguification in the patients.
Dr. Walshe prefers the iodide of Arsenic to any other remedy
in this disease.

And now I must draw this long dissertation to a close. I
would only ask you to note, in conclusion, the striking testimony borne by the drug to the validity of the method of
Hahnemann. Because it is the greatest of poisons, it is the
greatest of remedies ; and its poisonous and remedial effects
go hand in hand. Every morbid condition in which it has
gained repute it has been seen to cause ; and, by working the
same method since, its therapeutic sphere has been widely
extended. To ague, cutaneous disease, chorea and angina
pectoris, we have added—among other diseases—typhoid and
hectic conditions, cholera, cancrum oris, gastritis, chronic
diarrhœa, scrofulous ophthalmia, asthma, chronic cardiac and
renal disease, and serous effusions and dropsies. Truly a
goodly list ; and it might be yet extended. For myself I can
say this, that were I reduced to two medicines only out of the
whole Pharmacopœia, the two I should choose would be
Aconite and Arsenic.

The action of Arsenic is so extensive, that it has points of
analogy with nearly every medicine in the Materia Medica.
Those which resemble it most closely are *Mercurius corrosivus*,
Kali bichromicum, and *Iodine*.

Like all polychrests, Arsenic must be given in various
dilutions to obtain its full efficacy. In cholera, typhoid conditions, cancer, chronic menorrhagia and cutaneous diseases
we may use the first trituration of arsenious acid, or (which I
prefer) the liquor potassæ arsenitis, which contains gr. j of
arsenious acid in ℳcxx. The 3rd decimal trituration is a very
useful potency for chronic diarrhœa, and for chronic inflammation of those tissues to which Arsenic is irritant. The 6th
dilution answers admirably for influenza, coryza, acute serous
effusion, and other acute inflammations to which the drug is
homœopathic. The potencies from the 6th upward have
proved most serviceable in .neuralgia, in chronic intermittents,
and in asthma.

A word as to compounds of Arsenic. The iodide—
Arsenicum iodatum—has been proved by Drs. Beebe and
Blakeley on their own persons, the 1st and 2nd decimal
triturations being used. No special effects were obtained.
Dr. Hale esteems it highly for catarrhs of any part with
" peculiar and persistently irritating, corrosive character of all
discharges." He reports a cure of a malignant-looking

axillary induration by it, and a similar condition of the cervix uteri, suggesting scirrhus, has more than once disappeared under its use. The arseniate of soda—*Natrum arsenicatum*— was very thoroughly proved in 1875 by the Alleghany County Society. The results obtained may be read in the *Hahne-mannian Monthly* for 1876 and 1878, and in Allen's *Encyclo-pœdia*. The effect of the drug on the mucous membrane of the fauces and posterior nares was extremely marked ; and I have followed some of the provers themselves in using it, with much satisfaction, in superficial inflammatory conditions of these parts.

LECTURE XVII.

ARUM, ASAFŒTIDA, ASARUM, ASCLEPIAS, ASTERIAS, AURUM, BAPTISIA.

We have to consider to-day a few medicines of small importance, along with two of higher rank in the shape of Aurum and Baptisia.

The first in order is

Arum.

Under this head I include both the Arum maculatum—the "lords and ladies" of our popular nomenclature—and the Arum triphyllum, or Indian turnip, which is its American analogue. Of the former we prepare a tincture from the fresh root : of the latter the best preparation seems to be a trituration of the expressed juice of the same part with sugar of milk.

Arum maculatum was proved by Dr. Hering, and Arum triphyllum by Dr. Lippe. Their results, with symptoms observed in poisoning by the former species, are given in Allen's *Encyclopœdia*, and their clinical applications are described by Dr. Hale in his *New Remedies*.

The one interesting point about Arum is the application which has been made of its local effects on the mouth to a corresponding condition when occurring in malignant scarlatina. The following description has been given of the former :—" After chewing a young leaf-stalk for a few seconds, a very intense, prickling, stinging pain was felt upon the tongue and mucous membrane of the lips and throat, accompanied with a flow of saliva, which seemed to relieve the pain a little —the pains were as if a hundred little needles had been run into the tongue and lips." This was from the Arum maculatum, but Dr. Lippe has found some excellent results from the Arum triphyllum when scarlatinal and other patients have shown great irritation of the buccal mucous membrane. "The most indicative symptoms," he says, "are the very sore feeling in the mouth, the redness of the tongue, the elevated papillæ, the cracked lips and corners of the mouth." The nose also may be sore, with or without much coryza. Dr. Guernsey speaks of raw, bloody surfaces on these parts as characteristic of Arum, with which there is much itching, so that children will often pick at and bore into the places, though so doing causes great pain, and makes them scream. He further indicates an acrid coryza as calling for it.

Dr. Lippe commends the drug also for clergyman's sore throat. He gives the dilutions from the sixth upwards.

I have next to speak of

Asafœtida.

The drug known by this name is the dried juice of the root of the Indian plant which yields it. From the Asafœtida of commerce a tincture is prepared in the usual manner for homœopathic use.

The chief proving of Asafœtida is that of Jörg, in which twelve persons took part. Some additional experiments are collated with his in Dr. Allen's article, which gives 585 symptoms to the drug.

Jörg's results are fairly summed up thus by Dr. Phillips. "The administration of small doses causes alliaceous eructations ; the digestion is impaired ; there are burning sensations in the fauces ; there is pain, fulness, and oppression of the stomach ; the abdomen becomes distended with flatus, which, when discharged, is of a very fœtid and disagreeable character ; there is frequent inclination to evacuate the bowels, and the discharge is thin and watery. The urine is not augmented in quantity, but becomes acrid, and communicates a sense of burning. The pulse is at the same time quickened the head becomes more or less affected with flying pains, often attended with much giddiness ; and various nervous and hysterical phenomena make their appearance. Like the pulse, the respiration becomes quickened, and the secretion of the bronchial membrane is promoted." Pereira adds that "the urino-genital apparatus appeared to be specifically affected, for in the males there was an increase of the venereal feelings, with irritation about the glans penis, while in the females the catamenial discharge appeared before its time, and uterine pain was experienced." Trinks mentions a case in which (in large doses) it caused nymphomania.

Our main use of Asafœtida is as a remedy for hysterical troubles. A symptom repeatedly observed by two of the provers strikingly resembles the globus hystericus ; and hysterical cough, tympanites and asthma (it constricted the chest in some) come within its range of influence. I confess that I myself rarely use it, preferring the more agreeable Moschus, whose action seems so very similar. It is only in tympanitic distension of the abdomen that I find it preferable. Dr. Ringer recommends it here, in doses, for children, of less than a drop of the tincture. Dr. Guernsey, however, thinks it quite the best remedy when hysterical symptoms manifest themselves in the œsophagus, and Dr. Hoyne confirms this experience. Quite another, and a very inexplicable action of Asafœtida, is its influence upon diseases of bone. Dr. Holcombe writes, " I have twice verified the value of this remedy in scrofulous caries of the bones. I used the 12th dilution. It is singular that a remedy, whose principal applications are to the most fugitive and sympathetic disturbances of the nervous system, should extend its curative power to the most deep-seated and chronic organic lesions." It is also highly commended in acute periostitis. I give you these facts as they stand. For myself, I have given Asafœtida very persistently in several cases of chronic caries, without being able to discern the slightest result from its use. I should say that it is from the old school that its repute here originates. Stillé quotes Neumann as speaking of its utility as " generally admitted." Dr. Hoyne cites several instances of its beneficial use in syphilitic disease. Asafœtida is also reputed of value when the milk of nursing mothers is deficient.* In all these affections, *hyper-sensitiveness* is said by Dr. Guernsey to indicate the drug.

The relations of Asafœtida as a nervine are with *Ambra, Moschus,* and *Valerian.* Its influence upon ·bone (if a fact) ranks it with the metals and metalloids *Aurum, Fluoric acid, Mercurius, Phosphorus,* and *Silica.*

In hysteric disorders, the dose should probably be from the 2nd downwards. In diseases of bone Asafœtida is praised in the dilutions from 12 to 30.

* *Brit. Journ. of Hom.*, ii., 417.

I am entering a region unknown to you when I proceed to speak of

Asarum Europæum,

or Asarabacca. A tincture is prepared from the entire plant.

Asarum was proved by Hahnemann and four others : the pathogenesis, containing 270 symptoms, is in the third volume of the *Materia Medica Pura.* There is a good article upon it (the last published, I am sorry to say) in the *New Materia Medica.*

That Asarum is a local irritant, of the Elaterium and Veratrum type, to the mucous membranes generally, acting as errhine, emetic, and purgative, is pretty well known ; but the fact has little bearing on practice. In Hahnemann's provings we are most struck by, as general symptoms, excessive sensibility and general chilliness without thirst : in particular regions, depression of the cerebral functions with heavy headache ; weak sight and twitching of the eyelids ; still more striking dulness of hearing, as though a pellicle were stretched over the meatus auditorius ; passing of much mucus from the bowels ;* marked stitching in the lungs ; a great deal of myalgia in the back and lower extremities. Asarum has hardly ever been used in disease : the above symptoms may occasionally help you to its phenomenal application. It is said to be suitable to chilly subjects ; and to remove darting pains after operations on the eyes. It has a great reputation in Russia as a remedy for the effects of excessive drinking.

I can say nothing as to the analogous medicines or the dose of Asarum.

Of the plants known by the name of Asclepias we have information as to three, the A. incarnata, A. Syriaca, and A. tuberosa. The first and second seem to have some uterine influence, and the latter of these is a potent diuretic, increasing the solid constituents as well as the fluid portion of the urine. This we learn from Dr. Hale's *New Remedies.* But the same author communicates facts about the

Asclepias tuberosa

which fairly give it a place among homœopathic remedies. It is used as a tincture or trituration made from the root.

* The symptom " scanty, yellow, mucous stool, in one string," has been verified by three cases of cure by Dr. E. M. Hale (*Brit. Journ. of Hom.*, xxvi., 331).

The significant point about this plant is that it is popularly known as "pleurisy root." Such terms usually have more or less warrant from fact, and that it is so in the present case appears from a proving instituted by Dr. Thomas Nichol, of Montreal. Large doses caused only colic and purging; but from the first decimal dilution he got decided pleuritic symptoms. Thus :—" throughout the evening the pains kept increasing, making respiration painful, especially at the base of the left lung, which is dull on percussion, while the cough is dry and spasmodic." " The pain is very acute on the right side, and seems to be seated in the pleura." The remedy deserves a trial.

The next medicine I have to introduce you to is a novel one. It is made from the star-fish,

Asterias rubens,

by bruising the dried fish in a mortar and triturating with milk-sugar.

Our sole knowledge concerning Asterias is derived from the proving and clinical cases furnished by the late Dr. Petroz. They are translated from the first volume of the *Journal de la Société Gallicane* in Metcalf's *American Provings*. Seven persons took part in the experiments; but no information is given as to the size or frequency of the doses they took.

Dr. Petroz makes the following remark :—" Experimentation on the healthy gives readily, and often in profusion, symptoms indicating disturbance of function; but it never goes on to alteration of tissue, rarely even to the earliest indications thereof. We must therefore have recourse to clinical experience. Its teaching is sure, when time has confirmed it." To no medicine does this statement apply better than to Asterias rubens. The skin symptoms alone are well marked; and these have led to its employment in chronic ulceration, even when of a cancerous nature, with reported success. Its action seems limited to the left side of the body. It has also cured a case of cerebral congestion with obstinate constipation in an old gentleman : I have myself found it of great use in a similar case. Asterias had a reputation among the ancients in epilepsy; and Petroz cites two cases in which much benefit resulted from its use in infinitesimal doses. I have little personal experience with this remedy.

Teste classes it (with Petroz' assent) in his group headed by *Sulphur*, and including *Bovista*, *Æthusa*, and *Cicuta*.

The higher dilutions (12 to 24) were employed in all cases on record of relief or cure by Asterias.

We now come to a medicine which homœopathy has done much to rescue from unmerited neglect, and to restore to a high place in therapeutics. I speak of gold. There is so little difference between the action of the metal and its salts that I shall speak of them generally as

Aurum.

We use the pure metal in the form of a trituration of the finest gold leaf, which was that employed by Hahnemann in his provings. The trichloride—A. muriaticum—is also used in homœopathic practice : its solution is aqueous at first and alcoholic afterwards.

The first proving of Aurum appears in the fourth volume of the *Reine Arzneimittellehre.* It contains 137 symptoms observed by Hahnemann himself ; 198 from 7 fellow-observers ; and 3 from authors. There are also a few symptoms from A. muriaticum and A. fulminans. Those of the metal itself were obtained from one or two hundred grains of the first trituration ; so that they have uncommon value. There is a second pathogenesis in the *Chronischen Krankheiten.* It contains 82 fresh symptoms, of which 75 are Hahnemann's own. The worth of these, according to the facts we have ascertained, is more than problematical. Dr. Allen gives symptoms, both of Aurum metallicum and of Aurum muriaticum, from additional sources ; and some provings of Aurum sulphuratum, and of the chloride of gold and sodium. A valuable monograph on the drug has recently been given us by Dr. Burnett,* which contains a further proving on his own person.

Hahnemann's preface to Aurum is very interesting. He tells us that the physicians of his time so unanimously proclaimed the inertness of metallic gold, that he was at first led to use the muriate. Subsequently, however, he found that the Arabian physicians had been in the habit of using the metal itself in a fine powder; and had praised it as remedial in those very affections for which he had found the muriate beneficial. He then prepared a first trituration of gold-leaf in the usual way, and proved it as described. From the symptoms produced he found that the drug was perfectly homœopathic to the maladies for which the Arabians had given it ; and,

* *Gold as a remedy in disease.* 1879.

guided by the same principle of similarity, he found it—in the
1st and 2nd triturations—curative in several other important
affections.

He could hardly have been aware, when (in 1818) he first
stated this in print, that in 1811 Chrestien had revived in Paris
the use of powdered gold. In his *Observations sur un nouveau
remède dans le traitement des maladies vénériennes et lymphati-
ques* he communicates a number of cases illustrative of its value
in syphilis, scrofula, and even in uterine scirrhus ; and states that
the finely powdered leaf has the same effect as the oxide or the
muriate. Niel and Legrand have handed on the tradition, so
that a considerable body of information relative to the action
of gold has accumulated, and may be read in the account of it
given by Trousseau and Pidoux.

The anti-syphilitic virtues thus ascribed to gold. though
only a revival of its former repute (as Dr. Burnett has shown),
and though for a time very generally acknowledged, meet with
little recognition in the old school at the present day. The
drug is not mentioned by Wood, Ringer, or Stillé. But
among homœopathists it holds a high place in many of the
tertiary manifestations of the disease, especially the sarcocele,
the osseous affections, and the cachexia. It does so because
the provings have revealed an elective affinity on its part for
the organs involved. The bones are affected with burning
and boring pain, sometimes—especially in the face and feet—
accompanied by redness and swelling, sometimes—as in the
head—with nodes ; and in one prover swelling and tenderness
of the right testicle came on for some hours daily. Dr.
Burnett also experienced its effect on these organs.

But the provings go farther than this. In the first place
they show a marked melancholia as produced by Aurum, and
this of a distinctly suicidal character. One of the experimenters
" imagined himself not fit for this world, and longed for
death : thinking of death gave him intense joy." Then they
show a strong action on the nose, which is inflamed without,
and blocked up with ulcers and crusts within ; with putrid
smell when blowing it. Dr. Morse records an interesting
case in which a syphilitic patient, being overdosed with gold
by a quack, developed both sets of symptoms.* These two
actions have led to the chief uses of Aurum in the homœopathic school. In suicidal melancholy Hahnemann himself
repeatedly extols its virtues ; and Drs. Chapman, Bayes, and
Sharp speak in the same sense. Whether this affection is one
primarily seated in the brain is doubtful, from the other facts

* *Hahn. Monthly,* xii., 506.

about the action of Aurum. I am myself inclined to think it a hypochondriasis having its seat either in the liver or in the testes.* Dr. Bayes states that the cases in which he has seen Aurum curative have presented indications of congestion of the head and liver, with fixed colour in the face, and a yellowish tinge. Suicidal melancholia, moreover, is not an unfrequent accompaniment of testicular disease. The nasal action of the metal has led to its successful use in chronic rhinitis, in crusts of the nostrils, and above all in scrofulous and syphilitic ozæna. Many testimonies to and illustrations of its value in this complaint are on record.

Again, one of the affections specified by Hahnemann as cured by him with gold was a mercurial caries of the nasal and palatine bones. The French experience has shown that the action of the metal is closely analogous to that of Mercury, causing—as it does—its salivation (without much if any affection of the gums) and its erethistic fever with diuresis and sweat. Thus Aurum has come to be reputed among us as a remedy for chronic hydrargyrosis; in which we have the support of Dietrich. It is an admirable medicine for those constitutions broken down by the combined influence of syphilis and Mercury which sometimes come before us for treatment. I once gave to a poor fellow thus afflicted the first trituration of gold. He came back to me in a week's time, looking quite another man, and exclaimed—"Surely you have given me the elixir of life!" Dr. Chapman has narrated a similar case in the seventh volume of the *British Journal of Homœopathy* (p. 396).

Once more. The action of Aurum on the nasal mucous membrane has naturally suggested its use in affections of that offset of it which we call the conjunctiva. Provings have not yet manifested the influence of the drug here; but there are a good many cases of chronic scrofulous ophthalmia on record in

* Dr. Burnett (p. 136) challenges this opinion of mine, which he is of course quite in his rights in doing. But he is in error when he discusses it as if it were a "theory" about the seat of hypochondriasis. It refers only to the form of this mental disorder to which Aurum is homœopathic, which I judge—from the concomitants and the general action of the drug—to be that connected with hepatic or testicular disorder rather than one purely cerebral. Dr. Burnett himself supplies an excellent instance of its efficacy in the second of the two connexions I have specified, when he recommends it for pining, low-spirited boys, and says that, in these cases, if we examine the testes, we shall "find them mere pendent shreds, just on the verge of atrophy." When under Aurum they have brightened up and become like other boys— "look again," he writes, "at the before-mentioned glands, and you will find them larger, firm, and well suspended."

which it has proved very effectual, even to restoring transparency to the opaque cornea. It seems to have a special action on this membrane, as Drs. Allen and Norton speak highly of it for interstitial keratitis, and Mr. Clifton has lately communicated a case of the syphilitic form of the disease, in which its beneficial effects were unquestionable.

In these regions of action—in affections of the bones and glands, and of the oculo-nasal mucous membrane, especially when of syphilitic, mercurial, or scrofulous origin—Aurum has made its mark among us. I may add to these that in the Leopoldstadt Hospital at Vienna it was the favourite remedy for periostitis; and cured one severe case of albuminuria, with general and local dropsy. If I am right, too, in referring its melancholia to the liver, it is but an action of the same kind when we hear of it as occasionally curative in ascites from hepatic disease—possibly cirrhosis; and in chronic icterus. But I think that the future use of Aurum will extend beyond this range. We have not yet utilised the rushes of blood to head and chest it so markedly causes, though Dierbach has recorded his experience of its value in disturbance of the pulmonary circulation after hæmorrhages.* We have not yet ascertained if it affects the female sexual system as it does the male; though the salacity and erections it causes in the latter are paralleled by the menorrhagia set up in the former. We have not determined the precise nature of the dyspnœa caused by it, or applied to practice its undoubted action upon the heart.† I think, too, that strumous and syphilitic keratitis are not the only affections of the eye it can influence. When we read of Herrmann—its most thorough prover—experiencing " excessive *tension* in the eyes," now making sight indistinct, as if a black crape were drawn before the eyes, now causing hemiopia, in which only the lower half of objects is visible, and now diplopia—I think that we may find some work for the drug in the treatment of glaucoma. The horizontal hemiopia of the drug has led Drs. Allen and Norton to its use in detached retina, and with great advantage. Aurum seems to me one of the medicines of the future.

The only writer in the English language who gives any independent account of Aurum is Dr. Bartholow; and he, drawing partly from French and partly from homœopathic sources, has made out a list of its applications not unlike those which I have now mentioned. He finds it—in fractional doses

* See also Burnett, p. 124—126.

† Dr. Burnett relates a case of rheumatic endocarditis, in which it seemed very effective (p. 127).

of the chloride—useful in the granular and waxy forms of Bright's kidney. He cites also the experience of Martini as to its favourable action in chronic affections of the uterus and ovaries. Dr. Tritscher, in our own school, has carried out this treatment, and reports excellent results in indurations of the uterus and ovarian tumours. He gives from one to six grains of the first trituration of the chloride of gold and sodium.

The effects of Aurum take long to excite (10-15 days), and they are slow to decline.

After Mercury, the most striking analogue of Aurum is *Platina*, which is to the female sex what gold is to the male. Its points of similarity and difference with Mercury, Arsenic, Silica, and Phosphorus are well brought out by Dr. H. Goullon in a paper on the drug translated from the *Allg. Hom. Zeitung* in the twenty-second volume of the *North American Journal of Homœopathy*.

Hahnemann's published experience with Aurum was gained with the 1st and 2nd triturations; but subsequently he resorted to the 12th and at last to the 30th. His disciples (including Dr. Burnett) seem to have followed his earlier rather than his later practice in this matter.

I would speak last of the

Baptisia tinctoria.

This is the "wild indigo" of North America. We make a tincture of the bark of the root.

Short provings of Baptisia, made by seven persons, may be found in the fifth and seventh volumes of the *North American Journal of Homœopathy*. These, with further pathogenetic and clinical facts, are collected by Dr. Hale in the article on the drug in the second edition of his *New Remedies*, and by Dr. Allen in his *Encyclopœdia*, where the drug has 367 symptoms. There are two monographs extant on the use of Baptisia in typhoid fever,—one, published separately, by Dr. Bayes (1872); the other, by myself, read as a paper before the British Homœo-pathic Congress of 1872, and printed in the *Monthly Homœo-pathic Review* of that year.

It is on this point that the interest of Baptisia is centred. I have collected, in the paper referred to, fifty-three recorded cases of continued fever, in all of which the effect of the medi-cine was either to induce a speedy crisis, or materially to abate and curtail the disease. In the discussion which followed its

T

reading at the Congress speaker after speaker rose up to confirm from his own experience this estimate of its value ; and there was not a dissentient voice. Two of those who spoke were from the United States ; and it was from thence that we first heard of its virtues and reputation. Among the reports examined in the paper is one of the treatment of the " colonial fever " of Melbourne ; and Dr. Kitching has since given us his experience of the corresponding disorder at the Cape, where he has found Baptisia as potent as Dr. Madden found it in Victoria.* So from four continents the fame of the medicine comes borne to us ; and we cannot but give it a full consideration and trial.

The first question must be as to the nature of the continued fever in which Baptisia has been found so effective. It is described in the records under several names—" typhus," " typhoid," " continued," " gastric," " bilious." Is it nevertheless in all the one essential fever we know as " typhoid " or " enteric ?" or do some of the cases come within other categories ?

The four distinct forms of idiopathic fever which the labours of Stewart, of Jenner, and of Henderson have defined, are so universally recognised that I need not dwell upon them. The only one which concerns us here is the so-called " febricula." This is described as a primary fever—not catarrhal or sympathetic—pretty closely resembling in symptoms the onset of the other forms, but differenced in this, that it rapidly reaches its maximum, and as rapidly subsides, within, at the most, five days. It has no local complication or specific eruption. Now it is quite possible that some of the *sporadic* cases where the disease has broken up under Baptisia have been instances of this disorder, and four out of the fifty-three cases I have collated are perhaps invalidated on this account. But no such explanation is admissible as regards the remainder of the single cases in which it displayed curative powers, as all these were of more prolonged duration ; while in the epidemics reported by two of the observers, it is noted that under old school treatment the fever lasted two, three, or four weeks, and in two cases under other homœopathic remedies (Aconite and Bryonia) for twelve days. That under Baptisia it terminated not later than the fifth day is therefore no proof that it was febricula.

But is there yet another form of continued fever, resembling typhoid rather than febricula in its duration and progress, yet specifically distinct ? and is it this disease in which the good

* See *Monthly Hom. Review*, xix., 207.

work of Baptisia has been done? This is a more difficult question. Jenner, Trousseau and Murchison seem to answer it in the negative : they think that all the varieties of fever described by the old nosologists—gastric, bilious, mucous, nervous, putrid, and so forth—fall under one or other of the four types now recognised. But the Nomenclature of our College of Physicians gives us a "common continued fever," as distinct from either typhus, typhoid, relapsing fever, or febricula ; and Dr. Aitken cites several testimonies, direct or indirect, in favour of the existence of such a species. The opinion of several of our own school who have expressed themselves on the subject is of the same tenor. Thus—Dr. Russell, in his *Clinical Lectures*, writes : " I mean by 'gastric fever' a non-infectious continued fever, which has no regular course ; in which there is no eruption, and which is not attended with diarrhœa or intestinal affection." Dr. Jousset also maintains the existence of a " fièvre synoque," specifically distinct from the "fièvre ephémère" and "fièvre typhoide" which occur in France as in this country. I have hitherto gone with the general current of doctrine in accepting the other view, and maintaining that—excluding febricula—there is but one endemic species of continued fever, and that the enteric. I must now, however, acknowledge a change of view. Watching my own practice, and examining the records of that of others, I have come to the conclusion that there is a true " common continued fever," a veritable "synochus," which, though it may run on from the " gastric" into the "typhoid" condition, never has the essential features or typical clinical history of typhoid fever proper.

Our decision of this question has an important bearing on the claims made for Baptisia. Typhoid is a disease of such frequent occurrence and such ghastly mortality : it invades such high quarters, and threatens, if it do not actually destroy, such valuable lives ; it has, even when not fatal, so lengthened a process, so tedious a convalescence, such frequent *sequelæ* of even direr import than itself, that any promising addition to our power of controlling it cannot but be welcomed. But especially would this be so, if the promise held out were of more than mitigation of severity only, more than sustainment of the patient ; if it were of actual abortion and breaking up of the disease. If Baptisia proved to be the Aconite of this fever, we should without controversy have gained a priceless remedy.

I regret that I cannot stand to the claim on behalf of it to this power which I have many times made during the last sixteen years*. Were there no other endemic continued fever but typhoid, my conclusions from practice would be unassailable, and instances where the disease seemed to elude the abortive power of the medicine might be regarded as exceptional. But I am driven now to consider such cases as of the true enteric type, and the rest as belonging to the "common continued fever" whose existence I have been led to admit. I cannot, therefore, any longer maintain that Baptisia is capable of breaking up a genuine typhoid, and must acknowledge that those of my colleagues who have questioned its power so to do have been wiser than I.

But has it therefore no influence on the progress of this disease? Far from it: it plays a most important part in its treatment. To ascertain the precise place occupied by it—its relation to the stages of the disease and the sphere of other medicines—let us first consider the experiments made to ascertain its pathogenetic action.

These show the following symptoms :—

After taking during the day (Feb. 5th) four drops of the mother tincture, Dr. Douglass awoke in the night with a feeling as if the room were insufferably hot and close, hindering respiration. His pulse was about 90, full and soft. There was most uncomfortable burning heat of the whole surface, especially the face. The tongue was dry, and smarted and felt sore as if burnt. The heat compelled him to move to a cool part of the bed, and finally to rise and open a window, and bathe his face and hands. With these symptoms there was, he writes, a "peculiar feeling of the head, which is never felt except during the presence of fever, a sort of excitement of the brain, which is the preliminary to, or rather the beginning of delirium, which with me never fails to occur if fever continues and increases to any considerable intensity." He at length got to sleep again, but awoke the next morning with the same dry and burnt tongue.

The same symptoms recurred on the night of the 7th, after four more drops of the tincture. The oppression of breathing was still more marked, and felt quite congestive. Flushed face and dulness continued during the next day. Each night while awake he had painful intolerance of pressure as he lay, especially in the sacral region, obliging him at last to lie on his face.

On the 10th, after a dose of three drops taken in the afternoon, the same symptoms rapidly supervened. It is added that the head felt large, and the eyes were shining ; the hands also felt large, and were tremulous.

* See *Brit. Journ. of Hom.*, xxi., 385.

He took no more medicine. The bowels had been constipated throughout the proving till the 12th, when they resumed their usual condition. He felt weak and tremulous, as if recovering from an illness, and was not himself again till the 15th.

The other provers had the same febrile symptoms, with hot and high-coloured urine. Dr. Rowley records vomiting and diarrhœa. Dr. Sapp, pain in the stomach, abdomen, and right hypochondrium, passing down to the right iliac region ; also soreness in the region of the liver. Dr. Smith had diarrhœa, followed by constipation and hæmorrhoids ; and constipation was present also in Dr. Hoyt.

Lastly, in a more ignoble prover, a cat poisoned by Dr. Burt, the small and large intestines were found congested and filled with bloody mucus.

From these symptoms two facts seem to stand forth with unmistakable clearness.

1st. Baptisia is capable of exciting true primary *pyrexia* in the human subject. This is no slight thing, for there are very few other drugs to which we can ascribe such power. And this pyrexia, in the case of Baptisia, is exceedingly like that of the early period of typhoid. The soft and full, yet quickened pulse, the headache and tendency to delirium, the soreness all over, and intolerance of pressure when lying, are marked symptoms of this stage of the disease.

2nd. We have no evidence that Baptisia affects Peyer's patches as they are affected in typhoid, nor even that it acts upon them at all as Arsenic and Iodine, and perhaps Mercury and turpentine do. But it is certain that it produces congestion and catarrh of the intestinal mucous membrane, with abdominal tenderness and diarrhœa. Now this again is the condition present during the first week of typhoid.* The Peyerian and solitary glands are, till the seventh day, involved merely in the general hyperæmia, but the latter then subsides, and they stand out alone.

We have, therefore, in Baptisia a medicine precisely homœopathic to the first stage of typhoid fever, *i.e.*, to the period antecedent to the full development of the intestinal affection. There is nothing, I think, to render it inconceivable that, administered early and persistently in this period, though it may not blight the growth of the disease, it may considerably abate its energy. There are two opportunities then afforded it for so doing. The *dothien-entérite*—as Bretonneau proposed to call the infarction of the intestinal glands—does not begin

* See Aitken's *Science and Practice of Medicine*, i., 397-8.

till about the fifth or sixth day of the fever, to which it is (as it were) secondary. Why should not its development be materially hindered? Again, on the tenth day there is a natural tendency to resolution in the local affection. "The turgescence," writes Trousseau, " of the aggregate and solitary glands of Peyer, and of the mesenteric glands, begins to decrease, and goes on gradually subsiding up to the fourteenth day, at which date the affected glands are still a little swollen, but by the end of the third week resolution is complete, excepting that the mesenteric glands do not quite regain their normal condition till a short time later." Why should not Baptisia, by abating the whole force of the malady, favour this tendency to resolution?

Of such an action as the latter, we have seen an analogous instance in the case of Tartar emetic in smallpox. It does not prevent the formation of the eruption; but it does strenuously promote its resolution in the papular or vesicular stage, so that the processes which end in pitting, and the concomitant secondary fever, are averted. There is no reason why Baptisia should not have a corresponding effect in typhoid, which is not a more specific process, having a definite clinical history, than variola. My own experience is that it has such an influence, and that typhoid when treated with it from the commencement rarely reaches any serious height or runs an unduly protracted course. Some of the cases recorded, moreover, seem to show that at no stage of the fever is it without beneficial influence, and to lead to the inference that, unless other remedies are better indicated, the patient should always have the advantage of what it can do for him. It might be alternated in the more advanced period of the disease with the Arsenicum, the Mercurius, or the Terebinthina we should deem it right to give for the intestinal affection, just as we sometimes alternate Aconite with the local specific in fully developed inflammations.

Nor has the relegation of the abortive power of Baptisia to common continued fever a merely negative significance. It is of no little consequence to have a remedy which shall break up this fever, on which typhoid symptoms are very apt to supervene if it is only treated with ordinary medicines. You have but to try it here to be satisfied of its surpassing value.

I have gone fully into this matter on account of its great practical importance. For another statement of the question, from the side of disease, I may refer you to the second edition of my *Manual of Therapeutics*, in the articles on typhoid and common continued fever. I hope that the facts alleged may induce some of those who hear me to test the remedy in their own sphere of work, and to report the results. It need not be given in infinitesimal quantities. Drop-doses of the mother-tincture, or small portions of an infusion, were administered in most of the published cases. Such doses, moreover, will probably ensure a wider range for the medicine. The tendency in America just now is to restrict its action in continued fever to cases in which its minuter symptomatology is reproduced—as soreness in lying, a sense of being all to pieces, and so forth. Dr. Chargé adds softness of the pulse in the first stage, and fœtidity later on : Jahr gives despair of cure and certainty of death. I do not doubt that in cases so characterised its curative action may be markedly exhibited. But it will be observed that those who write thus use the higher dilutions exclusively. For more substantial doses it seems only necessary that the patient shall be within the first ten days of the fever, or at any rate shall not have passed from the " gastric " into the " typhoid " condition (I use these terms phenomenally), to ensure excellent effects from the drug.

The action of Baptisia in continued fever, like that of Ailanthus in malignant scarlatina, ought not to be allowed to stand alone, but should lead to its application to similar pyrexial states elsewhere encountered. The thirty-first volume of the *British Journal of Homœopathy* contains reports of epidemics of relapsing fever and of smallpox, by Drs. Dyce Brown and Eubulus Williams respectively. In the former malady it acted at least as well as the Bryonia we generally give ; but in the latter it displayed really remarkable powers, enabling hæmorrhagic cases to recover, averting prostration, improving appetite, obviating decomposition (as shown by the absence of the usual offensive effluvia), and preventing pitting. Of 185 cases treated with ordinary homœopathic remedies, 19 died : of 72 treated with Baptisia alone, none.

Dr. Bayes, saying truly that the most marked action of the drug in fevers is to clean the tongue and enable food to be taken, recommends it in analogous gastric conditions, with much sinking at the stomach. I myself find much benefit from it in the feverish colds of aged people, which often assume a low type. I can, moreover, substantiate from experience the high commendation given to it by Dr. Mitchell, of Chicago, as a reducer of the hectic of phthisis.*

The nearest analogue to Baptisia is *Gelsemium*, which takes its place in the " remittent fever " of childhood, now

* See *United States Med. and Surg. Investigator*, vi., 251-4.

maintained by most observers to be of the enteric type. It is
also allied, as an antipyretic, to *Bryonia;* and, more distantly,
to *Acidum muriaticum* and *Rhus.*

Of the dose I have already spoken.

LECTURE XVIII.

BARYTA—BELLADONNA.

I have to-day first of all to speak of the preparations of Barium. Of these we have information as to four, the acetate, the carbonate, the chloride, and the iodide. Let us take first the most important, the carbonate—

Baryta carbonica.

It is of course prepared for our use by trituration.

Baryta carbonica makes its earliest appearance in the first edition of the *Chronic Diseases*, where it has 286 symptoms. In the second edition the list has increased to 794, eight others contributing to it. Many of the additional symptoms, however, were obtained from the acetate. Dr. Allen judiciously isolates those of the carbonate, and, adding some other observations, gives it a pathogenesis of 674 symptoms.

The main interest of Baryta carbonica in my eyes lies in its influence on the *tonsils*. The muriate is, as we shall see, a powerful remedy for glandular engorgements; and the carbonate shares its virtues in an eminent degree when the glands affected are the tonsillar. In chronic enlargements of these organs there is general agreement as to this property of Baryta carbonica; but it is not so well known as a remedy for acute amygdalitis—for *quinsy*. Yet it is here, in my experience, the most potent of medicines. It was from Dr. Ransford that I first got the hint of its value; and he has recently given his experience on the subject.* It was suggested to him, he says, by Dr. Stens, of Bonn; and has since been of unfailing efficacy in his hands. I can speak almost as unreservedly. It is important to distinguish the precise form of angina which calls for Baryta. It is not the inflammation of the mucous membrane, where Belladonna is so potent, or, if there be much œdema, Apis; but it is when the parenchyma of the tonsils is the seat of the mischief. It has rarely occurred to me to see

* *Brit. Journ. of Hom.*, xxxi., 737.

suppuration follow when Baryta has been administered in good
time for this disorder.

It is probable (as Dr. Berridge points out) that Dr. Stens
took the idea of this piece of practice from s. 279 of Hahnemann's pathogenesis, which runs thus :—" After chilliness and
heat and bruised feeling in all the limbs, an inflammation of
the throat, with great swelling of the palate and tonsils, which
suppurate, and on account of which he cannot open the jaws,
speak, or swallow ; with dark-brown urine and sleeplessness."
One would like to know under what circumstances this symptom (which is said to have occurred 18 days after taking the
drug) was observed.

Baryta is also considered a valuable remedy for senility, so
far as this is premature and therefore morbid. It has sometimes removed, in old men (to whom it seems peculiarly adapted), the after-consequences of apoplexy. Dr. Guernsey considers it especially suitable to dwarfish subjects, of stunted
growth both in mind and in body ; and thinks that its action
extends to the lymphatic and salivary glands in the neck.

The medium dilutions—as the 6th and 12th—of this medicine are most in credit, but Dr. Carroll Dunham told me that
he had obtained the effects of Baryta in quinsy from the
200th.

Baryta acetica was, as I have said, the form in which the
metal was proved by several of Hahnemann's fellow-observers. Their symptoms—indicated by Hahnemann with a line
—have been separated from the rest by Dr. Allen ; and, with
those of a recent case of poisoning, are 223 in number.

The poisoning case I have referred to, which was fatal, may
be read in the seventeenth volume of the *Monthly Homœopathic
Review* (p. 505). It revealed an activity on the part of the
salt hitherto unsuspected : the patient died in the full possession of his senses, but with absolute paralysis of all the
voluntary muscles. The observer, Dr. Lagarde, proceeded to
test its action upon himself. " After a lapse of three hours,
discomfort and general weakness with light-headedness set in.
In the upper extremities, and under the scalp and skin of the
face, formication was felt. After a second period of three
hours the weakness had perceptibly increased, and the left
arm could no longer be moved, although sensation was intact.
Dr. L. found it impossible to pull the bell or to leave the bed,
and eight hours after taking the dose the upper and lower
extremities were almost paralysed. The paralysis spread to
the abdomen, then to the chest and neck, and lastly to the

sphincters. Coughing, spitting, and even the uttering of polysyllables, became difficult; the respirations were laboured, and the urine and fæces were evacuated involuntarily. The pulse fell to 56."

Such facts explain the repute of Baryta carbonica in paralytic affections, and suggest the acetate as a still more potent form of administering the metal.

Baryta muriatica, the chloride of barium, was the preparation of the drug given of old in scrofulous disease. Its physiological action is little known; but it has occasionally been given with much benefit in disease of the mesenteric and other glands in the homœopathic triturations, as you may read in Dr. Goullon's treatise on Scrofula. Dr. Hammond, of New York, employs it largely, in doses of a grain or two three times a day, in sclerosis of the brain and cord, and professes to obtain considerable amendment from it. One of our own practitioners, Dr. Flint, of Scarborough, has recently obtained with it striking remedial effects, almost amounting to a cure, in a case of abdominal aneurism, which you may read in the *Monthly Homœopathic Review* for June, 1879, and in the *Practitioner* for July of the same year. He accounts for its effect from the irritating influence on the arterial system which Baryta salts are found, in experiments on animals, to exert. I shall have more to say on this point when I come to the action on aneurism of iodide of potassium.

On *Baryta iodata*, the iodide of barium, you may with advantage read Dr. Hale's article in the fourth edition of his *New Remedies*. He considers it our best remedy in indurated glandular enlargements, as of the tonsils, testes, and perhaps the prostate. Dr. Liebold recommends it in strumous ophthalmia, where the cervical glands are consentaneously affected, and the patient is of stunted growth.*

We now begin the consideration of one of the most important remedies in homœopathic practice—another apt illustration, with Aconite and Arsenic, of the maxim *magis venenum, magis remedium*—the Atropa

Belladonna.

We prepare a tincture from the entire fresh plant in the usual manner.

* Trans. of Amer. Inst. of Hom. for 1874, p. 768.

Hahnemann early devoted attention to the pathogenetic effects of Belladonna, publishing in his *Fragmenta de viribus medicamentorum positivis* (1805) a list of 99 symptoms observed by himself, and 304 taken from records of poisoning and overdosing. In the last edition of the first volume of the *Reine Arzneimittellehre* (1830) the list has swollen to 1440, of which 390 are his own, 585 from thirteen fellow-provers, and 475 from seventy-two authors. Since that time observations of the poisonous effects of the plant have multiplied ; and fresh provings of it, in small doses of the extract, have been made by the Vienna Provers' Society.* These I have myself collated with Hahnemann's pathogenesis, after revising the cited symptoms of the latter from their originals, in an arrangement of the drug for the *Hahnemann Materia Medica* (part iii.). I have included many of the observed effects of atropia, the alkaloid contained in Belladonna, to which most, if not all, of its active properties are due. Among these are some excellent provings conducted under the superintendence of Dr. E. M. Hale, and recorded in the Transactions of the Homœopathic Medical Society of the State of New York for 1868. The provers—four in number—took doses of from the hundredth to the fifth of a grain. The results of recent experimentation with atropia on animals, which has been very extensive, are well summed up by Dr. Horatio Wood ; and to his article, to the chapter on Belladonna by Dr. John Harley in his *Old Vegetable Neurotics,* to the *Etude de la Belladonne* of Dr. Meuriot, and to the essay upon the drug in Hartmann's *Principal Homœopathic Remedies* (translated by Dr. Okie), I shall frequently refer in the course of my remarks. I should say that Dr. Allen gives separate pathogeneses of atropia and of Belladonna itself.

Belladonna is an excellent illustration of the fruitfulness of the Hahnemannian as compared with the ordinary method of studying medicines. The traditional plan has been to find out by a few experiments in what class or classes a drug is to be ranked—whether it is emetic, purgative, sudorific, narcotic, and so forth ; and then to use it in disease when it is thought desirable to obtain such effects from it. But Hahnemann taught that every drug must be studied as a separate individual ; that no general expression or classification can describe its action ; and that a complete register of the effects it produces is indispensable for its use as a medicine. The result of the former course of proceeding has been to class Belladonna as a narcotic and sedative, and to use it in a few

* See *Brit. Journ. of Hom.,* vi.

forms of pain and spasm. To these, previously to the
endosmose from homœopathy which has set in during the last
twelve years, the employment of the drug was restricted, save
for its old employment as a " resolvent," and when Trousseau
gave it empirically in constipation and acute rheumatism.
But the symptoms obtained from it by Hahnemann and those
who have followed him display its influence on well-nigh
every part of the organism ; and suggest its application to a
great variety of morbid phenomena.

But now in applying, as well as in studying our medicines,
the method of Hahnemann is the only one largely available.
What use can be made of the information obtained except
upon the principle of *similia similibus?* What avails it to
know that Belladonna disorders perception, ideation, and
emotion in the hundred and more various ways I have exhibited in my arrangement ? There is no malady in which it
can be desirable to set up such disorder. But the rule, " let
likes be treated by likes," at once lays hold of the whole body
of morbid phenomena induced by a drug, and applies it to the
treatment of disease. Because Belladonna has this vast range
of poisonous action, therefore and just so far has it power to
cure. It thus sprang rapidly, in the hands of Hahnemann
and his disciples, into the first rank of polychrests. The
observations of Hartmann well exhibit its estimation and employment in the homœopathic school. His catalogue of
disorders in which it has been found beneficial includes the
great majority of fevers, inflammations, congestions and
neuroses. It is probably more frequently prescribed in
homœopathic practice for acute disease than any other medicine save Aconite.

Let us first consider the traditional knowledge and use of
the drug, and see how far it can be recommended as worthy
of imitation.

1. It had long been noted, as Pereira says, that Belladonna
relieved external pains rather than internal. Physiological
experimentation has now explained this, by showing that the
extremities of the sensory nerves are affected by it before
their trunks, which indeed require large doses to influence
them. Thus çutaneous anæsthesia is most readily induced by
the local application of the drug ; but it occasionally appears
after its ingestion. It was a prominent symptom in Dr. Hale's
provers; and the amaurosis which we shall see caused so
often by Belladonna is of a piece with it.

Belladonna is thus a strictly local anæsthetic, acting as such
even when introduced into the general circulation. The only

truly analogous morbid state, as a whole, to that induced by
it is the absence of sensibility which sometimes exists in
mental disorder.   But the antipathic action of the drug may
here find a legitimate sphere of usefulness, and it may be employed—locally applied in ointment, liniment, and plaster—as
an anodyne for external pains.   Perhaps we homœopathists
do not avail ourselves sufficiently of such palliative aids,
which, with proper precautions, are as harmless as they are
comforting.

2. Belladonna affects the motor just as it does the sensory
nerves, *i.e.*, paralysing their extremities first, and then (if in
sufficient quantity) their trunks.   Its action on the motor
centres is, as we shall see hereafter, somewhat different.   But
this power of causing peripheral paralysis is turned to useful
account when the drug is employed locally as an anti-
spasmodic, as (for instance) in rigidity of the os uteri during
labour.   Such a use of it is probably seen in its control over
the nocturnal enuresis of children.   The bladder is one of the
few organs which it paralyses when taken internally ; and to a
lesser degree of the same influence must generally, I think, be
referred its power in this malady, which implies excess of
irritability rather than want of power.   The main proof of
this position is that large doses are required—ten or twenty
drops of the tincture ; and homœopathic records are signifi-
cantly silent on the practice.*   I have never seen any benefit
from the doses we ordinarily use ; and in this case we need
not fear the production of physiological effects from the
internal administration of the drug in substance, as children
below puberty are singularly insusceptible to its disturbing
influence.

3. Almost the same remarks may be made as to the action
of Belladonna on the sympathetic nerve-fibres, only that here
(with a not uncommon antagonism) it excites instead of
depressing.   But here also it affects primarily the extremities
of the nerves ; and its influence is only certainly manifest
when it is locally applied,—the dilatation of the pupil being the
sole witness to it after internal administration.   In this sphere,
too, we avail ourselves of the physiological action of the drug,
using it locally as a mydriatic.   I shall return to this subject,
when I come to its action on the eye.

4. There is yet another power of Belladonna which may

---

* Dr. Claude records two cases of cure by it in the homœopathic
attenuations ; but he admits that he has generally been disappointed
with it (*L'Art Médical*, xlviii., 345).

often be usefully employed, but which as yet is difficult of explanation ; I mean the arrest of secretion it causes, notably in the salivary glands and the skin. That this action is exerted through the nerves is pretty certain, both from the rapidity with which it is induced, and from the antagonism displayed in regard to it by such pure neurotics as pilocarpin, muscaria, and physostigma. But it can hardly be brought about by vaso-motor excitation, as the dried surfaces are congested rather than anæmic ; nor will the depression of the chorda tympani which is proved to exist account for its action on the sudoriparous glands, which have not (as far as we know) any such excitor nerves as have the salivary. But, however caused, the arrest of secretion which Belladonna brings about may not unfrequently be induced with benefit to our patients. We have probably better ways of checking the sweats of phthisis or other such fluxes, which require the internal administration of the drug. But its local application in hidrosis of the hands or feet, in salivation, and—above all— to check the secretion of milk in sudden weaning or threat- ened mastitis, is a practice often fraught with advantage.

I have willingly dwelt on these actions of Belladonna, as in them we are on common ground with our brethren of the old school, and in our frank acceptance of such practices lies one of the hopes of a better understanding in the future. The local and functional influence of the drug herein displayed can be better utilised in the way of antipathic palliation than in that of homœopathic cure. But it would be a great error to suppose that in such physiological effects and their applica- tion on the antipathic principle we have the whole sphere of the drug. When we look a little farther, we see behind these phenomena of the periphery central disturbances of a very different kind. While the retina is insensible to actual objects, visual hallucinations throng about the subject of Belladonna's influence. While the dilated pupil would indicate that the brain was suffering from anæmia or effusion, its actual condi- tion is that of active congestion and often furious excitement. These phenomena—as also the dry throat, the scarlet skin, and the conjunctival and vesical irritation which so often appear—point to properties of another kind. Now, although writers on Materia Medica treat of Belladonna as a pure nar- cotic, a toxicologist like Christison does not hesitate to class it among the narcotico-*acrids*, adducing several instances in which inflammatory irritation—as of the throat and bladder— has resulted from its ingestion. We have only to suppose that it exerts this influence upon the cerebro-spinal centres also—that it irritates nervous tissue besides disordering nervous function ; and the whole problem is solved. The symptoms of tissue-irritation are seen at the centre, those of functional excitation or depression at the periphery of the nervous system ; and hence the double set of phenomena manifested.

Let us now consider, in this light, the disturbances set up by Belladonna in the brain and cord; and the therapeutic applications to which they have led under the guidance of the law of similars. We may divide our matter according as the phenomena are those of sensibility, of motility, of the cerebral functions proper, or of the brain as a material organ.

1. The sensory disturbance caused by our drug varies according as the centre or the periphery is most affected. In the latter case we have the anæsthesia which has already come before us ; in the former we have such a condition as this, reported by Hahnemann, and confirmed by Harley—"great irritability and impressionableness of all the senses ; he tastes and smells everything more acutely ; the sense of taste, of sight, and of hearing is keener, and the mind is more easily moved and the thoughts more active." Such hyperæsthesia is always found to be an indication for Belladonna in homœopathic practice. To this point the statements of Pereira are singularly though unconsciously pertinent. " In the first degree of its operation," he writes, " Belladonna diminishes sensibility and irritability. This effect (called by some sedative) *is scarcely obvious in the healthy organism*, but is well seen in morbid states, when these properties are preternaturally increased."

2. The central motor disorder caused by Belladonna is quite analogous to its sensory disturbance, but is of more varied character. Now we see twitchings, jerkings, and jactitations like those of chorea, to which in one case of poisoning they were compared by the reporter.[*] Now the symptoms are tetaniform ; the animals experimented upon, says Dr. Fraser, appear as if suffering from strychnia.[†] Still more frequently, in severe cases of poisoning, clonic convulsions of epileptic type appear.[‡] Again, there may simply be great restlessness and bodily inquietude.[§]

All this is of a piece with the hyperæsthesia we have seen in the sensory sphere, and, like that, indicates the homœopathic

* See *Hahn. Mat. Med.*, part iii., s. 22.
† *Ibid.* s. 28, 29.
‡ *Ibid.*, s. 36-43.
§ *Ibid.*, s. 44-47.

use of the medicine. In chorea and tetanus we have scant records of its employment. Dr. Hoyne relates an instance of its favourable action in the latter disorder (1, 39); and Dr. Croucher has lately communicated a case in which a Belladonna plaster along the spine seems to have been the curative agent*. But in eclampsia, infantile and puerperal, it is largely and successfully used among us; and in epilepsy itself has no mean reputation. It probably acts here by modifying the irritability of the medulla oblongata, to which Schroeder van der Kolk has taught us to look as the centre of the epileptic convulsion. By the same action it influences hydrophobia, whose phenomena seem to depend on inflammatory irritation of the medulla and its issuing nerves; and thus also it occasionally benefits laryngismus, whooping-cough, and asthma. If it is to do good in affections like these, the patients must (as a rule) be young and impressionable subjects, of sanguine-nervous temperament; and, in epilepsy, the malady should be of recent origin. The use of the remedy on a large scale in this last disease—as by Greding,[†] Grandi,[‡] and Michéa[§]—where all sorts of cases are taken together, has not yielded any great percentage of cures. But Trousseau, after thirty years' experience, declared the Belladonna treatment of epilepsy the least inefficacious he had known; and speaks of having obtained a certain number of solid cures. Dr. Echeverria finds it beneficial in epileptic vertigo. As to hydrophobia the question is still more doubtful. But it is impossible to read the mass of evidence collected by Bayle[||] without concluding that Belladonna must sometimes have cured, and has often prevented, this dire disease, to which it is confessedly homœopathic in the first degree. Youatt had no small confidence in it as a prophylactic in dogs themselves.[¶]

So far the motor disturbance of Belladonna has been obviously connected with its irritant influence on the nervous centres. But now a glance at its pathogenesis will show a good many symptoms of loss of power over the extremities; and this not from exhaustion only, but occurring comparatively early in the poisoning. Sometimes, from atropia especially, the limbs are heavy and helpless: the condition is compared by one observer to the first stage of the progressive paralysis of the insane. More commonly, with Belladonna

* *Brit. Journ. of Hom.*, xxxiii, 266.
† *Adv. Med. Pract.*, ed. Ludwig, vol. i.
‡ *Gaz. Méd. de Paris*, 1854, p. 757.
§ *Gaz. des Hôpitaux*, 1861, p. 563-578.
|| *Bibl. de Thérap*, ii., 502.
¶ See Watson's *Lectures*, 4th ed., i., 629.

itself, there is a loss of co-ordination, resembling that of locomotor ataxy. I have pointed out in another place* that the poison causes nearly all the apparently incongruous symptoms which characterise this singular disease. In the eye it produces the injected conjunctiva ; the dilated, sometimes varying pupils ; the ptosis ; and the diplopia and amaurosis so often observed in ataxy. It develops incontinence of urine and tactile anæsthesia ; and (according to Brown-Séquard) depression of reflex excitability. Since, moreover, the pathological basis of the phenomena of this disease is in the first instance of inflammatory nature, it would be the truest homœopathy to give Belladonna as a remedy in its early stages. I have had one well-characterised though incipient case, in which a complete cure has been effected by the 1st decimal dilution of the drug. And such an application of the remedy should not stand alone. It has been ascertained that a morbid process similar to that of locomotor ataxy, but occurring in other tracts of the cord—a slow inflammation going on to induration or softening—lies at the root of many other diseases. This has been well shown by Dr. Jousset in respect of the muscular tremblings of *sclérose en plaques*, of spinal paralysis, of general paralysis of the insane, of the glosso-laryngeal paralysis of Duchenne, of infantile palsy, and of progressive muscular atrophy.† I should myself be inclined to extend it also to such affections as neuralgia, glaucoma, and exophthalmic goitre, in all of which we shall find our Belladonna in repute. It is of course in the incipience of these maladies—in their stage of excitement—that the remedy is indicated. Trousseau and Pidoux speak of Bretonneau as having obtained in several cases of paraplegia a cure as unexpected as inexplicable by the use of the drug.

3. We come now to the action of Belladonna in the mental and moral sphere, which is one of the most potent it exerts. Perception, ideation, and emotion are equally affected ; and in a manner similar to that which we have seen in the regions of sensibility and movement. The drug excites and at the same time perverts their function,—blunting their reaction to real impressions while quickening in them a feverish automatic activity, spurring them on in a rapid and disordered course until they fail for exhaustion. Hallucinations (Stillé says that the spectral illusions of Belladonna are all of a bright gleaming character), delirium (often compared to delirium tremens), insane talking and acting, melancholy and rage are

---

* *On the Various Forms of Paralysis*, 1869.
† Translated from *L'Art Médical* in *Brit. Journ. of Hom.*, xxxiii., 577.

the features of this part of the pathogenesis of Belladonna; and are present in the same degree and variety in that of no other drug save its congeners, Hyoscyamus and Stramonium.

Correspondingly, Belladonna occupies in homœopathic practice the first rank among the remedies for cerebral disturbance. It is best indicated in the sthenic and congestive delirium of the fevers and exanthemata; in mania-a-potu; in *furor transitorius;* and in acute maniacal delirium, the *délire aigue* of the French. A case of this last kind, related by Dr. Maudsley, resulted from transfer of erysipelas from the leg to the brain; and to this disease we shall hereafter see Belladonna strikingly homœopathic and curative. It should also be serviceable in acute melancholia; and in the alternation of epilepsy with insanity. Hitherto, indeed, homœopathy has had little opportunity of proving its powers in the treatment of mental disease. But now that the New York State Asylum has been erected for carrying out our method in the care of the insane, we shall soon learn what we can do in this direction, and how to do it. Dr. Butler tells me that Belladonna has been one of the medicines most largely and beneficially used there; and Dr. Talcott, the present superintendent, speaks warmly of it in acute mania.* In the ordinary practice, Belladonna was of old time often employed with success in mania and mental disorder generally. Trousseau and Pidoux justify this use of the drug, naïvely remarking that "experience has proved that a multitude of maladies are cured by therapeutic agents which seem to act in the same manner as the cause of the disease they oppose."

4. Throughout these pictures of sensory, motor, and mental disorder we continually have more or less evidence of the co-existence of active determination of blood. The disturbance set up is indeed, as I have argued, *inflammatory* in essence. Still more marked is this feature when we come to the symptoms of the head itself. The vertigo, intoxication and headache so constantly occurring in the provers are all hyperæmic in character; and in poisonings we have phenomena of acute cerebral congestion, going on sometimes nearly to phrenitis, more frequently to apoplexy. For the evidence of this I must refer you to my arrangement of the drug in the *Hahnemann Materia Medica :* I must here pass at once to its therapeutical applications.

The vertigo of Belladonna is, as I have said, hyperæmic; it is worse on movement and relieved in the open air. In Dr. Harley's experiments its development seemed to coincide

* *Homœopathic Times,* vii., 1.

with the rise of the pulse. Such congestive vertigo, when
occurring in subjects not too advanced in life, yields readily
to the drug. Of its headache I have been able to collect no
less than seventy-eight instances, including almost every
variety of the affection. Its most frequent seat is the forehead and the temples. Belladonna is, from these effects, and
from clinical experience, our chief remedy in headache. It is
suited both to the nervous or neuralgic form, and to the
congestive. Heavy, drooping eyelids, and blindness or flashes
of light before the eyes, point to it; also flushed face, hot
head, and sense of burning in the eyeballs. Secondary vomiting does not contra-indicate it; but in true gastric headache it
is of no use. The Belladonna headache is always aggravated
by light, noise, and movement, and also by lying down; it is
easiest in a quiet sitting posture. Its essential characters,
indéed, are hyperæmia and hyperæsthesia.

It is but a step farther to say that in arterial congestion of
the brain, from almost any cause, Belladonna is an invaluable
remedy. The only instance in which it is outrivalled is the
cerebral hyperæmia of sun-stroke, where Glonoin takes its
place; though not necessarily to its exclusion. Nor does it
cease to be of avail when the congestion runs on to inflammation. I must agree with Bähr that its action does not
reach to meningitis, if the meninges he has in view are the
dura mater and arachnoid. Over the inflammatory results of
injury to the skull it has thus little power. But in ordinary
phrenitis or encephalitis, such as we meet with in the course
of reaction from concussion, and as the result of mental
excitement, intemperance, and such-like causes, Belladonna
is (with or without Aconite) the main remedy; that is, if the
patient is in the first stage of the disorder, and not in that of
effusion or collapse. It is no less valuable in apoplexy, as
long as cerebral hyperæmia is present, whether before or after
extravasation has occurred. Here, too, it is useful to check
the tendency to secondary inflammation.

Before leaving the sphere of the nervous system, I must
speak of the action of Belladonna in neuralgia. Its causation
of this phenomenon is doubtful,—only one symptom of the
kind being on record, in the fourth of Dr. Hale's provers.*
But Dr. Anstie has argued (mainly on the ground of the
numerous complications so often present in severe cases—as
spasms, paralyses, inflammations, disorders of nutrition, secretion, and sensation) that true neuralgia is always of central
origin. The particular seat of it he thinks the posterior root

* See *Hahn. Mat. Med.*, part iii, s. 438.

of the spinal nerve in which the pain is felt. In reviewing Dr. Anstie's admirable treatise in the *British Journal of Homœo-pathy** I have suggested that it is rather to the grey nucleus we should look than to the issuing fibres. I have also pointed out that the analogy of locomotor ataxy, whose pains Dr. Anstie characterises as truly neuralgic, indicates that the central mischief is primarily at least of an inflammatory nature. If these things are so, we have no difficulty in understanding how Belladonna cures neuralgia homœopathically, though it has not time enough to set it up. The neuralgia which indicates it is of comparatively recent origin, and occurs in young or middle-aged persons. It is associated with marked symptoms of hyperæmia, and differs from that of Aconite—which otherwise it so closely resembles—in having hyperæsthesia present. It is usually situate in the trigeminus (especially the right one),—the drug having little influence over sciatica or other neuralgiæ occurring below the head and neck. This is also the experience of Trousseau.

Dr. Bayes says that a characteristic symptom here is accession or aggravation of the paroxysm at about 5 P.M.; while Dr. Guernsey notes of the pains that they come and go with great celerity, and are made worse by the least jar. Dr. Dunham considers the remedy not less indicated when the pains, though suddenly disappearing, gradually increase to their acme.

I have now concluded what I have to say of the action of Belladonna upon the nervous centres. We have seen it everywhere inducing excited but perverted functional activity, increased manifestation of energy with diminution of real power and effectiveness. Such are the hyperæsthesia in the sensory sphere, the jactitation in the motor, and the delirium in the ideational, which it confessedly developes. The phenomena precisely correspond with the more active production of cells of a low order—the "increased attraction" of nutrient fluid with "diminished selection"—displayed by the non-nervous tissues when inflamed. I have accordingly suggested† that they imply inflammatory irritation of the nervous substance on the part of the drug, and have supported my view by pointing to the active hyperæmia which is always more or less manifestly present. This doctrine has indeed long been tacitly accepted in the school of Hahnemann, as shown by the universal recognition of the homœopathicity of

* xxx., 367.
† I first did so—as a result of a study of the drug carried out with Dr. Madden—in the *Brit. Journ. of Hom.* for 1862 (vol. xx).

Belladonna to cerebral inflammation : I have only put it into the language of modern pathology. We are glad to receive for it the support of Dr. Harley. At the end of his analysis of the effects of the drug he concludes that " the whole of the phenomena may be attributed to excessive stimulation of the nerve-centre. attended by increased oxidation ;" and that " hyperoxidation of nerve-tissue " is the essential action of the poison. This is but the same thing in other words.

But observe the difference in practical results. Dr. Harley's conclusions lead him to no therapeutic application of the drug ; while ours, by the way indicated by the rule *similia similibus*, have made it the prime remedy for all disorders of the nervous centres in which hyperæmia is associated with hyperæsthesia or pain, disordered co-ordination or clonic convulsion, hallucination, excitement, or delirium. It is in such conditions a remedy most highly prized by all who practise homœopathically ; and by none more so than those among them who most habitually employ infinitesimal doses. The remedy thus reflects confirmation and honour on the method that created it, and adds another and no insignificant leaf to Hahnemann's laurel crown.

LECTURE XIX.

BELLADONNA *(continued)*.

At our last meeting we made a full study of the action of Belladonna in the sphere of the nervous system, where we meet with its most prominent effects and frequent uses. But we have yet to see it operating as a potent agent in several other regions. I shall speak of it to-day as it affects the circulation and temperature, the mucous membranes and skin, the eyes, the urinary organs, and the uterus ; concluding with some miscellaneous applications which it has received.

I. Belladonna, in not too excessive doses, increases the action of the heart both in force and frequency. The latter phenomenon seems due to paresis of the inhibitory fibres of the vagi,—the drug acting (as we have seen it do elsewhere) on the extremities of the nerves in the heart.* But were this its only property, there would be no increase of the force of the circulation ; and for this we must invoke the stimulant action on the sympathetic which we have already seen it displaying, and which—if exerted—would make the heart's beats stronger as well as more rapid. Thus also we account for the fact that the arteries are contracted under its influence, and the blood-pressure increased. Such arterial contraction was long ago ascertained to follow its application to the frog's web by Mr. Wharton Jones,† and the same thing has been observed as a consequence of its internal administration by Hughes Bennett‡ and by Harley. Many years ago, before I knew anything of homœopathy, I made an attempt to account for its whole action on the body by means of this influence ;§ and, though the generalisation was unwarranted, the fact remains established. Dr. Handfield Jones, it is true‖ —and also Dr. Dyce Brown¶—has assumed an opposite action on its part, on account of the hyperæmia manifested in

---

* A full account of the experimentation by which this action of atropia is ascertained is given by Dr. Lauder Brunton, in his *Experimental Investigation of the action of Medicines*, part i., p. 60.

† *Brit. and For. Med. Review*, xiv., 603.

‡ *Researches into the Antagonism of Medicines*, 1875, p. 41.

§ See *London Med. Review* for 1860.

‖ *Functional Nervous Disorders*, sub voce.

¶ *Monthly Hom. Review*, xv , 353.

the head and on other surfaces by the subjects of its influence.
But it must be remembered that there are two ways in which
the circulation in any part may be increased,—the one by
relaxation of its blood-vessels, the other by irritation of its
tissue. Opium, Amyl nitrite, and Glonoin, which primarily
dilate the arteries, may well be conceived to act in the first of
these two ways : Belladonna, which contracts them, can only
congest a part by irritating its substance, and so compelling a
larger afflux of blood. In this way—as we have seen in the
nervous system, and as we shall see in many other parts—I
account for the hyperæmia manifested under the influence of
our present drug.—Belladonna of course conforms to the law
of other stimuli, and in excessive quantities exhausts the susceptibility of, and so paralyses, the organs it naturally excites.
But such actions are, as I apprehend, beyond the sphere of
true pharmacodynamics, as available for therapeutic purposes.

The above phenomena, which I have expressed as obtained
by modern experimentation, have many prototypes in the
symptoms of poisoning and proving collected by Hahnemann.
Moreover, the febrile condition so repeatedly recorded by the
latter as resulting from the drug has now been demonstrated to
be a true *pyrexia*. "The similarity," writes Dr. Harley, "of the
general phenomena which attend the operation of Belladonna
and those which accompany pneumonia, enteritis, the development of pus in any of the tissues and organs of the body, &c.,
arrests attention ;" and again—"an infinitesimal quantity of
atropia—a mere atom—as soon as it enters the blood, originates an action which is closely allied to, if it be not identical
with, that which induces the circulatory and nervous phenomena accompanying meningitis, enteric, or typhus fever."
Other experimenters also have found a considerable elevation
of temperature—from 1 to 4 degrees centigrade—under the
action of atropia. The fever induced differs considerably from
that of Aconite and Arsenic. The chill is slight, and sweating is rare after the heat : the heat itself is very decided, the
surface feeling burning, but there is no great thirst, nor is
there either the prostration of Arsenic, or the restless,
uneasy, anxious condition especially characteristic of Aconite.

We of the homœopathic school have long ago drawn from
such facts the inference that Belladonna has an important
place in the treatment of the primary fevers ; and that where
pyrexia accompanies inflammation of parts which it specifically
irritates (as the brain or throat) it suffices to control both the
general and the local phenomena. It is interesting to
find Dr. Harley coming to the same conclusion. "It appears,"

he writes, "that the stimulant action of Belladonna is converted in great measure in febrile diseases into a tonic and sedative influence." He gives it largely in the continued fever to which he likens its action ; and in the pyrexia symptomatic of inflammations explains its *modus operandi* thus — " two similar effects, the one arising from a local irritation and the other from the presence of Belladonna, like spreading circles on a smooth sheet of water, interfere with and neutralise each other." He believes that " it has not yet attained to its legitimate place as a therapeutic agent," and anticipates that " its sphere of usefulness will be acknowledged before long to be co-extensive with acute disease itself." If he would look into homœopathic literature he would find that Belladonna had attained this its " legitimate place " among those whom he stigmatises as " blindly led by an unscientific dogma " at least fifty years ago ; and that the analogy by which he explains its action is a household word among them.

The kind of fever to which Belladonna is specifically applicable is that in which the excessive oxidation in which the febrile process may be conceived to exist falls chiefly on the nervous centres. The type to which it conforms is that which our forefathers described as " typhus nervosus." The most familiar example of the kind is the " brain fever" of over-excitement ; but a similar condition is often presented by the toxæmic fevers. It is where there is too much blood-poisoning for Aconite to act, but not enough to require Arsenic, and where the disorder of the vegetative life for which Baptisia is indicated is less prominent than that of the nervous centres, that Belladonna finds its sphere. It is thus very frequently our main antipyretic in the earlier stages of continued fever, especially when presenting the form which used to be called " cerebral typhus." Turgor of the face, often with shining eyes, is characteristic for it here. It also supplants Aconite in puerperal fever, and in the more profoundly penetrating exanthemata. In the initial fever of variola it has received high commendation in both schools.* With scarlatina its name is inseparably connected, from the virtues claimed for it by Hahnemann as a (temporary) prophylactic against the disease. His account of how he arrived at this estimate of it is very interesting : you may read it at p. 466 of Dr. Dudgeon's translation of his *Lesser Writings.* Much controversy has raged on this subject, and very different results have been obtained by different experimenters. I think (as does Dr. Stillé, no favourable judge) that the conclusion must be in

* See *London Med. Record,* Feb. 15, 1879.

favour of its pretensions; and that we do well in administering it—according to the custom of most homœopathists—whenever scarlatina breaks out in a household. The analogy of the prophylaxis of ague by quinine makes strongly in its favour.

It was the homœopathicity of Belladonna to scarlatina which led Hahnemann to it; and, though some rash controversialists have questioned the fact, it is generally admitted. Not merely has the cutaneous irritation of the drug (which sometimes ends in desquamation) been compared by many observers to the scarlatinal eruption, but we have also in the disorder the fever, the angina faucium, and the delirium also induced by the drug. It thus naturally plays an important part in our practice in the curative as well as the prophylactic treatment of scarlatina. Hahnemann lays much stress on its being the " smooth " scarlatina in which Belladonna is so potent to prevent and cure : disappointment, he says, has commonly proceeded from confounding this with the *rothe Friesel*, which is a different malady. It is the smooth scarlatina which we ordinarily see in this country.

II. Together with its pyrexia, Belladonna congests the mucous and cutaneous surfaces throughout the body. " The mucous membranes," writes Dr. Meuriot, " ten minutes after the injection of atropia, are red, injected, and dry." This seems to be the rationale of the well-known dry mouth of the drug. It is not the mere result of diminished saliva, nor of occluded arteries : " the blood-vessels of the part," says Dr. Harley, " are congested, and the blood is arrested." After a time, the dryness is relieved by a secretion of mucus, foul and viscid; and therewith the pulse falls. In fever, as the same author states, atropia will moisten the dry tongue, moderating the circulation at the same time.

This condition of mucous membrane is probably induced by the drug throughout the body : it explains many of the symptoms it causes, and warrants the use of the medicine in similar dry catarrhs wherever occurring. At some points, however, the action runs on to actual phlegmonous inflammation. Besides the conjunctiva (of which I shall speak hereafter), this condition is best seen in the throat, which is one of the cardinal centres of the action of Belladonna. Dryness, dysphagia, constriction, soreness, painful deglutition, swelling and burning, are the sensations experienced here by the subjects of its influence ; and the physical signs of inflammation are often evident. Correspondingly, for acute sore throat Belladonna is as complete a specific as medicine can present. It is specially indicated where there are much heat and pain on swallowing, bright redness of the affected parts, flushed face, and headache. When the parenchyma of the tonsils is involved—when we have true quinsy—I confess I prefer Baryta carbonica. But Hahnemann himself extols Belladonna here ; and cites a case* where quinsy supervened during the treatment of jaundice by Belladonna—whether *post* or *propter* can hardly be decided. Elsewhere the signs of its tonsillar influence are not very prominent.

III. The skin is affected with Belladonna much as are the mucous membranes ; it becomes dry, red, and hot. Sometimes, especially in the face,† the action goes on to inflammation ; and we have the condition which makes it as similar as it is potent in the treatment of erysipelas. Every one who has adopted this bit of homœopathy from us—from Liston of old down to Ringer to-day—speaks highly in its praise. Here, as in the throat, it is the smooth, tense, bright-red surface which calls for it ; when much œdema exists, Apis is considered preferable, and when many vesicles form, Rhus— though Dr. Yeldham would have us rely upon Belladonna in every variety of the disease. Boils and carbuncles, which bear so close a relation to erysipelas, may generally be helped— the former often blighted—by our medicine.

IV. I come now to a very important and interesting sphere of the action of Belladonna,—I mean the eye. The points which here arise for physiological discussion would well-nigh occupy a lecture of themselves : I must sternly confine myself to a statement of the facts and to practical conclusions.

Belladonna displays in the visual apparatus nearly all the actions of which we have seen it possessed. It anæsthetises the retina ; it depresses the motor oculi, and excites the sympathetic fibres which animate the iris ; it frets the visual centres to hallucinations, and inflames the conjunctiva. Let us consider,—first its inflammatory effects ; secondarily, its influence upon the pupil ; thirdly, the disorder of vision produced by it.

1. That Belladonna inflames the eye is very obvious. The injection of the ocular membranes present during its action is not merely symptomatic of cerebral hyperæmia, but is a direct tissue irritation, which has often gone on to conjunctivitis. Evidence of a similar condition in the sclerotica, iris, and even retina, is not wanting in the pathogenesis of the drug ; and the same may be said of the lachrymal sac and canals.‡

* S. 507.—See *Brit. Journ. of Hom.*, xxxi., 476.
† *Hahn. Mat. Med.*, part iii., s. 424-7.
‡ *Ibid*, s. 449, 458, 472-3, 502, 508-9, 532-4, 538-44.

Belladonna is, accordingly, a prime remedy in homœopathic practice for inflammatory affections of the eyes. It is indicated in the severer forms of catarrhal ophthalmia, and in strumous ophthalmia when of inflammatory type; also (say Drs. Allen and Norton) in the acute exacerbations of chronic disease, as granular ophthalmia. Sense of burning and dryness in the eyes is characteristic of it here. I have seen it act admirably in two cases of iritis of traumatic origin. Its use as a mydriatic in iritis generally is well known and universally adopted : I am not sure but that part of the good it does is due to its specific operation. Dr. Anstie thinks that he has seen incipient glaucoma checked by the subcutaneous injection of a minute dose of atropia in the neighbourhood of the eye, whilst not uncommonly, in chronic glaucoma, its employment has been known to cause an inflammatory attack. The fact that this peculiar affection is often a trigeminal neurosis, of cerebral origin, and liable to complicate neuralgia of that nerve, would also suggest the possible usefulness of Belladonna in it, as we have seen in the case of Aconite. Our remedy is suitable to retinal hyperæmia,—especially (Drs. Allen and Norton say) if a red conjunctival line is very marked along the line of fissure of the lids ; and even to retinitis when acute and recent. A good cure with it of the latter affection is recorded by a son of the Hartmann whose monograph on the drug I have mentioned,* and another by Dr. Norton. It has also cured optic neuritis.

2. The dilatation of the pupil so readily and uniformly caused by Belladonna has long been a subject of great interest. I have always been one of those who have maintained that the phenomenon is due to excitation of the radiating fibres of the iris through the sympathetic.† Dr. Harley has reinforced our side,—advancing against the opposite hypothesis of mere paralysis of the third nerve the very different effects of Conium (which undoubtedly causes such paralysis) and Belladonna on the eye. Dr. H. Wood, after reviewing all recent experimentation, concludes that here (as also in the heart and intestines) both kinds of influence are at work—the cerebro-spinal fibres being depressed and the sympathetic excited. But the most important fact he brings forward is that the whole action is a local one, even when the drug reaches the eye through the general circulation. For thus is explained that to which I have often called attention,—that the dilated pupil of Belladonna is quite unconnected with its cerebral

* *Brit. Journ. of Hom.*, xxxi., 182.
† See *Ibid*, xxii , 435.

effects, which indeed, when occurring idiopathically, are associated with contraction rather than expansion of the iridal aperture. Dilated pupils, therefore, are at least no necessary homœopathic indication for the use of Belladonna in cerebral disorders; and often tell of a condition of exhaustion or effusion to which the drug is quite unsuitable. Mere phenomenal homœopathy would demand their presence to make up the totality of symptoms; but here, as in so many places, physiology enables us to correct the impressions of our senses, and to obtain *similia* which shall be real and not apparent only. On the other hand, when Graves recommended the administration of Belladonna in the head affections of fever, when the pupils were contracted, although he thought himself acting upon the old principle of antipathy, his remedy was really homœopathic to the morbid condition present.

I do not of course deny that a dilated pupil may be one of a group of symptoms to which Belladonna is homœopathic and curative. It is a part of the general influence of the drug on the sympathetic (and perhaps musculo-motor) nervous system, though not of that which it ordinarily exerts upon the brain-substance. Thus Dr. Harley, when speaking of its action in fever as just the opposite of that which it exerts in health, says—" it may happen, if we give a dose of atropia to a patient with a pulse of 120 or higher, a dry and hard tongue, and pupils measuring the ¼", that after ten, twenty, or thirty minutes, when the action of the belladonna is fully developed, the pulse will be decreased, the tongue be moist, *and the pupils contracted.*" So von Graefe has sometimes observed ephemeral mydriasis as a premonitory symptom of insanity, especially of ambitious monomania.

3. The impairment of vision caused by Belladonna is of two kinds. That which is produced by its local application is *far-sightedness.* It is hardly correct to call it either hyper-metropia (as Dr. Harley does) or presbyopia (as it is generally styled); for both these names connote substantive alterations in the refracting media of the eye, while all that atropia produces is loss of power of accommodation for near objects. That it effects this by paralysing the ciliary muscle, through the nerves from the third which supply it, seems abundantly proved; and I must abandon the view which, in agreement with Dr. Harley, I formerly held as to the part played by the iris in the process.

No therapeutic inference, upon the homœopathic principle, is deducible from this action of the drug. But Pereira is mistaken in supposing that the impaired vision of Belladonna is

" chiefly or entirely presbyopia." It has been noted when no mydriasis has been present, and therefore presumably no paralysis of the accommodation.* I must, therefore, explain some at least of the blindness so often noted from its ingestion by a direct anæsthetic influence exerted by it upon the retina, analogous to that which it displays at other points of nerve-termination. Whether its occasional curative power in "amaurosis" is due to such an action I cannot say. Symptoms of hyperæmia, with photopsies and chromopsies (as red sparks, flames, bright spots, lights, &c.), or chromatic appearances of bright objects, have generally been present in such cases ; and suggest, as they do in the pathogenesis of the drug (where they frequently appear), congestion of the retina.

V. I have now to speak of the action of Belladonna on the urinary organs. Passing out with the renal secretion, it excites the circulation of the kidneys on its way ; causing either diuresis, or—if the dose be large—congestion and stasis, with diminution or even temporary suppression of urine. It seems to be the primary or Malpighian circulation of the kidneys which is influenced by Belladonna : there is no reason to suppose that it has any direct action on the secreting cells of the convoluted tubes. Belladonna, therefore, does not accompany the scarlatinal poison the whole length of its course. When tubal nephritis has been set up, it cannot neutralise the mischief; though it may (like Terebinthina) do good by unloading the Malpighian capillaries, and so setting free a copious flow of urine to flush the ducts. But if renal hyperæmia, whether from scarlatina or from cold, go no farther than to produce defective secretion, hæmaturia, or even albuminuria, Belladonna may be all that is required. Dr. Harley thinks highly of it in the last-named condition ; and himself points out that the quantity of albumen is liable to be increased " unless the dose is a very small one." That is, he admits its action to be homœopathic.

Descending from the kidneys to the bladder, we find the latter powerfully affected by Belladonna. The condition most frequently set up is well illustrated in a case seen by Sir William Jenner, where a Belladonna plaster had been placed on a somewhat abraded surface of the body. Two hours after the first appearance of the symptoms, " the patient was affected with an extreme desire to micturate, though he could pass only a few drops of perfectly colourless urine. From this time till he lost consciousness, his desire to pass urine was constant :

* See *Hahn. Mat. Med.*, part iii., s. 545-6.
† *Ibid*, s. 553-4.

whenever he could retire, he did so, but succeeded in expelling from the bladder, with considerable effort, only a few drops of colourless fluid." I cannot agree with Dr. Harley that this frequent and urgent micturition is "the result of repeated calls to empty a distended and weakened bladder." It seems to me a true strangury, by which phrase it is described by Christison as occurring, with even bloody micturition, at the close of poisoning cases.* No spasm, indeed, is present, and the absence of pain forbids the supposition of inflammation; but I think that *irritation* to no slight extent is set up. Böcker states that the vesical mucus in the urine is increased by Belladonna. Correspondingly, for simple irritation of the bladder, short of actual inflammation, I know of no medicine so valuable as Belladonna.

Of course in thus venturing to differ from Dr. Harley as to the ordinary action of Belladonna on the bladder, I have no thought of denying that in large doses it may paralyse this organ, both in its detrusor and in its sphincter fibres. I have already ascribed to such an action its power of breaking the habit of nocturnal incontinence of urine in children.

6. I would finally speak of the action of Belladonna on the uterus. Of this, from the physiological side, we have very little evidence. Nearly all the symptoms (which are but twenty out of a pathogenesis of 2680) given by Allen as belonging to the female sexual organs are from Houat or Greding,—either, though for different reasons, an impure source. The residue enable us to affirm two things only. The first is, that the drug is capable of producing a sensation of pressing and urging towards the sexual organs, as if everything would fall out there.† The second is, that it tends to promote and increase the menstrual flow. It is also said, in a quotation which I am unable to verify,‡ to have caused, in one case, "badly-smelling metrorrhagia." It is, however, in high esteem as a therapeutic agent in uterine congestions and inflammations. Hartmann writes—"that Belladonna exercises a decided influence upon the uterus is proved by the essential aid it affords

---

* See s. 2635 in Allen's Supplement.

† From the arrangement of the sexual symptoms in Hahnemann's pathogenesis, it would seem that this symptom had been observed by Stapf on his own person; and also by Hahnemann on a woman, under dubious circumstances, indicated by its being bracketed. Dr. Allen gives the latter under the head of "abdomen," and includes the former in his symptoms of the female sexual organs.

‡ Dr. Allen gives this symptom twice, ascribing it in the second case to Gross, as contained in Hahnemann's pathogenesis. I can find no such observation from him there.

in that terrible disease, uterine cancer, and in not merely the palliation, but the cure it effects in relaxation of the uterus, or even the prolapsus which results from that disease. In all of these affections, the sensitive urging and pressing downward, as if all the deeper-seated viscera would protrude at the genitals, exists, with which there is generally united a sensitive pain in the sacrum, all of which symptoms characteristically indicate Belladonna." He also recommends it for uterine congestion, "manifested particularly by a violent burning, stinging, fulness, tension and urging, deep in the abdomen and the sexual organs generally, with which there is often conjoined a dragging, lancinating sensation around the loins, and heat in the region; also sensitive pressure and constrictive pain in the small of the back, which causes the patient to walk slowly and carefully." Dr. Matheson* speaks in the warmest terms of the value of the drug in congestive and inflammatory conditions of the uterus. He gives the lowest decimal attenuations; but Drs. Leadam and Guernsey, who use the higher, seem no less appreciative of it. The former speaks warmly of its power to relax rigidity of the os uteri during labour; and the latter mentions hot discharges as indicating it in both menstrual and lochial derangements.

Dr. Dunham, in his *Lectures* (I, 262), has some valuable remarks on this subject. "No remedy," he says, "is more frequently and successfully employed for affections of the genital organs of women." He, with Hartmann, praises it in prolapsus, when this is (as it were) active, rather than the passive relaxed condition indicating Sepia and Stannum. The bearing down is worse when the patient sits bent over, and when she walks, but better when she sits erect or stands. I should call it a kind of tenesmus of the cervix. He describes a form of dysmenorrhœa connected with ovarian congestion, in which he has found its repetition just before each menstrual epoch for several months completely curative. He has also removed with it offensive odour of both catamenia and lochia, being led to it by the symptoms of Hahnemann's pathogenesis which I have mentioned.

In the observations I have now made, the main action of Belladonna, both as poison and as remedy, has been brought before you. There are yet a few other applications of it, however, which must be noted before I leave it.

1. The first is its use in exophthalmic goitre. Dr. Kidd

* *On Some of the Diseases of Women* (1876), p. 40.

long ago put on record a case cured by it,* and it has since become a favourite remedy in the hands of many homœopathists, as you may see from a discussion on the subject at the British Homœopathic Society, reported in the thirty-third volume of the *British Journal*. Dr. Jousset is one of those who esteems it here. Its employment is now gaining ground in the old school, as Dr. Ringer tells us—candidly admitting at the same time that the practice was initiated among homœopathists.

2. Belladonna does not play such an important part in aural as it does in ocular disorders ; but its applicability to inflammation of the middle ear, especially when brain symptoms coincide, is obvious. Hartmann writes—" Although I am convinced, from repeated experience, that Pulsatilla is almost specific in otitis interna et externa, still cases do occur in which it is not sufficient, but must give way to Belladonna. This occurs where the internal inflammation is more vividly developed than the external, or where the consensual cerebral symptoms are prominent phenomena." This expresses the general experience of homœopathists.

3. We should hardly have known that Belladonna had any action on the teeth and gums, had it not been for Hahnemann's provings. They, however, show it to be eminently suitable to inflammation of the dental pulp. Whenever the burning, throbbing and swelling indicative of this condition are present in toothache, Belladonna should be given, especially when the pain is worse at night.† It will often, especially if aided by Aconite, arrest an incipient gumboil. In this category, too, I must speak of its great value in the dentition troubles of children. It is when there is both the febrile condition of Aconite and the nervous erethism of Chamomilla, with marked cerebral excitement and tendency to convulsions, that Belladonna exceeds either medicine as a remedy. The higher dilutions generally answer best.

4. Belladonna plays but little part in the treatment of disorders of the digestive organs, though it affects the whole alimentary mucous membrane somewhat as it does the mouth and throat. It has been recommended in peritonitis, in inflammatory ileus, and in colic when a spot is as if griped with the nails, or when the transverse colon is felt through the abdominal walls distended like a pad. A corresponding action on the respiratory mucous membrane makes it very useful in dry, irritating laryngeal coughs, worse in the evening

---

* *Brit. Journ. of Hom.*, xxv., 187.

† See cases by Mr. Harmar Smith, *Brit. Journ. of Hom.*, xxv., 624.

X

and early night; also in incipient laryngeal and bronchial catarrhs, where congestive symptoms are marked. Dr. Dunham's comparison between it and its cognate remedies here should by all means be read (*loc. cit.*, p. 267).

5. Lastly, there seems little doubt of the influence of Belladonna upon the lymphatic and mammary glands. It will often subdue the beginnings of inflammation in the former,—best, Dr. Jousset says, when given in the mother tincture. In mastitis it is much praised when the mischief has got beyond the point at which Bryonia checks it. "The breasts feel heavy, and appear hard and red, the redness often running in radii; flushed face and injected eyeballs; full, bounding pulse; drowsiness; throbbing headache; sensitiveness to noise and light,"—these are Dr. Guernsey's indications for it.

I have yet to say a few words about the celebrated alkaloid of Belladonna,

Atropia. Being unable to discover the least difference in kind between the poisonous effects of the drug and its product, I have spoken of the two interchangeably. Dr. Allen, however, has given a separate pathogenesis of atropia, containing upwards of 500 symptoms. I too think that therapeutically we should keep them distinct. In all that I have said hitherto about treatment, I have been speaking of the administration of Belladonna. Whether atropia should ever be used in its stead has been inquired into by the late Dr. Caspar, of Vienna.[*] He treated more than a hundred cases,—at first by giving atropia after Belladonna, though apparently well indicated, had failed, and afterwards, as his knowledge grew, by prescribing it in the first instance, following it up, if ineffectual, by Belladonna. His main conclusion is that, as a therapeutical agent, atropia occupies the purely neurotic sphere of Belladonna, having no place in its tissue-irritations and vascular excitements. He has cured with it idiopathic and post-febrile headaches of long standing, hallucinations, epilepsy (in three instances), irritable throat and larynx, whooping-cough in the convulsive stage, and asthma. He thinks that it has little or no action below the diaphragm. But Dr. Kafka, after a proving of the sixtieth of a grain of the *sulphate* of atropia upon himself, was led by the symptoms induced to give it in chronic affections of the stomach attended with much pain and vomiting, and with very satisfactory results.[†] Dr. Bähr recommends it to relieve the pain of gastric

---

[*] See *North Am. Journ. of Hom.*, vi., 457.
[†] *Brit. Journ. of Hom.*, xv., 238.

ulcer; and in a case recently reported from America it seems
to have effected a complete cure.*

The second trituration has generally been that employed.

* *Amer. Journ. of Hom. Mat. Med.*, Nov., 1872.

LECTURE XX.

BERBERIS, BISMUTH, BORAX, BOVISTA, BROMINE AND THE
BROMIDES.

I shall begin this lecture with a sketch of the action of the
barberry,

Berberis vulgaris.

We make a tincture from the small branches of the root, or
the bark of the larger roots.

An excellent proving of Berberis, made upon five persons,
mainly with infusions of the root, was published by Dr. Hesse
in the first volume of the *Journal für Arzneimittellehre*. Its
symptomatology is reproduced by Dr. Allen, who gives 1262
symptoms to the drug. A study of this pathogenesis, by Dr.
Edward Blake, may be read in the thirty-third volume of the
British Journal of Homœopathy.

From some remarks of Dr. Hering's in the sixth volume of
the *American Homœopathic Review* (p. 48), we learn that the
symptoms of Berberis have led to its successful use in several
affections of the biliary and urinary tracts. Mr. Clifton has
commended it to relieve pain in the passing of gall-stones,
and in hepatic congestion ;* while Dr. S. E. Newton, following
up a previous experience of Dr. Lippe's, praises it in the
sufferings attendant on the passage of urinary gravel.† These
actions are in perfect accordance with its pathogenesis, which
shows a marked influence on the two tracts now specified, with
alteration in their secretions. I am inclined to think that the
hepatic is the primary action ; and that the urinary symptoms
are due to a change in the renal secretion secondary thereto,
setting up irritation of the mucous membrane along which it
passes. But, however this may be, whenever you meet with
pain, soreness, and burning in the biliary or urinary tracts
(especially when, in the latter case, there is much pain in the

* *Monthly Hom. Review*, xii., 405.
† *Brit. Journ. of Hom.*, xxxiii., 362.

hips), with tendency to gall-stone and gravel, you will do well to think of Berberis.

Some attention has of late been directed to an alkaloid found in Berberis, and present also in Hydrastis, Podophyllum, and Calumba, which is called berberin. Experiments on animals prove it a very mild poison, such symptoms as it does produce being those of gastro-intestinal irritation. "Given to fowls," writes Dr. Phillips, "in pills amounting to a quantum of four to eight grains with each day's food, the drug produced progressive loss of appetite, to the extent of causing marked inanition." These effects may throw some light upon the "stomachic" virtues ascribed to Calumba ; but they do not hint at the special virtues of Berberis. Berberin has also been credited with anti-periodic properties, but recent trials have resulted negatively.*

Berberis may be compared with *Nux vomica* and with *Capsicum.*

The dilutions from six to eighteen were used in the cases Dr. Hering reports ; but the later experience I have mentioned was gained with more substantial doses—Mr. Clifton getting no good effects until he resorted to the mother-tincture. Dr. Blake's experience, and (I may add) my own, is to the same effect.

My next medicine will be the familiar

Bismuthum.

Hahnemann called his preparation an oxide, and under this name its symptoms appear in Allen's *Encyclopædia.* But I think that if you read his directions for making it you will agree with me that the resulting salt is identical with that which chemists now style the subnitrate, and which is the bismuth of ordinary practice. This is the conclusion also of the British Homœopathic Pharmacopœia, which directs the officinal subnitrate to be used, and prepared of course by trituration.

The primary proving of Bismuth is in the sixth volume of the *Reine Arzneimittellehre,* where eleven symptoms are given by Hahnemann, and ninety-seven by three others. Some additional experiments with full doses are recorded by Wibmer, and given in symptom-form by Allen under the head of Bismuthum subnitricum.

* See *Brit. Journ. of Hom.,* xxxi., 190. *Practitioner,* xi., 333.

Bismuth has long been known as a remedy for gastric pain and vomiting. Hahnemann thinks that the symptoms obtained from it show it to be homœopathic enough to such conditions; and Pereira speaks to the same effect when he says that "in large doses it disorders the digestive organs, causing pain, vomiting and purging." But recent experience with it in chronic diarrhœa, such as that of phthisis and of unhealthy children, has elicited the fact that it may be given in enormous doses with nothing but benefit. The conclusion has hence been reached that the irritant effects ascribed to it of old were due to the Arsenic so often present in it, or to the development of an irritant nitrate; and that in its pure state it has no more active properties than chalk, and produces its good effects by a local "sedative and desiccant" action on the alimentary canal.

If this were so, Bismuth would lie outside the sphere of homœopathy. But Drs. Chapman* and Bayes have each put on record several cases in which, from the first to the third trituration, it proved curative in gastralgia, and my own experience is of the same tenor; while Dr. Jousset finds it quite effective, in similar forms, in the diarrhœa for which it is in repute. Prepared by our processes, therefore, Bismuth is not without dynamic action; and Dr. Horatio Wood shows that it is not so insoluble as is commonly supposed. It would probably repay a more thorough proving, directed to ascertain the precise form of gastralgia to which it corresponds. It seems indicated when there is sympathetic "stomach-cough," which is worse when the stomach is empty.

Bismuth seems also to exert a marked action on the heart, though this again may have been due to Arsenic. "Violent beating of the heart" appears in Hahnemann's pathogenesis;† a contracted pulse is several times noted by the provers; and in the post-mortem examination of the only case of poisoning on record the inner surface of both the ventricles was found very red. Arsenic can produce such effects, as we have seen; and we must not hastily use Bismuth in cardiac affections on the strength of these observations.

Teste states that he has used the drug with brilliant results in phlegmasia alba dolens.

Bismuth resembles, besides *Arsenic, Argentum, Hydrocyanic acid*, and perhaps *Zinc.*

Hahnemann recommended the 2nd trituration to be used for medicinal purposes; and in about that strength the drug has

* *Brit. Journ. of Hom.*, vii., 504.
† Dr. Allen (S. 61) has accidentally omitted the "violent" *(starker.)*

generally been given in homœopathic practice.   Dr. Yeldham, however, states that he has been compelled to give up all attenuations, and resort to five-grain doses of the pure substance, with which he has " met with almost unfailing success in that form of gastralgia to which females in particular are liable."*

I have again a well-known drug to bring before you in the sodic biborate,

Borax.

It is prepared for homœopathic use by trituration, or solution after 1ˣ.

Hahnemann gave in the second edition of the *Chronic Diseases* a pathogenesis of Borax, containing 460 symptoms ; nearly all of which are contributed by Dr. Schreter, and are stated to have been observed by him on several persons. These were evidently patients, and some of them infants, to whom he was probably giving the medicine for thrush.   Dr. Allen adds reports from two other experimenters ; but their results are so meagre as only to afford twenty-one additional symptoms.

Borax is best known as a local remedy for thrush.   Whatever the rationale of its action, we cannot but continue to employ a medication so simple and so effectual.   Yet it is of interest to inquire whether there is anything specific in the practice, and anything which illustrates the homœopathic method.   At first sight Hahnemann's pathogenesis would seem to show that Borax can produce thrush.   "Aphthæ in the mouth," "an aphtha inside the cheek, which bleeds when eating," "an aphtha on the tongue"—these symptoms from Schreter should be proof positive of homœopathicity.   But when we examine them closer, we find that they occurred from four to five weeks after the administration of the drug. Better evidence than this must therefore be given, ere we can affirm the thrush-producing power of Borax.   At the same time there can be no doubt that small doses—say grains of the first trituration, given internally, will cure the disease nearly if not quite as rapidly as when local application is employed ;—a fact which speaks strongly in favour of the dynamic action of the medicine.

However this may be, the local use of Borax in aphthous and also in pruriginous affections is of undoubted value.   To

* *Brit. Journ. of Hom.*, xxviii., 745, 757.

these its employment is at the present day well-nigh entirely
restricted. But in old times it was, as Pereira says, "regarded
as an agent exercising a specific influence over the uterus;
promoting menstruation, alleviating the pain which sometimes
attends this process, facilitating parturition, diminishing the
pain of accouchement, and favouring the expulsion of the
placenta and lochia." This use of the drug has been continued
in the homœopathic school. Schreter speaks of ready conception having been observed in five women under its use;
and mentions one case where a woman who had been sterile
fourteen years on account of an acrid leucorrhœa, after other
remedies at last took Borax, whereupon she became pregnant,
and the leucorrhœa improved. Dr. Middleton, of Philadelphia,
reports a similar experience in several cases of dysmenorrhœa
with sterility. He gave a grain of the crude salt night and
morning.* Dr. E. M. Hale has put on record a case of membranous dysmenorrhœa radically cured by it.† This piece of
practice, however, is not of homœopathic origin; for the physician who first recorded the successful use of the remedy was
Dr. Henry Bennet.

Dr. Guernsey lays much stress on "fear of downward
motion" as an indication for Borax. An ɲdult, he says,
dreads going down stairs, or the downward movement of the
rocking-chairs so much used in his country; a child seems
ever in dread of falling, and if the nurse attempts to lower it
from her arms while asleep, it will cry out and throw its hands
up as from fear. This feeling is part of a general nervous sensitiveness, especially to noise; but is peculiar to the present
drug.

Dr. Hale gave five-grain doses of the pure substance; and
neither for the uterus nor for the mouth does Borax seem to
need much dilution.

My next medicine is probably known to you by its poisonous
effects only. It is the "puff-ball," Lycoperdon

Bovista.

It is prepared by trituration.

Bovista was proved by Nenning and two others; 640

* See *Hahn. Monthly*, xi., 523.
† *Brit. Journ. of Hom.*, xxix., 746. There is another in the tenth
volume of the Transactions of the N. Y. State Hom. Society (p. 279),
where the first attenuation was employed; and two in the *New
England Medical Gazette* for December, 1879.

symptoms from this source appear in Hartlaub and Trinks' *Arzneimittellehre*. It was little used in practice until attention was called to it by Petroz in the fourth volume of the *Journal de la Société Gallicane*. The additional observations he communicates are combined with those of Hartlaub and Trinks by Allen.

The puff-ball has been found by Dr. Benjamin Richardson to be capable of producing anæsthesia in animals exposed to the fumes of its combustion. This anæsthesia is of the nature of asphyxia, like that of nitrous oxide; it is not of the chloroform character. Petroz, finding a similar condition set up from simple olfaction of the mother-tincture, was led to administer it in a serious case of asphyxia. He does not relate the circumstances, but says that the remedy was given with great success. His experimenters, and those who took part in the German proving, experienced great pain and heaviness in the head. Their symptoms should be carefully studied in Dr. Allen's arrangement, and may lead to valuable results. Teste (who has a good article on the drug) says that it is especially indicated by a sensation as if the head were swelling up to a great size. He mentions in another place the cure of a chronic leucorrhœa by Bovista, chosen mainly because of the co-existence of this symptom; and Dr. Walter Wesselhœft has recorded a very interesting one of protracted metrorhagia, in which, after the failure of all measures, medicinal and mechanical, improvement set in immediately after the administration of this remedy, to which he was led by the co-existence of "severe neuralgic pains in the eyes and temples, accompanied by a sense of enlargement and fulness of the whole head."[*] Dr. Guernsey recommends it in leucorrhœa like the white of an egg.

But the chief use of Bovista is in the cutaneous sphere. The skin appears in the proving as much affected with itching pimples; and Dr. Guernsey speaks of "tettery" persons as special subjects of its beneficial use. It is said to be indicated when the irritation is brought on by washing. Drs. Frédault and Guerin-Ménéville commend it in the eczema of the back of the hands known as bakers' and grocers' itch.

Bovista is classed by Teste with *Sulphur, Asterias,* and *Cicuta.*

The medium dilutions have been those hitherto used; but Dr. Wesselhœft gave the 3^x trituration.

I now come to the *piéce de résistance* of this lecture, in the

shape of a discussion of the action of Bromine and its compounds. And, first, of

Bromium

itself. An aqueous solution (alcoholic from the 3ˣ upwards)
is directed by the Pharmacopœia. But, as bromic acid soon
forms in such a preparation, it is recommended to keep the
Bromine pure, and dilute it with distilled water when required
for use.

In the second volume of the *Neues Archiv* Dr. Hering
published a pathogenesis of Bromine. The symptoms supplied by himself and his fellow-provers were mainly obtained
from the 30th dilution ; but some are taken from observers
who used material doses. The experiments of Höring,
Butzke, and Heiemdringer—which are of this character—are
given by Frank (i, 386), and should be consulted ; as also
should be an Harveian prize essay on the subject by Dr.
Glover, published in the fifty-eighth volume of the *Edinburgh
Medical and Surgical Journal.* The symptoms from these and
other sources, as collected by Dr. Allen, amount to 821 in
all. Some additional memoirs on Bromine are ᵣₑ ₙtioned
by Dr. Ozanam in the *brochure* to which I shall ᵣ ᵢer, and
may be consulted by those desiring further knowlea ᵧe of the
drug.

The results of all these investigations are but scanty.
Bromine is unquestionably a powerful irritant ; more so (Dr.
Glover says) when diluted than when pure. Hence it inflames
every mucous membrane with which it comes in contact.
Being very volatile, moreover, its exhalations ascend from the
stomach after it is swallowed ; so that the coryza and salivation it provokes may not be more than local effects. Nevertheless, as, even when injected into the veins, it sets up
inflammation of the lungs and air-passages, we may fairly
credit it with a specific influence on the respiratory organs ;
and these have been the main sphere of its homœopathic use.
The rigors and prostration which accompanied its coryza in
one of Glover's dogs suggest it in influenza. Since in
Höring it caused difficult and painful inspiration, violent
stitches in the lungs, and cough in attempting to draw a long
breath, it ought to find a place in the treatment of pneumonia ;
in which indeed, and in phthisis, Dr. Hering praises it.
Dr. Kafka, also, esteems it highly in croupous pneumonia,
when Iodine (his chief remedy) fails. I often find it useful in

dry laryngo-tracheal coughs, with hoarseness, and pain and
burning behind the sternum. But its chief credit has been
gained in the treatment of membranous croup, of which there
are numerous instances on record in which it effected a cure.*
As it usually came in to reinforce the ordinary remedies, the
cases in which it was employed were severe and advanced ; so
that its potency is the more established. One of our latest
reports comes from Dr. Meyhoffer, who in a very able way
discusses the precise place of Bromine in the therapeutics of
this disease. He points to the prostration manifest in its
poisonous effects (which was also, I may say, noted by
Höring in his experiments on the human subject with
moderate doses) ; and decides that it is in extension of
diphtheria to the air-passages that it is indicated, while Iodine
—whose primary constitutional action is excitant—is better
suited to what is distinguished as true croup. He does not,
however, admit an essential, but only a phenomenal, difference
between the two diseases ; and the whole tendency of medical
opinion is now in this direction.

Dr. Ozanam, of Paris, assuming this doctrine (which has
always been held by French pathologists), has published
several interesting observations on the use of Bromine in
croup and diphtheria, which are summed up in a short
treatise on the subject dated 1869.† He has ascertained that
an aqueous solution of Bromine, of the strength of one part
in a thousand, disintegrates a false membrane in an hour.
He then points to the elective action of the drug on the air-
passages, and also (as he thinks) on the throat ; and to its
property, when inhaled by animals, of determining the formation of false membranes on these parts. He finally advances
its power—equal to that of Chlorine—of destroying contagious germs ; and concludes that on every ground it ought to
be a prime remedy for diphtheritic affections. He himself
has found it to be so. His first success was obtained in 1849,
and since then he has treated some 150 cases, with the loss of
only five, all of which were croupous. He gives every hour
one or two drops (in *eau sucrée* for children) of a freshly prepared aqueous dilution of 3^x strength, and adds inhalations of
a weak solution. Of late he has found a combination of
Bromine and Kali bromatum—*bromure de potassium bromé*—

* *North Amer. Journ. of Hom.*, x., 296. *Philad. Journ. of
Hom.*, i.,529 ; ii., 74, 565. *Brit. Journ. of Hom.*, xxiv., 625.
† *Mémoire sur les dissolvants et les désagrégeants des produits
pseudo-membraneux, et sur l'emploi du Brome dans les affections
pseudo-membraneuses* (Baillière).

still more efficient, both chemically and clinically. Other
authors are cited by him as confirming his results; and I
should have mentioned that Dr. Meyhoffer speaks of having
treated twenty cases successfully with Bromine alone, where
diphtheritic exudation in the throat or larynx was accompanied by great prostration. M. Teste communicated to the
Paris Congress of 1878* a very favourable experience with
this medication, which he reckons " the most precious acquisition that the art of healing has made for a hundred years past."
He also uses the *eau bromée*, but in a one per cent. solution,
giving from one to three drops for a dose, every hour in
anginose diphtheria, every quarter of an hour in croupous. He
forbids the use of milk, which his observations lead him to
consider destructive of the action of the Bromine.

Dr. Oehme,† summing up the evidence as to the anti-
diphtheritic virtues of Bromine, concludes that it is mainly
from its chemical action that it proves useful ; and M. Teste
agrees with him here. Himself in general an advocate of the
use of attenuated medicines, he finds that the present drug
cannot be so given with advantage. He thinks that it acts
by its great affinity for hydrogen, much as Chlorine does ;
and relates some curious observations as to the change which
eau bromée undergoes when exposed to the exhalations from
diphtheritic patients.

However it may be as regards diphtheria, the specific
action of Bromine on croup is unquestionable. In addition to
the reports of its value I have already mentioned, I may
mention that Dr. Kafka has contributed to the *Allgemeine
homöopathische Zeitung* for 1875 a severe case of membranous croup in which inhalations of Bromine (1st and 2nd
decimal on cotton wool) had a most beneficial effect. Dr.
Guernsey's indication for it in croup and laryngeal diphtheria
is " rattling of mucus in the windpipe when coughing."

Besides its use in croup, Bromine has retained among
homœopathists the place it has lost in the old school as a
reducer of enlarged lymphatic glands. Dr. Goullon, in his
excellent treatise on scrofula, gives several instances of cure
of strumous glands by means of it. Dr. Guernsey recommends it in idiopathic physometra.

Some curious sensations in the extremities are related by
Trousseau and Pidoux to have been caused by Bromine when
administered by Andral and Fournet to a number of sufferers
from arthritis. But as these phenomena are quite unique, and

* See its Transactions, p. 72.
† *Therapeutics of Diphtheritis*, sub voce.

were accompanied by great diminution of their pains, I think they must have depended on the morbid state of the patients, and cannot be used as homœopathic indications.

The chief analogue of Bromine is *Iodine*, as compared with which, however, it has a very limited sphere.

In croup, Bromine has been usually given in about the 3rd decimal dilution, in strumous glands in the 3rd centesimal.

Having spoken of Bromine itself, it becomes necessary to enquire into its action when in combination with an alkali. This at once gives it other features and a new range of action. Let us speak of the bromide of potassium.

Kali bromatum.—The history of this substance is a curious one. It was first used as an analogue of the iodide of the same metal, and introduced into the Pharmacopœia on the strength of the virtues ascribed to it by Dr. Robert Williams in chronic enlargements of the spleen. Its repute here soon waned, and it ceased to be officinal. In 1857 the late Sir Charles Locock called attention to its power of checking epileptic fits dependent upon irritations of the female sexual organs. It was soon found that epilepsies from other causes were amenable to its influence; and it rapidly acquired—at least in this country, in France, and in America—an estimation as an anti-epileptic far excelling all other remedies now in use, and capable of doing more for the disease than had ever been done or hoped for hitherto. "It has changed," Dr. Anstie quotes an eminent authority as saying, " the whole prognostic significance of epileptic attacks."

" Like that of all other drugs," writes Sir Thomas Watson, " its special virtue was discovered empirically, and could never have been reasoned out." But, attention being once directed to it, experimentation as to its physiological effects followed. Conducted in the usual gross way, and on the lower animals only, this seemed to prove Kali bromatum a pure sedative to nervous tissue, and it was used accordingly in every kind of irritation of brain, cord, and nerves. Disappointment naturally followed, and the employment of the drug is now, by good judges, restricted to true convulsions recurring paroxysmally, excluding all habitual spasms. As Dr. Ringer says :—" although convulsions may be excited by many causes, it is probable that the conditions of the nervous centres producing the attack are in every instance identical ; and it appears to be these conditions which the bromide controls." At the same time, more careful reading of the physiological effects showed that it was the reflex function of the nervous centres—the "true spinal cord" of Marshall Hall—to which the bromide so readily acted as a sedative : sensation and voluntary motion were only affected by toxic quantities.

As checking convulsions, then, by deadening reflex excitability, bromide of potassium has taken its place in general therapeutics ; and we of the school of Hahnemann have had to consider what to do with it. Our power over convulsive affections—especially over epilepsy—is not so great as to make us independent of further aid ; and the mere fact that we have here to do with an antipathic action would not keep us from Kali bromatum any more than from Amyl nitrite. But palliation of paroxysms, as with the latter, is a very different thing from their suspension by the continued use of the drug. Here the vices of antipathic medication become manifest. It is allowed that epilepsy is seldom or never *cured* by the bromide, so that the patient remains free from it after ceasing to take the drug : it is only kept in check while he remains under its influence. For this purpose, moreover, it is necessary to take large and frequent doses, so that the blood be kept constantly charged with it, and the nervous system never free from the sedation it causes. Even then it is confessed that it oftentimes loses its power through habituation of the tissue to its action,* and has to be suspended for a time, at the risk of the paroxysms returning, so as to start afresh on its work.

Before committing our patients to such a course of treatment, it is necessary to enquire whether no harm results to the organism at large from this constant saturation with a medicinal agent—whether, in fact, the remedy is not worse than the disease. The phenomena of "bromism" are now well known. I will cite Dr. Bazire's description of them as they appear in the nervous centres.†

"When given in large doses, such as thirty and forty grains two or three times a day, it produces very striking symptoms in about ten or fifteen days. The patient at first complains of a dull headache, becomes listless and apathetic, with an expressionless gaze and a lustreless eye. His intellect is clouded, his mind confused, and he is unable to concentrate his thoughts. There is slowness of perception, and questions have to be asked several times before their meaning is understood and an answer can be obtained. If, when these symptoms have begun to show themselves, the medicine be continued, hebetude follows, with inability to think, and a kind of stupor resembling that of the first stage of typhoid fever, together with drowsiness, somnolence,

* The last writer on the subject, Kunze, says—" The bromides only retard the attack of epilepsy for at most half a year ; after which it comes on with renewed energy." (See *Practitioner*, xxii., 222.)

† See his translation of Trousseau's *Clinical Lectures*, vol. i.

and constant dropping off to sleep. The pupils are dilated, and contract very sluggishly under the influence of a strong light; the sensibility of the conjunctiva is so deadened that a finger may be passed with impunity on the surface of the eyeball without producing winking. Hearing loses its usual acuteness, and it is only by speaking in a very loud voice that the patient can be aroused from his stupor.

"The sense of taste is probably impaired like those of hearing and of sight. The tongue is moist and red at first, but after a few days it has a tendency to drying and browning. There is anæsthesia of the velum palati, the uvula and upper portion of the pharynx, so that these parts may be tickled without producing nausea or involuntary movements of deglutition. Swallowing itself, however, is unimpaired, and strangely enough the appetite remains very good; the patient takes his food well, and dozes off immediately after. Digestion seems to be easy, and the bowels, although sluggish in their action, are not very confined. There is intense thirst, and a craving for cold drinks. The anæsthesia is not confined to the mucous membranes only, for the sensibility of the skin is diminished also, so that pinching and pricking are scarcely noticed by the patient. From the beginning, the sexual aptitude fails; erections become rare and imperfect, and cease entirely after a few days.

"Simultaneously with the impairment of sensibility, disorders of motility manifest themselves. Thus the patient is averse to taking exercise, sits and lounges about; by degrees, his gait becomes altered, he rolls and staggers like a drunken man, his limbs shake and bend under him. After a time, he is obliged to keep to his bed, and when he uses his hands, as in the act of carrying anything to his mouth, they are seen to tremble, as if he were suffering from delirium tremens. The respiration is calm and tranquil, with occasional sighing. The circulation is considerably slackened; the pulse at the wrist is weak and slow; the heart's beat lacking in energy, and its sounds distant and feeble; in fact, in its effect on the heart, bromide of potassium seems to resemble digitalis. If the drug be withheld, these symptoms gradually diminish and pass off of themselves, but they leave behind them for some time afterwards great feebleness, both physical and mental. The anæsthesia of the fauces seems to be the last phenomenon to disappear."

To these effects, sufficiently undesirable, must be added the well-known acne of the drug, whose pustules sometimes become boils, and end in large ulcers with conical scabs like rupia. I may also cite Dr. Clarke's* description of the symptoms of a toxic dose, which, as he says, "are only an increase or an exaggeration of those of a therapeutic one. "The fœtid breath becomes nauseous; œdema supervenes on congestion of the uvula and fauces; the whispering voice sinks into aphonia; sexual weakness degenerates into impotence; muscular weakness becomes complete paralysis; reflex, general, and special sensibility disappears; the ears do not hear, nor the eyes see, nor the tongue taste; the expression of hebetude becomes first that of imbecility, and then that of

* *Abstract of the Physiological and Therapeutical Action of Bromide of Potassium*, by Drs. E. H. Clarke and R. Amory. Boston, 1872.

idiocy; hallucinations of sight and sound, with or without mania, precede general cerebral indifference, apathy, and paralysis ; the respiration, without the stertor of opium or alcohol, is easy but slow ; the temperature of the body is lowered. As the bromism becomes more profound, the patient lies quietly on his bed, unable to move, or feel, or swallow, or speak, with dilated and uncontractile pupils, and scarcely any change of the colour of the skin or face ; the extremities grow gradually colder and colder; the action of the heart becomes feebler and slower, till it ceases altogether."

I confess that my own decision is against the bromidal treatment of epileptic and other convulsions, save when from their frequency they are threatening life or reason, and when careful homœopathic medication has failed. I think, more- over, that herein I am expressing the mind of most practi- tioners of our school. It is quite possible, indeed, that some true specific influence of an anti-epileptic kind may be ex- erted by Bromine itself. This is suggested by the efficacy ascribed by Dr. Hammond to the bromide of zinc, in quite small doses, and by others to the bromide of arsenic in quan- tities smaller still. I am speaking, however, of the usual practice with the bromide of potassium. But we may here be positively as well as negatively consistent with our principles, and find in the phenomena of bromism indications for the use of the drug according to the law of similars. This has al- ready been done for us in several instances.

1. The acne of Kali bromatum was first noticed by Höring, of whose experiments with Bromine I have already spoken. It became in his case—as not unfrequently—a crop of boils. It is common, but not constant—Dr. Clarke observing it in two thirds of the cases treated by him with continuous doses ; and it is not, as Dr. Russell Reynolds says, determined by the quantity of bromide that is taken. He has seen it follow a few five-grain doses, and it has been absent in many cases where thirty grains have been taken, three times daily, for periods of six or even of twelve months. It sometimes results in suppuration : sometimes the pustules die away without going through this process. Its favourite seats are the face, scalp, and back.

Here is a suitable starting-point for homœopathic medica- tion ; and Dr. Drysdale states that he has more than once cured such an acne with two- or three-grain doses of Kali bromatum. But he had been anticipated in his statement by a practitioner of the old school, Dr. Cholmeley. He states that he has seen an obstinate, long-continued acne disappear entirely while bromide of potassium was being taken for a nervous disorder.*

2. Kali bromatum has an unquestionable soporific effect, and is in large use as a hypnotic, though opinions seem much divided as to its certainty. It concerns us little in this capacity ; but we read with much interest the description of the kind of sopor induced given by M. Laborde from observations made on himself. " It is," he says,† "a state of heavy somnolence ; it is often suddenly interrupted, although there are, properly speaking, no dreams, or no dreams that take a definite shape ; it is rather a nightmare, and an indefinite one. Waking is accomplished with great difficulty." The indications for the drug in certain morbid conditions of sleep are obvious ; and we have the encouragement of Dr. Ringer, who finds it very useful in the night-screaming and somnambulism of children, and the nightmare of adults. We may remember, too, the connection between too profound sleep and nocturnal enuresis.

3. According to physiological experimenters, bromide of potassium acts strongly on the vaso-motor nerves, constricting (at least at first) the arterioles. They maintain that it is in virtue of this power that it proves sedative to the nervous centres generally. Dr. Russell Reynolds, however, takes just the opposite view, considering that it acts upon the vaso-motor system as a "sedative," i.e., that it reduces such morbid activity as would lead to the spasmodic narrowing of vessels, and the consequent induction of irregularity in the supply of blood. The principle *similia similibus* explains the apparent contradiction. He commends it accordingly in disturbances of this system elsewhere than in the head, and finds ten- or even five-grain doses sufficient for their removal.

4. We shall probably find a place for Kali bromatum in some functional paralytic conditions, as tabes dorsalis from sexual excess, idiopathic aphasia, and simple dementia. Two local paralyses are mentioned as having been cured by it—dysphagia of liquids in infants by Dr. Ringer (I have had the same experience once myself), and incontinence of urine by Dr. Warburton Begbie.‡ The latter has been caused by the drug.

There are a good many other points of interest about bromide of potassium ; but I cannot do more than indicate them. There is the question of the source of its efficacy, whether

* *Med. Times and Gazette*, Dec. 11th, 1869.
† See *Practitioner*, xii., 9.
‡ *Ibid*, xii., 98.

Y

this be from its bromine, as maintained by .Dr. Richardson, or from its potassium, as suggested by Professor Binz, or whether (as Dr. R. Reynolds thinks) it is a *tertium quid* distinct from either.   Then there is its action on the sexual organs, whose activity it seems—in large doses—to diminish even to abolition : this being due, according to some observers, to a local action on the extremities of the excitor nerves, according to others, to its depressing influence on the spinal cord.   Dr. Anstie thought much of it in insomnia, and even neuralgia, from sexual worry ; and it seems effective in nymphomania. This, of course, belongs to its antipathic action ; for I do not think we can make capital out of the single observation of Laborde in which sexual excitement seemed to follow upon its use.   But it is here, perhaps, that I must mention the action of the drug on ovarian cysts.   A case of this kind is recorded in the *Edinburgh Medical Journal* for 1868, in which, after a single tapping, the continuous use of the bromide, in doses of five, ten, and fifteen grains, effected a complete cure.   In the twenty-seventh volume of the *British Journal of Homœo-pathy* Dr. Black records an equally satisfactory case, where grain doses sufficed for the cure ; and in the twenty-eighth volume you may read one of my own.*   There is much encouragement here for future trials.   Other applications of the drug may result in time from a consideration of the 444 pathogenetic effects of Kali bromatum recorded by Dr. Allen under that heading.

Of the other alkaline bromides, I may mention that that of ammonium has been proved by Dr. Cushing, of Lynn, and you will find his pathogenesis in Allen's first volume.   Its chief effect on him seems to have been the production of much white, sticky mucus about the upper part of the digestive and respiratory tracts.   Dr. Hale praises it in the treatment of chronic catarrh of the posterior nares.   This writer has some remarks on the dynamic action of other bromides, which you will do well to read.   The field is too little worked for me to adventure upon it at present.

* In my case the cyst seems to have ruptured into the peritoneum. Dr. Helmuth, in his *System of Surgery* (3rd ed. p. 106), relates a curious case of cysto-sarcoma of the breast, of many years standing, in which, under the influence of two-grain doses of the bromide, three times daily, the larger cysts broke and discharged, and a number of the smaller ones disappeared.

LECTURE XXI.

BRYONIA.

I shall devote this lecture to a medicine which, more than any one which has yet come before us, therapeutics owe entirely to Hahnemann.   I speak of

Bryonia.

A tincture of the root of the Bryonia alba is the ordinary homœopathic preparation; but the British Homœopathic Pharmacopœia allows the indigenous species—the Bryonia dioica—to be substituted. Mr. Turner tells me that now and then the tamus communis is brought to chemists by mistake for the bryony root, and might be incautiously used by them.

Bryonia was early proved by Hahnemann : the pathogenesis occurs in the second volume of the *Reine Arzneimittellehre*. It consists (in the latest edition) of 781 symptoms, two thirds of which are contributed by the master himself, and the rest by six fellow-provers. It was also one of the medicines selected for re-proving by the Austrian Society. Their results are published in the third volume of the *Oesterreichische Zeitchrift*. Eighteen persons took part in the proving, two of whom were females; and nearly all employed increasing doses of the mother-tincture. The symptoms obtained are amalgamated with Hahnemann's by Dr. Allen, forming a total of nearly two thousand; and the experiments on animals which were made have been translated for the *British Journal of Homœopathy* (vol. xxv). There are two interesting studies of Bryonia which I may commend to your notice,—the one by Dr. Hirschel, in that part of his *Pharmacodynamics* which has been translated by Dr. Hayle; the other by Dr. Dunham, in his *Lectures* (I. 89). It forms also one of the first series of "principal homœopathic remedies" on which Hartmann has made his *Practical Observations*.

I have said that therapeutics owe Bryonia to Hahnemann. Before his time it was known only as a drastic emetic and purgative, and very little used in practice. He proved it for the volume of Materia Medica which he brought out in 1816 ; and remarks there that " the symptoms it excites in the healthy correspond to many affections of daily occurrence," and that hence " its healing power must be of wide range." He had already found it very useful in the fever which ravaged Germany while the seat of war in 1813, as I shall tell you hereafter ; and he relates in the preface to this volume of the *Reine Arzneimittellehre* a case of gastralgia with water-brash cured by it in twenty-four hours, after the patient had been laid by for three weeks. He gave here a single dose of a drop of the pure juice, and at this time recommends the drug to be somewhat thus administered in maladies of some standing when the patient is fairly robust, but to be given in the 18th dilution in acute disease with much constitutional excitement. In a solution of about this strength he had employed it in the fever of which I have spoken. He compares it to Rhus (whose proving also first appeared at this time), giving as its distinguishing features its mental symptoms (of which immediately), and the aggravation of its pains by movement—those of Rhus being worse at rest. This last characteristic has proved of inestimable value in determining the selection of Bryonia. He further suggests its probable usefulness in certain abdominal spasms in the female sex, and (later) in some kinds of constipation and of menorrhagia.

In consequence of all this, Bryonia soon came to be largely used in homœopathic practice, and took that place among the polychrests of our Pharmacopœia which it has ever since retained. Of its high estimation and wide sphere of usefulness you cannot form a better idea than by reading Hartmann's *Observations ;* and I shall have to enlarge upon rather than detract from his recommendations of the drug.

As Bryonia will be a new medicine to most of my hearers, I must detail its pathogenetic effects with some minuteness.

Bryonia is a pure irritant. It has no neurotic or hæmatic power ; but sets up inflammation,—locally, wherever it is applied, specifically, in the serous membranes and the chief viscera they contain, some of the mucous membranes, and the muscles.

I. No poison (not even Aconite or Arsenic) affects the *serous membranes* so certainly and powerfully as Bryonia. If you will read the autopsies of the animals poisoned at Vienna, this fact will abundantly appear. In the first the pleuræ were injected and full of serum, and the peritoneum and arachnoid injected ; in the second, third, and fifth the arachnoid only was reddened; but in the sixth the pleuræ were as in the first, and the pericardial vessels were injected. Correspondingly, the provers have the characteristic pleuritic pains with fever; and although the symptoms of the head, heart, and abdomen are undecisive, they at least do not forbid the supposition of an affection of their respective serous membranes. Moreover, those close allies of the serous sacs—the synovial membranes, which are more easily affected by drug action, give plain indication of suffering from Bryony. The joints swell and become tender, especially those of the fingers.

Since all the parenchymatous organs influenced by Bryonia are enclosed in serous membrane, I used to try to account for their symptoms by the primary action of the drug on the investing tissue. I cannot, however, ask you to accept this doctrine now. I must describe the effects on the viscera as they exist, and leave their relation to the disorder of their envelopes for further investigation.

1. It is curious, nevertheless, that as of all the serous membranes the pleuræ are those most readily influenced by Bryonia, so of all the viscera the *lungs* are those which suffer most from its action. The short, quick, and oppressed breathing, heat and pain in the chest, cough and bloody expectoration, and fever, experienced by the provers, find their interpretation in the phenomena presented by the poisoned animals. In these, with similar symptoms during life, the lungs were always of deeper colour and diminished crepitation, while in two the lower lobes were hepatized.

2. Next to the lungs, the *brain* is the organ which shows most signs of being affected by Bryonia. There is no perversion of the sensorial functions, as with Belladonna; and the determination of blood does not pass beyond the stage of congestion. But up to this point it is very well marked; and the provers get a hot and red face, with headache (generally frontal), sense of weight and fulness, and vertigo. Epistaxis also is frequent.

3. Of the two chief viscera enfolded by the peritoneum, the *liver* is much more affected by Bryonia than the kidneys. It causes tensive and burning pain in the hepatic region, which is sometimes also sensitive to pressure. In one prover, the skin over the whole body became yellowish. In the animals the liver was always found gorged, and sometimes friable.— In two animals the kidneys also were found congested; but I think the scanty, hot, and high-coloured urine so often passed by the Austrian provers a symptom of general fever rather than of renal implication.

II. I now come to the action of Bryonia on the *mucous membranes*. It is interesting to observe (in connection with its relation to the rheumatic poison) how much less powerfully it influences these than it does the serous and synovial membranes. It is an acrid, and hence large doses cannot but irritate the alimentary canal as they go down. Accordingly, we have in the provers sore throat, vomiting, and diarrhœa with colic and flatulence; and in the animals an aphthous mouth, and ulcers in the stomach and intestines. But the essential phenomena of Bryony in the gastro-intestinal sphere do not seem to depend upon irritation of the mucous membrane. They are,—water-brash (with this there is the characteristic contractive pain at the lower end of the œsophagus), bitter risings and vomitings, pressure on the stomach, feeling of load as if a stone were there, and constipation. These await their physiological expression; but they have received, as we shall see, their full therapeutic application.

The respiratory mucous membrane is unquestionably affected by Bryonia, though I doubt whether the irritation extends lower than the first division of the bronchi. The symptoms of the provers (pain, cough, &c.), whenever localised, are referred to the trachea and its bifurcation; and these parts only were found injected in the poisoned animals. The pneumonia set up by Bryony was never associated with bronchitis, in this strikingly different from that of Tartar emetic and Phosphorus. If Bryonia causes any nasal catarrh, it is dry; and the cough also has little expectoration, and is continuous, irritating, and violent, often causing retching and pains in the walls of the chest. Of late, our knowledge of the action of Bryony on the air tubes has received a novel extension from an experiment of M. Curie's.* By administering to a rabbit gradually increasing doses of Bryonia during eight months till he came to 250 drops of the mother-tincture daily, he developed in the animal a firm pseudo-membranous tube, extending from the larynx to the third ramifications of the bronchiæ. While this fact is of great interest, I do not think it proves that the action of Bryonia on the air-passages is either profound or extensive. Pseudo-membranous formation on their surface is a pathological fact *per se*; and has no necessary relation to the amount of affection of the subjacent mucous membrane.

Upon the urinary mucous membrane I should have said that Bryony had little or no action, but that several of the provers experienced considerable vesical tenesmus, with a

* See *Brit. Journ. of Hom.*, xix., 455.

feeling after micturition as though all the urine had not been expelled.

III. In one of the animals poisoned with Bryony at Vienna, where a very minute autopsy was made by a practised pathologist, it is noted that the substance of the heart and the muscles of the neck were intensely red. Putting this together with the soreness and pain on motion experienced by the provers in so many parts of the body, even to the production of pleurodynia and lumbago, I venture to set down our drug is a specific irritant of muscular fibre. As we have no other medicine with such an action, we must not lose even the hint of it supplied by these facts.

Under these headings I have given you the main pathogenetic effects of Bryonia. I have only to add that in the female provers the menstruation was premature and excessive; and that in all febrile symptoms were frequent.

Let us now enquire what have been the clinical results of these very extensive provings.

To Bryonia, as to all the great Hahnemannian medicines, a special constitution and disposition has been assigned as that to which it is most suitable. It is said to act best in persons of firm and fleshy fibre, of dark hair and complexion, of "bilious" tendency and choleric temperament, and where much irritability and irascibility are present. You must not lay too much stress on such indications; nevertheless, they sometimes guide us to the true remedy. Still more characteristic are its pains, which are always of a shooting or tearing kind.

I shall begin by characterising the relation of Bryonia to fever. It is especially suitable to two great types, the rheumatic and the typhous.

I. After Aconite, Bryonia is incomparably the best remedy for *acute rheumatism*. In its whole pathogenetic action it reminds one of the rheumatic poison. Its feeble affinity for skin and mucous membrane, and its powerful influence over serous and synovial membrane and muscular fibre, with its fever and sour sweats, point unmistakeably to this disease. Accordingly, most of us employ it throughout rheumatic fever, generally in alternation with Aconite, unless the symptoms call urgently for some other medicine. But we need a series of comparative experiments which shall demonstrate what part the Aconite and what the Bryonia takes in controlling the disease. Bryonia appears equally suitable for articular and for muscular rheumatism: it is least fitted for affection of the fibrous tissues proper. It continues, of course, to be a

homœopathic remedy when any of the serous membranes are
inflamed in the course of rheumatic fever; though it may
yield in importance to some other medicines. It is a capital
remedy (at any rate after Aconite) for rheumatism attacking
particular muscles, as those of the loins or neck, or the diaphragm; particularly when brought on by cold draughts. In
chronic rheumatism it is specially indicated when the pain is
increased by motion, i.e., when the affection is sub-inflam-
matory in character.

II. The great campaign of 1813 in Germany, which ended
at Leipsic, left—after the war had rolled away over the Rhine
—a woeful legacy behind it in the shape of an epidemic fever.
Of this malady Hahnemann gives a graphic account in a
paper which you will find in Dr. Dudgeon's translation of his
Lesser Writings (p. 712). Bryonia was the remedy he most
frequently employed, being indicated by shooting pain, worst
on movement,—Rhus and Hyoscyamus also being given accord-
to the symptoms; and he treated 183 cases without a single
death. Bryonia has hence acquired among homœopathists a
large reputation in the treatment of the essential fevers. The
head symptoms and the bilious disturbance of the drug frequently find their antitypes here; and Hahnemann's pathogenesis adds the dry mouth and tongue, and the nocturnal
delirium. One of his symptoms, indeed, if a pure pathogenetic effect of the drug, would make it perfectly homœopathic to low fever :—"She sleeps the whole day, with dry,
great heat, without eating or drinking, with twitching in the
face; she has six involuntary passages, the stools being brown
and smelling badly." Hartmann characterises the fever of
Bryonia as one that often suggests Aconite, but wrongly; in
the old nomenclature, it is a synochus, not a synocha. The
patient, he adds, is often cold externally, though hot within.
Dr. Dunham attempts a detailed picture of the Bryonia fever.
"The headache," he writes, "is a splitting pain through the
temples, and at the same time, and more severely, in the
occiput. Oppression at the pit of the stomach, and tenderness
there; vomiting of food, mucus, and bile, stitches in the hypochondria, and soreness and tension in the hypochondriac
region, along with dry cough and decided constipation, without any desire for evacuation of the bowels, are present.
Together with these local symptoms, there are frequent short
chills, alternating or mixed up with heat of the body; a pulse
small and frequent, but somewhat hard. Add to the above,
a slimy and bitter taste, aversion to food, pains in the back
and limbs, much aggravated by touch and motion, together

with dulness of the sensorium and aversion to noises and to mental exertion, and we have a picture of the form of fever for which, whether remittent or intermittent, Bryonia is appropriate." You will find its symptomatic indications in typhoid very minutely detailed by Dr. Wolf in the eighth volume of the *British Journal of Homœopathy.*

Nosologically, Bryonia is especially suitable for *relapsing fever.* Dr. Kidd, who saw so much of this malady in Ireland in 1847, considers Bryony the best medicine for it ;* and Dr. Russell thinks that the fever treated by Hahnemann was of this nature. Its place in typhus and typhoid is more difficult to determine. There seems a general concurrence among the older homœopathists as to its power of modifying favourably the erethism of the first stage of "typhus abdominalis," our enteric fever ; and Trinks even claims for it the capability of aborting the disease.† He commends it also for the rheumatic pains and the bronchitis which occasionally complicate the course of fever. It has long been the favourite remedy in this country for " common continued fever "—the " gastric fever " of popular nomenclature ; but in my own hands Baptisia has quite dethroned it here.

III. I will now speak of the power of Bryonia in affections of the serous membranes and of the viscera which they enclose.

Dr. Trinks, than whom we have had no better practical physician among us, thus characterises the place of Bryonia in serous inflammations.‡

" From no small number of cases which I have carefully marked down, the fact comes out that Bryonia is the sovereign remedy in all inflammations of the serous membranes which have advanced to the stage of serous effusion. This action of Bryonia extends all over the serous membranes which cover the thorax and abdomen, and the organs situated in these cavities, and which are so often attacked by inflammation.

" As long as the local inflammatory condition had not reached this stage, the fever being still of a sharp, well-pronounced synochal character, the Bryonia was of no use, but at this time Aconite and Belladonna were the specific medicines which arrested the inflammation before it had been developed to the stage just specified. But when on the other hand the inflammation had advanced to the stage of serous exudation, then in all cases Bryonia showed itself a medicine of quick and certain operation, which not only removed the still-existing local inflammation, but also with the least possible delay effected the absorption of the serous effusion which had already taken place.

" I find in my journal many cases of inflammation of the pleura, as

* *Annals,* iv., 181.
† *Brit. Journ. of Hom.,* xxix., 303.
‡ *Ibid,* viii., 482.

they occur **very** frequently in Dresden in the beginning and end of winter, during the prevalence of strong east and north-east winds, in persons disposed to tubercular phthisis ; then two cases of inflammation of the pericardium with serous exudation ; and two very noteworthy cases of inflammation of the peritoneum, with very copious effusion of serum into the abdominal cavity.''

These doctrines of Trinks' about the place of Bryonia in inflammations of serous membranes have been confirmed by all subsequent observers. Aconite should be given at first, and continued (with aid from Sulphur) should the exudation be plastic ; but if serous effusion occur, its place must be taken by Bryonia. It is especially in *pleurisy* that this treatment has become accepted. You will find some good cases illustrative of it by the late Dr. Beilby, of Glasgow, in the tenth volume of the *British Journal of Homœopathy.* For *pericarditis* you should read Dr. Russell's *Clinical Lectures.* I myself greatly prefer in this disease Aconite or Colchicum. In *peritonitis* from exposure to cold I have seen Bryonia act exceedingly well after Aconite : there are two capital cases in Trinks' paper. It is recommended also for the puerperal form of this disease. *Arachnitis* is the only form of serous inflammation in which Bryonia has not proved curative ; but since this malady, as occurring (where we most frequently meet with it) in children, is generally tubercular, the failure of any given medicine to cure it reflects no discredit on the remedy. In non-tubercular cases in these subjects it would probably repay the confidence which is generally placed in it ; and in the acute meningitis of adults it is of unquestioned value.

Of the viscera enveloped by the serous membranes I shall only speak here of the brain, as the lungs and liver will come in under the head of the respiratory and digestive organs respectively. I will just say, however, that Bryonia is frequently indicated in inflammations of parenchymatous organs on which it has no direct action, when it is their serous envelope which is affected. Such maladies are the diaphragmitis, the lienitis and the ovaritis for which Hartmann commends it. Returning to the brain,—Bryonia is of great value in simple non-inflammatory *congestion* of this organ. Cases are on record in which such a condition arising from suppressed menstruation, from exposure to intense cold, and from seasickness with long-lasting constipation, was promptly dissipated by the medicine. It is also frequently useful in congestive headaches, with feeling of bursting or splitting, which are seated in the forehead, relieved by pressure, and much increased by stooping, which causes a sensation as if the brain would fall out. If—as it often is—giddiness is present, the patient feels as though he would pitch forwards. Another kind of headache for which Bryonia is useful is a form of hemicrania : the pain is generally on the right side, and is accompanied by retching and bilious vomiting.

Before leaving the serous membranes, I must refer to their synovial analogues ; only to say, however, that Bryonia has proved as useful in idiopathic synovitis—when caused by cold or injury—as when the affection is the local manifestation of rheumatism.

IV. I have now to speak of the power of Bryonia over affections of the digestive organs. A form of *gastralgia* for which it is suitable is again most excellently described by Trinks. " The pressure on the stomach, a much more frequent affection in the female than in the male, generally caused by irregularity in diet, eating indigestible food, bread not enough baked, coffee, brandy, or bad beer, finds for the most part its radical cure in Bryonia. It comes on when the stomach is empty as well as when it is full, but more frequently immediately after it has been emptied of its contents : the patients complain of a pressure at the pit of the stomach, *as if they felt a heavy annoying stone there ;* it lasts from two to four hours, sometimes longer, and goes off with much eructation. In worse cases, the so-called water-brash is an accompaniment, or there is a great deal of acidity generated, which shows itself by sour risings, heartburn, and vomiting of a very sour and acrid mucus. In the severer degrees of this pain of stomach, the epigastrium becomes extremely sensitive to external touch and pressure, and the patient cannot bear the clothes to be firmly put on." Teste notes of the Bryony dyspepsia, that beer disagrees or gives no satisfaction to thirst, and that water is absolutely required as a *dissolvent.* As with Nux vomica and Lycopodium, gastric disorder requiring Bryony is generally accompanied by *constipation ;* but whether for this malady occurring independently it is ever better than the other more important medicines we have, I cannot say. Hahnemann ranks it with Nux vomica and Opium. Dr. Dunham considers that Bryonia is specially adapted to torpor of the bowels, as distinguished from the ineffectual urging of Nux vomica ; and Dr. Guernsey indicates dryness of the fæces, as if burnt, as calling for it.* Dr. Bayes recommends it in the constipation of children, where the fæces are so large and hard as to cause pain in passing. The

* See cases in *Hoyne,* i., 80, and *Amer. Homœopathist,* ii., 43.

diarrhœa of Bryonia also must not be forgotten as a possible indication for its therapeutic use. I have heard of its doing much in America for cholera infantum. Causation of diarrhœa by dry, hot weather is always regarded as indicating it.

In affections of the liver, Bryonia frequently comes into play, often in association with Mercurius. It hardly reaches to true hepatitis ; but in congestive states of the organ, with pain in the right shoulder, giddiness, and slight yellowness of the skin and eyes, it is very useful. It is pre-eminently a gastro-hepatic medicine, and constantly finds place when the digestion is impaired in consequence of the imperfect action of the liver.

V. We come now to the action of Bryonia in affections of the respiratory organs, which from its pathogenesis should be rather extensive. It is the best medicine—after Aconite— for what is known as a " cold on the chest," *i.e.*, where a nasal catarrh has run down the air-passages, as far as the first or even second division of the bronchi. Heat, soreness, and pain behind the sternum, and an irritative shaking cough with scanty expectoration, make up the Bryony picture. Or, in Trinks's words, there is " dry, more or less severe cough, often rising to the point of retching, which is excited and maintained by a constant ' tickle ' in the lower part of the trachea or under the breast-bone, which is more severe by day than by night, and forces up only a very small quantity of clear, sometimes blood-streaked, expectoration ; gives rise to pain of being shaken in the abdomen, or in the chest and head, and makes the patients often complain of an extremely annoying pressure under the sternum, which confines the breathing. These states occur frequently in elderly persons with stuffing of the nose, running from the eyes, and derangement of the stomach, at the beginning and end of winter. For this condition Bryonia effects all that can be expected from a medicine, and that very speedily." Another of our veterans, Dr. Schrön, has some valuable remarks on the action of Bryony in the respiratory sphere.* Among other things, he says, " In chronic cough, which becomes very violent at the least excitation of the lungs, as speaking, which is worst morning and evening, and which is accompanied by very little expectoration, as we observe in individuals whose lungs have suffered from previous inflammation and frequent attacks of hæmoptysis, I have seen Bryonia administered with the best effects. I had such a case in which the patient coughed for whole nights together. Bryonia 6, given for some length of time, not only produced perfect night-rest, but favoured the process of nourishment in such a manner, that the patient, who was formerly quite emaciated, picked up flesh, and her appetite improved." Dr. Dunham notes of the Bryonia cough that the patient often presses on the sternum to support the chest during the exertions he makes.

But besides conditions such as these, Bryonia has obtained reputation in the treatment of the three great affections of the respiratory organs, croup, bronchitis, and pneumonia.

1. For *croup* Bryonia had been recommended by M. Teste (in alternation with Ipecacuanha) long before M. Curie ascertained its power of developing false membranes. He speaks very confidently of the certainty of this treatment. M. Curie himself relies upon Bryonia in the treatment of croup and laryngo-tracheal diphtheria. We have as yet no differential diagnosis between it and Iodine, Bromine and Kali bichromicum as anti-croupous remedies.

2. In most of our text-books and domestic treatises, Bryonia occupies the first place among the remedies for acute *bronchitis*. I myself am quite unable to see its homœopathicity to this disease, when the smaller bronchiæ are involved; and I have never been able to trace any good effect from it in practice. I said so much in a paper which I read on bronchitis before the British Homœopathic Society; and found that my colleagues generally had met with the same disappointment in the use of the drug.* Bryonia, therefore, must no longer stand at the head of the medicines curative of this disease. Dr. Jousset, indeed, praises it in capillary bronchitis; but he always gives Ipecacuanha in alternation with it, and I should be inclined to ascribe most of the benefit observed to the latter drug.

3. It is otherwise with *pneumonia*. From what has been said, indeed, Bryony can obviously do no good in the bronchopneumonia so common in children and aged persons, where a catarrh begins in the bronchial mucous membrane, and probably affects the air-cells rather in the way of œdema and collapse than of actual inflammation. But to primary "croupous" pneumonia Bryonia is perfectly homœopathic, even more so than the Phosphorus which in this country (at least) usually plays the chief part in the treatment of the disease. Its power of developing a false membrane in the air-tubes, which makes nothing in its favour in bronchitis, is all-important here, where we have to deal—not with catarrh of a mucous membrane (which is absent in the air-cells proper)—

* See *Annals*, v., 193.

but with fibrinous exudation. To convince yourself of its
power you have only to read Tessier's cases treated in the
Hôpital S. Marguerite, in which Bryonia was the chief
remedy employed.* Dr. Jousset continues to express unbounded confidence in it, giving it (like his master) in the
higher attenuations (12-24). I am myself in the habit of
administering it in the first decimal dilution ; and think I can
claim for it, thus given, the power ascribed by Kafka to
Iodine and Bromine, but refused by Jousset to any medicine,
of aborting the disease. Pleural complication would of course
confirm the indications for it in any given case ; and in
pleuro-pneumonia proper—if you ever encounter such an
affection in the human subject—you will find it specific. It
has been found curative of the epidemic pleuro-pneumonia of
animals.

There are yet a few residuary phenomena to be noted in
the action of Bryonia.

a. The first is the power which it exerts over the *mammary*
glands. Whenever, from the first coming in of the milk, from
catching cold while nursing, or from abrupt weaning, the
breast becomes swollen, tender, knotty, and painful, Bryonia
will almost certainly resolve the inflammation and prevent the
formation of abscess Dr. Dunham advises it in milk fever.

b. Secondly, Bryonia is of such high popular repute in the
scleroderma of horned cattle—*Haningkrankheit*—that it has
acquired the name of *Haningwurzel.* Dr. Mayrhofer proved
it on three oxen, and in each the primitive symptoms of the
disorder were developed—the skin becoming dry, creaky, and
adherent, and the hair bristly and knotty. It is thus suitable
in scleroderma neonatorum. It is occasionally praised by
homœopathists in dropsical conditions—as, for instance, in
the œdema of the legs which comes on in some pregnant
women without the intervention of renal mischief. It would
probably be suitable to the condition lately described as
" skin-dropsy," where anasarca occurs independently of disease
of the heart or kidneys, and is supposed to depend upon insufficient performance of their functions on the part of the
sudoriparous glands.—It is also possible that these effects of
the drug indicate a specific action as exerted by it on the
subcutaneous cellular tissue, and that it may prove useful
where inflammation and induration occur herein. Jahr considers it the most effective medicine we have for absorbing or
promoting the rapid maturation of carbuncle.

c. Bryonia has not much influence on the eye (at any rate

* *Recherches cliniques sur le traitement de la Pneumonie, &c.,* 1850.

it is not much used in its diseases), though it would seem suitable enough to rheumatic ophthalmia. Drs. Allen and Norton say :—" It is rarely, if ever, indicated in diseases affecting the external tissues of the eye, its great sphere of usefulness being in diseases of the uveal tract." They commend it in iritis, choroiditis (especially the so-called " serous " form), and ciliary neuralgia, where the pains are of its shooting character, and have its aggravation from motion. They add amelioration from pressure as a characteristic condition for it here. Dr. Vilas commends it in scleritis and episcleritis.

4. Several of Dr. Guernsey's indications for the drug I have already mentioned. I may add—dry, parched lips and mouth ; thirst for large draughts of water; nausea and faintness on sitting up ; vomiting of food soon after taking it. It is commended by some in vicarious menstruation, and is particularly good, Dr. Guernsey says, when this takes the form of epistaxis.

I mentioned at the outset of these remarks the kind of patient for whom Bryonia is suitable. I conclude by saying that it is well indicated for morbid states brought on by that very anger to which he is prone, and also to those resulting from the dry east winds of our climate. This last point gives it another feature of differentiation from Rhus, which rather meets the consequences of damp.

From its extensive range Bryonia cannot but have many analogues. In its relation to rheumatism, it compares with *Aconite, Rhus*, and *Colchicum ;* in fever it acts like *Baptisia* and *Eupatorium.* It affects the serous membranes like *Aconite, Arsenic,* and *Mercurius corrosivus ;* the synovial membranes like *Pulsatilla ;* the alimentary canal like *Nux vomica* and *Lycopodium ;* the liver like *Mercurius* and *Chelidonium ;* the air-passages like *Nux* and *Senega ;* the lungs like *Phosphorus, Chelidonium,* and *Tartar emetic.*

The dose of Bryonia, like that of all the polychrests, varies widely. As a rule it may be said that the lowest potencies act best in rheumatism and dyspepsia, and the medium and higher in respiratory affections. But even to this rule there are exceptions ; and in its other applications it is equally in favour with those who use the high and with those who prefer the low dilutions. That is, I believe, its action is qualitative rather than quantitative.

LECTURE XXII.

CACTUS—CALCAREA.

Our first medicine to-day comes to us—as a medicine—from Italy.

There are, I do not doubt, many excellent homœopathists in that country; but hitherto they have contributed little to our literature or to our Materia Medica. Dr. Rubini, of Naples, has come forward to redeem the credit of his countrymen in this matter, and has given us a new and valuable medicine in the night-blooming cereus,

Cactus grandiflorus.

A tincture is prepared from the young and tender branches and the flowers.

Dr. Rubini, after observation of the physiological and therapeutical effects of the Cactus for ten or twelve years, published a pamphlet containing the results of his experience. It was translated by Dr. Dudgeon for the *British Journal of Homœopathy*, in whose twenty-second volume it may be found. It contains numerous symptoms observed on the healthy (subjects and doses not specified), and as many cured in the sick. Some later provings, from four sources, are incorporated with Dr. Rubini's results in Allen's *Encyclopædia*; and Dr. Hale, in the article on the drug in the second edition of his *New Remedies*, has collected all the clinical experience with it which had appeared in print up to that time (1867).

From Dr. Rubini's proving it would appear that Cactus has a very powerful action upon the heart and arteries, closely resembling that of Aconite. General rigor, followed by much heat and sweat, even recurring daily at the same hour, and symptoms—as pain and hæmorrhage—of acute congestion in the head and chest, attest its action on the arterial system; while the heart gives evidence in pain, palpitation, oppressed breathing, and constriction about the chest, of being unusually affected. The pulsation in the scrobiculus cordis so characteristic of cardiac disorder is markedly produced by Cactus. It causes also painful pressure on the vertex; acid risings from the stomach, with sense of weight there; severe twisting colic, with heat (external and internal) of the abdomen; bilious diarrhœa, with pain before the stools; inflammatory strangury, followed by copious urine loaded with lithates; and painful menstruation. There is great prostration; and the mental condition is one of profound melancholy.

From such a pathogenesis as this brilliant results might be anticipated. Dr. Rubini assigns to it a wide range of curative power. "The characteristic feature of the Cactus consists in this, that while it developes its action specially in the heart and its blood-vessels, dissipating their congestions, and removing their irritations, it does not weaken the nervous system like Aconite;" so he writes in the preface to his proving. I must differ from him about Aconite weakening the nervous system. It need never do so, if the dose be not too large. But if Cactus acts in this manner, it may be a formidable rival to Aconite, as it would obviously be used in the same class of cases. It is said to have cured with striking rapidity acute otitis, acute and even chronic bronchitis, pleurisy, pneumonia, hæmoptysis, hæmatemesis, gastroenteritis, hepatitis, hæmaturia, and a quotidian ague. These experiences have yet to be confirmed. For my own part, when I meet with these acute fevers, congestions, and hæmorrhages, I seem quite content with my tried and valued Aconite, and am loth to experiment with any other medicine. It is otherwise in affections of the heart, where Cactus appears to exert a power beyond that of Aconite, and to fill a place hitherto vacant. It seems beneficial in all over-actions of this organ, from nervous palpitation to acute carditis. In the distress arising from hypertrophy; in the severe sufferings incident to valvular disease* (perhaps also in angina pectoris); and in chronic palpitation, it generally gives rapid and lasting relief. The feeling as if the heart were grasped and compressed as with an iron hand (probably spasm) is very characteristic of Cactus in these cases, and is well-marked in its pathogenesis. It would probably be beneficial, at least to relieve pain, in internal aneurisms.

* See an excellently narrated case by Dr. O'Brien in the tenth volume of the *Monthly Hom. Review.*—Dr. Meyhoffer's experience with Cactus in cardiac affections, as related in his contribution to the Transactions of the Paris Congress of 1878, is also worth consulting.

Dr. Lippe states that he has frequently cured with Cactus the pressive headache in the vertex so often met with as a result of menorrhagia. I myself place much reliance on it in the similar headache of the menopausia. Dr. Guernsey says that the constrictive sensation—as of an iron hoop—caused by Cactus in many parts of the body is an unerring indication for it in practice. This statement has been confirmed by many observers. Among them is Dr. Wallace McGeorge, whose communication on the subject may be read in the eleventh volume of the *Hahnemannian Monthly* (p. 507). He relates an instance of vaginismus in which, led by this characteristic, he prescribed Cactus with success. Dr. Farrington mentions another of rheumatism of the diaphragm, where the same constrictive sensation was prominent, and where the remedy proved equally potent.

The great analogue of Cactus is obviously *Aconite*. Its influence on the heart resembles that of *Naja*.

Dr. Rubini recommends the mother-tincture in acute inflammations and organic diseases of the heart. In its nervous affections he states that the higher dilutions act well.

The remainder of my lecture to-day will be occupied with the subject of the action within the organism of the preparations of lime—

Calcarea.

Hahnemann has proved two of these—the *acetate* and the *carbonate ;* and some later work has been done with *C. caustica, fluorata, iodata, phosphorica,* and *sulphurica,* and some knowledge attained of the virtues of *C. arsenica* and *muriatica.* I shall speak of each of these separately, in its distinctive characters. But, first of all, there is a good deal to be said upon lime as such, without reference to the peculiarities of its several salts.

Lime differs from all the substances which have hitherto come before us as medicines, in that it is a normal constituent of the animal body. It enters, as you know, into the composition not only of the bones and teeth, but into that also of muscle, nerve, and nearly every other solid and fluid portion of the organism. It may hence be thought doubtful, at the first blush, if such a substance can have pathogenetic properties beyond those belonging to any local influence it may exert. When absorbed into the blood, it must surely be taken up by the tissues which it goes to constitute, and welcomed instead of resented by them. It would seem, moreover, to act in disease as a food rather than as a medicine ; so that its remedial use belongs to dietetics, and finds no place in a course of Materia Medica.

I have no doubt that there is some measure of truth in such arguments, especially on their therapeutic side. That, in cases of deficiency of lime as of iron, these elements can be given as food and so appropriated by the hungry tissues, I have no doubt ; and the practice which results from the conviction is daily supported by success. But this does not warrant the inference that such substances can have no operation as poisons and no use as medicines. Consider what must happen if they are administered in excess—if more is introduced than the tissues require for their health and integrity. Elimination will doubtless dispose of some of the superfluity. But the affinity of the substance for certain parts of the organism will still be attracting it thither ; and, while its *quality* determines its destination, its *quantity* will prevent its acting as a food and being wholly assimilated. You cannot make perfect health more healthy ; and if you continue to ply a part with its natural stimuli and aliment beyond the point of perfect health, you necessarily produce disease.

Now it has been fully ascertained, and is well set forth by Dr. von Grauvogl in his *Text-Book of Homœopathy*, that the kind of disease produced is just that which ordinarily results from deficiency of the substance in question. Thus the habitual drinkers of chalybeate waters become anæmic. On the other side, it is a fact—and upon the principle *similia similibus* should be so—that these elements of the tissues, when given as medicines, promote the assimilation from the food and blood of the very material of which they consist. We shall see, when we come to Ferrum, that in this way anæmia may be cured by doses of iron far too small to have any nutritive value. Substances of this kind are called by von Grauvogl "nutrition-remedies," as distinguished from the "function-remedies," which are alien from the composition of the body.

A Dr. Schussler has lately caused some sensation by proposing to treat all diseases with such medicines as form part of the organism, and so to limit our Materia Medica to a dozen constituents. This proposition, indeed—commended to us strangely enough by Dr. Constantine Hering—we cannot for a moment entertain ; but the importance of the remedies in question is undoubted.

The question then arises—is lime one of them ? To answer it we must go, as with iron, to places where it is habitually introduced in excess as a constituent of the food or drink of the inhabitants. What do we find there ? In the first instance, *bronchocele*. An overwhelming mass of evidence has now been collected in favour of the opinion that "the endemic prevalence of goitre is connected with the use of water impregnated with calcareous salts." I quote Sir Thomas Watson, who himself endorses this view. But what does bronchocele mean ? Is it a mere local, perhaps mechanical, effect of the circulation of particles of lime through the gland ? Nay; for if we look a little farther—at the children of goitrous parents, at those whose thyroids are enlarging under unfavourable hygienic circumstances, we get a more general condition ; we have *cretinism*. Cretinism essentially consists in defective growth ; imperfect ossification of the skull, with hydrocephalus and imbecility ; and enlargement of the mesenteric glands. Here we have the ultimate pernicious effects of the introduction of lime in excess into the system; and they are obviously the same as those which follow its deficiency. Dr. Beneke has well pointed out the importance of phosphate of lime to cell-growth, as illustrated by agriculture ;* and no cells can need it more than those which are concerned in ossification. It only requires to be established that lime dynamically cures what dynamically it causes ; and this, I think, is fully substantiated by experience. It is apparent from the high repute which—as we shall see—the carbonate enjoys in homœopathic practice, when given for those very conditions in doses of the utmost minuteness. "Where we find," says Dr. Guernsey, "a large head, large features, pale skin with a chalky look, and (in infants) open fontanelles, we should think of Calcarea carbonica." It is hardly less apparent in the excellent results which Dr. Ringer reports from grain doses of the phosphate, of which he admits that only a small proportion can be dissolved in the gastric juices, and enter the blood.

I hold it established, therefore, that we have in lime a medicine as well as a food ; and that in the former capacity it acts, like all its congeners, according to the principle *similia similibus*. I pass, now, to consider the ascertained usefulness of its several salts.

Calcarea acetica was proved, in a saturated solution of oyster-shells in vinegar, by Hahnemann and four others : their

* See *Brit. Journ of Hom.*, xvii.

results, making 270 symptoms, appear in the fifth volume of
the *Reine Arzneimittellehre.* We count his solution our first
decimal potency, and make subsequent attenuations with
alcohol.

The pathogenesis of C. acetica deserves moie study than
it has received, as it supplies almost our only certain knowledge of the finer actions of lime. The salt has been mainly
used in the bowel affections, acute and chronic, of children
to whose general diathesis lime is suitable. Dr. Clotar
Müller says that it was the remedy in one of the only two
cases of migraine he ever succeeded in radically curing.
The symptoms indicating it were a feeling of great coldness
in the head and much gastric acidity.

It is usually given in the lowest attenuations.

Calcarea arsenica, the arsenite of lime, has not been proved,
but appears to possess the virtues of its constituent elements.
Dr. C. Hering commended it many years ago in epilepsy,[*]
and Dr. H. Nankivell has praised it in tabes mesenterica
and chronic pneumonic phthisis, with hæmoptysis,[†] while Dr.
Hilbers esteems it highly in dyspnœa from a feeble heart.
I can confirm the last-named indication.

Calcarea carbonica is the salt of lime which has found chief
use in homœopathic therapeutics. The form in which we
employ it is not chalk or marble, but the soft white substance
which is found between the external and internal hard layers
of the oyster-shell. This is triturated in the usual way. Its
pathogenesis appears in the first edition of the *Chronic
Diseases,* where 1090 symptoms are ascribed to it—all (as we
know) observed on patients taking it in the attenuations
from the 3rd to the 12th. In the second edition the list is
increased to 1631. Two hundred and seventy of the additional
symptoms are those of the acetate, which Hahnemann has
thought well to incorporate, marking them by a line—a sign
of distinction which Dr. Hempel's translation too often omits.
The remainder are from Hahnemann himself and from fresh
fellow-observers, all of course experimenting with globules of
the 30th. Dr. Allen's arrangement of the drug contains some
additional symptoms obtained from an alcoholic solution of
the precipitated carbonate by Dr. Koch on himself and four
others.

Hahnemann, in choosing this animalised form of carbon-

* *Brit. Journ. of Hom.,* vii., 564.
† *Monthly Hom. Review,* xvii., 631.

ate of lime for homœopathic purposes, was in harmony with all tradition. From early times similar natural products have been employed in medicine, such as " crabs' eyes," crabs' claws, coral, egg-shells, and powdered human cranium ; and have acquired no small reputation. Modern therapeutists, supposing themselves wiser, have substituted a more purely mineral form of the salt, but with the result of losing all but its chemical and mechanical qualities. A practitioner of the old school, who knows chalk only as a means of neutralising acid in the stomach, or of plastering over the intestinal surface to check diarrhœa, naturally ridicules us for counting it a polychrest remedy. But he forgets that our Calcarea carbonica is something more than his " creta preparata," and that it inherits an ancient and widespread renown. Stillé follows Richter in thinking that an error has been made in substituting mineral for animal preparations of lime, and says that the latter are certainly better borne by the stomach. Our fullest information on this subject, however, is given us by Dr. Imbert Gourbeyre, in his " History of Calcareous Preparations," which has been translated from *L'Art Médical* in the thirty-fourth volume of the *British Journal of Homœopathy*.

Of the symptoms of Hahnemann's pathogenesis I have nothing to say. But, taking the phenomena of cretinism as our best proving of lime, we have in the virtues of Calcarea (so called among us *par excellence*) their truly homœopathic application. It is in the large class of diseases due to derangement of the secondary assimilation that it finds its curative place. The three great forms of assimilative derangement are rachitis, scrofula, and tuberculosis ; and in all of these Calcarea is a principal remedy.

1. First, of *rachitis*. " If a child cuts its teeth late, if it does not walk so early as other children, if the fontanelles are late in closing, the probability is that it is the subject of rickets :" so writes the late Dr. Hillier, in his excellent *Clinical Treatise on Diseases of Children*. Well, then, when rachitis thus manifests itself, you will find Calcarea an invaluable aid in its treatment. But when the diathesis is more pronounced, when its phenomena reach beyond those of deficient supply of lime-salts, you will have to look farther for your medicinal remedies. I shall have more to say upon this subject when I come to Silica, which I believe to be the most potent of anti-rachitics. Let me notice here, however, that head sweats in the evening are noted by Hahnemann as an especial indication for Calcarea, and have lately been mentioned by Jenner as pathognomonic of rickets.

2. Regarding Calcarea in *scrofula*, I will begin by citing our latest writer on the disease, Dr. H. Goullon, of Weimar. " Water," he says, " that contains the salts of lime in excess is accused by some of producing scrofula. Thus it is said that the inhabitants of Rheims owe the large number of persons affected by scrofula among their population to this circumstance. If this be so, does there exist a greater triumph for Hahnemann's principle ? Certainly the Hahnemannian school, if it were without the salts of lime, would not wish to treat scrofula. Calcarea carbonica performs wonders in scrofulous ophthalmia ; like Sulphur, it removes scrofulous pot-bellies, if I may be allowed to use this expression ; like Phosphorus, it cures scrofulous diarrhœa." Dr. Goullon then cites cases of tabes mesenterica ; of strumous ophthalmia and otorrhœa ; and of disease of the joints and vertebræ in such subjects, where Calcarea has proved curative. Dr. Gourbeyre shews that scrofula was one of the chief maladies in whose treatment the animalised forms of carbonate of lime gained their ancient repute. My own experience with it is especially in the treatment of mesenteric disease, in which—if not too far advanced—it is an invaluable remedy. You will remember the enlarged abdomen of cretinism. This brings us also to bronchocele, of which Goullon writes : " The swelling of the thyroid gland is so intimately connected with scrofula that its former name—struma—has been applied to the diathesis." He gives three cases of the disease cured by Calcarea. They were all simple hypertrophies ; but the power of the drug over cystic growths—of which we shall speak presently—would encourage its use in the cystic form also of goitre. Dr. Gourbeyre relates the favourable experience of a French practitioner (Chlyssiol) in this disease with powdered egg-shells, and a case of his own, in which a large but soft goitre of many years standing disappeared in seven months under Hahnemann's Calcarea carbonica in the fourth trituration.

3. I cannot speak with any certainty of the action of Calcarea in *tuberculosis.* At the British Homœopathic Congress of 1873, Drs. Gibbs Blake and Wynne Thomas brought forward some evidence of its power over chronic maladies associated with high temperature, some of these being certainly and others presumably of a tuberculous nature.* But I have most confidence in it here as a preventive. There is a peculiar form of dyspepsia which often precedes the development of tuberculosis. Indicated more or less precisely by Drs. Tweedy Todd, Clark, Bennett, and Ancell, it has been most fully characterised

* *Monthly Hom. Review,* xvii., 683.

by Mr. Jonathan Hutchinson. Its special feature consists in
acid eructations after food : "everything the patient takes
'rises acid,' as he expresses it, but more particularly everything
containing fat, oil, or sugar." There is a special dislike to
fat present.* Now in this acid dyspepsia Calcarea proves
itself an excellent remedy. I know not whether the fact that
two of Hahnemann's provers of the acetate had constant sour
eructations has any bearing on the point, since they were
taking vinegar ; but of the value of the carbonate, in the
minutest doses, there is not the least question. I have myself
cured with it a most obstinate case, in which the fount of acid
seemed inexhaustible, and even gouty symptoms were set up
in a patient the most unlikely to be attacked with such a
malady.

In all derangements of nutrition, whether rachitic or not,
when occurring (as they generally do) in children, Calcarea is
indicated where the profuse perspiration of the head which I
have mentioned is present.

The powers of our drug seem moreover to extend to the
new products which result from disorders of growth. It has
repeatedly been reported as causing the disappearance of
warts, polypi, and even benignant tumours of the encysted
kind.† In this connexion it must not be forgotten as a possible aid against cancer. In the _Lancet_ for 1868 Dr. Peter
Hood published two cases in which the daily administration
of small quantities of powdered oyster-shell effected a cure of
this dire disease. Mr. Spencer Wells, who authenticated his
observations, suggested that the rationale of the cure was that
the lime caused ossification of the blood-vessels of the diseased
part, and so starved it out. The process is one not easy of
conception ; and a specific curative power is at least as
tenable a theory.

This is the great sphere of the action of Calcarea. But it
has other uses, which seem independent of its power over
assimilation. One of these is of a very curious kind ; and, if
I had not repeatedly seen it (and also felt it) myself, and had
it vouched for by excellent observers like Drs. Dudgeon,
Drury, and Bayes, could hardly have credited it. It is its
power, when given in repeated doses of the 30th dilution, of
relieving the pain attending the passage of biliary (Dr. Bayes
says also of renal) calculi. It has for me quite superseded the

---

* Aitken, _Science and Practice of Medicine_, 5th ed., ii., 206; to
whom I am indebted for these facts.

† See Goullon on Scrofula, art. _Calcarea_, and _Brit. Journ. of Hom._,
xxvi., 31.

need of chloroform and even of the hot bath. Hahnemann, moreover, insists much on the relation of Calcarea to the menstrual function. " It is indispensable and curative," he says, " when the catamenia appear a few days before the period, especially when the flow of blood is considerable. But if the catamenia appear at the regular period or a little later, Calcarea is hardly ever useful, even if the catamenia should be rather profuse." In these cases, says Dr. Guernsey (who has a great *penchant* for out-of-the-way symptoms), the patients often complain of a sensation as if cold, damp stockings were on their feet : whenever they do, we may think of Calcarea. Again, the medicine has a considerable reputation in epilepsy* (Dr. Gourbeyre mentions the high ancient repute of powdered human cranium in this malady) and in migraine,† when these affections appear in the natural subjects of its influence, *i.e.* (as I might have said from the first) in unhealthy women and children, of leuco-phlegmatic temperament, and with tendency to corpulence. In these subjects it will remove many anomalous symptoms and local troubles, as headache with sense of coldness, toothache (especially that of pregnancy) caused by the slightest cold, leucorrhœa, deficiency of milk while nursing ; and so forth. The sensitiveness to cold mentioned in connexion with the toothache of Calcarea is noted by Dr. Guernsey as characteristic of the general morbid condition calling for it ; " every current of cool air," he says, " seems to go through and through the patient." Vertigo on ascending, I may add, is another of his " keynotes " for it.

Jahr says that, after failing in acute hydrocephalus with the ordinary remedies, he took to treating the disease with Calcarea 30, and with very different results. I have mentioned in my *Therapeutics* a favourable result obtained by myself in this way. Still more decisive is its action in chronic hydrocephalus, where its power as a nutrition remedy comes into play. Perhaps C. phosphorica, as recommended by von Grauvogl, may be still more effectual here.

I have quoted Dr. Goullon's commendation of it in strumous ophthalmia. It is highly esteemed in the homœopathic treatment of this malady, especially when the cornea is involved. Hitherto, we have supposed it to act here by modifying the constitutional diathesis. Dr. Mc Dowell, of Baltimore, however, has recently described‡ what he calls " oyster-shucker's

* *Brit. Journ. of Hom.*, xxii., 246, 258.
† See *Ibid*, xxi., 282.
‡ See *N. York Medical Record*, xvi., 83.

corneitis." He is " disposed to attribute the disease to a specific toxic element contained in the slime and dirt which coats the oyster-shell ;" but I think we may fairly prefer to trace it to emanations from the shell itself.

The analogues of Calcarea carbonica are *Baryta, Iodium, Phosphorus,* and *Silica.*

The higher dilutions, from the 12th to the 30th, are those which appear to be most in favour, and which I myself use ; but the 3rd is undoubtedly efficacious. Calcarea seems seldom or never employed by the exclusive adherents of mother tinctures and crude drugs.

Calcarea caustica.—Lime in this form, in which we have it in the ordinary lime-water, can have but slight pathogenetic properties, as we give the latter freely, even to children, as an antacid. But provings made with it by Koch, Keil, and Liedbeck on thirteen persons give it in Dr. Allen's *Encyclopædia* a list of 342 symptoms. These seem but trivial ; and I have no knowledge of their having received any application to practice. Dr. Wyld speaks highly of it as a resolvent application to boils and carbuncles.

Calcarea fluorata has been proved on three persons, in the 15th dilution, by Dr. J. B. Bell. It is one of Schussler's "tissue remedies," introduced into the series because of its presence in bone and the enamel of teeth. It seems several times to have removed exostoses in the human subject, and is recommended for the spavin of horses.

Calcarea iodata, the iodide of lime, has been proved by Dr. W. S. Blakely and another in the crude substance and the lower triturations ; 47 symptoms of it are given by Allen. These, too, are of no very definite character ; though, as with C. caustica, the head is the part most affected. Dr. Meyhoffer thinks the iodide the best form of lime in the chronic bronchitis of scrofulous children, when in a thin subject (in the last point distinguished from the carbonate) the cervical glands are much swollen, the cough rather dry, and there is ground for suspicion of enlargement of the bronchial glands. It is soluble in water, and with this the lower attenuations are made ; but Dr. Sherman says that in this form it is readily decomposed, and that triturations are preferable.

Calcarea phosphorica..—Dr. Hering has justly taken me to

task for having said, in the first edition of my Manual, that this salt of lime had never been proved. He refers me to some provings of the 1st and 2nd triturations made under his superintendence, which I ought to have known of, as they were in Jahr's *New Manual.* He speaks also of yet more extensive provings still unpublished. Dr. Allen gives all that are now extant. It has not been largely used in homœopathic practice. Dr. von Grauvogl relies much upon it in chronic hydrocephalus, both to cure the already existing disease, and—by giving it to the mother during pregnancy—to avert the tendency to its recurrence in future children. Dr. Cooper* speaks highly of it for chronically-enlarged tonsils in strumous subjects; and Dr. Verdi, of Washington, has much confidence in it in phthisis.† Dr. Guernsey gives as a great indication for it that every cold causes rheumatic pain in the joints and in various parts of the body. It, too, is one of Schussler's twelve remedies, and is given by him to promote the nutrition of the tissues into whose composition it enters, especially the blood corpuscles and the bones. Dr. Hering long ago used it on the same principle to favour the union of fractures and the closing of open fontanelles, and also to aid in dentition. But the main use of phosphate of lime is as a food in the same class of cases in which we use the carbonate as a remedy, and perhaps in others. Dr. Dusart, of Paris, is a well-known advocate of its use in this way, and his syrup of the lacto-phosphate is a convenient form for its administration to children. Dr. Ringer gives us the latest estimate of its efficiency. He recommends it in most forms of mal-nutrition and defective cell-growth ; in anæmia from growing fast, rapid child-bearing, prolonged suckling, or excessive menstruation ; in chronic discharges ; in rachitis ; and for the bad effects of town life, including brain-fag. He gives one or two grains of the salt three times a day. The homœopathic uses have been made with the lower triturations.

Calcarea muriatica (the chloride of calcium) has not been proved. I find it extremely useful in the moist porrigo capitis of children, giving it in the first attenuation. Some use it in solution as an abortive local application for boils ; it is said to ease the pain also.‡ It has lately been recommended in the old school as an anti-scrofulous medicine.§

* *Monthly Hom. Review*, xi.
† *Brit. Journ. of Hom.*, xxix., 749.
‡ *Ibid*, xix., 498.
§ *Lancet*, Aug. 28, 1877.

Calcarea sulphurica, the sulphate of lime, has been proved (in the higher attenuations), as you will see from Allen ; but here too we owe any knowledge we possess of the drug to Dr. Schussler.   He says that it is present in connective tissue, and acts chiefly on this part, being thus valuable in suppurations. " It acts," he says, " with more intensity in most cases where Hepar sulphuris, the sulphide of lime, has heretofore been given."   Quaglio and Kock support this statement ; and " it is willingly confirmed," says Dr. Hering, " by the one who introduced the old Hepar in suppurations."

CALENDULA, CAMPHOR, CANNABIS SATIVA AND INDICA,
CANTHARIS.

I begin to-day with the common garden marigold—

Calendula.

This plant owes its place in the Materia Medica of Homœopathy to its power as a *vulnerary*. Dr. Allen gives a pathogenesis of it obtained by two provers, but the symptoms are
few and insignificant, and it is rarely given internally.   One
of our German practitioners, however, Dr. Thorer, becoming
acquainted with the virtues ascribed to the marigold by the
common people, endeavoured to ascertain by experiment its
exact place in the treatment of injuries.   You will find his
paper translated in the fifth volume of the *British Journal of
Homœopathy*.   His cases show that Calendula has a most
beneficial influence over wounds, especially incised wounds,
promoting union by first intention, or, where that is impossible, favourable cicatrisation with the least possible
amount of suppuration.   From that time to this Calendula
has always been used in homœopathic practice to promote
the healing process in wounds, ulcers, burns, and other
breaches of surface.   You may read instructive comments on
its virtues by Dr. Yeldham in several papers in the *British
Journal* and the *Annals*.   It was used on a large scale by our
American colleagues in the treatment of the injuries arising
in the course of their civil war ; and it obtained (as you may
see, for instance, from Dr. Franklin's book on surgery) their
warmest commendations.   No suppuration seems able to live
in its presence.

Of course there is nothing homœopathic about Calendula,—
its working, that is, is no instance (so far as we know) of the
operation of the law of similars.   Nevertheless, it is homœopathists only—at least in England and America—who give their
patients the benefit of this precious vulnerary. You will find it

invaluable in surgical, and also in gynæcological, practice. Dr. Ludlam, our foremost authority in the latter sphere, has just made some remarks on its value herein, advising its use in all solutions of continuity of the sexual passages, and even commending its internal use in chronic endo-cervicitis and scrofulous ulceration, with much purulent leucorrhœa.

I have now to speak to you of

Camphor,

of which we make an alcoholic solution. The proportion of drug to vehicle in this mother-tincture has ranged in homœopathic pharmacy from one eighth to one twelfth. The British Homœopathic Pharmacopœia makes it one tenth. The preparation sold as " Rubini's Camphor " is a saturated solution, as used by that physician in the treatment of cholera. Some alarming accidents have lately occurred from persons employing this tincture with the freedom to which they have been accustomed in the use of the ordinary preparation, which can do no harm. There has been a very absurd and unfair attempt to make capital out of these occurrences as against homœopathy.[*] A few minutes thought and inquiry would have shown that the only blame rested with the carelessness which ignored an obvious and reasonable difference of strength in the two solutions.

A proving of Camphor appears in the fourth volume of the *Reine Arzneimittellehre.* It contains 105 symptoms from Hahnemann himself, and 240 "observations of others," of which 93 are from twenty-one authors, and the rest from four fellow-provers. Camphor was also one of the medicines proved by Professor Jörg: his results, obtained upon himself and ten of his pupils, are given in Frank's *Magazin* (iv. 482), and related by Hempel, who adds some further pathogenetic records. Dr. Allen, combining these materials, gives 916 symptoms to the drug.

The action of Camphor on the organism has been a matter of dispute from early times. The old physicians were divided into two camps on the question whether it is a "hot" or a "cold" remedy. Hahnemann recognises the variable character of the facts before him, and suggests their explanation. "The action," he says, " of this substance on the healthy body is extremely problematic and difficult of definition, for this reason, that the primary action of Camphor alternates so

[*] See Transactions of Clinical Society of London, vii., 28.

suddenly, and is so easily confounded, with the reaction of the vital principle." He explains farther on that he agrees with those who consider chill and depression to be the first effects of Camphor, and refer the symptoms of stimulation so often observed to a secondary reaction. He is supported herein by the weighty authority of Trousseau and Pidoux. After a full survey of the evidence, they conclude that the essential action of Camphor is " refrigerant and sedative," and describe its full poisonous effects as those of collapse with chill. Stillé (who has an exhaustive article upon the drug) takes the same view *as regards large doses*—from thirty to sixty grains. But he thinks, on the other hand, that all the evidence goes to show that "the direct and primary action of small or medicinal doses—from one to fifteen grains—of Camphor is to stimulate and excite the nervous and vascular systems, and through them the whole organism." If he is right—and I myself think that the facts bear him out—Camphor conforms to the view of drug-action maintained by Dr. Sharp. It has an opposite action on the healthy body in large and small doses respectively ; and its effects in cold and depressed conditions of the system are due to the direct stimulant influence of the moderate quantities in which it is administered. I have already explained to you why I am unable to accept this law as true of medicinal action in general ; and I think that the exceptional character of the dosage of Camphor shows that, where it does apply, it leads to a mode of practice peculiar to its operation, and different from that which obtains in homœopathic treatment generally.

It was not many years before Hahnemann had an opportunity of giving his views about Camphor a practical application, and thereby of making a most important contribution to therapeutics. In 1831 Asiatic cholera for the first time invaded Europe. The few physicians then practising homœopathically sought diligently for its *similimum*, that they might be ready to encounter it. Several medicines were suggested ; but when Hahnemann spoke out from his retreat at Coethen, he pronounced the one great remedy to be Camphor. He described the well-known features of the first stage of the invasion,—the sinking of strength, the coldness, the anxietas ; all these occurring before the vomiting, purging, and cramps have set in. Here, Hahnemann said, Camphor is a potent and certain remedy. It should be given freely—by the mouth, by inhalation, by friction, by clyster ; and persevered with till the patient recovers. Nor, though the second stage has supervened ere the treatment has begun, should Camphor be neglected. But here, unless improvement set in within a couple of hours, it is of no use to persist, and recourse must be had to other remedies, of which he specifies Cuprum and Veratrum.*

Hahnemann had the gratification of hearing of the great success which attended all who followed this advice of his, and of numerous instances in which the family use of Camphor had checked the earliest symptoms of the prevailing scourge. In the epidemic of 1849, British physicians had an opportunity of testing the value of the remedy: and Dr. Drysdale in Liverpool † and Dr. Russell in Edinburgh vied in their praises of it. The latter, who has written a book on the disease, ‡ says: " It is our firm belief that Camphor is an almost infallible remedy for cholera, if given from the very outset." In 1854, the same testimony was given to its value in England; and from Italy still more striking evidence was adduced as to what it can do. Dr. Rubini, of Naples—he who has given us Cactus grandiflorus—states that during this epidemic he treated, together with his colleagues, 592 cases with Camphor alone without a single death. He gave it in the spirit of Hahnemann's instructions—*ad libitum* doses of a saturated tincture, and relied upon it to the exclusion of all other medicines in every stage of the disease. You will find a full account of his observations in the tenth volume of the *Monthly Homœopathic Review.* Much exception has been taken to his statement of results, as exaggerated; but I think without just cause. Dr. Rubini is a physician of undoubted experience and judgment, not to speak of trustworthiness; and his published affirmations have never been contradicted. He does not mean to say that all his cases were in collapse: on the contrary, of a set of 200 treated in one institution, it is expressly mentioned that collapse occurred in fifteen only. What our colleague wishes us to understand is, that in an epidemic of Asiatic cholera in which 377 cases came under his own treatment, and 215 more under that of his fellow-practitioners, they gave nothing but Camphor, and lost no patient. There must have been the usual proportion of severe cases among these; so that the results are most gratifying. We have hitherto been jubilant about reducing the ordinary 50 per cent. mortality from cholera to one half; but 26 per cent. of deaths is a melancholy rate after all. We are bound

---

* His paper may be read in Dudgeon's *Lesser Writings* of Hahnemann, p. 845.

† *Brit. Journ. of Hom.*, viii., 149.

‡ *On Epidemic Cholera*, p. 211.

to look in directions which promise something better still; and Dr. Rubini's extension of Hahnemann's Camphor-treatment deserves our most respectful attention. Mr. Proctor, indeed, reports less favourably of it in the Liverpool epidemic of 1866 ;* but further experimentation is required. In the same epidemic Dr. Rubini treated 123 cases, and again his mortality was nil.†

It is natural to inquire whether the report of the anti-choleraic virtues of Camphor has spread beyond homœopathic regions, and whether any trial has been made of it. This might well be, as in its case there are no posological prejudices to be overcome. I am only acquainted, however, with one miserable instance of its use in the last epidemic, where it was given to a few patients at the London Hospital. The physician did not deign to follow our method of administration, viz., dropping it on sugar, but gave it suspended in water. He thus nauseated his patients, and burnt their throats ; and consequently, instead of exhibiting it in a better form, thought fit to abandon its use altogether. Both Ringer and Wood, however, now recommend it ; and the latter states that it forms the chief ingredient in the popular cholera-mixtures sold in America.

A similar action to the foregoing, though on a humbler level, is the power which Camphor has of checking an incipient "cold." Hahnemann, in the preface to his proving, commends it in the influenza then first known as an epidemic ; and Dr. Ringer has lately extolled its virtues in the chronic paroxysmal coryza from which some people suffer. In all these nasal defluxions Camphor should be taken by olfaction as well as internally. It is also of much repute in summer diarrhœa. I think that Dr. Phillips well characterises the condition which calls for it here as one of exhaustion with irritability of the intestinal nerves resulting from high summer heat ; but Dr. Ringer finds it useful also in diarrhœa resulting from cold.

A few words must be said on the symptoms of re-action which sometimes occur after Camphor poisoning, where the primary effects have been sedative. They are those of fever, with much confusion and oppression of the brain, and even disorder of its functions. The fever, as in a case recorded by Dr. Hempel, may take on a typhoid form and be of some duration. I cannot say whether these facts have any relation

* See *Brit. Journ. of Hom.*, xxv., 92.
† See his *Statistica dei colerici curati colla sola Canfora in Napoli negli anni* 1854, 1855, 1865. 3rd edizione, ampliata. Napoli, 1866.

to the antifebrile and antiseptic powers ascribed to Camphor
by the physicians of the last century, or to its occasional
successful employment in mania. It was chiefly administered
in fever when an ataxic condition was present, and phenomena
of this kind are frequent in the Camphor re-action. But I do
think they are closely connected with another use made of it
in homœopathic practice, viz., to recover the patient from the
state into which he is thrown by the retrocession of measles
or scarlatina. There is here the same cerebral disturbance
and oppression ; and the patient, though hot within, is cold
without. He has that characteristic of Camphor noted by
Dr. Guernsey, that, though cold to the touch, he will not
remain covered. I know the value of cold affusion in these
terrible cases ; but it is 'at least *jucundius*, if not also *tutius*, to
effect what we want by the administration of Camphor.

The only marked local action of Camphor is on the genito-
urinary organs, which is all the more interesting, as it cannot
be detected as passing off by the urine. That it causes
strangury is undoubted, and is admitted both by Pereira and
by Ringer. The former is naturally astonished at a power of
diminishing irritation of the urinary organs being assigned to
Camphor. But that it has this power, whether the strangury
is idiopathic or the effect of Cantharides or other drugs, is
the testimony of all the old physicians. I have myself twice
seen patients in this agonising condition translated, as it were,
from hell to heaven in less than an hour by repeated small
doses of the drug. This action, therefore, is not antipathic, as
supposed by Stillé. As with Cantharis, the urinary irritation
of Camphor sometimes extends to the genitals, causing
priapism and such-like phenomena. But the ordinary and
permanent effect upon these organs (probably through the
nervous system) is of a depressing character. "Camphora per
nares castrat odore mares" is quoted in all books on Materia
Medica ; and Hahnemann cites an observation from Loss, in
which impotence thus produced lasted a considerable time. I
do not know whether much homœopathic use has been made
of this action of Camphor. Stillé mentions several striking
instances of its value as an antipathic palliative. Dr.
Hirsch has recommended it for irritable weakness of the
sexual organs, with nocturnal emissions. Dr. Norton mentions
a similar case.*

Besides these uses in disease, Camphor is reputed by Hahnemann an antidote to most vegetable and to some animal and
mineral poisons. Against the majority of these it probably

* In an article on the drug in *Brit. Journ. of Hom.*, ix., 407.

has no true antidotal power, and it would hardly neutralise their effects in poisonous quantities. But for the more delicate disturbances produced by minute doses Camphor may be a capital remedy, by substituting a more potent impression than theirs upon the nervous centres. This is probably what he meant.

Dr. Holcombe* thus sums up the action of Camphor : " It is antidotal to almost all the drastic vegetable poisons—relieves strangury—procures reaction from cold, congested conditions —is the great anti-choleraic—and quiets nervous irritability sometimes better than Coffea, Ignatia, or Hyoscyamus. This is its whole clinical value—and a great one it is—in a nut-shell."

I must not leave Camphor without referring to Dr. Harley's communication regarding it in the ninth volume of the *Practitioner*. He finds that in medicinal doses—from five to thirty grains—its effects are but slight, being chiefly those of sedation of the motor and ideational centres of the cerebrum, with much giddiness. These results are somewhat different from those of other observers, and can only be provisionally accepted at present. An epileptic fit has twice been observed as a result of an overdose of our concentrated solution.

In its influence over the circulation Camphor resembles *Aconite, Arsenic,* and *Veratrum album.* Its power of causing strangury is like that of *Cantharis* and *Terebinthina,* less like that of *Belladonna.*

The drug does not seem to bear attenuation. The primary solution is that always in use.

I will now give you some account of the medicinal virtues of *hemp.* Unlike the ordinary practice, we use not the Cannabis Indica only, but that also which grows in colder climates. Let me speak of the latter first—

Cannabis sativa.

Our tincture is prepared from the flowering tops and upper leaflets.

A proving of hemp, by Hahnemann and eight others, appears in the first volume of the *Reine Arzneimittellehre.* It contains 330 symptoms, 47 of which, however, are from authors. The severity of some of these is puzzling, when we consider how mild a poison the plant is. But the mystery is explained when we examine the originals of the two principal groups— those of Morgagni and of Ramazzini. The former consists of

* *United States Medical and Surgical Journal,* vol i.

cases of disease recorded in various parts of his *De sedibus et causis morborum,* and mentioned as occurring in hemp-dressers; but rarely traced or traceable to their occupation. The latter are symptoms occurring in workers in hemp *and linseed*—the connexion, as well as the nature of the phenomena, showing that they are mere local effects of the dust. These, therefore, must be eliminated from the pathogenesis of the drug. But in their place we have five more recent provings to put, all instituted with substantial doses, which are duly incorporated with Hahnemann's by Dr. Allen. There is an interesting study of the drug by the late Dr. Norton in the ninth volume of the *British Journal of Homœopathy.*

It would appear, from Hahnemann's preface to his proving, that Cannabis was in common use at his day as a remedy for acute gonorrhœa. It was supposed to act as a "demulcent;" but he is well warranted in saying that its curative powers depend upon the faculty it possesses of producing a similar morbid condition in the urinary organs Its pathogenesis shews excessive irritation of the mucous membrane of the bladder and urethra, and of the prepuce. The latter is dark red, hot, and inflamed ; there is much burning in the urethra, painful and difficult micturition, chordee, and mucous discharge. It has been customary to add the observation of Morgagni, in which the urine was so full of mucus and pus that the catheter became clogged, and failed in its office. This, however, is not to the point, as the case was one of paraplegia from spinal disease, and the state of the bladder (noted eight days before death) was only that incident to such affections. But there is amply sufficient evidence besides this to prove the homœopathicity of Cannabis to urinary inflammations ; and it continues to be in the school of Hahnemann the favourite remedy for gonorrhœa after the most urgent symptoms have been subdued by Aconite and (if necessary) Cantharis. Even when the inflammation is not so acute, I think we do well to commence the treatment with a more vascular medicine, which in such a case had best be Gelsemium.

A good deal of use has been made of Cannabis in affections of the eyes, owing to the symptoms in Hahnemann's pathogenesis—"the cornea becomes opaque ; pellicle before the eyes" and "cataract." For the first he himself vouches ; and though one would have liked to know under what circumstances it occurred, we cannot but accept it, and it is certain that the medicine has some effect in removing corneal opacities left behind after strumous ophthalmia. The symptom "cataract" is referred to Neuhold. This author is recording effects of the effluvia of hemp before drying, so that his symptoms are valid enough. Nor is there any doubt that his "suffusiones oculorum," which Hahnemann renders cataract, *may* mean this. Celsus* uses the phrase in this sense; and we cannot but remember Milton's

> "So thick a drop serene hath quenched their orbs,
>   Or *dim suffusion* veiled;"

though it is possible that by suffusion he means opacity of the cornea as distinguished from the "gutta serena" of cataract. At the same time, when we find the phrase occurring in a list of the observed effects of hemp without special mention or warrant, it becomes very unlikely that the author meant to hazard in this manner so startling an assertion as that the herb can cause cataract. We must wait for further information on this head.

Hahnemann's pathogenesis credits Cannabis with a power of causing inflammation of the lungs, with delirium and vomiting of green bile. Some recommendations and applications of it in pneumonia have followed, but I think without warrant. The observations in question are cited from Morgagni; and he is evidently speaking of the irritating effect of inhaling the hemp-dust on the workers in it.

In the fourth volume of the *British Journal of Homœopathy* Dr. Quin has recorded an excellent case of hemicrania cured by Cannabis. It was primarily coincident with the catamenia, which were far too copious. I think I have seen the medicine useful in menstrual headache.

The action of Cannabis on the urinary tract assimilates it to *Apis, Cantharis, Copaiba*, and *Terebinthina;* that on the eyes to *Euphrasia*.

There is a general agreement that for gonorrhœa the mother-tincture of Cannabis is required, in frequent doses of from one to ten drops; though Dr. Helmuth says that a tolerably large experience leads him to prefer the 12th. In the other affections mentioned the medium dilutions have been efficacious.

And now of the

Cannabis Indica.

The peculiar properties of this variety of hemp exist in a resin which is developed in it by climatic influences. This,

* Seventh book, vii., 13, 14.

when presented separately, is the substance known as has-chisch, bhang, gunjah, and churrus. A tincture is prepared from it for ordinary practice by dissolving one part in twenty of rectified spirit. One part of this tincture, therefore, to four of alcohol will make our first centesimal dilution.

Some provings of the Indian hemp, made upon seven persons with the tincture and lower attenuations, were published by the American Provers' Union in 1839. Since then scores of persons have tested its curious effects upon themselves ; and the experiences of haschish-eating have been put on record,—by one writer with a descriptive power and gorgeousness of diction hardly inferior to that of the " English Opium-eater." Of the results thus obtained Dr. Allen has made an exhaustive collection ; and 918 symptoms of the drug, including the mental phenomena described at full length, stand in his *Encyclopœdia*.

To possess yourselves of the characters of the haschish intoxication, it is necessary that you should study it thus in detail. No outline can adequately present it. It is a condition of intense *exaltation*, in which all perceptions and conceptions, all sensations and emotions, are exaggerated to the utmost degree. Distances seem infinite and time endless ; pleasure is paradise itself, and any painful thought or feeling plunges at once into the depths of misery. Hallucinations of the senses are common ; and the least suggestion will set going a train of vivid mental illusions. All the time a dual consciousness is present : the experimenter feels ever and anon that he is distinct from the subject of the haschisch dream, and can think rationally. The bodily sensations accompanying these phenomena are not many. Headache, sense of dryness of the mouth and throat, and anæsthesia of the surface, are not uncommon. The headache is very commonly a sensation as of the brain boiling over, and lifting the cranial arch like the lid of a tea-kettle. The anæsthesia may be preceded by sensations over the body like those produced by slight electric sparks. In the motor sphere there is experienced at times the peculiar condition known as cataleptic. Dr. O'Shaughnessy thus describes the effect of the resin on a native of India :—" At 8 p.m. we found him insensible, but breathing with perfect regularity, his pulse and skin natural, and the pupils freely contractile at the approach of light. Happening by chance to lift up the patient's right arm, the professional reader will judge of my astonishment, when I found that it remained in the posture in which I had placed it. It required but a very brief examination of the limbs to find that the patient had by the influence of this narcotic been thrown into that most strange and most extraordinary of all nervous conditions,—into that state which so few have seen, and the existence of which so many still discredit,—the genuine *catalepsy* of the nosologist."

Such application of Cannabis Indica to practice as has been made has been in perfect homœopathic *rapport* with these effects. Dr. Handfield Jones naïvely describes it as "physiologically a nervous stimulant, and therapeutically a nervous sedative." Dr. Ringer and others recommend it in headache, the former esteeming it the most useful medicine we possess for diminishing the frequency of the paroxysms of migraine. It seems, he says, to act on the nervous centre whence they spring. It is probable, however, that this effect is obtained by inducing the physiological action of the drug, as croton-chloral —which is a pure anæsthestic—produces similar results. It should be remembered if we ever come across a case of catalepsy. I myself had a patient in whom attacks, probably hysterical at bottom, assumed a cataleptiform character, and here Cannabis Indica proved rapidly curative. The exaltation of ideas it causes reminds one of the first stage of the general paralysis of the insane. It could not control the meningeal inflammation said to be always present in these patients; but it might benefit the excited nervous centres while other remedies were striking at that essential element of the malady. Its power of causing general anæsthesia adds another to the few remedies we have for this condition when occurring idiopathically. Dr. Gray reports its successful use in dissipating spectral illusions, without terror, occurring in the course of fevers, &c. Indian hemp is found to be almost entirely without effect in graminivorous animals. If Teste be right, this indicates it as specially suitable in sthenic constitutions and disorders.

The effects of Cannabis Indica on the brain may be advantageously compared with those of *Agaricus*, *Belladonna*, *Camphor*, *Crocus*, *Hyoscyamus*, *Opium*, and *Stramonium*. In its power of causing catalepsy its only rival is the chloride of tin.

In the case mentioned I gave the second dilution.

I have last to speak of the Spanish fly,

Cantharis,

of which we make a tincture by percolation.

There is a short pathogenesis of this substance in Hahnemann's *Fragmenta de viribus medicamentorum positivis*, consisting of 30 symptoms observed by himself, and 75 from
nineteen authors. He did not, however, take the medicine
up again; and its full proving appears in the first volume
of Hartlaub and Trinks' *Arzneimittellehre*. It contains 952
symptoms, many of which are citations from records of poisoning and overdosing, and the rest obtained by five provers.
Dr. Allen adds experiments made by Giacomini on his pupils,
and observations from many other sources, making a total of
1651. Some very complete studies of the action of the
Spanish fly on animals have lately been made by Dr. Cantieri,
of Milan, and published in the Italian journal *Lo Sperimentale*
(xxxiv, 9, 10). I take the account of these from the abstracts
which have appeared in English periodicals.

The primary interest of Cantharis arises from its local use
as an epispastic. The theory of the " counter-irritation " thus
practised has been much discussed of late; and Drs. Anstie*
and James Ross† have revived the doctrine of Fletcher‡ on
the subject, and (as I think) have demonstrated afresh its
soundness. We have but to go here as elsewhere to pathogenetics, and there we shall find the explanation and guidance
of our therapeutics. It appears, accordingly, that " blisters
applied to the thorax and abdomen of dogs and rabbits will
produce redness and absolute inflammation of the pleura and
peritoneum, in patches distinctly corresponding to the vesi-
cated surface of the skin."‖ Hence blisters when used (as
they principally are) for chronic inflammations are homœopathic agents, though acting by local absorption instead of
by elective affinity. We have not yet the same experimental
proof in the case of neuralgia, for which blisters are now
being so freely employed. But I have shown in other places§
that Dr. Anstie's whole theory and practice on this point is
homœopathic in everything but name, and implies that here
also an irritant is being sent to an already irritated part, and
needs to be diluted (by distance) to obviate aggravation.

But, although we thus claim for homœopathy whatever
benefit blisters may effect in the majority of cases in which
they are applied, we do not as a rule employ them. We have

---

* *Practitioner*, iv., 156.
† *On Counter-Irritation* (Churchill).
‡ *Elements of General Pathology* (1842), p. 484 ; see also Dr. Drys-
dale's exposition of Fletcher's doctrine in *Brit. Journ. of Hom.*,
xxvii., 494.
‖ Inman, *New Theory and Practice of Medicine*, p. 322.
§ See *Brit. Journ. of Hom.*, xxviii., 326 ; xxx,, 373.

medicines which, given internally, seek out under the guidance
of elective affinity the part that may be inflamed or the nerve
that is aching, and there more pleasantly and at least as
effectually extinguish the fire. So far as this holds good,
blisters are put out of court. But it is a question whether
there are not gaps as yet unfilled by specific medication, where
judicious counter-irritation might supply what is missing.
Should we desire to test this question the excellent account of
the value of blistering given by Dr. Ringer will help us. At
present we use Cantharis externally, not to produce blisters,
but to disperse them. In burns and scalds causing vesication,
in vesicular erysipelas, and in herpes zoster we have conditions
of the surface more or less resembling the local effects of
Cantharis ; and in all these affections the external application
of the diluted tincture has been attended with great advantage.
In burns and scalds I have often seen the best effects from it.
I once had a case in which both legs had been severely burned
by Phosphorus. Carron oil had already been applied to one
before I arrived, and I did not think it well to interfere with
the dressings : the other, however, I treated with rags dipped
in a lotion made with Cantharides. The difference between
the subsequent history of the two limbs was most instructive.
That to which the Spanish fly had been applied got well with
little trouble in a week : the other suppurated, and it was two
months before it had regained its integrity.

When introduced into the system, Cantharis acts as an
irritant poison, developing in all parts which it reaches either
by local contact or by elective affinity the same " pellicular
phlegmasia " (as Trousseau and Pidoux call it) which it
causes on the skin. The inflammation it sets up in the tract
from the mouth to the stomach seems purely local, but the
intestines are somewhat irritated even when it is introduced
directly into the blood. Under these circumstances it
quickens (while weakening) the pulse, and raises the temperature, thus producing a true (though only symptomatic)
febrile condition ; and it inflames, besides the genito-urinary
organs, the serous membranes throughout the body—peritoneum, pleura, pericardium, and the cerebral and spinal arachnoid. The first-named, however,—the genito-urinary organs—
are the chief seat of its action. The slightest effects are
increased quantity of urine and still more increased frequency
of urination, with heat in passing it in the case of men, in
women smarting. In higher degrees of its action it inflames
the whole mucous tract from the kidneys to the urethra,
causing pain in the loins ; scanty, high-coloured, bloody, and

generally albuminous urine, often loaded with tube-casts and sometimes with epithelial cells ; and burning pain and tenderness in the hypogastrium, with severe strangury.* The characteristic pellicle is sometimes found in the bladder, and has been voided (say Trousseau and Pidoux) into the chamberpot. With all this there is fever and great restlessness. The genital organs are similarly and considerably affected. With the slighter degrees of urinary irritation there is moderate erotic excitement ; but in poisoning by the drug this sometimes becomes painfully excessive, and is accompanied by priapism, inflammation (even to gangrenè) of the external parts, and of the uterus, sometimes causing abortion.

The nervous symptoms of Cantharis usually come on some days at least after the ingestion of the poison. They consist in delirium—which, with the local throat-symptoms, closely resembles hydrophobia, convulsions, and ultimately coma. They are possibly to some extent due to the meningeal irritation which Cantharis can set up : Dr. Cantieri also found softening of the nervous centres, especially in the cerebellum and the lumbar cord. ·But they are chiefly, I think, secondary to the renal mischief, i.e., they are uræmic.

It would seem that under favouring circumstances Cantharis can specifically irritate the skin. Pereira mentions a case in which the application of a blister to the pectoral region caused the development of ecthymatous pustules not only there, but all over the body. Occasional pimples, vesicles, and pustules are mentioned in Dr. Allen's pathogenesis as occurring in the provers, but the "psoriasis" and "eczema" which appear there are hardly to be depended upon.

Correspondingly with these physiological effects, the main homœopathic use of Cantharis is in inflammations of the urinary organs. This is no novelty as regards their chronic forms, for Groenvelt and Bartholin advocated the practice more than a century ago. The former was sent to Newgate for the offence† at the instance of the London College of Physicians ; but the practice has since had many upholders. To use the drug, however, in acute cystitis and nephritis, and in inflammatory strangury, was only possible upon the determinate method and with the small doses of homœopathy. In such affections we count it the chief remedy. Its renal symptoms show that it acts on the secreting tubes rather than, as turpentine, on the Malpighian bodies. It is hence inferior to that medicine in simple congestive suppression of

---

* See *Brit. Journ. of Hom.*, xvii., 548.
† *Ibid.*, x., 557.

urine or hæmaturia ; but when desquamation predominates
over congestion, as in the acute Bright's disease of post-
scarlatinal dropsy, Cantharis takes the highest place.* "There
can be no doubt," says Dr. Dickinson, "that the renal disorder produced by Cantharides is of the nature of tubal
nephritis." Its secondary head-symptoms are very significant
here. Dr. Ringer strongly recommends it in this malady in
minim doses of the tincture, after the first symptoms have
passed off ; and says that the discrepancy respecting the effect
of Cantharides arises probably from the difference of the dose
administered by different observers. He also recommends it
in the same quantities in diurnal enuresis in women—the
condition for which Dr. Cooper has established the use of
Ferrum. Pereira mentions a case of a boy of fourteen who
had been subject to incontinence of urine from infancy. By
means of gradually increasing doses of the tincture of Cantharides he was entirely relieved of the incontinence by
day, but the nocturnal discharge continued. It would seem
likely that some at least of the influence exerted by Cantharis
on the *functional* power of the bladder comes from the spinal
cord. Dr. Samuel Jones, in an exhaustive lecture on the
drug reported to the *American Observer* for 1879, puts in
juxtaposition cases in which paraplegia with cystoplegia were
caused by it, and in which its administration temporarily
restored power to a bladder paralysed in a corresponding connexion. The influence of Cantharis probably stops short of
the lower end of the urethra ; and it is not thought much of
in gonorrhœa, save where the inflammation extends so high as
to cause irritability of the bladder. But in those cases of
spermatorrhœa described by Lallemand, which depend on the
spread of gonorrhœal irritation through the ejaculatory ducts
along the spermatic passages, Cantharis is one of the most
homœopathic medicines ; and Dr. Kidd speaks well of its
efficacy in their treatment.†

As to the other parts irritated by Cantharis, we must note
the great success obtained by Cazenave and others in the
treatment of cutaneous squamæ and vesiculæ by small doses
(m iij—v) of the tincture.‡ We must also take into account
Dr. Jousset's estimate of the drug as the chief remedy for
pleurisy. As soon as effusion has taken place, he says in his
excellent *Eléments de Médécine Pratique*, we must resort to
Cantharis, in the third dilution, every two or three hours ; if
necessary (though he says he has rarely found it so) descend-

---

* See *Annals*, viii., 550, for two illustrative cases, † *Ibid*, v., 131.
‡ Trousseau and Pidoux; see also *Brit. Journ. of Hom.*, iii., 447.

ing to the second, the first, or even the mother tincture. In his hands it appears quite to take the place of Bryonia and Apis; but he mentions one case in which the last-named succeeded after it had failed. The original idea of using the Spanish fly in this disease was Giacomini's, and was an inference of his from the value of blisters therein, which he (rightly) conceived to act by the absorption of the Cantharis they contained.

Lastly, we must consider Bretonneau's comparison between the effects of Cantharis in animals and diphtheria. He describes the concrete exudation lining the mucous membranes, and the coldness and adynamia; to which Dr. Black, commenting on the point,* aptly adds the albuminuria of the two affections. This physician naturally suggests the trial of the drug as a remedy for the disease. I have rarely used it myself, and I believe that it has disappointed expectations. Dr. Ludlam, however, in his *Clinical Lectures on Diphtheria*, speaks highly of it for the prostration which often continues after the acuteness of the mischief has subsided; and Dr. Lawrence Newton communicates a similar experience.† The symptoms of Giacomini's provers establish its complete homœopathicity to this condition.

Dr. Guernsey says that it is often indicated (by the consentaneous urinary symptoms) in ovaritis. Dr. Jones lays much stress on external coldness, even with shuddering, coinciding with inward burning, as indicating it; and recommends it (in the tincture) for chronic ulcers of the legs.

In its action on the urinary organs Cantharis finds its nearest parallel in *Terebinthina;* but *Arsenic, Mercurius corrosivus, Scilla, Sabina, Kali bichromicum, Apis, Camphor, Cannabis sativa* and *Copaiba* coincide with it at some points of the tract.

The dilutions from the third decimal upwards have been those commonly used internally. For external application the lotion should not be stronger than one part of the tincture to forty of water.

* *Brit. Journ. of Hom.*, xvii.
† *Monthly Hom. Review*, xiv., 411.

LECTURE XXIV.

CAPSICUM, CARBON SULPHURATUM, CARBO ANIMALIS AND VEGETABILIS, CAULOPHYLLUM, CAUSTICUM, CEDRON.

My first medicine to-day is the Cayenne pepper,

Capsicum.

It is prepared by pulverising the ripe capsules of the Capsicum annuum, together with the seed, and from these making a tincture by percolation.

The pathogenesis of Capsicum is in the sixth volume of the *Reine Arzneimittellehre*, and contains 275 symptoms from Hahnemann, 65 from four fellow-workers, and four from authors. Dr. Allen has added a few later observations.

Capsicum produces its well-known burning in the mouth, throat, gullet, stomach, and intestines, along which it passes, and in the urinary passages by which it is eliminated. The condition set up is one of incipient inflammation, and is identical with that produced by the rubefacient action of the drug on the skin. Local application, moreover, is not always necessary to induce the latter effect. Dr. Allen's pathogenesis contains symptoms produced by repeated teaspoonfuls of a solution of Capsicum taken for a slight cold ; and among these are a papulo-vesicular eruption all over the body, with much itching and burning.

The common employment of Capsicum as a gargle in sore throat is undoubtedly an instance of homœopathic action. It used to be limited to relaxed conditions of the mucous membrane; but Drs. Ringer and Phillips concur to extend it to the early stage of acute inflammation. The latter recommends it in "throat-coughs," in which I have myself seen it of great service. Dr. Bayes says that an indication for it in coughs is when each paroxysm causes pain in the ear. Its usefulness in atonic dyspepsia, especially that of drunkards, is

well established.; but belongs to it rather as a condiment.* It
has been found of service in nervous irritability of the parts it
inflames, as hiccough, and tenesmus of the bladder and rectum ;
even in dysentery where the last symptom is prominent. A
sense of burning is of course another indication for it. It
should be useful in some irritations of the urinary tract : Dr.
Phillips speaks of having cured a chronic case of renal congestion with it. I am not aware of its having been used in
cutaneous affections, save as a local application to chilblains.

Hahnemann, in his preface, refers to Bergius' recommendation of the drug in intermittent fever. His own symptoms
present a very fair picture of the paroxysm of this disease.
He notes especially the chill, saying that he has seen it
gradually increasing for eleven hours after taking the medicine, and then declining for twelve hours more. Capsicum
has always occupied a high place in the homœopathic treatment of ague : it is found especially useful when the sweat
coincides with the heat, instead of following it.

It seems probable that Capsicum is capable of a more profound action than the sketch now given would suggest. Dr.
Houghton tells us that Dr. Allen directed his attention to one
of Hahnemann's symptoms—" a swelling on the bone behind
the ear, painful to the touch "—as suggesting its use in aural
inflammations, and that he has found it of the utmost service
in both chronic otorrhœa and acute median otitis, when the
mastoid cells are much involved. I have myself lately had a
case of the latter kind, in which I fully expected to have to
make a deep incision ; but complete recovery, with good
hearing power, has ensued upon the steady employment of
Capsicum. Again, Dr. O. R. Wright communicates a case, in
which, during pleuro-pneumonia, all the signs of abscess of the
lung supervened,—the cough becoming explosive, and the air
expelled therewith being intolerably fœtid, tainting the atmosphere of the room. Hahnemann's symptom, "the cough
expels an offensive breath from the lung," led to the administration of Capsicum in a high dilution, and under this remedy
rapid and complete recovery ensued.† Our French brethren
praise it in hæmorrhoids, for which cayenne pepper is well
known as a popular prophylactic.

* Dr. Ringer writes :—" I can endorse Dr. Lyon's strong recommendation of capsicum in dipsomania. Ten-minim doses of the tincture obviate the morning vomiting, remove the sinking at the pit of the
stomach, the intense craving for stimulants, and promote appetite and
digestion. It should be taken shortly before meals, or whenever depression and craving for alcohol arises."

† See *N. York State Hom. Soc.'s Transactions*, x., 123.

As an irritant of skin and mucous membrane Capsicum most resembles *Argentum nitricum Croton,* and *Euphorbium.*

Hahnemann recommends the 9th dilution, but nearer approaches to the crude drug have generally given complete satisfaction.

I have now to speak of the substance known since its discovery as Liquor Lampadii and Alcohol Sulphuris, under which latter name it stands in our Pharmacopœia. It is a bisulphide of carbon, CS_2. Pereira calls it Carbonei bisulphuretum, and it appears in Hering's *Materia Medica* as Carburetum sulphuris. I shall myself follow the analogy of similar compounds in styling it (much as Dr. Allen does)

Carbon sulphuratum.

Provings of this substance have been made by Knaf in the old school, and by Pemerl and Koch in the homœopathic ranks—altogether on thirteen persons. Its use in the manufacture of vulcanized india-rubber has led to many observations of the effects of inhaling its vapour. These have been collected by Delpech in the *Union Médicale* for 1855.* The materials thus specified, with others of like kind, have been worked up by Dr. Hering into one of the monographs of his volume of *Materia Medica,* and by Dr. Allen, who gives 750 symptoms to the drug.

Carbonic sulphide is a stimulant anæsthetic like ether, and can be given for this purpose by inhalation. It has too many inconveniences, however, to allow of its use in practice. If long inhaled it causes local irritation, besides headache and giddiness ; and the workers in it become impotent. The effect which most arrests my attention is the occurrence of long-lasting ringing in the ears, with or without deafness. This was experienced by one of those who took it internally ; but it is especially prominent in a record of the effects of inhaling the vapour given by Mr. T. Wilson in the seventeenth volume of the *British Journal of Homœopathy.* Neither Hering nor Allen has used this observation. It has led, however, to the only homœopathic application of the drug of which I am aware, Mr. Wilson stating that he has cured a case of tinnitus aurium of some standing with it in the first dilution. It is a medicine which ought to have a wider application.

* See an account of his observations by Dr. Jousset, in *Brit. Journ. of Hom.,* xv.

I should have mentioned that our preparation is a solution in alcohol, in which the drug is freely soluble.

I have now to speak of charcoal, animal and vegetable, which we will designate generically as

Carbo.

By all the writers on Materia Medica charcoal is regarded as utterly inert, and Hahnemann is laughed at by Pereira for filling thirty-five pages with the symptoms produced by the millionth of a grain. The learned writer has omitted to notice that this millionth of a grain was obtained by trituration, and that it is to this process that Hahnemann ascribes the development of such extensive powers in a substance inert in its crude state. This is a question of fact, and cannot be decided *à priori.* The same answer is to be made to Dr. Faivre, who, in *l' Art Médical* for 1869, relates some experiments with finely pulverized charcoal with negative results.* The division of the particles caused by his process is not to be compared to that of the Hahnemannic trituration. A more serious objection is raised by the results of the recent re-proving of Carbo vegetabilis by the American Institute.† The first, second and third centesimal triturations of this substance were tested upon nearly fifty healthy subjects, without producing any effect whatever. Nine other persons did report symptoms, which, arranged in schema form, number 327 ; but six of these had previously observed their health without taking any medicine at all, and under these circumstances had noted sensations and phenomena amounting to half as many again as those subsequently elicited by them. These results in no way disprove the medicinal value of the drug, especially when given (as it usually is) in the attenuations above the third ; but they render any pathogenetic effects ascribed to it (in the triturations) extremely dubious.

We will take first in order

Carbo animalis.—Hahnemann directs this to be prepared from ox-leather. Noack and Trinks recommend in preference meat—beef, veal, or mutton—as the substance to be carbonized. It probably matters little. The potencies are, of course, prepared by trituration.

A pathogenesis of Carbo animalis, made with the third

---

* *Brit. Journ. of Hom.*, xxviii., 232.
† See its Transactions for 1877, p. 181.

trituration, appears in the sixth volume of the *Reine Arznei-mittellehre*. It consists of 188 symptoms from Hahnemann himself and a Russian physician named Adam, with three from *Rust's Magazin*. Hartlaub and Trinks subsequently proved the drug, presumably in the same form; and gave their results in the shape of 254 symptoms in the third volume of their *Arzneimittellehre*. The final pathogenesis in the second edition of the *Chronic Diseases* incorporates these two series of symptoms. The remaining 283 of its 728 are from Wahle.

That *animal* charcoal, even in its crude state, is inert, can hardly be affirmed in the face of the observations cited by Hahnemann from *Rust's Magazin*, to which Dr. Hempel, in his article on the drug, adds some more of like tenor. Daily doses of from four to twenty-four grains have not only disordered the stomach and bowels, but have caused the breaking out of copper-coloured eruptions on the face, of acne, and of boils; and have developed painful swellings and indurations of the parotid and mammary glands. In these very glandular enlargements, especially when of a scirrhous nature, Carbo animalis has a repute of old which the homœopathic school has sustained,* extending it also to syphilitic glandular engorgements, as bubo.† It is also considered by some as having a dynamic controlling influence—distinct from its chemical action—over low states of the system characterised by putrescence of the fluids and secretions. Noack and Trinks, who praise it here, ascribe to it a deeper and more penetrating action than has its vegetable brother. Dr. Drury commends it, in a high dilution, against offensive lochia; and Dr. Allen emphasises "offensive night-sweat" as a symptom repeatedly verified.

Great lassitude, especially felt in the thighs, during and after the menstrual period, appears to be Dr. Guernsey's chief general indication for the remedy.

The action of Carbo animalis on the glands is somewhat like that of *Conium* and *Hydrastis*.

With the exception mentioned, the lower attenuations have generally been used.

Carbo vegetabilis is generally made from poplar, beech, or birch wood; and raised to the third potency by trituration.

Vegetable charcoal was proved, Hahnemann tells us, with doses of some grains of the third trituration. In the sixth

---

* See *Brit. Journ of Hom.*, xxxvi., 368.
† See *Ibid*, i., 300.

volume of his *Reine Arzneimittellehre* he gives 720 symptoms so obtained by himself and three others, which, on the grounds just stated, must be held of dubious validity. A later pathogenesis in the second edition of the *Chronic Diseases* extends the list to 1189; and, as no additional fellow provers are mentioned, the new symptoms must be understood as observed upon patients in the usual way. The symptoms obtained by Dr. Wesselhœft are given by Allen in his supplement.

Since the power of charcoal to check fermentation and to absorb gases has been known, it has been largely used in dyspepsia attended with acidity and flatulence. Dr. Madden, moreover, from experiments upon his own person, has been led to the conclusion that, swallowed in substance, finely-powdered charcoal acts as a mechanical detergent of the mucous membrane, dislodging any superfluous mucus it may have formed, and so aiding digestion.* All these are extra-medicinal effects of the drug, of which we may and do avail ourselves in common with our brethren of the old school. But, over and above them, we have dynamic uses of Carbo vegetabilis which make it an important remedy. One of these singularly coincides with its chemical action,—I mean its power over flatulence, whether existing alone, or associated with acidity and heart-burn. It is my own favourite remedy for this condition ; and I have seen the most distressing oppression and dyspnœa, recurring after every meal, removed by its use.† Dr. Guernsey's indication, " the patient wants to be fanned," belongs to this condition. I think it most suitable for cases where the gas distends the stomach more than the intestines, and where the tendency is rather to diarrhœa than to constipation—in this last feature contrasted with Lycopodium. Then there is an adynamia for which Carbo vegetabilis is specific. It is non-febrile, therein contrasted with that of Arsenic, and is attended by evidences (such as blueness and coldness) of defective circulation and imperfect oxidation of the blood. When such a condition exists in affections of the aged, and in advanced stages of typhus after the temperature has fallen, Carbo is an effectual rallier. But I cannot agree with those who see a Carbo adynamia in the collapse of cholera, and recommend it to be given therein.

* *Brit. Journ. of Hom*, xxvii., 64.
† Dr. Cooper prefers the C. animalis in flatulent dyspepsia ; and says that, given at night, it acts almost like an opiate in promoting sleep, by removing the gastric condition which prevents it (*Brit. Journ.*, xxxvi., 227).

There is, moreover, a good deal of evidence as to the power of Carbo vegetabilis over affections of the respiratory organs. Wurmb and Caspar esteemed it highly at the Leopoldstadt Hospital in chronic hoarseness (to which it is markedly homœopathic) and in emphysema. Bähr thinks it to be depended upon in chronic neglected bronchitis, with emphysema, and in the suppurative stage of pneumonia. Dr. Bayes says that in chronic bronchitis of aged people, with profuse expectoration or profuse accumulation of mucus, with imperfect power of expectoration, blue nails, and cold extremities, Carbo vegetabilis from 6th to 30th .is most useful. In all these affections of the respiratory organs a sense of weakness and fatigue in the parts is very characteristic for Carbo.

Dr. Thayer, of Boston, speaks highly of it in epistaxis, and Teste in soreness, itching, and burning of the female genitals with sexual excitement—both of which affections are recorded by Hahnemann (in the R. A. M. L.) as effects of the drug, and are in the list given by him of curative indications for it.

Lycopodium, *Veratrum album* and *Carbolic acid* are the medicines which may be most advantageously compared with Carbo vegetabilis. Carbolic acid has in the gastric sphere the same singular coincidence of chemical and dynamic action.

The sixth attenuation is that which I have almost always used, though I have found the third trituration act capitally in the dyspepsia of old people.

I have now to give an account of another of the many indigenous medicines with which our American brethren have of late years enriched the Materia Medica, the

Caulophyllum

thalictroides, popularly called " blue cohosh " or " squaw root." The former name hints at its similarity to Actæa racemosa (black cohosh); the latter points to its main sphere of action.

We prepare a tincture from the root. Caulophyllin' is also much used.

There is a proving of Caulophyllin by the indefatigable Dr. Burt in the second edition of Dr. Hale's *New Remedies*, together with all that is known regarding the drug. I do not find anything fresh about it in the fourth edition.

The " squaw root," as may be supposed, acts chiefly on the uterus. No woman having proved it, I am unable to state what are its physiological effects upon the organ. Dr. Hale

thinks that it is primarily excitant; and that it is homœopathic to dysmenorrhœa, uterine cramps, spurious labour-
pains, abortion, and after-pains.   It seems especially suitable
to affections of the motor nerves sympathetic with uterine
irritation (Actæa includes also reflex hyperæsthesiæ).   It has
been found useful in chorea, in spasms from suppression of
the menses, and in uterine paraplegia.   Cases are also on
record in which it has strengthened labour-pains, where ergot
could not be given on account of the rigidity of the os uteri;
and in which flooding after abortion and long-continuing lochia
after parturition have been checked by its use.   In "false
pains;" to avert threatened abortion; and to prevent premature labour, Caulophyllum is much recommended: also in
spasmodic dysmenorrhœa and after-pains, and as a preparatory
medicine for women who have difficult labours.*   It will probably continue to be given indiscriminately as a uterine
remedy, until a proving on a woman or the accumulation of
clinical experience enables its precise place to be fixed.   I
have myself had little experience with it.   The proving of Dr.
Burt reveals a marked power on the part of Caulophyllum of
causing acute rheumatoid affections of the small joints, especially those of the fingers.   Putting this and its uterine action
together, it becomes probable that Caulophyllum will rank
with Actæa, Pulsatilla, and Sabina, as a remedy for that peculiar form of chronic rheumatism described by Dr. Fuller as
secondary to uterine disorder.   It has made some brilliant
cures of inflammatory rheumatism of the hands and fingers,
and is said by Dr. Ludlam to be more effectual in females
than in males thus affected.

I have already pointed out the close relations of Caulophyllum with *Actæa racemosa*, *Pulsatilla*, and *Sabina*.   It has
some points of analogy also with *Secale*.

The Caulophyllin, in the triturations from the first to the
sixth decimal, has been most frequently used.

I have next to speak of

Causticum,

and, before I go any farther, must endeavour to satisfy your
natural curiosity as to what the medicine so named may be.

* "Dr. Helmuth informs me," writes Dr. Hale, "that he has used
the Caulophyllin successfully for the removal of those discolorations of
the skin of the face common in women with menstrual irregularities or
uterine disease."

Its history is as follows :—In the *Fragmenta de viribus* Hahnemann published thirty symptoms as obtained by him from a substance he called " Acris tinctura." He stated that it was an alcoholic solution of the principle to which quick-lime and the alkalies owed their causticity. He obtained it by digesting caustic potash in alcohol, and then saturating with vinegar to neutralise the potash. As he found (from its effects) a medicinal agent still present in the solution, he, strangely enough, considered this to be the caustic principle of the alkali. In the second volume of the second edition of the *Reine Arzneimittellehre* (1824) we find a more extensive pathogenesis of this preparation, now named " Aetzstoff-Tinctur—Tinctura acris sine kali." 106 symptoms have been observed from it by Hahnemann, and 201 from seven fellows ; and in a very long preface the chemical reality of the principle of causticity is defended. In the third edition (1833) the drug does not appear, for the reason that in the meanwhile Hahnemann had seen reason to class it among his antipsorics. Its pathogenesis had accordingly been transferred to the *Chronic Diseases*, in the first edition of which (1830) it appears with 1014 symptoms, including those which he had already published. It is now called simply " Aetzstoff" or " Causticum," and is directed to be prepared by adding to quick-lime a solution of some previously fused bisulphate of potash, and distilling. The product, he says, is hydrated causticum. In the second edition of the *Chronic Diseases* are incorporated some hundreds of symptoms communicated by Nenning to Hartlaub and Trinks, making a total of 1505.

What, then, is the real chemical nature of this preparation of Hahnemann's ? Dr. Black has had it analysed, with the result of finding it to be a weak solution of caustic potash of varying strength. He recommends that the dilutions shall in future be prepared from the liquor potassæ of the British Pharmacopœia. Twenty parts of this with eighty of distilled water constitute, according to him, the first centesimal dilution of what we might now more correctly style Kali causticum. You will decide for yourselves whether to adopt Dr. Black's suggestion, and will then look carefully to see if you get the same effects from his preparation as are ascribed to Hahnemann's. In the meantime, the British Homœopathic Pharmacopœia does wisely, I think, in adhering to the latter. It directs the attenuations to be made with rectified spirit.

Dr. Allen seems to agree with Dr. Black, for he incorporates with Hahnemann's symptoms " some effects of caustic potash."

The main sphere of the therapeutic action of Causticum has consisted in paralytic affections and laryngo-tracheal catarrhs. It was in facial paralysis that it first acquired reputation ; and as this affection, when local, readily admits of spontaneous recovery, it is not easy to prove that any medicine has cured it. But when so careful an observer as Bähr expresses no doubt of the anti-paralytic virtues of the drug, we may wisely avail ourselves of them ; and now with the more confidence that we have reason to believe that it is potash we are using. For it has been well ascertained of late years that potash has a poisonous action quite distinct from that of any alkali, and that this is especially seen in the way it paralyses the spinal cord and the heart.

What are the special paralytic conditions in which Causticum will prove efficacious has not been determined. I can speak with most certainty of it in local paretic states, whenever occurring. As regards the larynx we have the weighty testimony of Dr. Meyhoffer, "The absence," he writes, "of harmonious co-operation of the vocal cords is one of the most permanent and persevering symptoms of deficient innervation in laryngeal catarrh ; persons recovering from this affection cannot exert the vocal organ to the full compass of the voice, nor use it in all its modulations, for at least two or three weeks after every trace of capillary turgescence has subsided ; and any overstrained exercise of the vocal apparatus, or oratorical display, at this period tends to perpetuate the defect. This kind of diminished vitality is naturally of great consequence to singers and public speakers : fortunately, a specific remedy is at hand in what Hahnemann introduced into medical practice as *Hydrated Causticum* (Kali causticum), which often in a single dose removes this functional weakness of the glottis, as well as that resulting from over-exertion."* Of the same character is that which Dr. Guernsey notes of the cough of Causticum, that the expectoration only comes up far enough to be swallowed : there is no power to spit it out. In the bladder we have a similar condition. It is especially shown in that, when the patient coughs, there is involuntary emission of urine during the paroxysm. This is a well-known indication for Causticum. But it has also been useful when such paresis of the sphincter exists without cough, as in the enuresis of children and old persons ; and I have found it curative in a similar condition of the anus. In the eleventh

* *Chronic Diseases of the Organs of Respiration*, i., 56. See also a case of aphonia, with facial paralysis, by Dr. Kafka in *L'Art Médical* for June, 1875.

volume of the *New England Medical Gazette* (p. 491) a case is reported in which it had a decisive curative effect in post-diphtheritic paralysis of the fauces ; and Drs. Allen and Norton speak of it as the remedy *par excellence* for paralytic affections of the ocular muscles, especially if caused by exposure to cold.

Independently, moreover, of associated paretic symptoms (which may be absent), Causticum is a medicine of undoubted power in laryngo-tracheal catarrh. Dr. Black's experience is decisive here. He relates* cases of long-lasting catarrhal aphonia, and of violent and fatiguing cough, in which its administration effected speedy cure. It is especially indicated in coughs by the co-existence of a sore sensation in a streak down the trachea.

There is another property of the salts of potash which seems to have found its homœopathic application by means of Causticum. This is the increase of the urinary solids, first noticed by Golding Bird with the acetate, and since confirmed by Dr. Austin Flint with the nitrate, and by Rabuteau with the chloride. The late Mr. Freeman has put on record some cases where convalescence from typhoid fever was retarded by the passing of large quantities of urine loaded with lithic acid and lithates.† The excessive tissue waste revealed by this symptom was checked by Causticum, and the recovery went rapidly on. In a similar case occurring in my own practice, where after parturition this state of the urine was associated with debility, low spirits, anorexia, copious sour perspirations, and persistent aching of the mammæ, speedy change for the better ensued upon the administration of this remedy. It should be thought of for that rare form of disease, azoturia.

For possible further application of Causticum I may refer you to Hahnemann's list of morbid conditions in which it has been useful ; to a paper read upon it before the British Homœopathic Society by Mr. Nankivell, with the discussion following ;‡ to a study of it by Dr. Lohrbacher, now (1879) in course of translation in the *North American Journal of Homœopathy* ; and to Teste's article on the medicine, in which he lauds it in the treatment of smallpox. Some of the traditional uses of caustic potash and the liquor potassæ are, moreover, highly suggestive, especially Mr. Brandish's results from his alkaline solution in scrofula. He, indeed, gave the potash

* *Brit. Journ. of Hom.*, xxiv., 470.
† *Monthly Hom. Review*, x., 288.
‡ *Annals*, ii.

in large doses; but Sundelin's experience, which was equally favourable, was obtained by a preparation containing a drachm of the alkali to an ounce of water, of which he gave two drops twice a day, gradually increasing the dose. He " regarded the usefulness of potash as most striking in scrofula affecting persons of a soft but full muscular system, and a torpid phlegmatic temperament." Drs. Allen and Norton find frequent employment for it in scrofulous inflammations of the eyes. They also ascribe to it some power over cataract. " Several cases" they say "have been arrested in their progress, and the sight even improved, where, before its administration, they were rapidly going on to complete blindness." Dr. Bayes says that he has always found good results from Causticum in constipation, when the evacuation is very solid, is expelled with great difficulty and straining, and presents a shining appearance, as if greased.

Gelsemium corresponds best to the paralytic symptoms of Causticum ; *Bromine* and *Spongia* to its laryngeal action.

Dr. Black's success was obtained with the first and second decimal dilutions, and the anti-paralytic virtues of the drug have generally been elicited from the potencies just above these. In the higher attenuations, however, Causticum has played a prominent part in the treatment of chronic disease, as you may see from such a book as Jahr's *Forty Years' Practice*. It is especially esteemed in old rheumatisms, and is even praised by some in rheumatoid arthritis.

For my last subject to-day I have a drug which we know as

Cedron.

It is the fruit of a South American tree of doubtful species ; but identifiable through its extensive native use. Dr. Hale thinks there is no doubt of its being the Simaruba Cedron. A trituration of the seeds is the best preparation, according to Dr. Casanova ; but the British Homœopathic Pharmacopœia directs a tincture to be prepared from the whole fruit.

Cedron has been proved by M. Teste on three persons in the sixth dilution, and by Dr. Casanova on fourteen in the crude substance and first three decimal triturations. The full report of the former's experiments may be read in his *Matière Médicale :* the results of the latter are given by him, with much clinical observation, in a series of papers published in the fifth and sixth volumes of the *Monthly Homœopathic Review*. Dr. Allen adds symptoms from eight American provers, all using the crude drug or mother tincture.

It appears that in Panama Cedron is considered a specific for the bites of the venomous serpents of the country, and for its endemic intermittents. Teste's three provers each experienced a daily paroxysm closely simulating ague. The chills came on towards evening ; there was little or no sweat, but much cerebral congestion. Several of Dr. Casanova's provers had similar attacks, but there was no lack of perspiration with them. Teste reports brilliant results from Cedron in the intermittents of Martinique and Wallachia. A vial of the sixth attenuation, given by him without label to a friend visiting the island I have mentioned, attained quite a reputation as a secret remedy. Dr. Casanova's experiments, pathogenetic and clinical, point in the same direction. He considers Cedron a true anti-periodic, like Quinine and Arsenic ; and gives it in neuralgia and other disorders, as well as in ague, when appearing in regularly recurring paroxysms. The periodical ("almost clock-like," says Dr. Jones) recurrence of the symptoms in his provers led him to this practice. It checks, he reports, the tendency to miscarriage, when this repeats itself at the same epoch. He thinks it infallible in the endemic intermittents of damp, warm, and low marshy climates.

I am myself accustomed to use Cedron with success in obscure cases of recurring chills and fever, such as those we meet with in persons returned from tropical countries. I have generally used the second dilution. Dr. Casanova says that residents in hot climates are much more susceptible to its action, pathogenetic and curative, than others differently situated. Drs. Allen and Norton, guided by the severe shooting pain over the left eye experienced by one of the provers, have been led to use the drug to relieve the supra-orbital pains found in iritis, choroiditis, and other deep inflammations of the eye ; and have been frequently successful with it.

I should mention that the epithet I have cited as Dr. Jones' is from a study of Cedron by him in the seventh volume of the *American Observer*.

LECTURE XXV.

CHAMOMILLA, CHELIDONIUM, CHIMAPHILA, CHLORAL, CHLORUM, CICUTA, CINA AND SANTONINE.

I begin to-day with a humble and familiar plant, which, nevertheless, almost ranks with the polychrests of homœopathy,

Chamomilla.

By this we mean the common Matricaria Chamomilla, not the Anthemis nobilis. At least, so Hahnemann meant; but, if Stillé is right, the common wild camomile of England and America is the Anthemis nobilis, while in Germany it is the Matricaria Chamomilla. There is probably no essential difference between them.

Chamomilla early attracted Hahnemann's attention. A pathogenesis of it appeared in the *Fragmenta de viribus*, containing 272 symptoms observed by himself, and three from authors. In the second edition of the third volume of the *Reine Arzneimittellehre*, there are 189 additional symptoms of his own, and 30 observed by Stapf in a girl of nineteen, after drinking some large cupfuls of camomile tea. We have two later provings of the drug, one by Dr. Hoppe of Basel, on himself and two others, related in the thirteenth, fourteenth and fifteenth volumes of the *Vierteljahrschrift ;* the other by the Vienna Provers' Union.* Dr. Allen, incorporating the results thus obtained with a few others, gives us a pathogenesis of 1,446 symptoms. For the therapeutic action of Chamomilla, we have again the benefit of Hartmann's *Practical Observations* (first series).

Chamomilla, at times largely used by physicians, had in Hahnemann's day become practically a domestic remedy only. It was chiefly used in pains and difficulties of the uterus, from which action, it is said, its name Matricaria (from

* *Brit. Journ. of Hom.*, vi., 267, 270.

matrix) is derived. His proving, and the applications which have been made of it to practice, have given the drug a much wider range of action. I fully agree with one of the Vienna provers (Dr. Schneller) that Chamomilla affects the nervous system primarily. Its pathogenetic effects are faint and obscure ; but its curative power is well defined. It is when the sensory and excito-motor nerves are morbidly impressionable that Chamomilla is so valuable a medicine. Thus Hahnemann says— "Chamomilla seems, in the smallest doses, greatly to moderate excessive sensibility to pain and too great disturbance of the mind induced by much suffering, whence also it meets many of the troubles of coffee-drinkers and those who have been dosed with narcotic palliatives. It is on the other hand less beneficial to those who remain patient and composed during their sufferings,—an observation which I consider of the utmost importance." It has even cured rheumatism and neuralgia of the limbs where this great "nervousness" was present. Of its pains generally Hahnemann says—"It is their peculiarity that they are worse at night, when they often drive one to the border of distraction, not unfrequently accompanied with unquenchable thirst, and heat and redness of the cheeks ; also with hot sweat on the head and scalp. The pains of Chamomilla generally seem utterly intolerable." And again—"The paralytic sensation produced by Chamomilla in any part is always accompanied by drawing or tearing pain, and drawing and tearing pains rarely occur without the paralytic or numb sensation in the part." Dr. Dunham adds that the pains are made worse by warmth. "There must always be intolerance of pain, aggravation at night, and aggravation by warmth. This applies to the toothache, earache, facial and cervical neuralgia, and to the abdominal colic, and distinguishes it from the symptoms of Colocynth, which are diminished by warmth." The impressionability of the excito-motor nerves which Chamomilla so powerfully modifies shows itself in such clonic spasms as are apt to occur in women and young children. In the former, it effectually relieves the "false pains" and the cramps and painful twitches of the legs, which harass the later months of pregnancy ; it is good also for spasmodic dysmenorrhœa, for after-pains, and for metrorrhagia (whether in threatened miscarriage or otherwise) when there are forcing pains and the blood is dark and clotted. The presence in such patients of a "spiteful, sudden, uncivil irascibility," of which they are sometimes conscious, but say they cannot help it, is—according to Dr. Guernsey and others—a great indication for the remedy. In children it plays a most important part during the process of dentition. It probably has some specific influence on the pulp of the teeth itself in the gums, for it often gives great relief in ordinary inflammatory and rheumatic face-ache. Hahnemann gives* the following description of the symptoms which call for it :—" It is of service in those toothaches that occur in fits, most violently at night, with redness of the cheek, which during the fit seem to be quite unbearable, that do not affect any one tooth in particular, that in their slightest degree consist of formicating pecking pains, when more severe cause a tearing pain, and in their greatest severity occasion a shooting pain extending often into the ear, that most frequently come on soon after eating and drinking, are somewhat relieved by the application of a finger that has been dipped in water, but are much increased by drinking cold things, and that generally leave a swelling of the cheek." But when in dentition the nervous system becomes irritated, then for restlessness, fretfulness, and spasms there is no medicine like Chamomilla. Dr. Guernsey's indication for it in teething infants, that the child refuses to be soothed save when carried about, has often been verified. Hartmann recommends it for the sympathetic cough occurring at this time. Even the diarrhœa of teething will sometimes yield to it ; and when other remedies (as Mercurius) are strongly indicated, Chamomilla in alternation—by quieting the reflex irritation—will help them.

This application of Chamomilla to disturbance of the vegetative organs, when induced by nervous causes, finds another instance in its use in the effects of anger and active vexation, when showing themselves in " bilious fever " and jaundice, which was well known among the older homœo-pathists. Hahnemann himself wrote :—" The (sometimes dangerous) disorder, resembling an acute bilious fever, which is often brought on by violent angry vexation, with heat of the face, insatiable thirst, bilious taste, tendency to vomit, anxietas, restlessness, &c., has so much homœopathic similarity to the symptoms of Chamomilla that it can hardly fail to remove the whole sickness speedily and specifically : one drop of the juice diluted as before mentioned "—that is, to the twelfth degree—" cures as by magic." The occurrence of jaundice from such causes is well known, and always suggests Chamomilla. Dr. Hempel, however, maintains in his lectures that "the primary action of Chamomilla seems to be upon the functions of the biliary apparatus ; " and some recent obser-

* *Lesser Writings*, p. 641.

vations of Dr. Sharp's favour its direct hepatic influence. He found that, on a healthy person, the effect of the first dilution, in drop doses, was to produce motions like those of a baby : that is, as he thinks, to increase the secretion of bile. On the other hand, five and ten drop doses of the mother tincture made the motions scanty and dark in colour. He further relates one case of jaundice, and two of diabetes of hepatic origin, in which the action of Chamomilla was everything that could be desired. Another suggestion of its power of influencing the secretion of bile is supplied in a case of over-dosing observed by Dr. Burnett, in which the symptoms were diarrhœa of *white, putty-like stools*, white-coated tongue, and intense vertex headache, with a sensation of pressure from within the cranium.* This was from the Anthemis nobilis. Chamomilla, with Nux vomica, is Dr. Jousset's principal remedy for what he calls " ictére essentiel."

I can confirm from my own experience Hartmann's recommendation of the remedy in flatulent colic, where the flatus seems to collect in several spots in the abdomen, as if incarcerated.

The analogues of Chamomilla as a nervine are *Agaricus, Belladonna, Coffea, Hyoscyamus, Ignatia,* and *Stramonium.*

The facts about the dose of Chamomilla are very curious. I have hitherto been in the habit of stating as the general experience of homœopathic practitioners—as it was certainly my own—that the remedy begins at about the sixth potency to manifest its great curative powers, and may often be given with advantage as high as the 18th. I had in my mind recorded expressions of opinion on the part of Drs. Madden,† Bayes,‡ Hempel,§ and Holcombe‖—to say nothing of Hahnemann's own recommendation of the 12th as the best attenuation. Dr. Black¶ has since cited some testimonies on the other side ; but these, when examined, show that it is not the lower dilutions of the drug that give satisfaction, but the infusion, the mother tincture, or at the highest the first decimal. The only writer quoted by Dr. Black as using the 3rd decimal and centesimal is Dr. Clotar Müller, and he says that " the curative results were but seldom indubitable." The conclusion seems

---

* *Monthly Hom. Review,* xxi., 408.
† *Brit. Journ. of Hom.,* xxiii., 530.
‡ *Applied Homœopathy,* sub voce *Chamomilla.*
§ *Mat. Med.,* sub voce.
‖ *United States Med. and Surg. Journ.,* i., sub voce.
¶ *Brit. Journ. of Hom.,* xxix., 795.

to be that Chamomilla is one of those drugs whose crude and infinitesimal actions are about identical; but that there is an intermediate stage where dilution simply weakens. This is my reading of the facts; but the question is a difficult one at the best. It is, moreover, of Chamomilla as a nervine that the attenuations have found such favour. Dr. Sharp seems justified in saying that as an hepatic remedy the first dilution is preferable; and in its colic I have found the mother tincture most effectual.

I have now to bring before you a drug whose exhaustive proving of late years should give it a prominent place among our remedies. I refer to the greater celandine,

Chelidonium majus.

The tincture is prepared from the fresh plant in the usual manner.

The proving to which I refer is by Dr. Buchmann of Alvensleben. It appears in the seventieth volume of the *Allgemeine Homöopathische Zeitung*, and is translated in the twenty-third and two following volumes of the *British Journal of Homœopathy*. Hahnemann had previously given a short pathogenesis of the plant in the fourth volume of the *Reine Arzneimittellehre*, consisting of 28 symptoms from himself, 122 from eight fellow-observers, and 6 from authors. Teste also had contributed some provings on four persons with the sixth dilution, and the Vienna Provers' Union had experimented with the drug. All the results of the foregoing, and some symptoms from other sources, are incorporated by Dr. Buchmann with his own—making 1456 in all*—in the " schema " of the drug with which he concludes his record. I should have said that his experimenters were eighteen in number; and that nearly all took full doses of the mother tincture.†

Our knowledge of Chelidonium, which has been gradually building, is perfected by what Dr. Buchmann has now so ably done. Led by the doctrine of signatures, the Middle Age physicians supposed that the bitter yellow juice of this plant,

---

* Dr. Allen, though drawing from no other sources, gives (I suppose from difference of arrangement) 2428 symptoms to the drug.

† The fairness and impartiality of Dr. Phillips' book may be estimated by his statement that " exact experiments are altogether lacking as to the physiological action of the juice of Chelidonium." Yet he is acquainted with Dr. Buchmann's work, as he cites him as a therapeutic authority on the drug.

so nearly resembling bile, must be beneficial in disorders of the liver.   The disciples of Rademacher have shown that here at least the signature has proved a true guide, by adducing numerous cases of jaundice, gall-stones, and acute and chronic hepatitis cured by the drug.   Then comes Dr. Buchmann's proving to show that this remedial power obeys the law of similars.   The action on the liver is very strongly marked in his proving.   Pain, both acute and dull, and tenderness of the organ ; pain in the right shoulder ; stools either soft and bright yellow, or whitish and costive ; and deeply tinged urine, appeared in nearly every prover.   In three the skin became yellow or dark ; and in one regular jaundice was set up.   Correspondingly, Chelidonium bids fair to take high rank in our school as an hepatic medicine.   You will find a number of cases illustrative of its value at the end of the proving.   Further experience, however, is required to enable us to define its exact place here in relation to other hepatic remedies, as Mercurius, Bryonia, Phosphorus, and Podophyllum.   Dr. Guernsey says that a pain at the lower angle of the right scapula, running into the chest, is characteristic of it.   It has become my own stock-remedy for simple jaundice.

Next, the experiments instituted by Teste led him to credit Chelidonium with a specific affinity for the *respiratory organs*. The two disorders to which he thought its symptoms specially pointed were pertussis and pneumonia.   Subsequent experience has confirmed his predictions of its value.   In *whooping cough* it has been found to act specially well after Corallium, as indeed he recommends   And it really seems a most valuable accession to our remedies for *pneumonia*.   It is especially useful where the right lung is affected, and the liver involved.   Teste thinks it better than Bryonia in those cases where the patient is of blond complexion and placid temperament.   Dr. Ludlam praises it in the catarrhal pneumonia of young children, where there is an excess of the pulmonary secretion, with inability to raise or dislodge it.   All this you will find confirmed and made clear by Dr. Buchmann's experiments and observations.   He shows that in animals poisoned by the drug the lungs are found generally engorged, sometimes hepatised.   He developes in several of his provers all the symptoms of an incipient pneumonia.   And he contributes from his own practice cases of the disease, in which the beneficial action of the drug was most manifest.   He corroborates also its value in whooping-cough, and points to the spasmodic cough induced by it as showing its homœopathicity.

Lastly, the new proving of Chelidonium reveals a hitherto unknown influence exerted by it on the *kidneys*. Besides the general symptoms of renal irritation, an examination of the urine in one case showed the presence of tube-casts, of increased uric acid, and diminished chloride of sodium. The mischief in this case was so considerable that œdematous swellings of the extremities occurred. We have as yet had little or no experience with Chelidonium as a renal remedy.

Besides the facts embraced under the above headings, I would note in the proving the severe pains in the knee-joints, and the itching hæmorrhoids, developed in one prover (both occasionally symptoms of hepatic disorder); the dark redness so often appearing on the cheeks, hinting embarrassment of the pulmonary circulation ; the chills and fever ; the inflamed scrotum and eyelids ; the itching of the skin, generally in patches ; and the periodical toothache. Dr. Buchmann also points out a group of symptoms which show an action on the diaphragm. He esteems it very highly in all external neuralgiæ, and gives a good case of prosopalgia cured by it. In the twentieth volume of the *British Journal of Homœopathy* you will find some cases of supra-orbital neuralgia cured by Chelidonium, in which also its curious affinity for the right side of the body appears ; and in the twenty-eighth volume there is a case of my own, in which a migraine of this kind, evidently hepatic in origin, was removed by it. You will also do well to consult Mr. Clifton's graphic description of the form of dyspepsia calling for it in the seventeenth volume of the *Monthly Homœopathic Review.* I have only to add, that cases are appended to Dr. Buchmann's proving which hint at other fields of action for Chelidonium as yet unexplored. You must not suppose, from Hahnemann's 66th symptom, that gonorrhœa is one of these. It occurred in the case he cites only as a re-appearance after suppression, while Chelidonium was being taken for the swelled testicle which had resulted.

Bryonia and *Phosphorus* are the analogues of Chelidonium.

The dose for adults seems to range from the first to the sixth decimal ; from the sixth to the twelfth for infants.

I must now briefly mention one of the American indigenous remedies, the " Pipsissiwa," winter-green, prince's pine, or

Chimaphila.

A tincture is prepared from the fresh leaves, bruised.

Chimaphila has not been proved : all our information concerning it is derived from Dr. Hale's article in his *New Remedies*.

There is one and one only point of interest about this plant. It appears (besides being an active diuretic) to have a specific influence upon the urinary passages, like that of the Pareira brava and the Buchu, which ordinary practice knows well, but which we have hardly hitherto used. Dr. Hale has found it a valuable medicine in cases of dysuria with mucous sediment in the urine ; and has cured gleet with it. Dr. Holland relates a good case of chronic cystitis in which it proved curative after many medicines had failed.*

Besides Pareira and Buchu, Chimaphila may be compared with *Cannabis sativa, Cantharis, Copaiba, Eupatorium purpureum*, and *Uva ursi*.

From one to five drops of the mother-tincture appear to be the most suitable dose.

I have now to say something about the hydrate of

Chloral.

Into the use of this drug (obtained, as you know, by the action of chlorine upon alcohol) as a hypnotic I do not propose to enter. You can learn it from the ordinary text-books ; and you must use your judgment as to its adoption Chloral is unquestionably the least harmful agent of the kind we can employ, when we must employ them.

But our concern with the drug is to know whether we can utilise any of its physiological action homœopathically. Its influence on the system appears to be that of a pure nervous depressant. It acts very much as Opium does, only that it affects the cerebrum so quickly, that the so-called primary excitement of the latter, which I suppose to depend upon vaso-motor paralysis, is slightly and rarely visible. Every now and then, however, it does occur ; and the flushing of the surface is characterised by being accompanied with more or less eruption, most frequently urticarious or erythematous, but sometimes like that of measles or scarlatina, and always associated with great itching. The conjunctivæ, also, are not merely suffused, but hot, stiff, swelled, and tender (especially on the lids), and there is sometimes lachrymation. Dr. Allen gives a number of such phenomena in his pathogenesis of Chloral, which contains 281 symptoms from various sources.

* *Brit. Journ. of Hom.*, xxxii., 84.

Dr. Dyce Brown also has, in the fifteenth volume of the *Monthly Homœopathic Review*, related in detail many observations displaying its physiological effects ; and, in the thirty-second volume of the *British Journal of Homœopathy*, has shown us how to turn them to good account, by giving a series of cases of conjunctivitis, urticaria and pruritus in which, in grain doses or less, it proved very efficacious in his hands. In the former place he also calls attention to its disturbing and depressing influence upon the heart, showing this to be exerted through the nervous supply of the organ, and to indicate the drug when from nervous causes its action is disordered. The same thing may be said of its effects on the respiration.

Several corroborations of Dr. Brown's experience with Chloral in conjunctivitis and urticaria have been put on record. Among them I may mention that of Dr. Hale, who says that in two cases of conjunctivitis in his practice its effect was simply magical, and of Dr. Burnett, who communicates a case of nettlerash of four months' standing rapidly cured by it.* It is my own favourite medicine for chronic cases of this affection.

The drug has never been used above the first decimal attenuation.

And now for a few words about chlorine itself, which chemistry at the present day calls

Chlorum.

Dr. Allen gives a pathogenesis of this gas, embracing tne effects of its inhalation. The only one of these, however, which appears noteworthy is that twice observed by Dr. Carroll Dunham, viz : that while inspiration was easy enough, at most accompanied by a crowing noise, expiration became impossible, and asphyxic symptoms appeared. Now this, as you are probably aware, is the condition present in the spasmodic form of the disorder known as " laryngismus stridulus." I say, the spasmodic form ; for it not uncommonly comes before us as a consequence of pressure on the recurrent nerves by enlarged bronchial glands, and here the glottis is paralysed, and inspiration—always wheezing—sometimes becomes excessively difficult. Dr. Dunham at once perceived

* *Monthly Hom. Review*, xxi,, 341. See also two cases by Mr. Clifton in *Ibid*, p. 526.

its applicability to the first-named variety of the disease ; and both he and Dr. Searle have mentioned cases in which its administration, in a weak aqueous solution, effected a cure.*

Like its congeners, Iodine and Bromine, the combination of Chlorine with an alkali developes new features in its action. We know something of it as conjoined with lime and with soda.

Calcarea chlorata—as I suppose we must call the old "chlorinated lime," the "calx chlorata" of present nomenclature—is known to us only by Dr. Neidhard's strong recommendation of it in diphtheria.† He gives it in the form of the "liquor calcis chloratæ," a drop or less for a dose.

Natrum chloratum must be our title for Labarraque's solution—the "liquor sodæ chloratæ" of the British Pharmacopœia. It seems to be a complex preparation, containing the hypochlorite of soda with its carbonate and chlorate, and also hypochlorous acid. It has, however, been proved and used as a unity ; and this is all that we require to secure the "single remedy" of homœopathy. It has long been used in ordinary practice as a disinfectant; but Dr. Cooper, employing it on one occasion for this purpose in a case of leucorrhœa, was struck by the remarkable improvement in the patient's general uterine condition which ensued, and was led to test its internal administration. He found it, thus given, a most valuable remedy for congested and atonic states of the uterus and its ligaments, with their accompanying pains about the chest and hepatic disorders. Further experience has led him to regard it as a potent medicine in chronic catarrhal troubles of children, as in those of the middle ear ; and to have a general bracing influence upon the "flabby, debilitated, hydrogenic constitutions" to which he considers it best suited. You will find his original papers on the subject in the thirtieth and thirty-first volumes of the *British Journal of Homœopathy ;* and in the thirty-fifth volume he has given a complete list of its observed effects, pathogenetic‡ and curative.

In uterine affections, Dr. Cooper gives the liquor sodæ chloratæ with little dilution. For children he finds it act better in the (lower) attenuations.

---

* See *Hom. the Science of Therapeutics*, p. 493-501 ; Trans. of N. Y. State Hom. Med. Society, ix., 256, 262.

† *Diphtheria, its nature and homœopathic treatment*, 1867.

‡ Dr. Allen gives these in his supplement (vol. x.) under the heading of Natrum hypochlorosum.

Of the three very similarly acting Umbelliferæ, we have already discussed the Æthusa cynapium. The Œnanthe crocata is at present hardly used in our practice ; but we have some knowledge of the third, the long-leaved water hemlock, or

Cicuta virosa.

The tincture is made from the root.

Cicuta was proved by Hahnemann : the pathogenesis is in the sixth volume of the *Materia Medica Pura.* It contains 36 symptoms of his own, 168 from three fellow-provers, and 37 from authors—most of which were observed in eight children poisoned by the plant, as related by Wepfer in his treatise *De Cicutâ.* The poisonous effects of the plant are fully described by Hempel in his article.

From these cases of poisoning it appears that Cicuta causes tetanus as manifestly as does Strychnia. But it has this difference, that it affects the brain no less than the spinal cord. The cerebral symptoms are various ; but in their intensest form they approximate to those of epilepsy, which indeed in poisoning by Œnanthe crocata is exactly simulated. The proving adds little to the knowledge of Cicuta we thus derive from toxicology, save that it shows its power of causing local tonic spasms, as of the neck and jaw, and of developing pustular inflammation on the face and hands.

Cicuta has not been much used in homœopathic practice,— chiefly in epilepsy and pustular eruptions. Of the latter Hahnemann says—" I have cured chronic confluent impetigoes of the face, with burning pains, by means of one or two doses of a small portion of a drop of the juice, letting three or four weeks intervene ere I followed up the first (when necessary) with the second." Dr. Conrad Wesselhœft has recorded several cases showing its curative effects in eczema of the chin in the male subject.* Teste calls attention to its double action on the nervous system and the skin ; and suggests it as a remedy for cerebral and other nervous affections resulting from repercussion of eruptions. It is good for hiccough and belching when of a spasmodic character : I have myself cured an obstinate and long-lasting affection of this kind with it, and it has relieved such symptoms when occurring in cholera.

Dr. Lilienthal has a paper on Cicuta in the *Hahnemannian*
    * *N. Eng. Med. Gazette,* x., 505.

Monthly for 1875, in which he directs attention to the great hyperæmia of brain and cord found in animals poisoned by it, which die with convulsions, followed by paralysis. No wonder, he says, that so many of our practitioners consider Cicuta nearly a specific in (epidemic) meningitis cerebro-spinalis. He is referring especially to the results obtained by Dr. Baker, of Batavia, who reports sixty cases treated by this remedy without a single death.*

The analogues of Cicuta are *Aconite, Hydrocyanic acid,* and *Strychnia.*

It seems to have acted well in all dilutions.

I have last to speak of a medicine we call

Cina.

This is the "worm-seed" of commerce and domestic practice; and is said to consist of the unexpanded flower-heads of one or two eastern varieties of Artemisia. From it the now well-known Santonine is obtained. We triturate the latter, and make a tincture of the former.

The proving of Cina is in the first volume of the *Reine Arzneimittellehre.* It contains 290 symptoms from Hahnemann and five others, and 11 from three authors.

Cina has derived its reputation and its popular names from its activity as a vermifuge. That it does, especially in the form of Santonine, kill and expel the round-worm and occasionally the thread-worm, there can be no doubt. Hahnemann refers to this use of it; and very justly, as it was given in doses of from ten to sixty grains, warns against its danger. He adds, moreover, that worms in healthy children cause little inconvenience; while in the unhealthy they are a symptom of the morbid condition, and will continually recur after expulsion until this is remedied. He says nothing about the dynamic use of Cina in helminthiasis. But his experiments and citations revealed the curious fact, that Cina produces on the healthy body nearly, if not quite, all those symptoms whose presence leads us to suspect the existence of worms. There are the dilated pupils, with dimness of the sight and twitching of the eyelids, the ravenous appetite, the pinchings in the abdomen, the itching at the nose and anus, the frequent micturition, the spasmodic cough with vomiting, the restless sleep, the fever, and the twitchings in various parts of the body.

* N. Y. State Hom. Society's Transactions, x., 60.

General convulsions also have frequently resulted from the large doses of Cina or Santonine given as a vermifuge. Homœopathic practitioners thus came to give this drug in minute doses to children suffering from worm-affections. They calculated that, on the principle *similia similibus*, it might at least relieve the symptoms caused by the presence of the parasites, though they themselves remained *in situ*. It fully answered their expectations; and a curious result followed. By some inexplicable influence these infinitesimal quantities of Cina not only relieved worm-symptoms, but promoted the death and expulsion of the worms themselves. This occurred so often, that at length it became the recognised homœopathic practice to dispense with vermifuges, and to rely upon dynamic remedies alone. The pathology of the day was altogether favourable to this course, as it regarded worms as a morbid product of the organism.

The results of such practice have been partly beneficent, partly disastrous. It has saved thousands of children from nauseating and poisonous worm-medicines, which for them were quite needless, as Cina and similar remedies in minute doses did all that was required. But, on the other hand, by making treatment by the latter only a sort of orthodoxy in homœopathy, it has left hundreds of others unrelieved, when a few grains of Santonine, or an injection of salt or quassia, would have delivered them from their tormentors. With the demonstration, now fully made, that worms are in all cases introduced from without and act as foreign bodies, the reasonableness of destroying them directly, where possible, necessarily follows. This has been seen by most homœopathists; and our later Domestic Guides have ceased to display the helpless inanity into which Hering's falls on the subject.

Our wisdom, therefore, in the treatment of helminthiasis is first of all to give the patient the possible benefit of the dynamic action of medicines,—that is, unless any other be distinctly indicated, of Cina. It seems beneficial in all varieties of the malady, as Dr. Bayes says that he has repeatedly killed tapeworm with it, as well as the lumbrici and ascarides for which it is generally given; and it acts *omni dosi*, from the twelfth dilution of Cina of this writer to the twentieth of a grain of Santonine recommended by Dr. Dyce Brown. What the former will sometimes do is illustrated by an excellent case of Dr. Hamilton's in the thirteenth volume of the *British Journal of Homœopathy*, where chorea depended on the presence of ascarides, and was cured by their expulsion by this means. But, unless such measures speedily succeed, then—if the symptoms are at all urgent—we are bound to resort to the usual parasiticides, among which Santonine, especially against the round worm, holds a prominent place.

This is the most important sphere of the action of Cina. But Hahnemann, saying that it has more valuable properties than those which make it a vermifuge, indicates it in whooping-cough (in which Dr. Jousset esteems it the principal remedy), and in certain intermittents accompanied by vomiting and canine hunger. Teste commends it in the flatulent colic, without diarrhœa, of older children; and Dr. Bayes in the gastralgia of empty stomachs. Dr. Martin Deschere, who has recently given us a study of the drug,* justly says, that where symptoms like those of helminthiasis present themselves, Cina will cure, whether worms are present or not. Dr. Chepmell has pointed out that such a condition often occurs in lingering remittent fevers in children, and says that here Cina is quite specific.

Of the dose of Cina I have already spoken; and I am unable to mention any true analogue to it.

I must now dwell somewhat upon

Santonine, whose properties, though involved in those of Cina, are much more marked when it is administered separately. One of these is enuresis. As Dr. Ringer writes— "Santonine, if given frequently, is very apt to occasion a great difficulty in holding the water, and thus it is not uncommon for children, if they take much of this medicine, to wet the bed, and to be obliged to pass the water very frequently, or even to be unable to hold it during the day." He characteristically adds: "this remedy is sometimes able to stay the nocturnal incontinence of urine of children." I had suggested that it did so when, as often happens, worms were the cause of it; but in his later editions Dr. Ringer says that this is no necessary element in the cases.

A more important and interesting action of Santonine is that which it exerts upon the eyes. The xanthopsia caused by it has long been noticed, and has of late years been fully studied by Dr. Edmund Rose.† He finds the derangement of vision produced by it to be, in the first degree, "colour-blindness;" in the second degree, "colour-confusion," which he considers to be the condition known as Daltonism; and, in full intoxication, hallucinations. His inquiry into the causa-

* *North Amer. Journ. of Hom.*, xxvi., 115.
† See *Brit. Journ. of Hom.*, xxvii., 214.

tion of these phenomena leads him entirely to reject the theory —of which there is no proof—that the xanthopsia is due to a staining of the media of the eye. He sets it down rather, connecting it with the other phenomena, as a result of congestion of the retina, which the opthalmoscope demonstrates to be present. The colour-confusion and hallucinations he traces to a corresponding influence on the optic nerves and the visual centres respectively. The latter he connects with the hallucinations of other senses, the (evidently cerebral) vomiting, and the spasms of the cranial nerves, as showing that the drug acts directly on the brain.

Such investigations seemed at first sight to have rather a scientific than a practical interest. But Dr. Dyce Brown, whom we always find quick at seeing the therapeutic inferences to be drawn from physiological observations, has done this good work for Santonine. In conjunction with an ocuiist friend, Dr. Ogston, he put the drug to the test as a remedy for several of the deeper-seated affections of the eye. The results, which were published in the *British and Foreign Medico-Chirurgical Review* for 1871, are very striking.* Of the forty-two cases treated thirty-one were cured or improved; and these included choroiditis, retinitis, atrophy of the optic disc, pure amblyopia, and retinal anæsthesia. The ultimate influence of Santonine on the brain was manifest, for cerebral amblyopia and paralysis of the motor oculi were greatly benefited, and concomitant headaches removed. In one case, moreover, of undoubted double cataract vision was greatly improved after some months' use of the Santonine ; and with reference to this Dr. Brown tells us that in some experiments of Dr. Ogston's "it several times happened, especially when young kittens were employed, that within a few minutes after the animal was killed, a dense cataract developed itself in the lenses of both eyes. Within half an hour these parts became quite opaque, the opacity remaining very marked after the removal of the lens from the eye." "It seldom," he says, "occurred to any extent in the eyes of adult animals, nor has it ever been observed to occur during life." Nevertheless, unless cataracts are of spontaneous origin in recently defunct kittens, the tendency of Santonine to produce them is undoubted ; and that is enough for homœopathy.

I am not aware whether any further testing of the power of Santonine in eye disease has been carried out. But Dr. H. Wood reminds us that in 1862 MM. Guérin and Martin had recommended it in amaurosis, especially in that following

* See also *Brit. Journ. of Hom.*, xxix., 445.

acute choroiditis and iritis.* *Apropos* of this, it is worth mentioning that Stillé cites a case in which a child of six months took five grains of it, instead of three which had been ordered. It became amaurotic, and did not recover its sight for two months. I myself rely on it with much confidence in that hyperæsthetic and hyperæmic condition of the organs which comes on from continuous fine work, as in seamstresses.

The action of Santonine on the eyes is comparable with that of *Atropia* and of *Digitalis.*

In Dr. Ogston's cases a grain of the drug was given every night. But Dr. Brown's first patient, whose improvement in sight while taking Santonine for worms first drew his attention to the subject, had doses of the twentieth of a grain only. It must be remembered that two grains have proved fatal to a child.

* I had referred to the record of their experience in the second edition of this Manual.

LECTURE XXVI.

CINCHONA.

We will address ourselves to-day to the consideration of the famous Peruvian bark and its no less famous alkaloid, quinine. I have had some doubts as to the designation I should use for the bark itself. Cinchona is the scientific name of the botanical genus, and perpetuates the memory of its introducer into Europe : by this term it has always been known in England. But if you look into the continental medical Latin of the last two centuries you will find it called, if not " cortex Peruvianus," then " china-china." This is said to represent its native appellation, " china " meaning bark, and the reduplication implying that it is bark of barks. By this name it has passed into the nomenclature of other countries : it is still " china-china " in Italy, it is " quinquina " in France, and " china " or " chinarinde " in Germany. Under this last title it stands in the *Materia Medica Pura ;* and as China it is known in the school of Hahnemann throughout the world. I cannot refrain from using the familiar term when speaking of the special homœopathic uses of the drug ; though for historical and general purposes I shall best—lecturing as I do in England and for Englishmen—call it

Cinchona.

The homœopathic tincture is directed to be prepared from the yellow bark, which was that mainly used in the provings. It is richer in quinine than the other varieties.

Hahnemann has bestowed great attention on Cinchona. Its first pathogenesis appears in the *Fragmenta de viribus*, where it is credited with 122 symptoms of his own, and 99 from authors. In the last edition of the third volume of the *Reine Arneimittellehre* Hahnemann's own symptoms have increased to 427, and he has pressed no less than 21 provers into his service, obtaining from them 575 symptoms. There are also given 141 observations from authors, 35 in number. You may well be surprised at hearing that so many ill-effects have been ascribed by medical writers to a substance of by no means virulent nature; and an examination of the originals justifies the hesitation to accept them. A good many are the obvious mechanical effects of the large quantities of powdered bark in those days introduced into the stomach; and are often so represented by their reporters, and stated to have disappeared after an emetic. These are quite inadmissible as pathogenetic effects of the drug; and I think that the mass of those that remain are no less so, for another reason. The opponents of the use of bark in intermittents, and also those who maintained that it should not be given without the previous use of evacuants, alleged many instances of harm resulting from its administration. To all these phenomena (including asthma, jaundice, and dropsy), whether aggravations of the paroxysms, their transformation into other shapes, or results of their suppression, Hahnemann has freely helped himself to complete the Cinchona-pathogenesis. Influenced by his then theory of homœopathic cure, he considered all these to be symptoms of the Cinchona-disease, by the induction of which in a mild form even cases suitable for it were cured. The objection to such a doctrine is that no Cinchona-disease of the kind has ever been induced upon other than aguish subjects. So that the phenomena are at the utmost effects of the compound influence of the drug and the disease; and are more probably due to the latter alone, the bark acting only as a disturbing influence of no specific kind. I would therefore recommend you to expunge from the pathogenesis of Cinchona all the symptoms which Hahnemann has cited from authors, save the few I shall mention. For the study of the symptoms of his fellow-provers I can recommend you a paper by Dr. Langheinz, "On the relation of Peruvian bark to Intermittent Fever," which is translated from the *Vierteljahrschrift* in the twenty-fourth volume of the *British Journal of Homœopathy*. He arranges some of them according to the time of their occurrence after the ingestion of the drug, and so reconstructs a fair picture of the effects as they followed one upon another. He also relates the proving of Cinchona by seven of Jörg's pupils, and some other experiments with it.

Hahnemann found Cinchona in use for two great purposes, —as a tonic, and as a remedy for intermittent fevers. He proved it to discover on what principle it so acted. That it caused a febrile paroxysm was the Newton's apple which led him to formulate *similia similibus* as the law of specific therapeutics. Of this I will presently speak at length. But he also found that it produced in the healthy a peculiar kind of debility; and that its "tonic" properties in disease, when analysed, were demonstrably applicable to weakness of this very sort. When used with precision, under the guidance of the homœopathic rule, he stated that Cinchona would do all its strengthening work in infinitesimal doses, as high even as the twelfth dilution. The special kind of debility for which it is suitable he indicates as that which results from exhausting discharges or other loss of fluids. There is here emptiness of the blood-vessels and much loss of energy, but therewith considerable erethism of the nervous and even of the circulatory system. In this condition, where the weakness is itself the disease, Cinchona is curative, because homœopathic to it. Hahnemann reprobates in a forcible manner the pernicious practice, prevalent in his day, of giving bark for every kind of weakness, and where the disease which caused the weakness was still present. He acutely pointed out that the best results which were obtained from it were seen in the convalescence from acute disease, and were just correlative to the super-added debility caused by the depleting treatment then pursued. For all this you should read the preface to his proving, which is a master-piece of observation and reasoning.

This thought of Hahnemann's was as original as it was brilliant and fruitful. It was a pure induction from his provings. The only attempt made at precisionising the tonic properties of bark in former times was the doctrine that it acted best in a relaxed state of the solids. Here its large proportion of tannin may have come into play. But Hahnemann's doctrine was far more definite, and at once fixed its genuine and certain range of action. It will not cure anæmic debility like Ferrum, or nervous debility like Phosphoric acid. But in that occasioned by loss of blood; by diarrhœa, diuresis, or excessive sweating; by over-lactation; and by too great and rapid expenditure of semen, it is a most effectual remedy. Nor does it fail us when a discharge is a morbid one *ab initio*, as in excessive suppuration. "In all these cases," says Hahnemann, "the other symptoms of the patient generally correspond to those of China." In one particular especially they do so, viz., in their tendency to pass into a *hectic* condition. We have here the succession of chill, heat, and sweat which we shall see to be characteristic of the drug, and which gives it its place in the treatment of ague. It cannot be too strongly impressed on the mind that China is the great anti-hectic. It is to this febrile condition what Aconite is to the synochal and Arsenic to the typhoid form. But whether with hectic or without, remember that weakness from drain on the system is the sphere of the tonic action of Cinchona ; and within it you will find it manifesting some of the most beautiful curative powers known to the art of medicine. They are seen alike in the most acute and the most chronic forms of debility so induced. Thus, in the prostration, even to syncope, which follows upon puerperal hæmorrhages, Dr. Guernsey relies upon it with undoubting confidence ; and that in the minute doses he habitually employs. (Failure of vision and ringing in the ears are of course indications of this condition ; but I hardly think that Dr. Guernsey is warranted in pointing to the well-known tinnitus of quinine as proving the homœo-pathicity of China to the last-named symptom. It is generally, in quinic intoxication, associated with symptoms of cerebral hyperæmia ; whereas here we have present a precisely reverse state of things.) The virtues of the remedy extend, moreover, to other effects of the same cause—to headaches and various pains and neuroses, to hydræmia, and even to dropsy.

For want of such a defining thought, bark and its alkaloid, hitherto indiscriminately used as tonics, seem now falling out of favour. All recent physiological experimentation, moreover, has gone against the notion that the drug exerts any primarily roborant action on the system. Quinine was found by Briquet (as we shall see) to lessen the force of the heart's action and diminish the arterial pressure, and also to impoverish the blood. The latter action has been studied more fully by Binz, with the result of proving quinine to be the most potent of protoplasm-poisons, so that even in minute doses it kills the white corpuscles. While such facts indispose the practitioners of traditional medicine to use Cinchona as a tonic, they support its credit in the school of Hahnemann. They show also, as Dr. Drysdale has pointed out,* how just was Hahnemann's discernment of the precise kind of debility to which bark is homœopathic. To check the formation of the blood by killing its white corpuscles is to produce a similar effect on the system to that occasioned by actual loss of the vital fluid.

We enter upon a larger and more difficult question when we come to the action of Cinchona as a remedy for intermittents. Is it anti-periodic, whatever be the origin of the

* Brit. Journ. of Hom., xxvii., 283.

malady so recurring; or is it anti-malarial, whatever be the form assumed by the disorders so caused? What is the measure and extent of its efficacy, and what the dose and time of its administration? Lastly, what is the rationale of its action? These are some of the points presenting themselves for discussion.

And, first, as to the facts. There can be no doubt of the specific power of bark over ague. It was the one bright spot in the medicine of Hahnemann's day, which led him to believe that if he could find the rule of its action he would have the clue to a better therapeutics. It is still cited—as by Dr. Latham—as the cardinal instance of the "cure" as distinguished from the "treatment" of disease.* And it has been shown that "the disappearance of ague, as a cause of mortality in this country, exactly coincides with the introduction of Cinchona bark into general use;" so that while between the years 1653 and 1660 there died in England of ague 10,466 persons, in the corresponding septenary period from 1733 to 1740 the deaths from this cause were only 31.†

And now, how is this curative power of Cinchona and its alkaloids to be characterised? If it is anti-periodic, it will manifest itself more or less in all affections of periodic recurrence : if it is anti-malarial, it will hold good to some extent in all results (at any rate, all recent results) of malarial poisoning. The action will spread laterally along whichever plane it occupies in ague itself. Well ; the testimony to the general anti-periodic virtues of Cinchona is somewhat conflicting. Hahnemann says that "almost all typical diseases may be suppressed by powerful doses of China ;" and, though in his Materia Medica he condemns the practice as pernicious, it appears from some papers included in Dr. Dudgeon's collection of his *Lesser Writings* to have been formerly his own, and fairly successful. Pereira speaks of it as "beneficial" and "serviceable" in many cases where "a paroxysm (of pain, spasm, inflammation, hæmorrhage, or fever) returns at stated intervals ;" but he does not use such qualified language of its power over ague. Trousseau and Pidoux will not allow that it is an anti-periodic. If periodicity, they say, belongs to an affection which has not malaria for its cause, bark often fails to influence it. Of our latest writers, Horatio Wood states that quinine has no less power over non-malarial than over malarial periodic affections, so far as checking their recurrence

* *British Medical Journal*, Aug. 17, 1861.
† Russell, *Clinical Lectures*, p. 355.

is concerned; but that the benefit is often temporary only. Ringer speaks less distinctly on the subject. He commends it in periodic, but also in non-periodic neuralgia; and writes— "Quinia appears to be useful in some, but quite useless in other cases of intermittent hæmaturia." Phillips is decided on the other side. "It is a stereotyped remark in medical works," he writes, "that the more exactly a nervous (or indeed any other) disease conforms to a regular type of periodic exacerbations, the more surely will quinine prove useful. As a general proposition this is untrue. It is only when the neuralgia is due to actual malaria that the rule holds; and in the case of recurrent inflammation, or of hectic, there must be either malaria or else septic poisoning at work, or else we shall find this maxim fail us." It is evident from his whole work that our late colleague speaks from a survey of others' experience, and not merely from the brief space of his own in this field; otherwise his statements of fact could not be allowed much weight. He makes a good point, however, when he points to the inefficacy of quinine in migraine, however strictly periodic its recurrence.

On the other hand, the testimony to its efficacy in malarial poisoning, whatever form it may assume, is loud and uniform. To begin with, it is an almost certain prophylactic.* Its use renders possible the penetration into certain regions which would otherwise be deadly to the traveller. Then it is no less effectual whatever be the type of the malarial fever, whether intermittent, remittent, or continued. Dr. Maclean shows that by far the best treatment for the incessant vomiting and distressing pain in the head which occur in bad remittents is to give quinine freely. Again, when malaria manifests itself in quite different ways, as in dysentery on the one side, in neuralgia or even epilepsy on the other, quinine is the one and most effective remedy.

I think, then, we may conclude that Cinchona cures ague by its specific antidotal influence against the malarial poison. But what kind of antidote is it? Does it act after the manner of a chemical neutraliser? or does it set up in the parts affected an action incompatible with that of the poison, and is this action of a similar or an opposite kind? The former alternative has of late been widely advocated. Since the researches of Binz and others have shown how potent a poison quinine is to all protoplasm, the hypothesis has been framed that malaria consists of an abundance of low organisms, and that bark antidotes it by destroying these. I think that

* See Stillé, op. cit., i., 514; Ringer, 7th ed., p. 559.

several considerations concur to render such a theory untenable. One is that the dose of quinine which suffices to cure an intermittent is often far too small to affect the vitality of the supposed microzymes. I will not bring forward homœopathic experience, but will content myself with referring to the treatment of ague by subcutaneous injection of the drug. It is found that by this method doses of two grains each, repeated every fourteen or twenty days, are generally sufficient to check the paroxysms and prevent relapse : the maximum quantity required in the worst cases was from six to ten grains, and the maximum frequency of injection every day or two.* Still better results have been obtained ; but I give these as easily credible. On the other side, Dr. Buchanan Baxter has ascertained† that the vitality of microzymes is suspended only, not annihilated, by quinine in such proportions as the animal body can bear in its blood. But the crucial test is afforded here, as previously, by the extension of the plane of action. Quinine is not the only protoplasm poison. Strychnia and mercuric chloride have the same property in less degree ; yet they have little or no power over intermittents. So also bark is not the only febrifuge ; but the other substances which resemble it in this power exercise no common destroying agency over infusoria. Some have it, as Dr. Baxter has ascertained with regard to beeberine and picric acid, and as is now generally recognised in respect of willow-bark and its derivatives ; but no one would think of ascribing it to black pepper, chamomile, and cobweb, whose repute against intermittents is nevertheless considerable.

I cannot therefore assent to the hypothesis that bark cures ague by destroying in the blood the microzymes which cause it. My conclusion accordingly must be that it antidotes malaria by setting up, in the parts that are or would be affected by it, an action incompatible with its own. In this I am supported by the high authority of Bretonneau, of Trousseau and Pidoux, and of the elder Wood. " I know," the latter writes, " no better explanation of the anti-periodic property than that which supposes it to depend upon the powerful influence exercised by the remedy upon the nervous centres, through which probably the paroxysms are produced. Every consideration in connection with the peculiarities of regular intermittent diseases leads to the conclusion, that the paroxysms are produced by an influence acting through the cerebral centres, without which the result would not take place. Now,

* Lond. Med. Record, ii., 333.
† Practitioner, xi., 342.

if these centres can be preoccupied by a strong impression from some other source, they may be rendered insensible to the morbid influence, and the paroxysm, therefore, set aside. Quinia is characterised by its disposition to act energetically upon certain nervous centres, which are probably the same as those through which the cause of the disease operates. Quinia, therefore, interrupts the succession of the paroxysms ; and, as they are sustained, probably, in part at least, either by habit, or by some chain of morbid action passing insensibly from one paroxysm to the succeeding, the interruption is either permanent, or continues until the original cause may reassume, in some mysterious way, its original activity, and produce a relapse in the now unguarded system."

We are thus prepared for the question whether bark is homœopathic to ague, whether this prerogative instance of specific therapeutics conforms to the principle *similia similibus.* This question is sometimes put thus—Can the drug cause, has it ever caused, an intermittent fever? But even though we had to answer in the negative, the homœopathicity of the remedy would not be disproved. It is rare that drugs can excite concrete diseases ; and it is quite unnecessary for the practical carrying out of the rule " let likes be treated by likes " that they should do so. For this, and for the demonstration of similarity in a remedy, it is sufficient that it is seen working in the same direction as the disease ;—that it affects the same parts, and—so far as its action goes—in a similar manner.

Now of such homœopathicity of bark to ague we have abundant evidence. I will not dwell on mere assertions, though several of these might be cited from out of the ranks of the old school to corroborate that of Hahnemann.* But from the elaborate discussion of the question carried on by Dr. Langheinz, and also by Dr. Rogers in his tractate entitled *The Present State of Therapeutics,* I will cull two or three actual observations bearing on the point.

The first is a case of tertian fever in a child, which was treated by grain doses of quinine every two hours during the interval. After the third dose there appeared a rigor, followed by heat and sweat; the whole attack lasting forty-five minutes. The same thing happened after each succeeding dose ; and one of the attacks was witnessed by the reporting physician, who describes it. It was a typical ague on a small scale, with thirst during the heat. The tertian paroxysm recurred once

* See the testimonies of Auber and Goedorf in Langheinz' article, and of Weitenweber and Götz in *Monthly Hom. Review.,* x., 760.

at the expected time, but in less force; and then came no
more. The bark fever also, after growing slighter and slighter,
disappeared; and the patient became and continued well.
But it may be said that this was not a pure experiment, as the
patient was already suffering from ague; and if I were endeavouring to prove that Cinchona can cause intermittent
fever in the healthy, the objection would be valid. When,
however, my object rather is to ascertain the direction in
which it acts, the *modus operandi* of its curative working, then
such an observation is most illuminative. It shows the drug
at every dose exciting a miniature paroxysm of the disease,
until the susceptibility of the system for both bark and malaria
was exhausted. It suggests that a similar process, though
without such outward manifestations, is going on in all cases
where a single full dose is administered—as recommended by
Briquet and most therapeutists—some score or more of hours
before the expected paroxysm. It tells the same story as
that which we shall hereafter meet with when we speak of
Thuja; when we shall see this medicine, given continuously
to a sufferer from warts, excite two crops of new ones, whose
dying away is followed in a short time by the disappearance
of the old enemies.

But we have further testimony. In Dr. Langheinz' paper
you may read a case in which a patient convalescing from
typhoid, and taking half-grain doses of quinine, had what the
reporter calls "a well marked fit of ague" after each dose.
The medicine was omitted for ten days; but on its being prescribed again, in the form of decoction of bark, the same
phenomena followed. Three other cases are cited by this
writer in which quinine given to patients affected with other
diseases caused in them a single or (as in one of them) a
double paroxysm of fever, *i.e.*, of the typical sequence of chill,
heat, and sweat. If you will have experiments on the healthy,
you will find some there from Wittman, in which the same
phenomenon appeared; or I may refer you to Hahnemann's
provings of Cinchona and Noack's (of which I shall presently
speak) of quinine, in which it was of no unfrequent occurrence.
If you wish for such experiments on a larger scale, I may
refer you to the report—cited by the same writer—of the
health of the workmen in the quinine manufactory at Frank-
fort-on-Maine. From this it appears that most of those who
are much exposed to the dust of the bark sooner or later get
an attack of fever, consisting of one violent paroxysm of chill
and heat; after which they seem to become insusceptible.

I will sum up in the words of Trousseau and Pidoux.

" Daily observation, says M. Bretonneau, proves that Cinchona given in a strong dose determines, in a great number of subjects, a very marked febrile movement. The characters of this fever, and the epo̧h at which it manifests itself, vary in different individuals. Most frequently tinnitus aurium, deafness, and a sort of intoxication precede the invasion of this fever ; a light rigor then is added, a dry heat accompanied by headache succeeds the first symptoms, subsides gradually, and ends in moisture. Far from yielding to new and stronger doses of the drug, the fever caused by the absorption of the active principle of Cinchona does not fail to be exasperated." I am sorry to say that these authors do violence to history and truth by claiming this discovery for Bretonneau, instead of acknowledging it as Hahnemann's.

Now it is no answer to such facts as these to point to the exceptional nature of their occurrence,—to bring forward the number of patients, workmen, and even experimenters in whom Cinchona and quinine have produced no such symptoms. You will remember how Dr. Drysdale has shown that there are two classes of drug effects, which he names absolute and contingent ; the one resulting in almost every subject of the drug's influence, as the mydriasis of Belladonna, the other requiring for its development a special susceptibility on the part of the prover, and, like disease itself, not to be produced at will. It is symptoms of this contingent order which most closely resemble the phenomena of idiopathic disease, and avail best for the working out of the rule *similia similibus*. Of such kind is the fever of bark. I think that the evidence I have adduced is quite sufficient to show that the aguish paroxysm may be and has been induced by the drug ; and this is enough to outweigh hundreds of instances in which it has failed so to act. It is enough, moreover—since there are no opposite facts on record which suggest that it is antipathic —to justify the conclusion that it is homœopathic to the disease it cures ;* in further support of which we have the fact noted by several observers, that the first paroxysm occurring after quinine is begun is apt to be more violent than its predecessors. This invariably occurs when a full dose is given immediately before a paroxysm.

This question is of so much importance to the argument for and against homœopathy as a therapeutic method, that I have gone into it at greater length than I should otherwise

* The absence of subsequent periodical recurrence of the fever induced by bark is of no importance to the question. The deficiency can be supplied in treatment by the repetition of the dose.

have been justified in doing.   But its determination has also
a practical bearing on the use of the remedy.   If it cures
ague by destroying microzymes, it must be given in large and
frequently repeated doses, so as to saturate the blood up to
their perishing point.   If it acts by giving the nervous system
a substitutive shock, as Dr. Wood seems to suggest, it is best
administered in single full doses to cinchonism shortly before
each expected paroxysm.   But if " substitutive " here, as elsewhere, means " homœopathic,"* then no such violent measures are required ; and we need only proportion our doses to
the severity of the disease, giving them with moderate frequency during the interval.   And again, if Cinchona cures in
virtue of its homœopathicity, it will cure most effectually when
most homœopathic, and less so as the type of the fever
departs from that which it causes ; till at length we shall come
into a region where it will not cure at all, even though it may,
if given in sufficiently large doses, suppress the paroxysms.

Now these corollaries just express the experience of homœopathists in the treatment of intermittent fever.   Hahnemann says, in his preface to Cinchona, that, when all the
symptoms correspond, a single small dose of bark given
directly after the attack, previous to the elements of a new
paroxysm having accumulated in the system, will cure the
ague then and there.   He does not here specify what these
corresponding symptoms must be.   But from some of his
notes to the proving we may gather them to be—thirst just
before and after the hot stage ; commencement of the paroxysm with some accessory symptoms, as palpitation, anxiety,
nausea, great thirst, canine hunger, pressing pain in the hypogastrium, or headache ; distension of the external veins ; and
rush of blood to the head.   Dr. Bayes, who saw much of ague
in Cambridge, cured the majority of his cases with the third
and higher dilutions.   He states that " in intermittent fever
the symptoms which most strongly indicate China are where
the chills, the hot stage, and the perspirations are generally
evenly and well marked, and there is a distinct intermission
of comparative health.   There is a loud rumbling in the head,
sense of constriction from ear to ear over the vertex, great
sensibility to currents of air, sinking at the epigastrium, a
feeling of emptiness without hunger, or of hunger easily ap-
peased, contractive pain under the lower left ribs, sometimes a
sense of fluttering, mental depression with irritability."   Dr.
Chargé emphasises the absence of thirst during the actual
chill and heat, saying that its presence in either is a positive

* See p. 221.

counter-indication for the drug; he also notes the abundance, though slow development, of the sweat (which occurs mostly at night), and the frequency of gastro-hepatic disturbance during the intervals. I am speaking here, of course, of China itself; the minute indications for quinine as a distinctive remedy I shall specify hereafter.

I have entered into these *minutiæ* because it is by attending to them that the most brilliant cures are made, and with the smallest and least frequent doses. But I am bound to say that I think the good to be done by attempting such precise practice is far outweighed by the disadvantages it entails. In the pursuit of the exact *similimum* through an interminable list of not always trustworthy symptoms time is lost and disappointment incurred. Bark is passed by because the correspondence is not exact; whereas it is sufficiently close to enable it to cure quite satisfactorily, even if the doses must be a little larger and the repetitions rather more frequent than would otherwise be necessary. The result is that Dr. Rogers is able to make a point against homœopathy, that its treatment of ague is, by the statements and confessions of its own adherents, not so successful as that of the old school; and this simply through its neglect of quinine. It ought not to be possible to substantiate such a charge, as I must confess Dr. Rogers to have done; and I must again advocate, as I have often done before, the treatment of all recent and simple agues with quinine alone. When these display the regular series of chill, heat, and sweat, unmarked by any special phenomena, the remedy is pretty well infallible. The objection that it merely "suppresses the paroxysms," and does not really cure the disease, has no weight here; for in such recent cases the paroxysm is the disease, and in its repeated recurrence lies all secondary evil which may occur. Nor can any harm be done, even in case of failure, while moderate dosage is practised; and here, as quinine cures rapidly if at all, little time need be lost before resorting to other means.

I am glad to be supported in this position by one of the veteran homœopathists of the United States (now just lost to us), Dr. Jeanes. In a paper recently read before the Philadelphia Medical Society on "Intermittent Fever,"* he maintained that the power of Cinchona and its alkaloid to check the progress of ague is a great boon to humanity, and one of which we should not hesitate to avail ourselves, even though we have to use massive doses for the purpose. On the other side I fully concur in all that has been said, by Dr. Hirsch†

* See *Brit. Journ. of Hom.*, xxxii., 723. † *Ibid*, xxv., 406.

and others, on the evil of forcing a suspension of the paroxysms by needlessly large doses—using, as Dr. Drysdale puts it, a surplus of physiological action, instead of suffering the whole of this to be absorbed into the therapeutic operation. Such practice is especially to be reprobated in cases of long standing, where cachexia is established. Here the more minute and specialised homœopathic treatment has time to be carried out, and repays the trouble ; and in this bark is rarely indicated for chronic intermittents.

I have now said enough upon the two great actions of Cinchona, its tonic and its febrifuge properties. But, over and above all this, Cinchona does good service to us in several ways, most of which Hahnemann himself has pointed out. It appears from the pathogenetic symptoms, he says, that it will cure only a small number of diseases. He first specifies the kind of ague in which it is febrifuge and of weakness where it is tonic, as we have already seen. And then he goes on—

1. " The primary effect of China is to open the bowels ; hence it will cure certain kinds of diarrhœa, provided the other symptoms correspond."

This is a curious effect of a substance containing so much tannin, yet it occurred repeatedly, both in Hahnemann's and in Jörg's experiments, and has been observed also in the workers in bark at the Paris manufactories. I have repeatedly verified it in practice, both in acute and chronic diarrhœa. The latter must be of a passive and painless character to call for it ; when enteritic or ulcerative it requires Arsenic and remedies of that kind. But in acute *summer* diarrhœa—not that of autumn, which is more profuse and bilious—severe griping pain is nearly always present ; and the first effect of the China is to relieve this, after which the flux itself ceases. China is also one of the remedies for lienteria, —diarrhœa with undigested food having been noted from it by both Hahnemann and Herrmann.

2. " The too ready and frequent morbid excitement of the sexual organs, resulting in an involuntary emission of semen, and caused even by slight abdominal irritations, is permanently relieved by China."

Sexual excitement was noticed by several of Jörg's provers and by Hahnemann himself : Dr. Phillips says that all the alkaloids of Cinchona will cause it. The condition Hahnemann describes is just that left behind by a too frequent repetition of such excitement, especially of an abnormal kind.

3. " Pain which is excited by merely moving the affected parts, and which gradually rises to the most fearful height, has frequently been cured by a single drop of the twelfth dilution of China, even when the attack had returned frequently." In another place he notes of the pains of China, that they are " increased by motion, and especially by touching the affected parts ; and also characterised by this, that the pain, though it may have disappeared for the moment, may be excited again by simply touching the parts, when it frequently becomes horrid and intolerable."

Neuralgic and rheumatic pains, having these features, may be controlled by China ; they are said to be of drawing, tearing, or even jerking character.

Hahnemann indicates China also in certain forms of jaundice, in humid gangrene of the outer parts, and in suppuration of the lungs. And lastly he lays down that "bark will scarcely ever be useful except where the nightly rest of the patient is disturbed similarly to the disturbance which characterises China ;" of which disturbance he says : " China is characterised by restless night-sleep, with dreams causing anxiety and starting ; when waking from these dreams one finds it difficult to come to one's senses, or the anxiety continues." It is the best remedy when such disorder of sleep is readily brought on by drinking *tea*. It is, indeed, to the general effects of excess in this beverage what Nux vomica is to the corresponding evils of much coffee-drinking.

I have cited these remarks of Hahnemann's at length, a; he has evidently studied China very closely. Its pathogenesis abounds with references from one symptom to another, which only appear elsewhere under Ignatia and Pulsatilla. There is little to add to his enumeration of the curative powers of the drug. I may mention its value, however, in that relaxed state of the ligaments of the joints which makes them (especially the ankles) ache after any exertion. I may say, moreover, that it seems to excite the ovario-uterine functions so as to convert the existing catamenia into a hæmorrhage—the blood coming away in black lumps. It is thus homœopathic to a form of menorrhagia itself, as well as to the debility which it occasions. Dr. Guernsey considers it to be a " keynote "for the drug when the symptoms are aggravated every other day. He also lays much stress on distension of the abdomen as characteristic of it : " the abdomen feels full and tight, as if stuffed—eructations afford no relief." A similar feeling is experienced elsewhere, even in the limbs, so that the garters, as well as the clothes about the waist, must be loosened.   Dr. Thayer, of Boston—an old and experienced practitioner—esteems China very highly in gall-stones. Since 1854, he says (writing in 1874), he has "not failed in a single instance to cure, permanently and radically, every patient with gall-stone colic who has taken the remedy" in his manner; and he has treated many from all parts of the United States. He gives the 6th dilution, at increasing intervals, till only one dose a month is taken. Sometimes, he says, the first effect seems to be an increase in the frequency of the attacks, till (as he supposes) the gall-bladder is emptied; but then they subside and cease.*

As an anti-malarious agent, Cinchona compares with *Arsenic* and *Cedron*; as a tonic, with *Ferrum*.

For dose, Hahnemann recommends the 12th dilution. I confess, however, that save for nervous conditions I have never found it necessary to go above the 1st; and for the hectic of suppuration the mother-tincture seems to act best.

* See *Brit. Journ. of Hom.*, xxxiii., 345.

LECTURE XXVII.

CINCHONA ALKALOIDS, CISTUS, CLEMATIS, COCA, COCCULUS, COCCUS CACTI, COFFEA.

In connexion with Cinchona it is necessary to speak of two at least of its alkaloids. The first is the well-known quinia, which homœopathic nomenclature follows that of Germany in calling

Chininum, but which is better known by its popular name of quinine. It is, as you know, commonly used in the form of a sulphate, of which triturations or an alcoholic solution may be made.

Quinine has, since its discovery in 1820, gradually taken the place of the powdered bark as a remedy for ague. It has, moreover, manifested such decided physiological properties of its own, that it has been thought worthy of a special proving, which it has received at the hands of Dr. Alphonse Noack, of Lyons. Five persons took part in it; and its record is contained in the second volume of the *Journal für Arzneimittellehre.** Dr. Allen gives its results, together with those of numerous other experimenters (among whom I may especially mention our colleague, Dr. J. C. Morgan, of Phila-delphia), making a total symptom-list of 1076. Much infor-mation, moreover, as to the physiological action of quinine is contained in M. Briquet's *Traité thérapeutique du Quin-quina et ses préparations* (1853); and Binz's recent publication, *Ueber das Chinin und seine Wirkung* (1877), gives the latest researches on its action. I may also refer you to a useful collection of facts relative to its pathogenetic effects made by Dr. Ch. de Moor, and appearing month by month, since its commencement, in *L'Homœopathie Militante.*

So far as the pathogenetic properties of quinine have re-lation to its use in intermittent fever, they have already come before us. But experiment reveals other actions exerted by it, which have to be considered and utilised; while its ex-tensive use as a medicine makes it necessary that we should form a precise apprehension of what can be wisely and well done with it.

* See also vol. i. of the *Révue de la Mat. Méd. Spécifique.*

1. Let us first consider the group of phenomena entitled " cinchonism," and readily induced by full doses of quinine. Their seat is the head, with the eyes and ears. There is deafness, with tinnitus—the latter preceding and being more considerable than the former, and taking the form of buzzing, singing, roaring, or hissing ; there is disturbed visual function, even to blindness; and in the brain itself we have headache, with fulness, weight, and tension, vertigo, and sometimes epistaxis. When the headache is localised, the forehead and temples are its seat. Accompanying these phenomena are evident signs of congestion, as flushing of the face and redness of the eyes and ears. One of Noack's provers describes his headache as intense towards evening, when the arteries of the head began to beat with violence, as if the skull was about to burst. His face was burning ; there were noises in the ears and sparks before the eyes. Dr. Hammond has lately examined precisely into this matter, In a man who had taken ten grains the retina and tympanum were found sharing in the hyperæmia of the outward parts ; and in a cinchonised rabbit the same condition was seen in the brain, when a hole was made in the cranium.* In animals, and even in the human subject, meningitis may follow, with delirium and convulsions ; and with or without this complication collapse and coma succeed the stage of excitement when the dose has been large.

Such effects as these are in the ordinary mode of treatment simply an unpleasant, but to some extent necessary, evidence that the system is thoroughly affected by the drug. For homœopathy they are direct therapeutic indications. They should give us a valuable medicine for some forms of headache, and for congestive disorders of sight and hearing. We have yet to learn what is the pathological (or even the full symptomatic) condition of those eyes and ears, which are reported as having been rendered permanently amaurotic or deaf by the drug. In chronic congestive headaches it is a favourite remedy in my own hands.

2. Next, the survey of Noack's provings—in which full doses were taken—shows several pretty uniform effects of the drug. One of these was tenderness and pain in the vertebræ, especially in the dorsal region ; another was the pain and tension at

---

* It is fair to say that opposite results were obtained by Vicol and Mossop, who after five and ten grain doses found the disk and retina very anæmic. Here, however, no disturbance of vision was present, and the phenomena may have depended upon depressed general circulation.

the stomach which Trousseau and Pidoux also note. The most constant phenomenon was a highly lateritious state of the urine, which, on cooling, deposited numerous orange coloured crystals consisting of urate and purpurate of ammonia, with phosphates.

It is not easy to give these effects of the drug any physiological expression. But they must be borne in mind as indications for it in ague or other disorders to which it is found adapted. The state of the urine mentioned led me once to give it with striking success, though no stronger than the 3rd dilution, in a case of daily occurring supra-orbital neuralgia, as I have related in the twenty-sixth volume of the *British Journal of Homœopathy*.

3. M. Briquet, besides investigating fully the phenomena of cinchonism, ascertained by exact experiment the influence of quinine on the circulation. He found that while small and rare doses seemed to increase the force and frequency of the heart's action, the more intense and sustained effect of the drug was enfeeblement of the circulation, with diminished arterial pressure and lowered temperature. In this he has been supported by subsequent observers. He concluded that quinine could not have any of the tonic properties of Cinchona, but should rather be used as a " hyposthenisant" in febrile and inflammatory states. His conclusions have been carried out by his native *confrères*, especially in the treatment of acute rheumatism. That there is something specific about it here may be inferred from the fact that Dr. Jousset reports it very efficacious in the small doses of the school of Hahnemann; and that Sydenham is rightly cited by Hahnemann as stating that the continued use of bark sets up a sort of "scorbutic rheumatism," shifting in situation, and alternating with internal pains. It was in such rheumatic conditions that Cinchona in substance was so esteemed by the older physicians, and Stillé thinks that it is more effective than its alkaloid.

4. The ideas of those who use quinine as a tonic, supposing such to be its primary influence on the system, have sustained a still graver shock from the experiments of Binz, to which I have already referred. Briquet had found that quinine, while it increases the fibrin, diminishes the number of the red corpuscles of the blood. Binz has further ascertained that in virtue of its power as a protoplasm-poison it paralyses and kills the white corpuscles, so that they never become red : it also lessens the ozonising property of the blood. As a tonic, therefore, it is under a cloud ; but, on the other hand, German

and English practitioners are now following suit with the French, and, taught by Cohnheim the important part played by the white corpuscles in inflammation, are giving quinine in large doses to restrain their activity. Cinchonism, however, is not found a desirable addition to the patient's sufferings; so as alcohol is found to hinder its development, it is given simultaneously. Thus the unhappy subject of inflammatory fever, to whom Aconite and cold water would be the greatest of boons, is now to be dosed with quinine and brandy. I frankly say that for myself in such a case I should prefer the lancet. I am not objecting to using quinine in such disorders as pyæmia and leucocythæmia; and in the former of these it seems to have proved strikingly efficacious. The quantity given need not be very considerable, as Binz finds that one part in four thousand, or even less, will effect the purpose.

5. Another indiscriminate and, I think, unwarranted use of quinine seems to be receiving its death-blow; I mean its prescription for every kind of neuralgia. Dr. Anstie coincides with foreign observers in rejecting it in all but malarious neuralgia, making a doubtful exception in the case of the supra-orbital form when otherwise caused. It was this nerve which was affected in the case of my own which I have cited : it is probable that more extensive provings would show that the drug has an elective affinity for it. It appeared, indeed, to have such affinity in Dr. Morgan's proving, who, though experiencing some amount of neuralgiform pain everywhere, felt it far more frequently and acutely in the supra-orbital region. Dr. Ringer thinks that, therapeutically, this nerve is the special seat of the influence of quinine.

6. The power of quinine to arrest the paroxysms of pernicious malarial fever, otherwise almost certainly fatal, has been turned to good account by our French homœopathic colleagues in a similar condition which occasionally complicates any form of acute disease. It has best been studied by Dr. Frédault, under the name of " ataxy," in *L'Art Médical* for 1876-7. He describes it thus :—" There may present itself not so much a serious condition, permanent and established, as in simple *gravity ;* not so much a serious condition approaching to *malignity* by an increasing tendency to aggravation even till death ; but one characterised by disorders in its progress, and especially by relapses and amendments, remissions, and then again aggravations,—the phenomena having features which remind one of the *perniciosity* of marsh fevers, not indeed having their regularity and defined characters, yet resembling them though at a distance, and denoting a special gravity."

When this condition—whose three signs are gravity with incoordination of symptoms, temporary seizures resembling those of pernicious ague, and threatenings of a fatal issue—supervenes in the progress of any acute disorder, he thinks that it is best met by the administration of a *gramme* of quinine, either at once, or *in dosi refractâ*. He relates several cases illustrative of his remarks; and points to attacks of coldness of the extremities, especially of the hands and the nose, as very significant of this condition. Drs. Jousset and Cretin fully agree with him; and the occasional administration of quinine in this way seems to play no unfrequent part in the practice of our Parisian *confrères*. I am a little jealous lest it should be adopted too frequently, to the neglect of more purely homœopathic treatment; but I cannot doubt that it is a valuable piece of practice, and one which may at times render us serviceable aid. I have seen such phenomena occurring in acute disease, and know well their peril.

The only other alkaloid of bark which I shall mention is cinchonia—

Cinchoninum.—This has received a good deal of experimentation on the human subject in the old school, so that Dr. Allen can give a pathogenesis of 288 symptoms taken from fourteen observers. The most significant point is that noted by Bouchardat, that it is less liable than quinia to produce tinnitus and visual disorders, but that in smaller doses and more frequently it occasions a peculiar and pretty severe tensive pain in the forehead. In doses of twelve or fifteen grains, he says, it is much more apt than quinia to cause præcordial pain, and faintness even to syncope.

I pass now to some medicines of lesser note, beginning by giving you a short account of the rock-rose, or

Cistus Canadensis.

The tincture is prepared from the whole plant.

The Cistus has been proved, mainly in the tincture and 1st dilution, under the superintendence of Dr. Hering. His pathogenesis, with the medical history of the plant, is given entire by Dr. Hale in the second edition of his *New Remedies*.

It was the great popular reputation of the rock-rose in *scrofula* which led to its being proved. The symptoms (which we have only in schema-form) shadow forth, faintly indeed, the manifestations of the diathesis in the eyes, ears, nose, and lymphatic glands; and in such affections (especially in glandular enlargements) it has been used successfully by homœopathic physicians. Dr. Bradshaw has cured white swelling oʻthe knee-joint with it,* in which, and in the corresponding disease of the hip, it is in considerable old school repute. I am myself most impressed with its effects upon the *throat.* The sense of dryness there is more marked in the pathogenesis of Cistus than in that of any other medicine I know,—except perhaps Belladonna. The following symptom, too, looks very like *shingles.* "Below the right shoulder-blade, extending round to the front of the body, was a very much inflamed spot about the size of the palm of the hand, painfully sore to the touch; soon after pimples began to appear on this spot in a large group; they caused violent burning. Later, a pain went from this belt-like spot to the left hip, and into the groin; the pain was like rheumatism, motion increased it."

Cistus is said to require a magnesian soil; and Dr. Hering suggests that it may be related to that mineral as (for similar reasons) Belladonna is to lime and Pulsatilla to iron.

The 1st dilution has been used successfully in scrofula.

If the next name on my list were as valuable a medicine as its sister is a beautiful flower, it would be precious indeed.

Clematis

is prepared from the leaves and stems of the Clematis erecta.

A pathogenesis of Clematis, obtained by seven persons with substantial doses, was published by Stapf in his *Archiv* (vol. vii). Hahnemann subsequently included the drug among those of the second edition of his *Chronic Diseases*, but only added to Stapf's symptoms six from Stoerck, of which more anon. It was next taken up by the Austrian Society, where twenty-one persons proved it, nearly all using the mother tincture. The symptoms from all these sources, with a few others, are given by Dr. Allen, whose total amounts to 821.

I shall best bring the results of this extensive experimentation before you by connecting them with the therapeutic uses of the drug. Hahnemann says in his preface that "it will be found curative in a number of affections which have their origin in the abuse of Mercury and are complicated with

* *Monthly Hom. Review,* xiii., 38.

psora, in foul eruptions of the head and general surface, in several urinary troubles, in stricture of the urethra, and various kinds of very troublesome inflammation of the eyes." He goes on to state that Stapf has found it helpful in orchitis and indurated swellings of the testes following mismanaged gonorrhœa; and then refers to Stoerck's previous experiences with the drug.

This well-known physician published, in 1769, a tract entitled *Libellus, quo demonstratur, herbam veteribus dictam Flammulam Jovis posse tutó et magna cum utilitate exhiberi ægrotantibus.* His cases are given in the fourth volume of Frank's *Magazin;* and include ulcers and excrescences, secondary syphilis, "scabies humida," arthritis, and headache. The drug appears to act much like Dulcamara and Sarsaparilla in such affections, setting up diuresis and diaphoresis, increasing the circulation on the surface, and favouring the return of suppressed discharges; so changing chronic morbid conditions for the better. Full doses of course are required for such actions.

As regards orchitis, Dr. Desterne has criticised unfavourably the published experience with Clematis;* but such a case as that recorded by Dr. Ransford in the twenty-fifth volume of the *British Journal of Homœopathy* appears exempt from his objections, and bears out the credit of the remedy. There seems no doubt of its pathogenetic action upon these organs : the swelling and painful sensitiveness noted by Stapf's provers being reproduced in several of those of the Austrian Society. Its efficacy in urethral stricture is equally warranted by its effects in the healthy, and has received several testimonies in its favour besides that of Hahnemann. Hirsch† praises it in the spasmodic form, and Franklin‡ in the inflammatory variety. I have myself seen it act with rapid curative power in symptoms of commencing stricture supervening upon chronic gleet. It is only, of course, in such conditions that internal medication can be expected to do anything : you would not look for help from it in organic strictures of long standing. As to eruptions, the provers experienced several, of vesicular and even pustular kind; and Hempel gives one case and Hirsch another of eczema impetiginodes cured by it. Hahnemann's last recommendation speaks of several kinds of inflammation of the eyes as curable by it. Much burning and redness were developed in the provers; in one the pupils were contracted;

---

* See Hempel, *sub voce.*
† *Brit. Journ. of Hom.*, xxv., 612.
‡ *Science and Art of Surgery*, i., 428.

and in three the vision was indistinct, as if objects were seen through a gauze or fog. Hirsch recommends Clematis in "chronic inflammatory states of the borders of the eyelids, with soreness and swelling of the meibomian glands, such as we find in young scrofulous subjects." But the affection of the eyes in which Clematis has done yeoman's service is iritis. Drs. Allen and Norton do not seem to speak from personal experience of it here, but they mention the high praise it has received from many, among whom was my own teacher, Dr. Madden. They consider it indicated where great sensitiveness to cold is present, as is Mercury, to which they reckon it an analogue in point of its action in iritis. I myself have every confidence in it in both the rheumatic and the syphilitic forms of this disease.

All this evidence makes it probable that we have not yet sounded to the depths the virtues of Clematis, or assigned it its definite sphere of action. I know of no medicine presenting much analogy with it; nor has its use been extensive enough to enable us to fix its most suitable dose.

I have now to bring before you the Peruvian shrub known as the Erythroxylon

Coca.

The leaves are the officinal portion; a tincture may be made from them when fresh, or triturations when dried.

Coca has been proved by twenty-four persons in all (mostly homœopathists), besides the observations made by travellers of its effects on the natives. A full collection of all this information has been made by Dr. C. Hering, and published by him in his *Materia Medica*.

Coca is one of those substances of which we shall soon encounter a cardinal instance in coffee—substances which "cheer, but not inebriate," stimulating the nervous centres without engorging their substance and disordering their functions like alcohol, opium, and haschisch. It has been used from time immemorial by the natives of South America as we use tea and tobacco. Taken in excess, it causes mental excitement, palpitation, sleeplessness or vivid dreaming, sparks or flames before the eyes, and r nging in the ears, with increased susceptibility of the senses. It has in a marked degree the property belonging to this class of substances ("aliments d'épargne") of diminishing tissue-waste; so that, while under

its influence, there is little need of food, the bowels are costive
and the urine is deficient in solid matter. By acting thus, and
by diminishing the sense of fatigue, it proves invaluable to
the travellers in its native regions, who chew the leaves as
they go on. It has a further virtue, common to it with
Arsenic, of obviating the distress experienced in climbing
heights, and breathing

"the difficult air of the keen mountain-top."

This power of the plant is witnessed to by all observers.

Coca has found little use as yet in practice. Dr. Hering
recommends its employment in troubles coming on with a low
state of the barometer; and the analogy of Arsenic would
suggest its trial in asthma. Dr. Clotar Müller,* who was one
of the first to prove and discuss Coca, says that he has found
it useful to palliate over-action in cardiac disease. It may
occasionally replace Coffea in insomnia from nervous excite
ment.

And now, of

Cocculus Indicus.

This is unknown as a medicine save in homœopathic practice
where it is employed in the form of a tincture prepared from
the seeds.

Cocculus was proved by Hahnemann among his earliest
medicines; a pathogenesis of it appears in the *Fragmenta de
viribus*, containing 156 symptoms from himself, and 6 from
three authors. In the third edition of the first volume of the
Reine Arzneimittellehre the number has swelled to 557, of
which more than half are Hahnemann's, the remainder being
contributed by eight fellow-observers.

Hahnemann says in his preface that Cocculus had never
been employed as a remedial agent previous to the provings
instituted by him with it on the healthy. He commends it in
some lentescent nervous fevers; in abdominal and other
spasms, with depression of spirits, especially in women, and
in not a few paralytic affections and moral disturbances.
The experience of his disciples has verified especially the
second of these recommendations, and has established it as a
true anti-paralytic; while it has, with the aid of physiological
experimentation, both defined and extended its sphere of
action.

* See *Brit. Journ. of Hom.*, xv.

2 E

Cocculus is well-known as a poison for fishes, and as an agent used for the adulteration of beer. In both cases the intoxication it produces is manifest rather in the motor than in the ideational centres; and to the same effect is the testimony of those who have experienced its effects in their own persons. Hahnemann has related in *Hufeland's Journal* a case of poisoning by it, which may be read in English in Dr. Dudgeon's collection of his *Lesser Writings* (p. 377). Coldness; paralytic stiffness of the limbs, with drawing pains in their bones and in the back; and sullen irritability, with anxiety, were the prominent symptoms. The patient said that his brain felt as if constricted by a ligature. He wished to sleep, but a frightful sensation, as of a hideous dream, came over him directly he closed his eyes, and made him start up again. He had great repugnance to food and drink. This last is a frequent symptom of Cocculus, and is very characteristic of it.* The experiments which have lately been made on animals with the alkaloid contained in Cocculus, picrotoxine, show that convulsions, both tonic and clonic, are a special characteristic of its action. The latter present many of those singular features which have been observed as results of injury to the crura cerebelli, as semi-circular and backward movements, and rolling over on the axis of the body. With these there is great slowness of pulse and respiration, indicating disturbance at the origin of the vagi.

Cocculus thus appears to influence the motor nervous tract throughout the cranio-spinal axis. To such action is referable, I think, the whole range of its curative influence. It is of great service in certain kinds of vomiting. These, when analysed, appear to be of cerebral rather than gastric origin. They are such as occur in sea-sickness, and in some persons from riding in a carriage or any similar motion; they have another instance in the vomiting of migraine and of cerebral tumours. In the latter Cocculus yields to Apomorphia, but in the former it has no rival. Such sickness is usually accompanied with vertigo; and for this trouble, when thus associated or appearing independently, Cocculus is a principal remedy. You will recollect the constant association of vertigo with those movements of gyration of which I have spoken as caused by Cocculus: it is, Dr. Ferrier says, their subjective side. The abdominal spasms in which it is, as Hahnemann alleges, so frequently serviceable are not mere colic; they appear always to spring from the nervous centres either directly or by reflex irritation. They are generally accom-

* See Meyhoffer, *op. cit.*, i., 111.

panied by flatulence, which is not the product of fermentation, but seemingly generated by the intestinal walls. It is most troublesome at night, so that it wakes the patient, or prevents his sleeping. Such flatulent spasms are most frequently seen in the female sex, and especially when its characteristic functions are being performed, as during menstruation and pregnancy. " Menstrual colic " is an example, and here Cocculus is renowned : Dr. Edward Blake esteems it also our best remedy for pure dysmenorrhœa. It is also useful in other nervous affections occurring at these times, as in menstrual headache. The following case of Dr. Black's shows what it can do here, and illustrates also the nausea and vertigo characteristic of the drug :

" Miss H—, æt. 35, of a full plethoric habit, has suffered from her present headaches for now fifteen years ; they came on shortly after the catamenia appeared, and have ever since regularly occurred at that period. Violent headache—described as a dull pain affecting the whole head ; the patient has a difficulty in describing it minutely ; is unable to lie for a moment on the back of the head ; is forced to lie on the side ; unable to bear the least light; any noise excites nausea and vomiting. During the headache she feels as if suffering from sea-sickness, and, on sitting up, the objects around seem to move up and down. The headache lasts from thirty-six to forty-eight hours, and comes on the third or fourth day of the catamenial period. The catamenia are abundant, but unattended by local pain. General health good.
" March 16th.—Cocc. 18, m. et n.
" April 4th.—The headache has occurred at the usual time but not so severe as usual, for she was able to move about, and was not confined to bed, as she always was before. A dose of the 6th dilution was given from every half-hour to every six hours during the third and fourth days of her period with great advantage. Cont. Cocc.
" 20th.—Rept. Cocc. 18, as on March 16th.
" May 1st.—Has had a very slight headache at the usual period, which was again much relieved by frequently repeated doses of Cocc. 18 ; she was now ordered Bell. 6, alternately with Cocc. 18, m. et n. This was the last prescription ; for one headache occurring after that she took the Cocc. Since October, 1844, to July, 1846, she has continued free from those headaches.
" Remarks.—The principal indication in this case for the selection of Cocculus was the marked tendency to nausea resembling sea-sickness, as if the stomach heaved up and down. So great was this idiosyncrasy that she told me that travelling in a carriage made her feel ill, and that sickness has often been brought on by looking at a vessel pitching up."

The use of Cocculus in convulsive and paralytic affections is yet in its infancy. It is said to have removed hemiplegia following apoplexy ; and Trinks has recorded an excellent case of post-diphtheritic paralysis in which it was the curative

agent.* It might prove useful (perhaps in the form of picrotoxine) in some of the rarer forms of chorea, in which peculiar
and definite involuntary movements—like those it produces—
constitute the disorder. Dr. Phillips' recommendation of it
in hysterical paralysis seems well in accordance with its
general action; and from its pathogenesis it should be useful
in paralytic weakness of the cervical muscles.

A French physician, M. Felix Planat, has just published a
treatise entitled *Récherches physiologiques et thérapeutiques sur
la picrotoxine*. He states that he has, by the administration
of this alkaloid, brought on convulsions, with foam at the
mouth, in a rabbit, a kitten, and other animals of lower or-
ganization; and that, giving it persistently in epilepsy (in
the form of a strong tincture of Cocculus), on the prin iple
similia similibus curantur, he has obtained several undoubted
cures. The French Academy has awarded this writer a prize
upon the Barbier foundation.† I have recently had a case of
epilepsy, in which repeated drawing of the head to the right
side with temporary unconsciousness occurred. Cocculus has
completely removed this feature of the case, though the actual
fits have not been influenced by it.

The only medicine with which I can compare Cocculus is
Chamomilla, and this solely in regard of its abdominal symptoms.

The medium dilutions (as in Dr. Black's case) have been
those mainly used, Hahnemann himself recommending the
twelfth. But Dr. Phillips says he has got excellent results in
cerebral vomiting, flatulent distension and spasms, and menstrual colic—for none of which uses, however, does he credit
the school in which he learnt them—with doses of one to three
drops of a strong tincture.

We have next to consider the place and action of cochineal,

Coccus cacti.

This must not be confounded, as is sometimes done, with the
Coccinella septempunctata, the lady-bird. The dried insect,
powdered, is treated with alcohol for a tincture, or (better)
triturated with milk-sugar.

Cochineal has been proved by the members of the Austrian
Society in their wonted exhaustive manner. The experiments

* See *Brit. journ. of Hom.*, xix., 312.
† *London Medical Record*. May 26, 1875.

—in which twenty-eight persons took part—are related in detail in the fourth volume of the *Œsterreichische Zeitschrift ;* and the schema of the symptoms may be found translated in Metcalf's *Homœopathic Provings,* and by Dr. Allen, who adds symptoms from two other provers. Hempel's article, also, should be consulted.

The Austrian proving makes it evident that the virtues popularly ascribed to cochineal in whooping-cough spring from its homœopathic relation to the disease. Few of the provers escaped a cough ; and with Dr. Wurmb it was " so violent that it caused vomiting, and the expectoration of a great quantity of thick, viscous, and albuminous mucus." I am not aware, however, that the medicine has been much used by homœopathists against this disease, save in France, where Dr. Guérin-Méneville says that it is in daily employment. Jousset considers frequent micturition of pale clear urine, with tenesmus, an indication for it here. I myself gave it once, in the 1st decimal trituration, in a case where a father whose house was full of whooping-cough contracted just such a cough as that Dr. Wurmb describes. The curative effect was very marked. Again, this proving amply accounts for the reputation of cochineal in the school of Rademacher as a "kidney remedy." The urinary symptoms are numerous, and of a high grade of intensity. Nephritic colic and vesical and urethral tenesmus are plainly pictured therein ; and you may read in Hempel cases where affections of this kind and also acute renal dropsies have been cured by cochineal. I have little doubt but that the study of this beautiful proving will lead to a more extensive use of the medicine, especially in sore throat with great dryness (like Belladonna and Lachesis, which last was taken by one of the provers to relieve the symptom, and with immediate effect), in inflammation of the labia (like Apis), and in laryngeal irritation and hoarseness.

Cochineal has hitherto proved curative chiefly in tolerably material doses ; but, as the proving was mainly made with the dilutions, we ought to get more out of these than we hitherto have done. In whooping-cough, Jousset gives it from the 6th to the 30th.

We now come to one of those substances which stand on the boundary line between food and medicine,

Coffea.

We use the raw, not the roasted bean, preparing it either as a

tincture or by trituration. Hahnemann's caution in this respect is justified by the discovery that methylamine is developed
in coffee by roasting.

A full proving of Coffea—by five persons, one of whom was
Hahnemann—is recorded by Stapf in his *Beiträge;* and contains 246 symptoms.

Stapf well characterises the primary effect of coffee as " a
pathological excitation of all the organic functions. When
coffee acts moderately upon the healthy organism " (he says)
" the irritability of the organs of sense is morbidly increased,
the visual power becomes more acute, the hearing more sensitive, the taste is finer, the sensorium is more vivid (hence
increased susceptibility to pain), the mobility of the muscles
is increased, the sexual desire is more excited, even the
nervous activity of the digestive and secretive organs is increased ; hence a morbid sensation of excessive hunger,
increased desire and facility for alvine evacuations and for the
emissions of urine. To what an extent the nervous and
animal activity of the organism is increased by coffee appears
from the sleeplessness which it excites in various shades and
degrees, from the peculiar pathological excitation of the mind
and soul, and from the febrile warmth which it causes to a
considerable extent." This primary effect of coffee is made
use of in many ways, as you well know,—to arrest the paroxysm of ague and of asthma, to relieve headache, and to
antidote the depressing effects of vegetable poisons, such as
Opium. But it also points to several conditions in which
the drug may become homœopathically curative, as when
pain is felt excessively (in labour, for instance), in nervous
excitement, and especially in sleeplessness. For this last it
has a high repute in the school of Hahnemann ; and my own
experience with it makes me surprised to find Dr. Ker saying
that he has never known it to do any good.* Possibly he
used it in too low dilution. I find it particularly useful when
the patient cannot get to sleep because of ideas perpetually
forcing themselves upon his mind. Dr. Bayes says that the
insomnia cured by Coffea is that which is owing to excessive
agitation of mind or body.

There are two forms of neuralgia in which Coffea has often
proved beneficial. One of these is toothache. We are indebted to Dr. E. M. Hale for establishing as the characteristic
for it here (besides restlessness and great complaining) that
the pain is entirely relieved for a time by holding cold water

---

* *Monthly Hom. Review,* xviii., 744.

in the mouth, returning as this grows warm.* He has lately communicated a case in which strong coffee drunk to keep off sleep produced a toothache having this very feature.† The other Coffea neuralgia is a variety of migraine, which the excessive use of the beverage is so apt to occasion. Hahnemann, who wrote an essay on the injurious effects of this practice, so common in Germany in his time, thus describes the migraine it causes :—" It comes on in the morning shortly after waking, and increases little by little. The pain becomes intolerable, and sometimes burning ; the integuments of the head are very sensitive, and hurt when touched ever so slightly. Body and mind seem excessively sensitive. The patients look exhausted ; they retire to lonely and dark places, and close their eyes in order to avoid the light of day ; they remain seated in an arm-chair, or stretched upon a bed. The least noise or motion excites the pain. They avoid talking or being talked to, or hearing others talk. The body is colder than usual, although no chills are experienced ; the hands and feet especially are very cold. They loathe all food and drink, on account of a continual sickness at the stomach. If the attack is very violent, a vomiting of mucus takes place, which, however, does not diminish the headache. There are no alvine discharges. The pain scarcely ever ceases before evening. The attacks come on irregularly, and without premonitory symptoms."

I have given this description, because of late the alkaloid of Coffea—caffeine—has come into use, generally by hypodermic injection, as a remedy for migraine. This caffeine contains the toxic principles of coffee in a very concentrated form. In doses of from two to ten grains, it causes (according to Lehmann) violent excitement of the vascular and nervous systems —palpitations of the heart, extraordinary frequency, irregularity, and often intermission of the pulse, oppression of the chest, pains in the head, confusion of the senses, singing in the ears, scintillations before the eyes, sleeplessness, erections, and delirium. These phenomena seem to be the result of direct excitation of the heart and nervous centres, which latter (in animals) goes on to tetanus. The cardiac condition induced by it is described by Dr. Phillips as one of irritability, in which the slightest excitement is sufficient to bring on violent palpitations.

This keener action of the alkaloid should be utilised in practice according to the law of similars. That it can be we

* *Brit. Journ. of Hom.*, xxiii., 492.
† *Ibid*, xxxii., 546.

have the testimony of Dr. Anstie. His experience led him to hope that caffeine might prove a very valuable remedy, both in neuralgia and in alcoholic insomnia. And when a correspondent asked how an agent mainly employed for rousing the nervous system (as in opium-poisoning) can be effectively used as a calmer of pain and nervous irritation, his reply was just that which ours would have been—that " the dosage is wholly different in the two cases." Dr. Meyhoffer has made much use of the cardiac action of the drug. " Coffea," he says,* " is to the nerves of the heart what Cactus is to its muscle." In nervous palpitation, with abundant secretion of urine, he gives the 3rd or 6th dilution with rapid effect. In asystolia he finds caffeine, in doses of one or two centigrammes, to exert a most beneficial effect, very like that of Digitalis, but more completely ameliorative when sleeplessness is part of the patient's distress.

I have only to add that Dr. Bayes describes the hemicrania in which Coffea is useful as a kind of clavus ; and mentions a case in which spasmodic stricture of the rectum was remarkably controlled by the medicine.

Coffea admits of close and profitable comparison with *Chamomilla* and *Ignatia,* and (less so) with *Coca.*

The attenuations from the third upwards have generally been used. Dr. Bayes finds the twelfth most effectual; and with this my own experience coincides.

* *Comptes rendus du Congrés International d' homœopathie.* 1878, p. 60.

COLCHICUM, COLLINSONIA, COLOCYNTH, CONIUM, COPAIBA.

Our first medicine to-day is the meadow-saffron,

Colchicum.

We prepare the tincture from the fresh common bulb, by expressing the juice, and treating the residue with alcohol.

Colchicum has twice been proved in the school of Hahnemann, first by Stapf (*Archiv*, vol. vi.), and later by Reil (*Vierteljahrschrift*, vol. viii).* The two pathogeneses, with numerous observations from other sources, are combined by Dr. Allen, giving a collection of nearly 1,200 symptoms.

In poisoning by Colchicum, the gastro-enteric symptoms are very prominent. These are of specific nature, as they appear with hardly less severity when the poison is directly introduced into the circulation. They have two forms, or perhaps stages. In the first, there are constant and profuse serous evacuations, with collapse, blueness and coldness, hoarse voice, and cramps—the whole forming a vivid picture of Asiatic cholera. In the second the symptoms are those of gastro-enteritis, with especial dysenteric phenomena—the passing of shreddy mucus from the bowel being a constant feature. In both forms muscular weakness is very marked; and there is often deathly nausea.

Next to the stomach and intestines, Colchicum acts most powerfully on the kidneys. It is supposed to be diuretic; but I apprehend that the notion has arisen from observation of its action in disease. In a short proving of it which I made twenty years ago upon my own person the quantity of urine was very notably decreased; and Stoerck found the same thing.† Suppression often occurs in cases of poisoning, and is probably due to intense congestion of the Malpighian bodies, which lesion has been caused by the poison in dogs.

* See *Brit. Journ. of Hom.*, xix.
† *Libellus de Rad. Colch. Autumn*, 1759.

A more important question concerns its influence upon the elimination of the urinary solids. Some statements have been made to the effect that it increases the proportion of these, and especially of the urea and uric acid. Dr. Garrod* has analysed these statements, and made some careful experiments himself, with the conclusion that "there is no evidence that Colchicum produces any of its effects upon the system by causing the kidneys to eliminate an increased quantity of uric acid; in fact, when the drug is continued for any lengthened time, it appears to exert a contrary effect." He also says—"We cannot assert that Colchicum has any influence upon the excretion of urea, or the other solid ingredients of the urine."

A case of poisoning by Colchicum is reported in the *London Medical Gazette* for 1838-9 in which the symptoms assumed another character. There was intense gnawing, dragging pain in all the joints of the extremities, beginning in the hands and feet with numbness and pricking, with profuse acid sweating, and stiffness and pain in the occiput and nape of the neck. Such rheumatoid phenomena occurred in Stoerck's experiment on himself, and are very marked in Dr. Reil's proving. Here, however, they seemed seated in the muscles rather than the joints; and Teste's statement was borne out, that the neck is especially influenced by the drug. Several provers had decided pleurodynia.

There are three other statements to be made about the physiological action of Colchicum. The first is, that cows which eat it become affected with distressing and sometimes fatal tympanitic distension. The second, that it appears directly to slow the heart's action. The third, that in one case of poisoning by it the pleuræ were found inflamed.

We pass now to therapeutics. The gastro-enteric action of Colchicum has hardly yet been utilised in homœopathic practice. Its botanical congener, Veratrum album, has preoccupied any place it might have found in the treatment of cholera. I should suggest its substitution, however, in some cases, should great nausea be present, and should the cramps attack especially the soles of the feet. Stillé mentions its being recommended for cholera (to which he recognizes its homœopathicity) by a Mr. Cotter, who states that he used it successfully in eight cases. I once effected a rapid cure of an obstinate acute diarrhœa with Colchicum, guided to this medicine by the deathly nausea and prostration which were present. It ought to find an occasional place in the treatment of dysen-

* *Nature and Treatment of Gout*, 2nd ed., 1863.

tery and sub-acute proctitis, with much passing of mucus; and might be useful in relieving tympanites, as indeed in veterinary practice it has proved to be. Borborygmi are very marked in its diarrhœa; and the symptom, "He has appetite for forty different things, but as soon as he sees them, *or, still more, smells them*, he shudders from nausea, and cannot eat anything," has been frequently verified clinically.

But the main interest of Colchicum lies in its relation to gout and rheumatism. Its power of relieving the gouty paroxysm was renowned of old; and, since its revival in later times, has become firmly established and universally recognised. It is confessedly, moreover, of a "specific" nature. It is not an indirect result of evacuations caused by the drug, for it occurs just as surely when these are absent. It is not an ordinary "anodyne" effect, for Colchicum has no such property. Nor does the medicine act as an "antiphlogistic," for it subdues the pain before the heat and swelling begin to subside, and some time before the temperature falls; it, is moreover, inoperative in other than gouty inflammations. The term "specific" is accordingly used to denote its action; and pathogenesy shows that here, as elsewhere, "specific" means homœopathic. The anti-arthritic power of Colchicum would hardly, indeed, have been arrived at by the rule *similia similibus;* but, being empirically discovered, no other formula seems so well to express the relation of its curative to its physiological effects. So far as it influences healthy joints it is to cause inflammation and pain in them, and not any condition opposite to that which obtains in the gouty state.

If this be the rationale of its influence, Colchicum acts directly upon the affected joints in acute gout, and may have no power over the morbid diathesis. Pereira writes—"That Colchicum alleviates a paroxysm of gout I have before mentioned; but that alleviation is palliative, not curative. It has no tendency to prevent a speedy recurrence of the attack; nay, according to Sir Charles Scudamore, it renders the disposition to the disease much stronger in the system." Ringer says that a full dose may remove the pain in an hour, but Wood adds that by such practice the mischief is often transferred to the internal organs. It was supposed at one time that it might be of permanent benefit by increasing the elimination of uric acid by the kidneys; but Dr. Garrod's investigations seem to have barred this claim. It must thus be concluded that, in the ordinary dosage, Colchicum acts locally only upon gout; and, like quinine with ague, may by excess of action suppress it injuriously. It is a question whether homœopathy can make a better use of it. There must be something in the physiological action of the drug which makes it so effective specially against *gouty* pain and inflammation—something qualitative, as Drysdale expresses it,* in its relation to the disease. Whether the suggestion of Dr. Garrod's results is worth anything—whether Colchicum diminishes the renal elimination of uric acid, and is thus homœopathic and curative to gout at its possible fountainhead, remains to be investigated. However this may be, it is certain that in the various gouty neuralgiæ and inflammations Colchicum is more effective than any other medicine. Herein we agree with the late Sir H. Holland, who says that whether the gouty inflammation developes itself in the foot, the bronchi, the eyes, or the head, the specific virtues of the remedy are equally apparent. Several of these affections—especially the pleurodynia, the angina, and the ophthalmia—are figured pretty plainly in its pathogenesis ; and quite small doses are often sufficient to cure them. Dr. Dunham lays stress on the tendency of Colchicum to make the returns of gout more asthenic ; and, connecting this with the muscular weakness it causes, thinks it most perfectly homœopathic when gout presents the asthenic form in coming before us for treatment. The old-school writers of course present this as a counter-indication for the drug.

It makes for the purely local action of Colchicum in gout, that rheumatism—so similar to it in its arthritis, but so unlike it essentially—should be also under the control of the medicine. But it further strengthens the doctrine of qualitative relation, that rheumatic joints are not nearly so much influenced by it as gouty, and are most helped when the inflammation is, as there, purely synovial. It is, as its provings indicate, in muscular rheumatism—especially torticollis—that it shows itself most effectual. But in two published cases—one of Dr. Kidd's and one of Dr. Laurie's†—it displayed such remarkable power of controlling rheumatic pericarditis, that it ought to be more frequently used in the treatment of this affection. We have seen that it has inflamed the pleuræ. Teste says that the rheumatic pains to which it corresponds are generally *tearing*. In warm weather they are principally felt at the surface of the body ; as the air grows cooler they seem to penetrate the deeper tissues and the bones. Dr. Dunham says that they are worse at night.

A statement of the last-named author's I must cite without comment, for what it is worth. "I would draw attention,"

* *Brit. Journ. of Hom.*, xxvi., 313.   † *Ibid*, v., 314, and xiii., 198.

he writes, " to the fact that, in many cases of poisoning by Colchicum, cataracts have formed before death in the eyes of the sufferers. Professor Hoppe reports that with it he greatly benefited, though he failed to cure, three cases of soft cataract."

This is all I have to say about the therapeutic power of Colchicum. But I know of few drugs which seem to promise more extensive applications in the future.

Actæa racemosa, Arnica, Bryonia and *Veratrum album* seem to be its closest analogues.

The question of dose is a large one. Five drops of the mother-tincture every few hours seem to give speedy relief, without baneful consequences, in ordinary gout; but Dr. Dunham says that in the atonic forms to which he thinks it specially suitable, the 15th dilution is quite strong enough. There seems nothing gained by diluting the drug for its other applications.

Another valuable contribution to our Materia Medica from the indigenous plants of the American continent is the

Collinsonia Canadensis.

The tincture should be prepared from the root.

In the second edition of Dr. Hale's *New Remedies* may be found a short proving of Collinsonia, together with all that is known about the drug.

From this proving, and from the considerable clinical experience now accumulated, we are able to define pretty clearly the sphere of action of Collinsonia. It affects the whole gastro-intestinal canal, but especially the *rectum*. The presence of flatulence, spasm, and colic in the parts above confirms the indications for the remedy drawn from the condition of the rectum itself; but these last alone are decisive. From Dr. Burt's proving it appears that Collinsonia in small doses causes constipation, with straining and dull pain in the anus after stool. Here is shadowed forth the most important action of the drug. It is in *constipation* and *hæmorrhoids* from congestive inertia of the lower bowel that Collinsonia proves such a precious remedy. We frequently meet with such a condition in the middle and latter months of pregnancy; and here I have the greatest confidence in the drug. But it is also a most effective remedy for piles in general, when connected with constipation, and may be resorted to with advantage whenever Æsculus fails. Nor, though acting primarily on the rectum, does it confine its curative influence to that one only of the pelvic viscera. In many uterine affections connected with constipation it is of great value. Cases are collected by Dr. Hale in which dysmenorrhœa, pruritus, and even prolapsus uteri have under such circumstances yielded to its use. One of the cases of pruritus was a woman in the eighth month of pregnancy ; so that Collinsonia should be remembered when we meet with that distressing form of the affection. In larger doses, it irritates the rectum so much as to set up diarrhœa, soon running on into dysentery : there are severe colicky pains in the hypogastric region before and after the stools, and much tenesmus. It has not been used to any extent in complaints of this kind ; but in proctitis and rectal dysentery it should rival Aloes.

The rectum is thus the main field of action of Collinsonia ; but you will see from Dr. Hale's article that it is gaining considerable reputation as a cardiac remedy. Time will show its real place and value here, whether it is merely in the sympathetic cardiac disturbance of hæmorrhoidal subjects that it is effective, or whether it acts more directly on the organ.

Dr. Ludlam has lately borne a testimony to the virtues of Collinsonia, which, from the high estimate we all entertain of his judgment, is worth citing here. " We have often," he says, " used this remedy in hospital and private practice. It seems specially adapted to women, and to those women who have hæmorrhoids either during, or as a sequel to, pregnancy and parturition, or in complication with obstinate constipation or chronic inflammation with slight displacement of the womb. For the first of these cases, where the trouble dates from gestation or from labour, or from both, and the condition has become chronic, there is no remedy to compare with it for efficacy. We have cured a dozen cases of this kind that have been sent to us by physicians from as many states, with the *collinsonia* in the 3rd dilution. And the college class can bear witness to its remarkable efficacy in many such cases in our clinic at the Hahnemann Hospital. When the hæmorrhoids are associated with constipation, and with a mild form of retroflexion or retroversion, and especially with prolapse of the uterus, it will often relieve the whole difficulty."

I have already hinted that *Aloes* is a close analogue of Collinsonia. So also are *Æsculus* and *Podophyllum*, and—more remotely—*Hydrastis, Nux vomica*, and *Sulphur*.

I have nearly always used the 2nd dilution ; but others seem to have done as well with the 3rd, and others with more material doses. Herein also Collinsonia resembles Æsculus.

I now go on to speak of

Colocynth,

a drug which is a crucial instance of the fruitful results attainable by the Hahnemannian process of " proving " on the healthy body. Here is a substance which traditional medicine knows simply as a purgative. The modern experimentation on animals has done nothing for it : as a purgative and nothing else it still stands in the works of Ringer, Wood, and even Phillips. But a few physicians in Vienna agreed to test its effects on their own bodies ; and lo ! a range of action is revealed which at once puts it in a high place among specific remedies.

The dry pulp of the fruit is either triturated, or treated with alcohol to make a tincture.

There is a pathogenesis of Colocynth in the sixth volume of the *Reine Arzneimittellehre.* It contains 26 symptoms from Hahnemann himself, 195 from six fellow-observers, and 29 from authors. In the *Chronic Diseases* a second pathogenesis appears, but has only swollen to 283 symptoms in all, the additional ones being mainly Hahnemann's, *i.e.,* observed on patients. But our knowledge of the drug has been immensely increased, and, indeed, pretty well perfected, by an exhaustive proving conducted with it by the Austrian Society. Dr. Watzke's account of the experiments—in which seventeen persons, including two women, took part—is translated from the first volume of the *Œsterreichische Zeitschrift* in Metcalf's *Homœopathic Provings.* It contains also an analysis of Hahnemann's pathogenesis, and a complete account of all that is known of the drug, both as poison and as medicine. This monograph is indispensable for the study of Colocynth ; and so also is a commentary upon it by Dr. Pope, which you will find in the twelfth volume of the *Monthly Homœopathic Review.*

Traditional medicine, as I have said, knows Colocynth only as a purgative. It is aware, however, that this action is specific, and not merely local, being induced by its external application as well as by its introduction into the stomach. It seems most probable that thus, at least, it purges the lower bowel only, as the rectum is the only part of the alimentary tract found inflamed when a poisonous dose is injected into a vein. As under such circumstances there is no manifest irritation of the stomach, the vomiting which has been observed as a consequence of its external application would appear to result from an influence upon the (gastric) nerves. Still more certain evidence of such an influence is the severe colic which always accompanies the purgative action of Colocynth, and which is more marked with it than with any other cathartic. The pain is generally about the umbilicus, is of a twisting and burning character, increased by food, and relieved by the accompanying diarrhœic evacuations. Tenesmus also is a constant feature of the Colocynth diarrhœa. In one case of poisoning by it the intestines were glued together by recent lymph, showing its power to inflame the peritoneum.

The colic and diarrhœa so characteristic of Colocynth were experienced by all the provers. But in most of them other symptoms appeared, showing the power of the drug to act upon the nervous trunks on the surface as vigorously as upon the abdominal plexuses. The trigeminus is not uncommonly affected, causing toothache and hemicrania. But the nerves about the hip-joint suffer most severely, the pain darting sometimes down the anterior crural and sometimes down the sciatic trunks, even to the foot. The spermatic and ovarian nerves are also affected—the only two provers of the female sex complaining of deep stitches as from a needle in the ovaries; and one of the male provers experienced pain and swelling of the testicle and spermatic cord.

The therapeutical virtues of Colocynth are a true reflection of the pathogenetic powers now described as belonging to it. It is occasionally but rarely indicated in dysentery. It is homœopathic to this disease when the morbid process is confined to the rectum, the evacuations consisting chiefly of blood; or when severe colic is present. So also it may now and then be of service in peritonitis :* Dr. Ludlam recommends it especially when that portion of the membrane which envelopes the ovaries is affected. I may remind you that this trouble is often spoken of as "ovarian neuralgia." In both these inflammations, however, I prefer Mercurius corrosivus as a rule. The grand sphere of Colocynth lies among the *neuroses*, especially where pain is the most prominent feature. In Dr. Watzke's article you will find collected a number of cases in which neuralgiæ of the fifth nerve, of the solar and

* Dr. Watzke's case, in vol. xxv. of the *Brit. Journ.*, p. 561, looks like commencing peritonitis nipped in the bud by Colocynth.

other abdominal plexuses, and of the lumbar and femoral nerves, have been cured in a brilliant manner by this medicine. It is in colic and sciatica that its greatest triumphs have been achieved. I have myself found it curative only in recent cases of the latter disease, greatly preferring Arsenic and Rhus in those of longer standing. But for colic I rarely require any other remedy, save in those cases for which Plumbum is the obvious simillimum. Dr. Bähr thinks it is "rheumatic colic" for which Colocynth is suitable, and Plumbum for neuralgic. He describes a similar condition in the stomach, for which also he recommends this remedy. Both "are met with in the transition seasons when the air is cold, but the sun is still powerful enough to heat the blood; they likewise occur in summer, in consequence of sudden changes in the weather." In the colic most characteristic of Colocynth, the patient doubles himself up to relieve the pain, which he describes as very sharp. Dr. Carroll Dunham* mentions a case in which Colocynth, given because of the presence of its characteristic symptoms in the abdomen and about the hip, seemed to cause the permanent disappearance of an enlarged ovary; and Dr. Ludlam recommends it, under the same circumstances, in ovarian neuralgia. In one of the provers it removed neuralgic pain and swelling of the right testicle and spermatic cord—the result, as he believes, of his previous provings of Natrum muriaticum; and it has been found of service in the violent pains in the eye ball which precede the development of glaucoma.

I would add what Dr. Pope says of the Colocynth neuralgia in general. "It appears to me to be that of the rheumatic or gouty-rheumatic diathesis. The character of the pain, the fact that the joints are all prominently affected, that in the extremities motion so generally increases the suffering, that aggravation of it is so readily induced by cold and damp, all seem to indicate a dyscrasia of this nature." I may say in corroboration of this that Wurmb, who was subject to articular rheumatism and diarrhœa on the slightest chill, entirely lost this tendency after proving Colocynth.

The medicine which seems to me most closely allied to Colocynth is *Bryonia*. It has some points of analogy, moreover, with *Arsenicum*, *Chamomilla*, *Chelidonium*, *Cocculus*, *Gambogia*, and *Nux vomica*; Dr. Pope says also with *Staphisagria*.

It seems generally agreed that Colocynth must be somewhat diluted to obtain good effects from it in neuralgia. Even

* *Hom. the Science of Therapeutics*, p. 485.

2 F

Dr. Kidd advises the 3rd decimal here, and I myself prefer the 6th. But in colic he speaks of getting from the mother-tincture the same results for which Hahnemann recommends the 24th and 30th dilutions. I have myself always seen aggravation, where diarrhœa or dysentery co-existed, from any approach to this strength.

We have next to study the action of hemlock,

Conium.

Our tincture is, and always has been, made from the expressed juice of the whole plant. It is thus equivalent to the " succus " of the British Pharmacopœia, which Dr. Harley has demon-strated to be the only really active preparation of hemlock.

Conium is one of the medicines of the *Reine Arzneimit-tellehre*. Its pathogenesis appears in the fourth volume, and contains 89 symptoms from Hahnemann, 131 from 3 fellow-observers, and 155 from 30 authors. A later pathogenesis in the first edition of the *Chronic Diseases* adds observations by two others and by Hahnemann himself, swelling the list to 700 : and in the second edition Hahnemann supplies 212 more, which must have been observed upon sick persons while taking the 30th dilution. These new symptoms I have as usual to discard ; and I must do the same with nearly all those cited by Hahnemann from authors. They are, with hardly an exception, observations on patients taking Conium for cancer and other serious diseases : they profess to result from preparations and doses of the drug which later investi-gation has shown to be inert ; and they are but seldom put forth by the writers themselves as medicinal effects. It is Hahnemann who, unable to credit Stoerck's statement of the innocuousness of this renowned poison, chooses to set down to its action all phenomena appearing in the patients while taking it. Symptoms most obviously the result of the disease, or of an occasional cause—the cough of pulmonary cancer, the enteritis and death of a severe chill, the serous apoplexy of an octogenarian—are all set down as pathogenetic effects of Conium. Dr. Harley has now shown that Stoerck was quite right, and that hemlock as he gave it is incapable of pro-ducing its physiological effects. Unless, then, the cited symp-toms of Hahnemann's list are read in Allen, where they have been revised, you will do well to refrain from using them as instances of the action of our drug upon the healthy.

There has been so much confusion between Conium and the other umbelliferae and the extracts in which it has been given have been such bad preparations, that—save Hahnemann's earlier provings with the juice—nothing was certainly known of the real action of Conium till some thirty years ago. One description of poisoning by it, however, stood on immortal record. I make no apology for gracing this lecture with the passage from the *Pha'do* of Plato which contains it.

"Socrates, having walked about, when he said that his legs were growing heavy, lay down on his back for the man so directed him. And at the same time he who gave him the poison, taking hold of him, after a short interval examined his feet and legs and then having pressed his foot hard, he asked if he felt. He said that he did not. After this he pressed his thighs; and thus going higher, he showed us that he was growing cold and stiff. Then Socrates touched himself, and said that when the poison reached his heart he should then depart. But now the parts around the lower belly were almost cold; when uncovering himself, for he had been covered over, he said (and they were his last words) 'Crito, we owe a cock to Aesculapius; pay it therefore, and do not neglect it.' 'It shall be done, said Crito, 'but consider whether you have anything else to say'. To this question he gave no reply but shortly after he gave a convulsive movement, and the man covered him, and his eyes were fixed; and Crito, perceiving it, closed his mouth and eye".

If we needed any further demonstration that the *potion* with which the Athenians poisoned their criminals was our Conium maculatum, we should have it in the elaborate argument—philological, botanical, and physiological—which Dr. Imbert-Gourbeyre has given us in the pages of *L' Art Medical.**. But evidence of convincing force was afforded by the case of poisoning recorded by Dr. Hughes Bennett in his *Clinical Lectures*, *which revived* the interest in Conium in recent times. The identity of the phenomena he described with those recorded by Plato was obvious: both were speaking of a poison which caused paralysis from below upwards killing at last by gradual asphyxia. Dr. Christison began at once to experiment with it on animals, and got the same results, 'In various experiments," he writes, "with a very strong extract prepared from the green seeds with absolute alcohol, the only effects I could remark were palsy, first of the voluntary muscles, next of the chest, lastly of the diaphragm, —asphyxia, in short, from paralysis, without insensibility, and

* Trans. in Brit. Journal of Hom. xxxiii.

with slight occasional twitches only of the limbs." Similar conclusions have been reached by more recent experimenters, who have mostly used the alkaloid of hemlock, conia. But the most satisfactory observations with the drug are those of Dr. John Harley, who has followed (though without acknowledgment) the Hahnemannian method of proving on the human subject. It appears from the facts recorded in his *Old Vegetable Neurotics* that the main and only action of full doses of hemlock is upon the motor centres, which are—as it were—put to sleep. If the experimenter continues to use his legs the effect will most probably be earlier felt in these parts, after the manner seen in Socrates. If he remain in a state of comparative rest, the effects will be first declared in the eyes. There is here enfeebled power of accommodation of vision, with giddiness accompanying every fresh adjustment of focus; then ptosis, subjective or objective from fuller doses, a dull lazy or fixed expressionless stare and some dilatation of the pupils more rarely diplopia. These phenomena can imply paralysis of the third, fourth, and sixth cranial nerves. They come on, together with those of the legs, within an hour after the ingestion of the dose, and sometimes pretty suddenly: in another three hours they are gone. Consciousness is unaffected, and sensation slightly and rarely. No other effect on the system was observed.

It is a moot question whether Conium produces these results by affecting the intracranial motor centres, or by directly paralysing the peripheral extremities of the nerves. All agree that the cord is not involved, as it is only by poisonous doses that reflex function is affected. But on the former question Dr. Harley is on one side, and the Continental experimenters on the other. It is probably a matter of physiological interest only, so far as homoeopathic applications of the facts are concerned. For, even were its action primarily central, there is no general paralysis originating in the brain or cord which is merely functional, as that of Conium from its brevity must be. It might, however, be useful in local paretic conditions, especially of the ocular muscles. Given antipathically, and in doses large enough to produce its physiological effects, it has been reported useful by Dr. Harley in many forms of motor irritability, as chorea, paralysis agitans, infantile convulsions, and local spasms and cramps but the observations of others have hardly confirmed his results.

So far of the neurotic action of hemlook, which is all that is recognised by modern medicine. But we are now confronted with the fact that the plant was re-introduced into practice by Störck as a remedy for various profound derangements of the vegetative life, and that in this capacity it continues in high favour in the school of Hahnemann. (Its action on the nervous system was indeed hardly perceived by the older homœopathists. Caspar, in his lectures at Vienna in 1851, spoke of it as slight, mainly secondary, and displaying itself chiefly in spasms!) It is the fashion nowadays to reject all experience gained before the rigid experimentation of later times set in ; but it is a very unwise fashion. Trousseau and Pidoux set a much better example ; and profess to have verified to some extent the statements of Störck and his imitators. Such experiments as those of Harley, valuable as they are in themselves, prove no negative. They say nothing as to what the long-continued use of small doses of the drug might do, either pathogenetically or curatively. Hahnemann was led, from his provings of this kind, to conclude that Conium tended to engorge the glands, and recommended it in practice for such engorgements, especially when the result of mechanical injury. The experience of the old physicians went to prove it useful also when cancer or scrofula attacked these organs ; and this too has been taken up in the school of Hahnemann. Again,—that wasting of the mammæ and testicles has not uncommonly occurred (according to the same authorities) from its use suggests the glands of the reproductive system as especially under its influence, and warrants its use in ovarian affections also. Thus, in one way and another, an extensive homœopathic employment of Conium has grown up, as you may see from reading Noack and Trinks' recommendations of it, or the catalogue of its curative applications given by Dr. Carroll Dunham in an article upon it in his *Homœopathy the Science of Therapeutics* (p. 443). I may sum it up in the following propositions :

1. Conium is especially useful in the organic affections of lymphatic individuals, and among these to children and *old* women.

2. It is of frequent service in hypochondriasis starting from the sexual organs, as in that of uterine disease, and that which occurs (in either sex) in connexion with enforced abstinence from sexual intercourse. Its characteristic mental symptoms are depression, timidity, taciturnity, aversion to society, and, at the same time, a dread of being alone.

3. It is a genuine anti-scrofulous medicine, reducing swollen glands, especially when very hard, and especially removing the photophobia of strumous ophthalmia. This last property

is a very curious one, as it has never caused photophobia in the healthy and yet it removes it (and with it much of the co-existing malady) in strumous ophthalmia in doses far too minute for any primary physiological action to be exerted.

4. It had a great repute of old in "scirrhus." This term was often applied to all tumors hard enough to merit the name. Caspar commends it in the forming stages of fibrous tumour of the uterus, and two cases are mentioned treated by it in the Leopoldstadt Hospital at Vienna, the tumour in one disappearing, in the other becoming greatly diminished in size. But homoeopathy preserves to some extent the Storckian tradition of its efficacy in true malignant scirrhus. There appears no doubt of its having checked, if not cured, cancer of the breast, lip, and stomach in the small doses we employ.

5. It is very beneficial in indurations of glands or other soft parts caused by injuries, including in this category traumatic cataract.

6. It has a specific action on the female breast, dissipating its engorgements and tumors, and relieving its pains. Dr. Imbert-Gourbeyre cites some observations showing its homoeopathicity to the latter, though its action on the former is presumably antipathic.

7. It has hardly less influence on the ovaries, and on their homologues in the male—the testes. It is often beneficial in scanty menstruation and unready conception in the one sex, and in deficient virility in the other, resulting from passive engorgements of these organs and also in feeble but erethistic conditions of the male genitals.

8. It is of great value in a certain form of cough. Dr. Hirschel describes this as "periodical, dry, excited by itching, grating, tickling in the throat and behind the sternum; it comes in short bouts, and is especially evoked by lying down, talking and laughing." It is worse in the evening and at night.

These are the main uses of Conium among us, but every mans published experience adds to it. I may refer you to that of Dr. Baycs, who has much faith in it in hepatic and uterine derangements, with acrid secretions and to that of Teste, who thinks it a prime remedy in all chronic inflammations of parenchymatous organs. Dr. Guernsey gives as "key-notes" for it—intermission of the urine during its flow, vertigo on turning from side to side in the recumbent posture and swelling, pain, and hardness of the breasts (which at other times may be lax) at each menstrual period. This is the field which needs careful survey and fresh work. I believe that is the original experiments of Hahnemann and his disciples

were disengaged from their questionable surroundings, and
the outline filled in by some patient proving on the healthy
carried on for a length of time, we might have a valuable
pathogenesis for future applications.

In its action on the motor nervous system Conium resembles,
phenomenally at least, *Curare, Kali bromatum*, and especially
Gelsemium : in the vegetative sphere its analogues are *Iodine*,
Hydrastis, and *Baryta*.

The homœopathic uses of which I have spoken have been
obtained mainly with the medium and higher dilutions.

The medicine last on our list is

Copaiba.

Our tincture is a solution of this oleo-resin in absolute
alcohol.

A short pathogenesis of Copaiba appeared in the *Fragmenta
de viribus*, containing 12 symptoms from Hahnemann and
8 from authors. He did not again take up the medicine; and
the pathogenesis in Allen consists of these symptoms and
others observed as results of excessive medicinal doses, with
those of a proving made by Teste on himself and seven or
eight others with the 6th dilution.

The interest of Copaiba centres in its action on the urinary
mucous membrane. It is generally acknowledged that it acts
here as an irritant—the influence being strongest in the
urethra, and becoming weaker as it ascends towards the
kidney. Even on the latter, however, it acts as sometimes a
potent diuretic, sometimes a provocant of hæmaturia or
ischuria; and Bartholow says that he has reason to believe
that desquamative nephritis and fibroid kidney have resulted
from its free administration for a lengthened period. But the
urethral influence is most marked. Sometimes the irritation
travels along the seminal tracts, and the testicle swells and is
tender. Even rheumatism, according to Pereira, has been
ascribed to the use of the balsam. But without building upon
this last statement, enough has been said to show the perfect
homœopathicity of Copaiba to gonorrhœa, in the treatment of
which disease it has so high a reputation. This it enjoys in
the homœopathic school also, as you may see by reading Dr.
Yeldham's excellent treatise on *Venereal Diseases*. He professes to agree with Ricord that its local effect is indispensable
for cure to be wrought by it; but departs from this position in

recommending it also in the gonorrhœa of women, for which, and for some forms of leucorrhœa, it is of undoubted value. The truth is that Copaiba affects more or less all the mucous membranes, as well as their external continuation, the skin. An eruption—now measle-like, now urticarioid, now erythematous—often accompanies the action of the drug ; and not only is the digestive tube disordered, which might be from local action, but also the respiratory passages. Ricord has found it produce " irritation in the larynx and bronchi ; dryness also in the larynx, huskiness in the chest, and dry and painful cough, in connection with which there is expectoration of a semi-purulent, greenish, and nauseously-smelling mucus " (Phillips).

Thus the ancient repute of the drug—as well sketched by Teste—in bronchial affections is substantiated and explained. Stillé believes its value equalled by that of no other medicine in chronic bronchitis without fever. But, after all, it is as a remedy for urinary catarrhs that it must be chiefly used. I have found it specially valuable in irritation of the urethra and neck of the bladder occurring in old women. The cutaneous action of the drug has hardly been utilised among us ; but Dr. Guérin-Méneville mentions that on one occasion, when giving it to a lady in the 6th dilution for some urinary troubles, it caused the disappearance of an acne which had long and obstinately disfigured her face. Bartholow thinks that the eruption of Copaiba is only secondary to gastro-intestinal disturbance ; but Allen cites an observation of Hardy's, in which a sort of pemphigus was developed under its use, and this can scarcely be so explained. Moreover, it has been given with some advantage in the old school for psoriasis, and it is said that when it disagrees with the stomach, or purges, it does not benefit the disease,—its good effect on which is generally marked by the development of its own specific eruption on the skin. Even if Dr. Bartholow should be correct, it would only make Copaiba a better remedy for that form of urticaria which is owing to the ingestion of some offending article of diet. Dr. Dessau, an old-school physician of New York, in communicating to his colleagues some illustrations of " the value of small and frequently-repeated doses," mentions a very severe case following the eating of lobster-salad, which, after lasting three days and three nights, untouched by ordinary treatment, disappeared in twenty-four hours under the use of Copaiba. He speaks also of having had " most gratifying results " from it in chronic urticaria occurring in children. He confesses to having been led to the remedy by the principle *similia similibus*, and gives it in drop doses.*

Cannabis sativa, *Cantharis* and *Terebinthina* are the nearest analogues to Copaiba.

There seems nothing gained by raising the drug above the 1st dilution ; and in gonorrhœa Dr. Yeldham recommends from ten to twenty drops of the first decimal for a dose.

* See *New York Medical Record*, July 28, 1877.

LECTURE XXIX.

CORALLIUM, CROCUS, CROTON, CUNDURANGO, CUPRUM,
CURARE, CYCLAMEN, DIOSCOREA.

I have but a few words to say of the first name on my list
to-day—

Corallium rubrum.

It is prepared by trituration.

There is a short pathogenesis of coral, taken from the third
volume of the *Archiv*, in Allen ; it was obtained from four
persons, using the 3rd trituration. Our only therapeutic
knowledge about it is derived from Teste. " In the provings,"
he writes, " which I made with this drug on my own person,
some years ago, I elicited a few exceedingly characteristic
symptoms, which induced me to prescribe it, sometimes with
striking success, for nervous cough, asthma Millari, and
endemic whooping-cough." In his *Treatise on Diseases of
Children*, M. Teste places Corallium first among the remedies
for laryngismus stridulus and the spasmodic stage of pertussis,
and says that a patient, to whom he had given the medicine
for a chronic convulsive cough, said to him, " It is like water
thrown upon fire." I have myself once or twice given
Corallium in whooping-cough with very satisfactory results.
On February 1st, 1867, I was asked to see the daughter of the
Rev. S. E.—. In the previous November she had had a very
troublesome cough, which resisted all the treatment of the
ordinary kind directed against it. Change of air was at last
prescribed ; and immediately on arriving at Norwood the
cough ceased. She returned home at Christmas time ; but
the cough gradually reappeared, and had now assumed its
former intensity. I found her firing minute-guns of short
barking cough. This, I was told, went on all day ; and for
half-an-hour or so towards evening increased to a violent
spasmodic paroxysm. In other respects the health was fair.

She was nearly 13, and had not yet menstruated. The larynx and trachea were not tender, and the cough gave no pain. I ascertained on inquiry that she was of nervous temperament, and had more than once manifested hysterical symptoms. I gave her a drop of Corallium 30 three times a day. On the 5th I saw the patient again. The cough had steadily diminished since beginning the medicine. There had been no paroxysm for two evenings, and I heard not a single bark during my visit. By the 9th the cough had quite disappeared; and it did not return. Since this time Corallium has become quite a favourite medicine with me for hysterical and other spasmodic coughs; and I am rarely disappointed by it.

The provings in the *Archiv* developed much coryza and epistaxis, and even ulceration within the nostril. Balanitis also was set up. The last symptom has led to the recommendation of the drug in soft chancre; but I am not aware that any evidence of its efficacy has been adduced.

We have analogous medicines in *Nitric acid, Atropia, Drosera, Hyoscyamus,* and *Nux vomica.*

For dose M. Teste recommends for children the 30th potency, which led me to choose it in the case I have just related. I have since found the 12th to answer every purpose.

I come now to a medicine which Homœopathy has revived out of long neglect and disuse, the saffron,

Crocus sativus.

We prepare by percolation a tincture from the saffron of commerce.

There is a very fair proving of Crocus in Stapf's *Beiträge*. It was conducted on several persons, and with the mother-tincture. The articles of Hempel and Teste also should be consulted.

The ancient reputation of Crocus as an emmenagogue, though ignored by modern therapeutists, has been confirmed by our provings. We of course use the drug medicinally for precisely the opposite purpose, viz., to restrain *menorrhagia.* It is specially recommended where the menstrual blood is blackish and clotted, or (Dr. Guernsey says) of pitchy consistence. I have cured with Crocus many a case of menorrhagia so characterised, giving this drug during the period, and China in the intervals. In this, and indeed in other affections, the coexistence of a feeling as if something alive were moving about in the abdomen is said to be a special indication for Crocus. Its relation to such a symptom, which appears also in its pathogenesis, would make it suitable in cases of imaginary pregnancy, for which indeed Teste recommends it. Crocus has some power of affecting the brain, causing determination of blood thereto, with epistaxis (the blood having the same pitchy character as that before noted), and exciting in some persons immoderate fits of laughter. It might be useful in hysteria, or even in recent insanity, in which this symptom was prominent. I am myself most struck, in reading the pathogenesis of Crocus, with the eye-symptoms. It ought to be very useful in that form of weak vision in which the patient feels as if there were a gauze before the eyes, and tries to wink or wipe it away. It is, Drs. Allen and Norton say, asthenopia; and they have found Crocus of marked benefit in it.

The analogues of Crocus are *Belladonna*, *Platina*, *Sabina*, and (most complete of all) *Ruta*.

I have always given the 2nd dilution; and should prefer descending to ascending the scale.

Alphabetically, my next medicine would be the poison of the rattle-snake, *Crotalus*. But I think it more convenient to discuss this under the head of the serpent-poisons in general, which I propose to do when I come to the chief of them, Lachesis. I will, therefore, proceed to give you some account of the homœopathic uses of

Croton Tiglium.

The expressed oil may be triturated with milk-sugar, or dissolved in alcohol; but the officinal preparation is a tincture of the seeds.

A very full pathogenesis of Croton, taken from sixty-three different sources—a good many of which are provings, is given by Dr. Allen. It contains 815 symptoms.

Croton is another of those drugs whose use well illustrates the difference between Old Medicine and Homœopathy. It is found to have drastic and rubefacient properties. Hence, says Old Medicine, we will use it to purge and to counter-irritate whenever we think such processes likely to be beneficial. Nay, replies Homœopathy: Croton will rather be a remedy for certain forms of diarrhœa and of cutaneous inflammation, resembling those which it causes. And this we have indeed found it to be.

The purgation produced by Croton is specific, and seems not the result of inflammatory irritation, but rather of such a transudation of the watery part of the blood as is caused by Elaterium and Veratrum album, and obtains in Asiatic cholera. The accompanying symptoms in severe cases, indeed, are strikingly choleraic in character; and Croton might fairly take rank among the remedies for *choleraic diarrhœa*, for which indeed Dr. Jousset recommends it. Dr. Guernsey considers a sudden and forcible expulsion of the stool a leading indication for its choice: the liquid evacuation, he says, is poured as from a hydrant. It has not, however, been so much used in this sphere as in that of cutaneous disease. Teste was the first to call attention to the specific nature of its action on the skin,* and to recommend it as a cutaneous remedy. Later, Dr. Bähr has followed in the same track: you will find his observations translated in the sixteenth volume of the *British Journal of Homœopathy.* It is agreed that *eczema* is the special form of exanthem developed by Croton, and that the face and the external genitals are its favourite habitats. It is precisely in such eczematous rashes that both Teste and Bähr have found it curative; and I can add my mite of confirmation to their statements. The rapid and permanent manner in which Croton often relieves the itching attendant upon eczema is one of the prettiest things in medicine.

Dr. Guernsey says that Croton will remove the pain shooting through from the nipple to the shoulder of which nursing women sometimes complain.

The analogues of Croton as a drastic are *Elaterium, Veratrum,* and *Colchicum ;* as a cutaneous irritant it ranks with *Rhus, Apis,* and *Mezereum.*

The attenuations from the 3rd decimal to the 6th centesimal have been successfully used.

I have now to speak of the drug known as

Cundurango.

This a South American shrub, the bark of whose stem is used, in tincture or trituration. It has been proved by Dr. Burnett

* " Dr. Tilbury Fox states that Croton oil sometimes produces a symmetrical erythema of the face, lasting for a few days, where no direct application of the drug could have occurred " (*Ringer*, p. 281).

in this country, and Drs. Dinsmore and Dikeman in America ; so that Allen's *Encyclopædia* can give a pathogenesis of it, containing seventy-five symptoms.

Cundurango has been introduced as a remedy for *cancer*. You will find its history in various places in the volumes of the *British Journal of Homœopathy* from the thirtieth to the thirty-fourth. Dr. Clotar Müller was the first of the homœopathic school to test it. He found it powerless in scirrhous indurations ; but over malignant ulcerations, to all appearance carcinomatous, it exerted in his hands an un-doubted curative influence. The same experience is reported by Dr. Obolinski, of Cracow. Professor Friedreich, of Berlin, next followed with a case which his experienced diagnosis declared to be unquestionable cancer of the stomach, and which Cundurango cured in three months.* Dr. Fischer, from our ranks, communicates another instance of cure of what *seemed* the same disease. Lastly, Professor Nussbaum has has been able to say :†—" We have seen good results in cancer from Cundurango. Friedreich reports several perfect cures ; and I have seen good effects, though no cure, from its internal use. I applied locally only compresses moistened with a solution of sugar of lead, and still the internal use of Cundurango produced extraordinary and lasting amelio-ration."

In the view of these encouraging results, we disciples of Hahnemann naturally inquire what is the pathogenetic action of the substance. Dr. Burnett‡ made a full proving of the infusion. It congested his Schneiderian membrane, the effect extending into the frontal sinus ; caused pimples, pustules, and blotches on the skin ; and especially affected the lips, making them red, and giving rise to painful cracks in the corners of the mouth. This last trouble it caused also in two patients who were taking it for other affections ; and Dr. Burnett re-ports several cures by the drug of the same condition when occurring idiopathically, both in the mouth and at the anus. Mr. Proctor suggested to him the similarity between its effects and those of syphilis ; and it seems that it was an accidental cure of constitutional syphilis by the herb which first led to its use in Ecuador, and that it is as an anti-syphilitic that it there enjoys most repute. Dr. Dikeman§ took several five-

---

* See *North American Journ. of Hom.*, May, 1874 ; and Ziems-sen's *Cyclopædia*, vii., 252.
† See *Ibid*, August, 1875.
‡ See *Brit. Journ. of Hom.*, xxxiii., 400.
§ *New England Medical Gazette*, x., 486.

drop doses of the mother tincture, and found it act as a diuretic, causing also much cardialgia, and itching with brownish tint of the skin. Dr. Dinsmore experienced a curious derangement of the sight of the right eye, lasting some time, and appearing to depend upon congestion of the retina.

No inference seems deducible from such facts as to the relation of the drug to cancer, and its use must be, for the present, regarded as empirical only.* I can but suggest its comparison with *Hydrastis*, and mention that Friedreich gave it in tablespoonfuls of a decoction made with half an ounce of the bark to a pound of water. Dr. Müller used the 1st decimal dilution or mother tincture.

I have now to speak of a more important remedy, in the shape of

Cuprum,

by which I mean the salts of copper in general as well as the pure metal; for there seems no difference in their action, and they were used indiscriminately by Hahnemann in his provings and citations from authors. We triturate the metal, and make solutions of its salts.

A short pathogenesis of Cuprum, in the form of the sulphate, appeared in the *Fragmenta de viribus*. The acetate was then proved by Hahnemann and four others, and the results published in Stapf's *Archiv*. These and the foregoing finally appeared under the heading " Cuprum " in the third volume of the *Chronic Diseases*, with additional symptoms from Hahnemann himself, obtained doubtless from patients with the 30th potency of the triturated metal. If these last could be eliminated, we should have in the rest a very fair pathogenesis of Cuprum; the more so, as 154 of the 387 symptoms are from authors, nearly all being observations of poisoning with the various salts. A collection of cases of poisoning has been recently given us by Dr. Berridge, in the appendix to the *British Journal of Homœopathy ;* and these, with the symptoms of the *Chronic Diseases* and a few others, have been arranged by Hering in his *Materia Medica*. Dr.

* Dr. Gutteridge, in a recent summary of experience with cancer, says—" Cundurango relieves pain traceable to cancer; for example, patients sometimes complain that any movement of the thumb and fingers on the affected side gives pain, and Cundurango relieves this. I have found it of no further service " (*Annals*, viii., 172).

Allen divides his pathogenesis of the drug into three portions, headed Cuprum, C. aceticum, and C. sulphuricum respectively; but, with some inconsistency, gives to the first the symptoms recorded in the *Archiv* as produced by the acetate.

The poisonous action of copper, like that of most metals, is exerted primarily upon the alimentary canal, and secondarily, after absorption, upon the nervous centres. In these two spheres of action I propose to consider it.

I. The gastro-enteric symptoms induced by copper are those of acute inflammation, with severe colic and tympanites. That they are specific, and not local only, would appear from the sixth case of Dr. Berridge's collection, where they occurred in a lady who was in the habit of using vaginal injections from a brass syringe which proved to be coated internally with verdigris. They also appear in workers with copper. Their abdominal trouble is described by M. Blandet as " a form of enteritis of which the chief symptom is a colic, with remissions. The workman bends himself double to relieve it; the belly is tender on pressure; there is headache and inclination to vomit; diarrhœa or constipation; the vomit consists of bilious fluid; fever is present, and frequently lassitude."* The copper colic is thus different from that of lead, which is non-inflammatory.

Little or no use has been made of these effects of the metal in the school of Hahnemann; for the employment of the drug in cholera rests upon other grounds. We must go to the ordinary practice to find an instance of the homœopathic use of Cuprum here; and it at once meets us in the case of chronic diarrhœa with or without ulceration, for which the sulphate is in high repute. One of the latest writers on Materia Medica in the school, Dr. Bartholow, speaks highly of the sulphate in many acute and chronic inflammatory states of the stomach and intestines; and shows his sense of the kind of practice he is following by always advising minute doses—from $\frac{1}{12}$th to $\frac{1}{32}$nd of a grain. Dr. Wood speaks of its action as " stimulant and astringent ;" but in the face of toxicology this seems a mere evasion of the obvious inference from the facts. Vomiting and diarrhœa, to indicate Cuprum, should be spasmodic and painful.

II. The neurotic influence of copper is very decided. " The effects," writes Pereira, " produced by the long-continued use of small doses of the preparations of copper are said to be various affections of the nervous system, such as cramps and paralysis." Then he writes—" If the cupreous

* See Berridge, Obs. 37.

preparations be used in very small doses, they sometimes give relief in certain diseases, principally of the nervous system, without obviously disordering the functions ; in other words, in these instances the only apparent effect is the modification observed in the morbid condition." This is pretty good homœopathy, as far as it goes ; but we must individualise rather more closely.

1. The *cramps* mentioned by Pereira are especially characteristic of the action of Cuprum. We have seen an instance of them in its colic ; and you have only to read a few cases of poisoning by it to observe how readily they are induced elsewhere under its influence. They may be local or general, clonic or tonic ; they may be a simple trembling, or may go on to violent convulsions. Sometimes they occur in the air-tubes, as observed by Dr. Maissonneuve,* causing very intense dyspnœa with laryngeal and bronchial spasm.

Hence has arisen the first great homœopathic use of Cuprum, viz., to relieve cramp or spasm, and check convulsions. Its applications of this kind are very numerous. In cramps of the calves Dr. Jousset (giving it in the 12th dilution) has never known it to fail ; and Dr. Guernsey commends it in violent after-pains. In spasmodic affections of the respiratory organs it takes a high place. In prolonged laryngismus it may be given with great relief ;† though it is doubtful whether it can check the recurrence of the complaint in children, where deeper causes are usually at work. In whooping-cough it has been much praised by Drs. Neidhard‡ and Drummond ;§ and Bähr says that by giving it as soon as the spasmodic stage sets in he has succeeded so well that he has scarcely ever been obliged to resort to any other treatment. It is especially indicated here when the cough is so violent as almost to suffocate the patient, who remains stiff and motionless after it, or threatens to go off into convulsions. When these actually occur, Dr. Jousset esteems it highly. In pure nervous asthma Dr. Russell says‖ that there is no medicine on which we may rely more confidently to relieve the paroxysms : he says nothing, however, about checking their recurrence. Passing now to the heart, we find Dr. Bayes commending it highly in angina pectoris, and ascribing the suggestion to Dr. Holland. The experience of these practical

* See Berridge, Obs. 96.
† See *Brit. Journ. of Hom.*, xxiii., 675.
‡ *Ibid*, xii., 437.
§ *Ibid*, xxxi., 411.
‖ *Clinical Lectures.*

physicians should be borne in mind; I have more than once followed its guidance with advantage. Then we have the use of copper, common to both schools, in chorea and epilepsy. It is difficult to assign it its exact place in the treatment of either affection; but in epilepsy Dr. Bayes suggests that it is indicated by extreme violence of the convulsions. He thinks it (as also do Bähr and Jousset) one of our best medicines in this disease, and cites several cases in point. Many others are given by Dr. Baertl, in a collection of cures of epilepsy which is translated in the twenty-second volume of the *British Journal of Homœopathy*. In chorea Cuprum is very effective in giving the final steadying to the muscles, after medicines like Actæa, Agaricus, or Stramonium have quieted their excessive agitation. It has often been noted as characteristic of Cuprum in convulsive disorders that they begin with cramps in the extremities, especially in the fingers and toes. This would suggest the drug as a remedy in the " carpo-pedal spasms" of childhood—in a case of which lately seen by myself it proved speedily curative. Restlessness between the paroxysms is regarded by Dr. Guernsey as indicative of Cuprum in such affections.

It is, lastly, that feature in Asiatic cholera which has given it the name "spasmodic," which also gives Cuprum a place among its remedies. The alvine evacuations of cholera are altogether different from those produced by copper; yet the true correspondence of disease and drug was perceived by Hahnemann, and his discernment has been thoroughly warranted subsequently. In his original directions for the treatment of cholera* he put forth Cuprum as the specific remedy for the " second stage of clonic spasmodic character" if—as too often happened—Camphor failed to relieve. He stated that it was to be preferred even to Veratrum here; and recommended it also as a prophylactic. There is now abundant evidence of its efficacy in this last capacity, both among the workers in the metal and in those who have worn a plate of it next the body during the prevalence of the epidemic. Drs. Russell and Drysdale both had occasion to speak well of it in the epidemic of 1849 in this country,—the former commending it for the cramps, the latter also for the vomiting. In 1866 Mr. Proctor, who treated a number of fully developed cases with great success (he lost 14 only out of 98), writes†—" For the cramps it was unquestionably the best remedy, and I may say for the vomiting also. In the stage of collapse I

---

* *Lesser Writings*, p. 847.
† *Brit. Journ.*, xxv., 94.

gradually found myself trusting mainly to Cuprum, and the impression is very strong on my mind that in collapse it is the most reliable of our remedies. It appears to go deeper into the organism and to fasten upon the disease with a firmer and more tenacious grip. Certainly it accomplishes much by keeping the stomach quiet, and thus enabling us to introduce and retain what other medicine, or stimulant, or nourishment, we may desire."

2. The paralysis of Cuprum resembles that of Plumbum more closely than does its colic. It is one affecting the hands alone, or at most the arms. Here is a description of it in a copper-worker :—" Right forearm in constant pronation, hand bent at right angle to arm, thumbs drawn into palm, fingers flexed ; motion of elbow remains good, but in the hand, and especially in the joints of the fingers, extension is impossible, and flexion only partial ; upper extremities much emaciated, right more than the left ; right hand nothing but skin and bone." At one time I should have been unable to point to any application of such facts ; but if you will compare this picture with that given by Dr. Hammond in his *Diseases of the Nervous System* of " amyotrophic lateral spinal sclerosis," I think you will be struck with the coincidence. Cuprum may well have the same relation to " amyotrophy "—that is, the same morbid influence on the trophic centres—as Plumbum : the great emaciation so often noted in chronic poisoning by it involving the muscles.

3. A more important part of the neurotic action of Cuprum is its powerful influence upon the brain. Almost every form of cerebral disorder has been induced by its poisonous action ; at the same time autopsy shows no sign of organic mischief. The inferences deducible herefrom were well drawn out and set forth by Dr. George Schmid, of Vienna : you will find his paper on the subject translated in the first volume of the *British Journal of Homœopathy*. He was led especially to recommend the use of copper—in the form of the acetate—in the cerebral symptoms which result from the retrocession of any of the acute exanthemata, or from difficult dentition in children, when the condition is scarcely active enough to require Belladonna. These suggestions have been confirmed by the experience of most homœopathists ; and the use of Cuprum in such conditions may be considered established. Its last illustrator is Dr. Drummond, of Manchester, who in a paper published in the thirty-first volume of the *British Journal* relates cases of retrocession of eczema, measles, and scarlatina in which Cuprum aceticum was employed with most grati-

fying results. He speaks, also, of great benefit from its use in cerebro-spinal meningitis ; and in some recent experiments on animals related in the thirty-second volume of the same journal great hyperæmia of the meninges of brain and spine was noted.

The experiments just mentioned were made in view of an extensive proving of copper and its salts, lately set on foot by the Central Homœopathic Society of Germany, which promises greatly to enlarge our knowledge of the action of the drug. In two rabbits to whom the drug was administered by subcutaneous injection the urine became scanty and albuminous, and the kidneys were found after death with their tubes full of shed and degenerated ephithelium. The left ventricle of the heart was much hypertrophied and the liver granular. This is very suggestive, and connects Cuprum with Arsenic. It has been found of service in the uræmic cramps and convulsions of granular degeneration of the kidneys. Further indications for its use may be derived from the experience of the school of Rademacher, with whom it is one of the great systemic remedies. Dr. Heinigke states that Rademacher considered it indicated when there was premature exhaustion of strength in illness ; and that it rapidly showed when it was doing good by the sense of being better which the patient experienced. Another sign of the same meaning was that the urine became clearer and more plentiful when it was otherwise. A long series of cases of diseases benefited by it, related by Dr. Kissel, a prominent member of the school, is translated in the eighteenth volume of the *British Journal*. I should add that the jaundice which so often appears in copper-poisoning has not yet been accounted for or utilised in practice ; and that its effect on the skin deserves further notice. Patches of " lepra " have been observed as a result of the continued ingestion both of the acetate and of the metal ; so that the drug may prove curative in the squamous forms of cutaneous disease. Hahnemann recommends it in old ulcerations.

The chief analogues of Cuprum are its fellow-metals, *Arsenicum* and *Plumbum*. It has points of resemblance, moreover, to *Nux vomica* and *Secale*.

The higher potencies of metallic copper, the lowest of the acetate, have been most frequently given with success.

My next medicine is one of almost purely physiological interest, but which homœopathy has lately begun to employ in practice. It is the Indian arrow-poison, variously called wourali, woorara, or (as we have it)

Curare.

It is prepared for our use by solution in alcohol.

Our knowledge of the poisonous action of Curare is well put together by Dr. Carfrae in the fourth volume of the *Annals*. Cases illustrating its curative power have been given us by Mr. Freeman in the ninth volume of the *Monthly Homœopathic Review*.

The poisonous effects of Curare are very well ascertained. It seems to act purely and simply upon the motor portion of the nervous system, paralysing it, and doing so from the periphery towards the centre. It has very naturally been tried in tetanus ; but without success. If, however, the cure of hydrophobia recently obtained by it be repeated in subsequent trials, its antipathic action will have achieved a real triumph. We on the other hand have as naturally endeavoured to put it to use in the treatment of paralysis. Mr. Freeman's observations are the only records of its use which we have at present. He specifies his cases as—1. Paralysis of the parts supplied by the motor cranial nerves, pains being absent. 2. Lateral paralysis after apoplexy. 3. Paralysis from mechanical injury. 4. The class of cases known as nervous debility. 5. The debility of aged persons. 6. Debility after exhausting illness. Of the two cases cited under the first heading, one is briefly described as " general motor paralysis," and the action of the drug is dubious. The other seems an instance of temporary loss of motor power from repeated attacks of " apoplectiform congestion," which, according to Trousseau, is epilepsy. There was double facial and right lateral paralysis ; swallowing and articulation also were affected. Curare immediately restored the power of swallowing : and the other symptoms steadily subsided, whether *post* or *propter hoc* I cannot say. The cases of the second and third sections do not impress me with the power of the drug. Far more satisfactory is its action in the semiparalysis called nervous debility, and in that which results from over-suckling, or from exhausting illnesses. On the whole, it is in these last-named conditions that we may expect most benefit from Curare, as its action reaches only to functional changes.

I would add that Claude Bernard states that, Curare paralyses the vaso-motor as well as the musculo-motor nerves. The fact may bear fruit one day in our therapeutics.

A paper on Curare was presented to the World's Convention at Philadelphia, by Dr. Pitet, of Paris, containing some additional observations upon its therapeutic powers. It has not yet been printed ; but from my recollection of it I may state that he reported it of striking service in relieving some forms of paralytic dyspnœa. I hope that by the time I next lecture on the drug the Transactions of the Convention, containing this paper, will have been published.*

The dilutions from 3 to 12 were used in Mr. Freeman's cases.

Causticum, Conium and *Physostigma* are analogues of Curare ; and also *Gelsemium.*

The next medicine on my list is the common sowbread,

Cyclamen Europæum.

The tincture is prepared from the fresh root.

The original proving is in the fifth volume of the *Reine Arzneimittellehre,* where there are 5 symptoms from Hahnemann himself, and 197 from four fellow-observers. The medicine has since been re-proved in Germany, in the mother-tincture and lowest dilutions,—30 persons taking part in the experiments. You may read their results—originally published in the *Zeitschrift* of the Austrian Society—in Allen's *Encyclopædia,* where 753 symptoms are recorded.

Cyclamen was in ancient repute as an emmenagogue, and was accounted so potent an abortifacient that Gerarde, in his *Herball,* cautions pregnant women against walking over it in gardens. Our provings give evidence of the former property, and show the menstrual flow induced to be black, clotted, and even membranous, with violent labour-pains. Its most remarkable action otherwise is on the head and eyes, where it causes headache, with great dizziness, and flickering or obscuration of sight. Some remarks upon its sphere of influence, and cases illustrating its therapeutic virtues, by Dr. Eidherr, of Vienna, may be read in the tenth volume of the *North American Journal of Homœopathy.* He relates several instances in which such symptoms of the head and eyes co-existed with menstrual derangements, and in which Cyclamen proved a most valuable remedy. Dr. Dunham, moreover, mentions

* Still, alas ! (Feb., 1880) unpublished.

that these phenomena had led him to its use in similar cases before the Austrian provings had shown its action on the female sexual system ; and Dr. Merryman relates a good case of climacteric vertigo and mental confusion cured by it.*

I think, however, that the use of Cyclamen should not be confined to such purely sympathetic derangements of the head and eyes. I should suggest its trial in that form of migraine which begins with flickering before the eye of the side affected ; and Drs. Allen and Norton consider it as ranking among our most important remedial agents for convergent strabismus.

The resemblance to *Pulsatilla* is most obvious ; also to *Ruta* and *Crocus*.

In Dr. Eidherr's cases the 15th decimal attenuation was that employed.

My next medicine in regular course would be Digitalis ; but as I cannot begin this important remedy just as the hour is up, I will occupy our remaining time to-day with its nearest successor in alphabetical order. This is the wild yam root—

Dioscorea villosa.

A tincture (triturations would be better) is prepared from the root; but the special virtues of the drug appear to reside in the resinoid, Dioscorein, triturations of which are accordingly in most frequent use.

Our knowledge of this drug, first derived from Dr. Hale's *New Remedies*, has been greatly increased by Dr. Cushing, of Lynn, U.S., who has published a monograph upon it. To the four provings supplied by the former writer he has added some extensive experimentation on his own person, both with substantial and with attenuated doses.

Dioscorea is a medicine for one disease—a form of colic. This has hitherto been described—by the American " Eclectics," to whom we owe the drug—as " bilious," meaning thereby not the passage of gall-stones, but abdominal pain accompanied by vomiting of bile. Subsequent experience has shown that this last symptom is non-essential ; and also that the drug is homœopathic to the malady, and cures excellently well in the small doses we affect. Those who have proved it concur in reporting severe pain about the umbilical region as the most marked of their symptoms : it is from this

* *United States Medical Investigator*, iv., 576.

point that the colic demanding the medicine starts.   Dr. Helmuth, from clinical experience, considers that the colic requiring Dioscorea is more continuous than that to which Colocynth is suited : it is also described as "a constant pain, aggravated at regular intervals by paroxysms of intense suffering."   One of the best descriptions we have of its sphere of action is that given by Mr. Clifton.*   It is in "flatulent spasms," whether affecting the stomach or bowels, that he finds it especially useful.   There is frequent expulsion of wind, but little relief therefrom.   While the patient has a tendency to bend double, and feels as if pressure would relieve him, as a matter of fact it rather aggravates, and most solace is obtained by stretching the body out."   In these circumstances of amelioration and aggravation the drug is most distinguished from Colocynth.

From one to three grains of the first trituration of Dioscorein form the usual dose, but Mr. Clifton gives drop doses of the mother tincture of the root.

* See *Monthly Hom. Review*, xxi., 473.

LECTURE XXX.

DIGITALIS, DROSERA.

We begin to-day with a medicine of great interest and importance, the purple foxglove,

Digitalis.

The tincture of the British Homœopathic Pharmacopœia is made from the leaves. This is of consequence, as they are the only part of the plant which contains digitaline, and alcohol dissolves it freely.

Digitalis was proved by Hahnemann, with the expressed juice of the leaves, for the *Fragmenta de viribus*, where its pathogenesis contains 23 symptoms from himself, and 33 from ten authors. In the fourth volume of the *Materia Medica Pura* his own symptoms have increased to 73, and there are 224 from ten fellow-provers ; while he has gone to thirty-seven authors, and obtained from them 131 observations. These were mostly made upon patients taking the drug, but are not often vitiated on that account. The *Chronic Diseases* (in its latest form) gives us another pathogenesis, containing 702 symptoms. The additional 300 are furnished by three new observers, and by the experiments of Jörg and eight of his pupils, who proved the drug in small doses—one to three grains—of the powdered leaves. I should say that in the *Materia Medica Pura* Hahnemann directs the seeds to be used, in the *Chronic Diseases* the whole plant. The essay by Dr. Bähr, which obtained the prize of the Central Homœopathic Society of Germany in 1858,* adds several experiments of his own, and the drug has also been proved by Lembke,—both these latter observers using digitaline as well as the mother plant. The result of all these provings, with copious records of the effects of poisonings and over-dosings, is given us by Dr. Allen in his *Encyclopædia*.

* *Digitalis purpurea*. Leipzig, 1859.

Upon the facts as known in the time of each have been based two studies of the drug, one by Dr. Black in the fourth (1846), and another by Dr. Madden and myself in the twenty-first volume (1863) of the *British Journal of Homœopathy*. But even since the later date the literature of the medicine has immensely increased. It has been largely experimented with on animals both at home and abroad, and its effects and *modus operandi* have excited continual discussion. Its therapeutic applications, moreover, first made to scrofula, and then to phthisis, have received a wide extension in the sphere of cardiac disease and other disorders of the circulation. It therefore fills a large space in the treatises of Wood, Ringer, and Phillips, and has been made the subject of special monographs by Brunton,* Reith,† and Fothergill.‡ To the conclusions arrived at in our study of the drug I still in the main adhere ; but the whole subject needs fresh exposition as it has received renewed consideration.

I would first call your attention to the emetic effects of Digitalis. The drug is not used medicinally to excite vomiting, as its other workings are undesirable. But its emetic properties are undoubted, active, and specific. It sets up the condition of nausea—with its depression, salivation, sweating, and other phenomena—as powerfully as does Antimony ; and its vomiting is severe, and, when once excited, often lasts for days. When once excited, I say ; for it frequently does not come on for many hours after the ingestion of the drug.

We have already studied the nausea and emesis produced by drug-action when speaking of Tartar emetic. We have seen that it is brought about by an influence on the nervous centres at the base of the brain and in the medulla oblongata. We have also seen in the case of that drug a power to retard to a large extent the action of the heart and lungs, and have found such power explicable by a similar central impression, in this case transmitted by the pneumogastrics. Now the effect of Digitalis which most struck the older observers was its slow pulse. They found the rate reduced from its norm or higher to about 40, as Hahnemann shows by numerous citations. To the same effect is the testimony of all recent observation and experiment. Some indeed speak of a primary acceleration, and many more of the same thing occurring secondarily ; but nearly all agree that retardation is the characteristic and long-lasting effect of the drug. Analogy

* On *Digitalis*. Lond., 1868.
† On the actions and uses of Digitalis, *Edinb. Med. Journ.*, 1868.
‡ *Digitalis : its mode of action, and its use.* Lond., 1871.

would suggest that with Digitalis, as with Tartar emetic, the slow pulse is an effect of stimulation of the vagi ; and the balance of experiment is decidedly in favour of the hypothesis. The primary acceleration, noticed by several as an effect of small doses, is readily thus accounted for, as a very weak galvanic stimulation of the pneumogastrics is found to quicken the heart's action. It may be, however, a result of the un-opposed influence of the ganglionic excitation of which I shall presently speak. In the former case the pulse would be weaker, in the latter stronger ; and both characters have been noticed in it by different experimenters.

But now another fact encounters us. The retarded heart-beat of excitation of the vagi is always accompanied by diminution of arterial pressure, whereas this last is notably increased under the influence of Digitalis. We have thus to suppose a similar action exerted by it upon the arteries them-selves, through the medium of the vaso-motor nerves. Such an action is acknowledged by all observers ; and, with hardly an exception, is affirmed to be central rather than peripheral. That is, it is effected by an influence exerted by the drug on that uppermost vaso-motor centre which physiological research has discovered at the base of the brain, hard by the corpora quadrigemina.* By this influence the whole arterial system is thrown into a state of tension ; the vessels themselves are contracted ; and the heart is stimulated to beat forcibly, and would beat fast if the inhibitory power of the vagi would permit. Thus it comes about that the slow pulse of Digitalis is often a strong one.

These are the primary phenomena of the action of Digi-talis. It is seen to have just such a limited neurotic influ-ence as that which belongs to Tartar emetic (and also to Lobelia and Tabacum) ; an influence upon the group of centres at the base of the brain which preside over nausea and vomiting and control the circulation. It may either excite the first of these alone ; or, if this be avoided, it stimulates the whole nervous system—inhibitory and motor—of the circula-tion, holding heart and arteries in a firm grip. This increase of tension by excitation of the vaso-motor centre is peculiar to it among its cognate drugs.

But it is admitted by all observers that, after a time when moderate doses, at once if large doses are given, an opposite condition manifests itself. The pulse quickens, and becomes

* An interesting account of the process by which this centre has been discovered is given by Dr. Moreau in the *Revue Homœopathique Belge* for January and February, 1875.

weak, irregular, and intermittent; the arterial pressure, as measured by the hæmadynamometer, falls. The heart's action is still for a time forcible, but it is tumultuous. The general symptoms are those of depressed circulation, with lowered temperature : there is syncope, and—if the dose be large enough—death. It is the custom to speak of such phenomena as those of reaction, from exhaustion of the over-stimulated nerves. But I think that it is impossible to explain them all upon such an hypothesis. No nervous exhaustion can stop the heart's action, as long as the organ itself is healthy ; and after death thus induced the ventricles are found contracted and not dilated. These are insurmountable difficulties in the way of adopting it. Some recoil there doubtless is after over-stimulation ; but not to such an extent as that seen in the collapse of Digitalis-poisoning. I believe that we must look for an explanation of this to an action of the drug upon the heart itself. That it has such an action seems proved by the researches of Claude Bernard, which have been strangely lost sight of in the recent discussions about Digitalis. It is, according to him,* one of the poisons which act directly upon the muscular tissue, paralysing and killing it. It affects that portion of muscular tissue which constitutes the heart earlier than any other, so that in cold-blooded animals like frogs the heart's action may cease four hours before general death ensues : there is (as has been said) a dead heart in a living body. Rigor mortis sets in exceedingly early; and on opening the thorax immediately after death the heart is found contracted, rigid, motionless, and totally empty. A further examination discloses remarkable chemical and electrical changes in the heart and other muscles. The muscular juice is acid instead of alkaline; and the external surface is electrically negative to the cut surface, instead of (as normally) positive.

I am glad to find these views, in maintaining which, as I have done since 1863, I imagined I stood alone, supported by Dr. Stillé. "It is evident," he says, "that the increased power of the heart under the influence of Digitalis is not identical with that which it acquires from the use of diffusible stimuli or hæmatic tonics, but, on the other hand, may co-exist with an impaired muscular energy." By them, as it seems to me—and recent experimentation is in accordance with them—all the phenomena before us are elucidated. While Digitalis stimulates the nervous supply of

* See *Med. Times and Gazette*, Sept. 29, 1860. Dybkowsky and Pelikan have been led (according to Stillé) to the same conclusion.

the circulation, it kills its muscular apparatus. The latter action is slower than the former, and is for a time masked by it. But that, while pneumogastrics and sympathetic are acting upon the heart, slowing and at the same time urging its beat it is nevertheless losing its inherent vigour, is shown by a remarkable fact. It is often noted by the older observers that though the pulse under the influence of the drug was slow while the patient retained the recumbent posture, it became enormously quickened—often to double its rate and more— when he stood up. This could only be from enfeeblement of the muscular walls of the heart, which endeavoured by increased rapidity of action to answer the additional call made upon it. Thus rightly was the fact explained.* The same account must, I think, be given of the irregularity of pulse so characteristic of the drug's action. The rhythm of the heart's alternate contractions and expansions is a property of its tissue. It cannot be altered by any modification of its nervous supply : it fails only as the muscular substance itself loses its integrity. As Dr. Fothergill says,—" Irregularity of rhythm is not due to disordered innervation, but to obvious debility." Lastly, the symptoms and post-mortem appearances which show the heart dying in systole instead of diastole, which are thought to prove the drug a cardiac stimulant to the last receive their explanation. The heart poisoned by Digitalis is contracted and not dilated ; but the contraction is the *rigor mortis*. The immediate cause of this phenomenon has been shown to be the change of the muscular juice from alkaline to acid ; and this very change is involved in the destructive action of the drug upon the integrity of the muscular tissue.

It will be well, while these facts are before us, to speak of the therapeutic virtues of Digitalis in the sphere of the circulation. Its power of slowing the heart's action was early made use of in the treatment of phthisis, where rapidity of circulation is so obvious and exhausting ; and subsequently by the Rasorists in Italy, and again of late years in Germany, it has been largely employed in the treatment of fevers and inflammations. In the former it certainly retarded the pulse, but rarely checked the progress of the disease : in the latter it effectually reduces the temperature, but does nothing to abate—if it does not actually increase—the mortality. It is

* Of the same character is that which von Boeck (Ziemssen's *Cyclo - pædia*, xvii., 710) remarks, that even in the stage of recovery from the effects of the poison, very slight causes suffice to bring on cardiac paralysis.

abandoned in phthisis; and will inevitably share the same
fate in fever. Such primary actions of drugs are rarely available for true curative purposes. The only really valuable
application of this property of Digitalis seems to be in cases
where the orifices of the heart are narrowed, and the frequency
of its contractions prevents it from returning to a functionally
normal state, and keeps up the disturbance of the circulation.
It was in this cardiac condition that Digitalis was most frequently used of old; and the physicians of the first half of
the present century speak in high terms of the benefit obtained by the temporary retardation of the heart's action
induced by the drug.

But it had early been noted by several—and notably by
Pereira and Sir Henry Holland—that, though it seemed
strange, a weak heart would grow strong and an intermittent
pulse become regular under the action of the foxglove. Such
experiences accumulated; and, when physiological experiments
began to be made, it was thought that the facts were well
accounted for, and that Digitalis was after all a stimulant and
not a depressant of the heart. A rush was made in the opposite direction, and Dr. Handfield Jones gave utterance to the
general impression when he proclaimed the drug " our cardiac
tonic κὰτ' ἐξοχήν, specially to be resorted to in cases of
asthenia and peril from failing circulation." That such
effects can be produced by utilising the sympathetic channel
of the neurotic stimulation induced by Digitalis is, I think,
undoubted It is surely this which is brought into play
in such cases of collapse as that recorded by Dr. Fothergill.
The patient—after a labour with twins—was apparently *in
articulo mortis :* the limbs were cold, the body in a state of
deathly clammy sweat, the face livid, no pulse could be felt at
the wrists, and a mere fluttering was heard when the ear was
placed over the region of the heart. Brandy and ether had
been given without any good effect; and, as dissolution was
every moment expected, it was decided to try Digitalis.
Half-a-drachm of the tincture was given every hour; after
four doses reaction set in, and after three more recovery was
complete. Digitalis acts here on the hollow muscle of the
heart as it does on that of the uterus, stimulating it to contract ; and through the same ganglionic nerves. By a similar
process mainly it is, as I shall argue presently, that it promotes
the action of the kidneys and drains the water-logged tissues
in cardiac dropsy. But, if Digitalis acts upon the heart only
through its nerves, it is difficult to see how it can exercise
more than a temporary stimulant influence upon it. A drug

can surely give strength to a tissue only by acting directly upon the tissue itself, or upon the blood which nourishes it. The theory is seen by many to be fallacious; and Brunton gives warning that a fragile heart may easily rupture under stimulation, while Reith asserts that sudden death is no uncommon result of the practice, accounting for this by the anæmia of the organ caused by the contraction of the coronary arterioles. Ringer finally argues that the "tonic" theory fails to explain the benefit wrought by the drug in cardiac disease, and asserts that in simple debility of the heart it is useless and even hurtful.

While these variations have been going on in the ranks of the old school, Homœopathy has been pursuing with Digitalis, as with other medicines, the even tenor of her way. I know not how it has been with my colleagues, as there has been little published on the subject: but for myself Digitalis has always been a valued remedy in weakness of the heart. I have regarded it as a cardiac tonic in disease because it is a cardiac debilitant in health; and have used it accordingly. Simple enfeeblement of the muscular walls of the heart has seemed to me a very common condition. Vertigo, tendency to syncope, breathlessness on exertion, and palpitation—some or all of these are its symptoms; and it finds in Digitalis a potent and rarely failing remedy.* Again, the slow pulse of the drug, seized upon by Hahnemann's penetration as the characteristic feature of its action, has often led to its successful use in cases where it was present.

The use of Digitalis in organic disease of the heart is a larger subject. The old view of its operation led to its being given in hypertrophy and over-action of the organ: now it is prescribed for dilatation and debility—and in both one and the other with good effects. From what I have said you will infer that I regard the benefit wrought in the former class of cases to be due to its primary action in slowing the heart through the vagi; while in the second class there may be a combination of primary sympathetic stimulation, which would account for any speedy results manifested, and homœopathic strengthening of the enfeebled muscular tissue. Upon these principles I should judge the virtues now ascribed to it as a remedy. Dr. Ringer has furnished a most elaborate and practical survey of all the facts; and comes to the conclusion

* The hypothesis of direct action upon the substance of the heart thus implied is supported by what Trousseau and Pidoux note, that Digitalis is less useful in functional (that is, nervous) than in organic disease of the organ.

that Digitalis is useful in proportion as the symptoms depend upon irregularity of the heart's action. As such irregularity prevails throughout the action of the drug, Digitalis would seem homœopathic to it whenever present. So also as regards the conditions which Dr. Phillips postulates for it, viz., a general venous hyperæmia—Dr. Ringer meaning the same thing when he says that it is in heart disease with lividity and jugular fulness, not in that with waxy pallor, that it is available. Here again the *modus operandi* of the drug, and therefore the manner of its administration, must depend upon whether we have only enfeebled or also obstructed circulation to deal with.

This brings us to the action of fox-glove in cardiac dropsy. It is confessedly by no direct diuretic operation that it benefits here, as its effects of this kind under other circumstances are very uncertain. It only certainly increases the flow of urine when dropsy is present, and that from imperfect action of the heart. By removing the weakness or irregularity of the organ on which the œdema of the limbs depends it allows of the re-absorption of the effused serum into the relieved veins ; and then the kidneys take on the work of pouring the fluid out from the body. This is Dr. Ringer's explanation ; and it seems to me in perfect accordance with the observed facts,—especially in these points, that Digitalis is most effective in dropsies occurring in relaxed and debilitated subjects, and that its diuresis coincides with increase of arterial tension. " The same kidneys," writes Bartels, " which for months had secreted small quantities of dark albuminous urine of high specific gravity, as long as the tension in the general arterial system remained far below normal, and the cyanotic colour of the patient demonstrated the serious over-repletion of his veins, secrete ample quantities of urine free from albumen, clear, and of normal specific gravity, so soon as, in consequence of some spontaneous process of cure, or by interposition of medical skill, the distribution of the blood is once more equalised, the natural blood-pressure being restored to the arterial system, and the abnormal increase of tension in the veins being subdued."

But here once more we have to consider what is the cause of the deficient arterial tension,—whether it is due simply to enfeeblement of the cardiac muscle, or to embarrassment of its (otherwise normal) action through alteration of the valves. In the former case Digitalis would be truly homœopathic ; and, given in our usual doses, may prove permanently curative. But the evidence goes to show that the latter alternative more frequently obtains; and here we can only increase the lacking tension by stimulating the vaso-motor nerves, which act directly upon the arteries as well as on the heart itself. We can do this with Digitalis, but it must be by inducing its primary physiological action, for which purpose larger doses are required.*

I have dwelt thus fully upon the principal sphere of the action of the drug, as it was necessary to clear it from misapprehensions, and to ascertain the exact *modus operandi* of the benefit it affords. Beyond this sphere Digitalis is hardly used in ordinary practice. Its occasional success in hæmorrhages seems to belong to it, as it is supposed to check them by contracting the arterioles, as Secale does. But pathogenetic experiment reveals a much wider range of influence on the part of the drug; and homœopathic therapeutics have done much to utilise the same for the benefit of suffering humanity. I will try to indicate the salient points.

1. The influence of Digitalis upon the *brain* is evidenced by various cerebral symptoms, and by consentaneous subjective disorders of the sight and hearing. Headache, chiefly frontal, heavy and throbbing in character, has often been observed: the drug, when pushed in experiment, has threatened to set up meningitis, and in poisoning by it delirium and mania are not uncommonly observed. There is buzzing in the ears; and the sight is affected in a remarkable manner. The colouring of objects is altered; they appear blue, yellow, or green, or all faces seem of a corpse-like whiteness. Motes float before the sight, which on covering and pressing the eyes appear as sparks; then flashes and balls of fire are seen, and objects appear brilliant, with a fiery halo round them. Last, amaurosis sets in; which has been known to last for a month after omitting the drug. With these disorders of vision there is at first pressure in the eyeballs; later, throbbing pain and sense of fulness and enlargement.

The clue to all these phenomena (which remind one of those of quinine) seems afforded by the highly injected state of the cerebral meninges which was found in the only post-mortem examination of Digitalis-poisoning Christison was able to discover. The visual symptoms, like those of Santonine, suggest congestion of the retina and incipient glaucoma. For these the drug has not been, to my knowledge, used therapeutically; but Hahnemann says that "hardness of hearing, with hissing as of boiling water, has been frequently cured by

* Dr. Kidd, in his *Laws of Therapeutics,* has some very instructive cases illustrating this practice.

Digitalis, when the other symptoms corresponded likewise to that drug." The head-symptoms have led to its use in acute hydrocephalus, for which it already comes to us with high repute, Pereira accounting it "a most valuable agent in the arachnitis of children." He, and Bähr with him, thinks this a part of a general specific influence it exerts upon inflammation of serous membranes : the latter considers it applicable not only to the serous pleurisy for which Wurmb and Fleischmann commend it, but to all forms of the disease, and extols its virtues in pericarditis with much serous effusion. As regards hydrocephalus, there are two instances of its successful use in the seventh and twelfth volumes of the *British Journal of Homœopathy*, which are encouraging to further trial of the drug in this fatal disease.

2. Of the mucous membranes, the stomach and descending colon are specifically inflamed by Digitalis. It causes ash-coloured stools ; but not, I think, from any influence on the liver. Dr. Inman has shown that the fæces do not become brown until they reach the colon, and that the green stools of infants assume their peculiar colour at this point also. It would appear, therefore, that the secretion from the follicles of the colon has an important influence on the colour of the fæces ; and through these I conceive that Digitalis whitens the stools, for it causes no other element of jaundice or sign of hepatic disorder. Now it is no uncommon thing to be consulted about children whose liver is said to be locked up, because they are passing white chalky stools. There is no jaundice ; and I do not believe that the liver is here in fault at all, but that the secretion of the colon is deranged. Digitalis is a capital remedy for this condition, as pointed out by Drs. Chapman and Black.* I must tell you, however, that true jaundice is said to have been occasionally cured by it.

3. Although in cardiac dropsy Digitalis is only secondarily diuretic, yet I must agree with Dr. Brunton that it has a direct irritant action on the kidneys. In Jörg's provers, and in Bähr, decided diuresis was set up, and in acute poisoning by the drug suppression is often present. It diminishes the urinary solids, and this not merely relatively but absolutely. It is thus decidedly homœopathic to the granular degeneration of the kidneys in which Christison praises it so highly. Dr. Clifford Allbutt writes accordingly :—" In granular kidney the one drug which of all others seems least appropriate, but which is, on the other hand, most beneficial, both temporarily

* *Brit. Journ. of Hom.*, iv., 279.

and permanently, is Digitalis." He is thinking especially of the high arterial tension common to drug and disease. Dr. Dickinson esteems it the best medicine in the acute Bright's disease which follows scarlatina.

4. Considerable influence is exerted by Digitalis on the male sexual organs. In Jörg's provings these were uniformly excited,—one prover having to leave off after three days on account of the extent to which the irritation proceeded. Bähr found similar effects. The fact that other observers have found it to exert an anti-aphrodisiac effect must not be allowed to prejudice these undoubted facts. It is possible that the large doses taken by them exerted the contracting influence of the drug upon the arteries, and thus rendered erectile processes and the venereal *nisus* impossible, while smaller quantities may excite the nervous centres of the function. It is certain that it is not only from the old school, and in the mode of administration recognised there, that we hear of the medicine being given to diminish venereal excitement, and in spermatorrhœa. Dr. Bähr has the highest opinion of its value in the last-named malady, and in nocturnal emissions. He gives here a grain of the third decimal trituration of digitaline every second morning, saying that if taken at night it is liable to disturb the sleep. I have often confirmed this experience.

These are the main points of the action of Digitalis. If you would enlarge them, I would refer you to Teste's article on the drug—who says, by the way, that *sadness* is a characteristic feature of its action, both in men and animals; and to Dr. Bähr's excellent treatise, most of the recommendations of which he has reproduced in his no less excellent *Science of Therapeutics.*

Digitalis finds a good many parallel medicines in its many-sided action. As a myotic, its only fellows are *Arnica, Arsenic,* and *Physostigma ;* myalgia, cramp, and fibrillary contraction being to these drugs respectively what paralysis is to Digitalis. In its influence on the pneumogastrics Digitalis resembles *Tartar emetic, Lobelia,* and *Tabacum ;* as a renal poison its analogues are *Colchicum* and *Scilla.* In its action on the heart it stands quite alone—*Arsenic* and *Kalmia* only approaching it at all in character.

The question of dose as regards Digitalis has some interesting points about it. It seems strange that a drug so perfectly and primarily homœopathic to weakness of the heart should not aggravate rather than improve this condition in the full doses prescribed in the old school. Yet they seem to obtain none but beneficial results from doses of the tincture varying from 5 to 15 minims. Lately, a still more surprising administration of the drug has taken place. The tincture has been given in *half-ounce* doses, several times repeated, as a remedy for delirium tremens, and does not seem to have done any harm. Any attempt, however, to give the same quantity of the infusion will bring on distressing and some-times alarming symptoms,—while yet the tincture is eight times stronger. It is a fair inference from these facts, that the presence of alcohol—as in the tincture—directly opposes the action of the drug : which in its turn may be antidotal to alcohol, and perhaps in this way be beneficial in delirium tremens. If, then, the tincture be used for homœopathic purposes, the counteracting influence of the alcohol must be borne in mind, and the lowest potencies selected. I have never seen any benefit from the dilutions above the 1st centesimal, and generally use the 1st decimal or mother-tincture ; which also seems to be the general practice.

A word in conclusion about

Digitaline, which appears to possess at least the cardiac and renal influence of the mother-drug. It has occasionally been used in heart disease with dropsy instead of Digitalis, as in a case recorded in the seventh volume of the *North American Journal of Homœopathy.* Dr. Meyhoffer highly esteems it here. It would be a suitable form of the drug when given to check its characteristic vomiting. Digitaline may be triturated, or dissolved in alcohol of 90° ; or it may be given in the granules of Homolle and Quevenne, each of which contains a milligramme, *i.e.*, about the sixty-fifth of a grain. These have to be used cautiously, however, if the assertion of their designers is correct, that digitaline is a hundred times as strong as the powdered leaf of the plant.

Dr. Allen gives a separate and very full pathogenesis of this alkaloid, and a single experiment with "digitoxine," which seems more potent still.

We will occupy the remainder of our time with the sun-dew,

Drosera.

The tincture of homœopathic practice—in which alone Drosera is used—is prepared from the entire fresh plant.
The pathogenesis appears in the sixth volume of the *Rein*

Arzneimittellehre, containing 132 symptoms from Hahnemann himself, 152 from three fellow-observers, and 3 from authors.

The most significant fact in this pathogenesis is the spasmodic cough induced by the drug. Hahnemann's wonted sagacity led him to perceive this ; and he recommended the medicine accordingly in *pertussis.* If after-experience has not quite verified his statement that a single dose of Drosera 30 will cure whooping-cough in a week,* it has nevertheless sustained the drug in the first rank of remedies for the disease. The common experience is that of Dr. Bayes, that repeated doses of the first or first decimal dilution will bring most uncomplicated cases of whooping-cough to an end within two, three, or four weeks, greatly mitigating the severity of the paroxsyms meanwhile. I myself prefer Aconite and Ipecacuanha in the catarrhal stage ; but quite agree in the praise given to Drosera when the cough has become spasmodic.

The virtues of Drosera in whooping-cough have formed one of the recent discoveries (save the mark !) of the old school. At a meeting of the Société Thérapeutique of Paris, on April 10, 1878, Dr. Lamarc reported his favourable experience with the remedy, and several other members present corroborated him. As with all thefts (I must call them so, as long as the borrowing is unacknowledged) from homœopathy, the small dose goes with the similar remedy : the tincture is administered " goutte par goutte " †.

It is of course not essential that a spasmodic cough should be true pertussis for Drosera to cure it : in sympathetic and nervous coughs of this kind it often acts admirably. Dr. Jousset‡ considers its power here one of the best illustrations we have of the efficacy of infinitesimal doses. " Cough from tickling in the larynx, with vomiting of food," being the precise definition of its sphere of action, he communicates 107 instances of it, of which 101 were relieved or cured by the medicine. The 3rd, 12th, and 30th dilutions were found alike efficacious, and superior to the mother-tincture.

One of Hahnemann's provers had a hoarse voice and expectoration of yellow mucus with his cough, which suggested to him its use in laryngeal phthisis when he remem-

---

* Dr. Buchmann has recently affirmed the correctness of this observation of Hahnemann's, and adduces several other testimonies in its support. See *Brit. Journ.,* xxxvi., 268.

† See *Bull. de Thérapeutique,* 8° livraison, 1878, p. 381 ; and *L'Art Médical,* xlvi., 457.

‡ See *Brit. Journ of Hom.,* xxvi., 210.

bered the statements of the herbals and of the country people,
that the sundew causes a violent cough in sheep, under which
they waste away.   He says that some of the older physicians
have cured certain kinds of malignant cough and purulent
phthisis with it; but that in modern times its acridity has
caused its disuse.   Influenced by such facts, Dr. Curie, of
Paris—whose doings with Bryonia have already come before
us—determined to ascertain by experiment its real action.
He reported to the French Academy of Sciences* that he had
slowly poisoned three cats with daily doses of Drosera.   Diarrhœa at the commencement, and weakness of voice about six
weeks later, are the only symptoms mentioned as observed
during life.   But, on post-mortem examination, the trachea
was found unchanged, while the pleural surface of both lungs
was studded with what the microscope decided to be true
tubercle.   In one cat the mesenteric glands were much
enlarged ; in another the submaxillary glands, with the solitary
glands of the large intestine and Peyer's patches.   Now as
cats are not at all liable to tubercle, I think it cannot be
doubted that Drosera here caused the deposit, with the consentaneous enlargement of the lymphatic glands.   Putting
this together with the effects ascribed to it in sheep, it looks
very much as if Drosera would turn out a true *simile* for
phthisis pulmonalis.   Dr. Curie, indeed, asserts that in the
incipient stage of the disease a cure may nearly always be
brought about by Drosera, given in doses of from four to
twenty drops of the mother-tincture in the twenty-four hours.
I can only say that I once gave drop doses four times a day,
with the effect of setting up a most violent spasmodic cough,
which subsided to the ordinary cough of phthisis when the
medicine was discontinued.   Dr. Jousset found a similar
aggravation in two cases out of six which he treated on Dr.
Curie's plan.   In two others the effect was *nil,* and in the
remaining two a primary amelioration did not last.   I know
of no other trials of the remedy.

   Acidum hydrocyanicum, Acidum nitricum, Belladonna, Che-
~~*lidonium, Cina, Corallium, Cuprum, Hyoscyamus,*~~ *Ipecacuanha,*
Nux vomica and *Sambucus* should be compared with Drosera
in their relation to spasmodic coughs.

   I suspect that Dr. Curie's mother-tincture will have to be
modified no less than Hahnemann's 30th.   I myself have been
very well satisfied with the 1st dilution.

                    * See *Brit. Journ. of Hom.,* xx., 39.

LECTURE XXXI.

DULCAMARA, ELATERIUM, EUPATORIUM PERFOLIATUM AND PURPUREUM, EUPHORBIUM, EUPHRASIA, FERRUM.

My first medicine to-day is the bitter-sweet or woody night-shade, Solanum

Dulcamara.

We use a tincture prepared from the leaves and green shoots.

The proving of Dulcamara appears in the first volume of the *Reine Arzneimittellehre*, where the drug has 318 symptoms from Hahnemann and ten fellow-provers, and 83 from authors. Most of· these last are taken from Carrére (of whom more anon) and his German editor, Starke, and are nearly always critical and curative effects of the medicine when given to patients. They cannot, therefore, without great caution be used as pathogenetic phenomena. The proving in the *Chronic Diseases* has only 8 additional symptoms. Dr. Allen, how-ever, is able to give some valuable new observations of the effects of the plant, both when proved and when taken in excess.

Hahnemann found Dulcamara in use for a variety of affec-tions supposed to depend upon a vitiated state of the blood, which it seemed to benefit by determining to the periphery or increasing the secretions. The fullest account of its applica-tions is that published by Carrére in 1789.* He relates many cases of gout, rheumatism, and cutaneous disease, and of suppression of the latter or of the secretions, in which it proved very effectual, always, however, by inducing some critical evacuant phenomena. Hahnemann, whose numerous citations show how largely he has used Carrére's work, cites these phenomena—eruptions, diarrhœas, sweatings, and urinary depositions—as pathogenetic effects of the drug. This I con-ceive to be unwarrantable, unless the same results can be obtained on the healthy, of which (save as regards the

* *Traité des propriétés, usages, et effets de la Douce-Amère.* Paris, 1789.

diarrhœa) there is no evidence. It is therefore very doubtful whether its benefit in the squamous forms of cutaneous disease, so largely vouched for by the older physicians, is of a specific and homœopathic nature. It neither causes such affection of the skin in the healthy,* nor does it cure without evacuation. It does, however, excite erythematous and urticarious rashes, and pruritus ; and it is in urticaria, and in such forms of eczema as crusta lactea, that it has found place in homœopathic practice.

But there are other effects of the drug observed by Carrère which Hahnemann has incorporated into his pathogenesis, and which seem to be truly physiological. This author says that, after seventeen years' use of the drug, he has seen no inconvenience from full doses, save occasionally some twitching of the eyelids and lips, and slight convulsive movements of the hands ; heat and itching, with desire, in the genitals ; heaviness of the head, with dimness of sight ; and sore throat. The critical eruptions, moreover, were often preceded by restlessness, insomnia, and even a febrile state. Of the first-named phenomena—those of the eyelids, lips, and hands—he makes the curious observation that they only occurred when the patient was exposed to cold, damp weather, and that they could be readily removed by external warmth. Hence has arisen one of those happy defining rules which abound in homœopathic therapeutics, viz., that Dulcamara is indicated for the result of exposure to damp. It is certainly an excellent remedy here. I am myself very liable to catch cold if I get at all wet ; but since I have (acting on a suggestion of Dr. Chapman's)† taken Dulcamara on such occasions as a prophylactic, I have hardly ever suffered. Twice, too, I have arrested in myself incipient results of moist air by Dulcamara ; the first time it was angina, the second time stiff neck. The medicine is also useful in diarrhœa resulting from a chill in damp weather ; in catarrh of the bladder from the same cause—even, Dr. Drury says,‡ when chronic, with much mucus and offensive urine ; and indeed in almost any mild catarrhal irritation of the mucous membranes owning this origin. Its influence extends also to subacute articular rheumatism in this way set up,§ and indeed to any malady not utterly beyond its range of influence, when there is a marked

* The symptom assigned to it in Allen's Supplement, "in some cases *lepra*, nausea, and headache" would seem to say otherwise; but "of" should have been inserted before "lepra."
† See *Brit. Journ. of Hom.*, viii., 33.
‡ *Ibid*, xxviii., 174.
§ *Ibid*, xxiii., 630.

aggravation of the symptoms at every change of the weather to damp and cold. Hahnemann, who was the first to indicate these anti-catarrhal properties of Dulcamara, says also that it is specific in some epidemic fevers, but does not identify them.

Of the genital irritation ascribed by Carrére and Starke to Dulcamara Stillé writes—" Should this statement be correct, as well as the one made by several physicians, that it has the power of *subduing* the sexual appetite of maniacs and others in whom this propensity is morbidly active, both facts should be borne in mind as illustrating the opposite effects sometimes produced by medicines when administered in health and disease." Dr. Guernsey commends the remedy when the slighter forms of nymphomania in women are associated with heat, itching, and herpetic eruptions about the genitals. Stillé further mentions the paralysis of the tongue which is said to have resulted from its protracted use, but which also occurred in three of the poisoning cases cited by Allen. I am not aware of any therapeutic use having been made of this effect of the drug.

So far extended our knowledge of Dulcamara before its active principle was isolated. This is known as *solania*, and is found to be common to it and the Solanum nigrum, though Dulcamara possesses it in much smaller proportion. Solania has now been pretty fully tested by experiments on animals, of which the most satisfactory are those of Professor Clarus, who also took it himself : you may read them in English in the eighteenth volume of the *British Journal of Homœopathy*. Two very important phenomena were observed, the one neurotic, the other of irritant character. The first was that the respiration became much slower, the heart's action much quicker (though at the same time feebler). Since this curious antagonism is also caused by division of the vagi in the neck, Professor Clarus infers that solania acts by depressing these very nerves. Such depression is further indicated by the filling of the pulmonary tissues with a serous exudation, and the emphysematous distension of isolated portions of the lung, which were observed in the rabbits killed by solania :—these phenomena having resulted from division of the vagi. Other symptoms also indicate an action on the medulla oblongata, as vomiting long after taking the drug, spasms of the thoracic muscles extending to those of the extremities, snapping of the jaws, and a pendulum-like motion of the head. After death, the membranes of the medulla oblongata, and of the parts just above and below it, were found highly injected, but the nervous substance itself healthy.

Subsequent experimentation (of which a good account is given by Dr. Phillips) has confirmed this neurotic action of solania, only giving as its first effect a hurried state of the respiration, which is probably the earliest response of the medulla to the disturbing influence of the drug.* It supports, moreover, Clarus' second observation, viz., hyperæmia of the kidneys with albuminous urine, and shows the engorgement sometimes going on to inflammation, and involving the liver also. The effects of the alkaloid on the human subject have been ascertained by Schroff. Giving it to healthy persons in various doses, from one thirtieth of a grain to three grains, he observed "increased cutaneous sensibility, itching of the skin, gaping, general numbness, sleepiness, slight tonic cramps in the legs, and increasing frequency of the pulse, which at the same time grew feeble and thready; there was some dyspnœa and oppression in breathing, with nausea and ineffectual efforts at vomiting; the head was hot, heavy, and dizzy, with drowsiness, yet with inability to sleep; the extremities were cold, the skin dry and itching, and there was marked general debility. The pupil remained unchanged: the sleep was restless, and disturbed by frightful dreams" (Stillé).

I know of no application to practice of the effects of solania on the kidneys, though it might seem indicated in the first stage of Bright's disease. But I have now for years been in the habit of relying upon it in the threatening paralysis of the lungs which we often encounter in the bronchitis of old people and young children. It has several times done me excellent service in this condition; and not less so in a minor form of the trouble in the aged, when from weakness they have to cough a long time to expel the phlegm.

After the facts now brought forward, especially as regards solania, you may estimate the value of Dr. John Harley's recent experiments, which lead him to consider Dulcamara altogether inert! It proved so, indeed, in his trials of it, as it has before in other hands;† but it would be wiser to seek to ascertain the cause of this occasional absence of activity, instead of dismissing the counter-observations of so many competent persons. Dr. Harley's iconoclasm will not exclude Dulcamara, any more than it will Æthusa, from our Materia Medica.

* "It is a general principle" says Dr. Burdon-Sanderson "applicable to most toxical action, that paresis of a central organ is preceded by over-action." (See p. 74)
† See Stillé, *sub voce*.

Dulcamara has so very unique an action that I hardly see my way to putting down any other medicines as true analogues of it.

The medium dilutions have seemed to answer very well. Solania I have always given in the second attenuation of the acetate.

We now come to an old acquaintance,

Elaterium.

The dried sediment of the juice is triturated for our use.

There is a short proving of Elaterium, made with the second dilution, in the *Materia Medica of American Provings*. Dr. Allen adds several other observations.

It is needless to describe to you the physiological action of Elaterium. Nevertheless, it has been so graphically put by Dr. T. K. Chambers, that I cannot refrain from quoting his account of the drug. "It causes," he says, "an enormous flow of watery serum from the first mucous membrane that absorbs it. If its vapour be drawn up into the nostrils for a short time, it is a powerful errhine, and is followed by the secretion of floods of water from the Schneiderian membrane : —if it is dissolved in the œsophagus it causes such a deluge of the gastric fluids that the stomach cannot contain them, and they are rejected by vomiting : if it succeeds in passing the pylorus, a choleraic diarrhœa gushes forth, stripping the membrane of its epithelium, just like its morbid prototype." Elaterium would thus seem homœopathic to choleraic diarrhœa and vomiting. There is this difference, however, that the prolonged action of Elaterium sets up gastro-enteritis, which the cholera poison never does. I think that nevertheless I should be disposed to try it where the excessive *quantity* of the evacuations was especially noticeable. There are several cases of endemic cholera reported at the end of the proving, in which Elaterium was successful after Veratrum had failed. It might be useful in "cholerine," which seems to be the ordinary cholera nostras modified by the presence of the Asiatic variety. Some well-marked rheumatico-neuralgic pains, also, appear in the proving, and have led to a cure of one case of rheumatic sciatica. Intermittent fever, too, counts Elaterium among the numerous medicines which at various times have cured or seemed to cure it.

Elaterium forms a group with *Colchicum, Croton,* and *Veratrum.*

The 2nd dilution was given in nearly all the cases reported in the proving.

We have next an American medicine, the thorough-wort, bone-set, ague-weed,

Eupatorium perfoliatum.

The tincture is prepared from the whole plant.

The original proving of Eupatorium, also, is in the *Materia Medica of American Provings.* Cases of cure with it are there given; and a full account of its virtues is to be found in Dr. Hale's *New Remedies.*

Eupatorium has long been highly esteemed on the American continent as a remedy against intermittent fever; hence its popular name among the Indians, " ague-weed." Its other appellation, " bone-set," is obtained from the remarkable power it showed in relieving the bone-pains of dengue in an epidemic of this disease. The pains were so severe that the malady was spoken of as the " break-bone fever." The provings of Homœopathy have enabled us to define the precise sphere of Eupatorium in the treatment of these maladies. In intermittents the setting in of thirst before the chill, which usually occurs in the morning, bilious vomiting during the paroxysm, and scanty perspiration at its close, are characteristic symptoms calling for its use. If, also, the peculiar bone-pains are present, the medicine is doubly indicated : you may read a case of this kind by Dr. Bayes in the first volume of the *Annals* of the British Homœopathic Society. I have no experience of Eupatorium in intermittents or dengue ; but can bear my testimony to its extreme value in relieving the bone-pains of influenza. Dr. Carroll Dunham directed attention to the marked *hepatic* action of Eupatorium, which he compared with that of Bryonia.* The group of symptoms to which he referred are—intense headache with soreness of the scalp, soreness of the eyes, redness of the face, nausea and prostration, soreness in the region of the liver, constipation, and high-coloured urine. He gives a capital case of " bilious fever," in which these symptoms, with violent bone-pains, were present, and which was broken up by Eupatorium 3 with marvellous rapidity.

Besides the *Bryonia* already referred to, I do not know of any true analogue of Eupatorium. Dr. Dunham points out

* *Amer. Hom. Rev.*, vi., 229; and *Lectures*, sub voce.

as elements of distinction between these two—first, that the perspiration is free with Bryonia, deficient with Eupatorium; second, that Eupatorium pains make the patient restless, those of Bryonia make him keep very still.

The range of recorded use has been from the 3rd dilution to the mother-tincture.

More recently, another species of Eupatorium has come into notice, the

Eupatorium purpureum.

A tincture is prepared from the fresh root.

A capital proving on a woman, and some cases of cure, are given in the second edition of Hale's *New Remedies.**

The interest of E. purpureum centres in its action on the urinary organs. In moderate doses, it acts as a powerful diuretic; and the frequent emptying of the bladder which is necessary seems almost entirely due to the excess of urine secreted. But even thus there are some symptoms of vesical irritation; and, when larger doses are taken, these unmistakeably increase. Micturition now becomes more frequent, urgent, and painful: the urine is scanty, mucus appears in it, and later on it is high-coloured and dense. The reading of these phenomena is plain; and the therapeutic indications are easily perceived. Three good cases of inflammatory irritation of the bladder are given in Dr. Hale's article, and others are referred to. The drug has become my favourite remedy for vesical irritability in women: I have not tried it upon men. It has effected a cure of some intermittents. Their characters, according to Dr. Hale, are—irregular advent of the paroxysms, chills beginning in the small of the back, and running upwards and downwards; lips and nails blue, violent shaking, with comparatively little coldness; during the sweat, any attempt on the part of the patient to change his position ever so little causes a chilliness to pass through the body. In other respects, the symptoms are like those of the E. perfoliatum. These characteristics are clinical only, no fever-symptoms having appeared in the solitary prover the drug has yet had. Dr. Bayes has communicated to the *Monthly Homœopathic Review* for January, 1878, a case of chronic Burmese fever somewhat of this kind, in which E. purpureum

* Arrangements of the symptoms, pathogenetic and curative, of both species of Eupatorium are given by Dr. Hering in his volume of *Materia Medica.*

proved curative, the chief indication for it being the presence
of a somewhat hysterical condition during the attack, which
was developed by the drug in its (feminine) experimenter.
Dr. Bayes seems to consider that the strictly mental symptoms
also of patient and prover coincided. But I can hardly think
that "first the brain became very active, the mind apparently
exceptionally clear, and of greater capacity for work than
ordinarily," with which the paroxysms began, is represented
by "the mind is possessed by various delusions" of the
pathogenesis.

The chief analogues are *Cantharis, Copaiba,* and *Ferrum.*

The second dilution was used in the cases on record; and I
have myself never required any other.

My next medicine,

Euphorbium,

is, according to Dr. Allen, the gum-resin of the Euphorbia
resinifera, commonly called E. officinarum. Of late, the
American Euphorbia corollata has been introduced into practice; it is prepared by triturating the dried root. Other
varieties of the spurge are being proved, as Allen's *Encyclopædia* shows.

Euphorbium was proved by Hahnemann: its pathogenesis,
containing 281 symptoms from himself and two others, is in
the second edition of the *Chronic Diseases.* There is an article
on Euphorbia corollata in Hale's *New Remedies.*

Euphorbium, belonging as it does to the family which includes Croton, Ricinus, and Jatropha, is another instance of
the drastic purgative, and gives us another remedy for endemic
cholera and choleraic diarrhœa. The E. corollata has been a
good deal used in America in cholera infantum. It is much
less liable to cause inflammation than the other Euphorbiæ,
and is accordingly better suited to these non-inflammatory
disorders. When applied to the skin, Euphorbium, like Croton,
causes an eczematous inflammation; but it is not known
whether this is a specific effect of its action.

Dr. Chapman* relates a case of spasmodic cough, characterised by accompanying stitches from the pit of the stomach
to both sides of the chest, in which Euphorbium proved
rapidly curative. He (as also Noack and Trinks) commends
it for red inflammatory swelling of the cheek, with sensation
of burning heat.

* *Brit. Journ. of Hom.,* viii., 34.

Besides the members of its own family already mentioned, Euphorbium is closely allied with *Veratrum* and *Colchicum*, with *Elaterium*, and with *Tartar emetic*.

We have no records in any degree fixing its dose.

We now come to a medicine for which I confess an especial *penchant*, the eye-bright,

Euphrasia.

The homœopathic tincture is prepared from the whole plant.

Hahnemann has given us a pathogenesis of Euphrasia in the fifth volume of the *Reine Arzneimittellehre*, containing 37 symptoms from himself, 58 from three fellow-observers, and 2 from authors. A proving by four other persons is translated from the *Allgemeine Homöopathische Zeitung* in the sixteenth volume of the *British Journal*, and yet another—by six more —is added by Allen.

The great charm of Euphrasia as a medicine is that it has a distinct and limited sphere of action, beyond which it advances no pretensions, but within which it manifests virtues which are as unvarying as they are potent. It acts upon the upper portion of the respiratory mucous membrane, *i.e.*, upon its conjunctival and nasal portions, only just reaching the larynx. It developes in this region a catarrhal inflammation, generally characterised by profuse secretion. Hence it takes a first place among the remedies for *fluent coryza*, when this is a local affection, and not a symptom of general influenza, in which latter case Arsenic is preferable. The involvement of the conjunctiva in the catarrh is a special indication for Euphrasia ; and sometimes the secretion from the eyes is acrid, while that from the nares is bland,—the opposite condition obtaining with Arsenic. The coryza which accompanies the commencement of *measles* is one to which Euphrasia is well suited :* and I nearly always give it in this stage in alternation with Aconite, and have reason to believe that the eyes are the better for it at the time and afterwards. The *eyes* themselves, indeed, are the special seat of the influence of Euphrasia. Its name in most languages refers to its healing power over these organs (in English it is eye-bright ; in German, Augen-trost ; in French, casse-lunettes) : and you know

* *Brit. Journ.*, xi., 484.

how the Archangel in Milton, when he would clear the vision of our first parent,

> " purged with *euphrasy* and rue
> The visual nerve, for he had much to see."[*]

This is one of the many instances in which Homœopathy has revived and confirmed, while defining, the old traditions about herbs. Conjunctivitis is very marked in the provings, especially of the palpebral margins, with photophobia, and there are even indications of affection of the deeper tissues, and of vision, which is dimmed. Correspondingly, Euphrasia is among the chief of our eye-medicines. In simple acute conjunctivitis it is rare that any other remedy is required ; and in the chronic stage it has often effected cures. Given at the commencement of strumous ophthalmia, it will nearly always check incipient ulceration ; but its action needs sustaining by constitutional medicines, especially Sulphur. It comes in again later to remove specks on the cornea, for which it is very efficacious. Dr. Dudgeon has communicated two cases to the *British Journal of Homœopathy*,[†] in which a rapid cure of rheumatic ophthalmia (sclerotitis and iritis) was effected by Euphrasia, after other remedies had failed. There is, moreover, an interesting communication by Dr. Robert Jackson in the twenty-third volume of the *Medical and Physical Journal* (1810), in which he relates several cases where chronically impaired vision, coexisting with signs or feelings of disorder in the eyeballs, was greatly benefited by an infusion of the plant. Used in this manner, I know of no medicine which will less frequently disappoint expectation than the little eye-bright.

Drs. Allen and Norton say of it—" Euphrasia is one of our most important remedies in diseases of the eye, especially superficial." Profuse acrid and burning lachrymation they find a good indication for it in conjunctival disorders. They have also found it curative in paralysis of the oculo-motor nerve, coming on after exposure to cold and wet. They say that its characteristic discharges are thicker than those indicating Arsenicum and Mercurius, which otherwise it much resembles in its action upon the eye.

The analogues of Euphrasia are *Æthusa, Allium Cepa, Apis, Argentum nitricum, Arsenicum, Hepar sulphuris, Kali bich-*

---

[*] I might also quote Shenstone :

> " Yet euphrasy may not be left unsung,
> That gives dim eyes to wander leagues around."

[†] Vol. xxii., p. 355.

romicum, Kali iodatum, Mercurius solubilis and *corrosivus,* and *Pulsatilla.*

Small doses of the mother-tincture, as recommended by Hahnemann himself, appear to answer all purposes excellently well.

We have, in conclusion, to consider the action and uses of one of the most celebrated of medicines,

Ferrum.

For the preparation of the salts of iron used in homœopathic practice I must refer you to the Pharmacopœia. Our only peculiarity is the frequent use of the acetate, as with this were made nearly all the provings of the metal we possess.

Ferrum was proved by Hahnemann and three others : their 261 symptoms, with 37 from seven authors, appear in the second volume of the *Reine Arzneimittellehre.* Dr. Hempel has accidentally omitted this pathogenesis in his translation ; but the deficiency has been supplied in the thirty-second volume of the *British Journal of Homœopathy.* In the ninth volume of the same journal may be read another proving of the metal by five of Rademacher's followers, where the blood was examined before and after the experiments ; and Dr. Allen supplies a third, conducted by the American Provers' Union. His supplement also contains some experiments made with Ferrum phosphoricum by Dr. J. H. Morgan, of Philadelphia.

The primary interest of iron lies in its remedial power over anæmia. Whether this condition arise as the chlorosis of defective menstruation, or the simple " poverty of blood " induced by hæmorrhages, by deficiency of air, light, and suitable food, or by exhausting diseases—iron is its one great remedy. It so rarely fails to cure, and its action is so *tuto, cito, et jucunde,* that it would be unpardonable to deprive any patient of its benefits, whatever be our theory of its action or the manner in which it must be given. The treatment of anæmia by iron is one of the few satisfactory and certain things in modern medicine, and we who believe in the supreme value of the homœopathic method may not neglect it because it does not seem conformable thereto, unless we can do better. That we cannot is the general confession ; we must, therefore, give our anæmic patients the iron they need, in whatever quantity may be necessary.

2 I

But while we follow facts rather than theory, it is nevertheless of considerable importance that we understand the
theory of our facts, that we may know what we are about.
How does iron act in the treatment of anæmia ? Is it a food
or a medicine? and, if a medicine, is it homœopathic or
antipathic to the condition present ? These are questions
which have been largely discussed in both schools of medicine,
and which can hardly be said to be closed. I shall submit to
you a few facts and considerations bearing upon them, which
may help us to come to a decision.

First of all we notice that iron, like lime, is a normal constituent of the body, and is continually being supplied with
the food. It is, again, in the red corpuscles of the blood that
the metal finds its *habitat* and performs its functions. Now
it is the deficiency of these very corpuscles wherein the " poverty
of blood " we call anæmia consists. It is impossible to deny
the significance of such facts, or to resist the conclusion that
the relation of iron to the blood is a fact of the same order as
that of lime to the bones.

You will perceive that, in so speaking, I am identifying
anæmia with oligocythæmia. I am well aware that, in many
cases, this deficiency of the red corpuscles of the blood is
associated with a similar poverty in the solid constituents of the
plasma—with hypalbuminosis, and that we may even have
such a condition existing alone, or almost so. Etymologically,
this is anæmia, or oligæmia ; but practically we call it rather
impaired nutrition. We need a term for that peculiar state of
system showing itself in pallor of skin and mucous membrane,
with breathlessness, palpitation, cardiac and venous murmurs,
&c., and which may exist without any marasmus. We have
long had it in " anæmia," and with this meaning we shall (I
think) continue to use the term. When hypalbuminosis is
present, hygienic and dietetic treatment is of paramount importance ; and medicines like Argentum nitricum, Calcarea
phosphorica, Natrum muriaticum, Zincum and Plumbum, are
of most service. But when oligocythæmia shows its existence,
all the food and air in the world yield in value to the suitable administration of iron.

Is iron, then, a direct food ? Is it merely by supplying a
want of its normal proportion in the body that it cures
anæmia ? This position cannot, I think, be sustained. The
malady does not ordinarily arise from any failure in the
quantity of iron supplied in the food : if the element is
deficient in the blood, the fault lies in the assimilative processes. But Reveil, according to Trousseau and Pidoux, has

ascertained that in anæmia there is no change whatever in the amount of iron present in the blood. However few the corpuscles, they contain within them the full proportion of the metal normal to health; and, though under the influence of iron itself they increase to double and treble their number, they yield no more of it.

Not, then, from want of their metallic constituent, but from deficiency of the red corpuscles themselves, is the blood poor in the condition we call anæmia. And why are the corpuscles few? Their development is the ultimate result of the elaboration of the vital fluid: their defect must be owing to a fault somewhere existing in the blood-making processes. Can we remedy such fault merely by giving an increased quantity of one constituent of the pabulum from which they are built up? It can hardly be so. If the parts concerned in sanguification have proved unable to perform their task hitherto, they will not work the better because more material is supplied for their operations. What is wanted is a *stimulus*, elective in its affinity for the parts concerned, and specific in its correspondence with the morbid condition induced.

That we have such a stimulus in iron appears from two classes of facts—first, its effects on the healthy; second, its operation in small doses in disease.

1. The hæmatic effect of iron on the healthy does not appear with any distinctness in the provings of Hahnemann. The pale face and lips he cites from Ritter were the result of metrorrhagia induced by iron, not its primary effect. But in the experiments conducted by Löffler, the Rademacherian, the blood itself was examined before and after the experiments. In all cases there was increase of the water, and a corresponding diminution of the dry residuum. The general condition and appearance, moreover, which at first improved during the ingestion of the medicine, rapidly fell off afterwards, and assumed all the characters of debility and hydræmia. It is a fair inference that Ferrum, when given in health in quantities beyond those required for nutriment, disorders the very processes of sanguification in which it takes part as a food. We need yet more precise experimentation as to its effect on the number of the red corpuscles, which can now be counted without difficulty. If, as has been shown with Mercury and syphilis, it is found to reduce their number in health while augmenting it in chlorosis, its homœopathicity to anæmia will be established. In such experimentation, however, it must be borne in mind that few persons are in such perfect health that a small addition to the

pabulum of their tissues is needless and injurious. It is only when these are as it were saturated that morbid phenomena can be expected to appear.

Our only other source of information as to the effects of iron on the healthy is the condition of people who habitually drink ferruginous waters. Hahnemann gives a grievous list of maladies as those to which they are subject, all implying great depression of the nutritive powers. But I know not on what authority he makes his statements, nor am I acquainted with any careful observations on the subject. Brandis, indeed, "states that the waters of chalybeate springs are habitually drunk by man and beast without the slightest injury" (Stillé).

2. But, in the next place, we have evidence that iron, in doses far too small to be of any use as pabulum, has proved curative in anæmia. Dr. Russell relates one case in the twelfth volume of the *British Journal of Homœopathy* (p. 376). Dr. Drysdale, in his excellent discussion on the action of iron in the twenty-seventh volume of the same journal, cites another. But the most forcible testimony is that of Dr. Bayes, who speaks of one or two drops of the first dilution of the acetate as an excellent chalybeate ; and writes—"The exhibition of iron in doses of the thousandth of a grain (the third decimal dilution) has been, very generally, followed by more rapid amendment in the ferruginising of the blood (and the consequent cure of diseased conditions and states of parts and organs) than I have hitherto seen result from the gross and material doses of the chemical physicians." Such experience (and I myself have lately had some of the same kind) may be exceptional, but it could not have been gained at all had Ferrum no action as a specific stimulus on blood-making over and above that which makes it a food.

The conclusion, then, I think must be that the metal has such action—that it probably hinders the formation of red blood in health and certainly promotes it in disease in the same manner in which other drugs affect the functions. But while this is true, and Ferrum may be given for anæmia in small doses as a homœopathic medicine, it must not be forgotten that it is also a food, and is required as such. Doubtless a larger supply of nourishment would meet the want ; but this is not always possible to obtain, or even then to digest. Iron may therefore with advantage be given as food in most cases of anæmia, even though itself or some other medicine should be administered at the same time. The latter should be given on an empty stomach, that it may act as a stimulus; the former should be taken at meal-time, since it is part of the pabulum of the body. These conclusions are the same as those of Dr. Drysdale, whose exhaustive paper on the subject I would strongly urge you to read.

The conclusion to which I am led as to the treatment of anæmia by iron is that it should always be commenced after a dynamic fashion, *i.e.*, by giving such small doses as I have mentioned. If the improvement be not rapid, it may be hastened by administering the metal as a food also. By this method the risk will be avoided of producing those disastrous results in the production of hæmoptysis and subsequent phthisis with which Trousseau has to reproach himself.

I should say that in that idiopathic anæmia lately described, and bearing the ominous titles of "pernicious" and "progressive," iron has proved of no service. In chlorosis, moreover, it is less suitable in the febrile form, and where there is much debility and œdema. In all these cases its place is taken, as we have seen, by Arsenic.

But now, over and above the hæmatic action of iron, it has properties, pathogenetic and curative, of no mean importance. In the infinitesimal doses of the older homœopathists, it did little save occasionally check vomiting of the ingesta and lienteria. But, given in a less attenuated form, it has received strong testimony to its value in many disorders of the head, the lungs, and the pelvic organs in general.*

1. The determination of blood to the head which follows overdosing with iron is well known, and ought to be utilised in our practice. Dr. Kidd has found the pyrophosphate (first decimal) very useful in the headaches of passive congestion ; I have also learned to depend upon it, in preference even to China, in the pseudo-hyperæmic headaches following large losses of blood. Dr. Cooper (and my own experience confirms his) has much confidence in it in recurrent *epistaxis*, giving the first trituration of the phosphate.

2. The provings of iron show that it determines blood to the lungs no less than to the head. It has accordingly become a favourite remedy in our school for *hæmoptysis*. Drs. Kidd and Pope concur in esteeming the acetate, in the first decimal dilution, above all other remedies for this accident, especially when a tickling cough and oppression of the chest are present. Trousseau has pointed out (as I have said) how often the in-

* Statements made without references in what follows are mostly taken from a paper by Dr. Cooper " On the Action of Iron," with the discussion following its reading, contained in the fifth volume of the *Annals.*

cautious use of the drug causes this hæmorrhage, and so leads
on to phthisis. On this subject I refer you to Dr. Cl. Müller's
remarks in the eighteenth volume of the *British Journal*. He
recommends it from experience in the so-called "phthisis
florida," in the form of the chloride, from 1^x to 3.

3. Iron is a decided irritant of the urethra and neck of the
bladder, and the chloride has some repute in the treatment of
vesical catarrh and of gleet : Dr. Kidd also speaks highly of it
in urinary irritation. But we owe to Dr. Cooper a very pretty
bit of precisionising, which indicates the especial sphere of
action of Ferrum in this region. You will find his original
paper in the fifth volume of the *Annals* of the British
Homœopathic Society, and his more detailed observations in
the twenty-eighth volume of the *British Journal*. The enuresis
calling for it is characteristically *diurnal*,—depending on an
irritability of the trigone and cervix vesicæ, which diminishes
when the pressure of the urine is taken off by the recumbent
posture. He gives ten well-marked cases of this affection
cured by the phosphate in the 1st or 2nd decimal trituration.
I have verified his suggestions with much success. But iron
has been also found curative, especially in the form of the
iodide, in nocturnal incontinence of urine ; and here too it is
homœopathic, three of the American provers having experienced this casualty under its use. There is some reason to
think that iron acts also on the kidneys. Its repute in Bright's
disease is well known, and it is admitted (by Dr. George
Johnson) that the urine may become more scanty or more
deeply coloured and albuminous after its use. In the discussion on Dr. Cooper's paper, Dr. Metcalfe mentioned a case in
which from a single overdose of iron suppression of urine
occurred, with head-symptoms like those of uræmia,
relieved as soon as the secretion was restored, and the iron
eliminated.

4. The pelvic symptoms of Ferrum are analogous to those
of the head and the thorax. Dr. Kidd recommends it in
uterine congestion and menorrhagia : Dr. Cooper in tenesmus
of the cervix uteri similar to that of the bladder in diurnal
enuresis. But the strongest testimony to its value as a uterine
remedy comes from our American colleague, Dr. H. C. Preston,
to whom we owe Hamamelis. He tells us that the first
trituration of the iodide has proved a most useful medicine in
his hands in uterine displacements, including retroversion and
prolapsus. You will find his observations in the twenty-fifth
volume of the *British Journal of Homœopathy*.

5. When, as in one of his cases, the rectum is much irri-

tated in sympathy with the womb, Ferrum will set it right. But the provings evidence an independent action on this part in the male subject also, showing itself mainly by tenesmus. Dr. Cooper finds it the best remedy for prolapsus recti in children. Dr. Markwick has put on record a case in which its over-use caused dysenteric symptoms*—a fact which may find practical applications.

Dr. Cooper, who has done much useful work in enlarging and defining the applications of Ferrum, has lately given us† another paper on the subject. In this he lays down "painless irritability of fibre" as the condition especially calling for it, thus giving it place as a remedy for some forms of cough, as well as for those other expulsive actions whose impatience and excess it has already been seen to moderate.

Another advocate for a more extensive use of Ferrum is Dr. Schussler, of whose "tissue remedies" I have already spoken to you. The presence of iron in the blood, and its power of causing congestions and hæmorrhages in divers places, make it—according to him—the prime remedy in all active hyperæmic conditions, even in inflammations before exudation has taken place. He gives the phosphate, in the 12th decimal trituration.

Dr. Guernsey considers the most suitable subjects for Ferrum to be weakly and complaining women and children whose faces nevertheless tend to be fiery-red.

As a hæmatic, Ferrum has no true analogue, unless it be Manganese. The medicines which act like it on the head are *Belladonna, Nux vomica,* and *Quinine;* on the lungs, *Millefolium* and perhaps *Arnica;* on the bladder, *Cantharis, Copaiba,* and *Eupatorium purpureum;* and on the uterus and rectum, *Sabina.*

The best doses have been mentioned as we have proceeded. As a chalybeate food I like nothing so well as the Ferrum redactum of the British Pharmacopœia, of which a grain or two daily answers every purpose. The pyrophosphate is an elegant preparation when a liquid form is preferred.

* *Brit. Journ. of Hom.,* xix., 309. † *Ibid,* xxxii., 409

LECTURE XXXII.

GAMBOGE, GELSEMIUM, GLONOIN, GRAPHITES, GRATIOLA, GUAIACUM.

I begin this lecture with a drug which generally appears in homœopathic works under its old name of " Gummi guttæ," but which may as well stand here as

Gambogia.

The Siamese resin so called is dissolved in rectified spirit to form a tincture for our use.

There is a pathogenesis of Gamboge in Allen's *Encyclopædia*, chiefly taken from an unpublished monograph by Cajetan Nenning, the " Ng." of Hahnemann's provings.

There is no evidence, here or elsewhere, of any action of Gamboge beyond that which belongs to it as a drastic purgative ; and in this sphere only has it received homœopathic applications. Dr. Hilbers has much esteem for it in summer diarrhœa accompanied by severe colic ; and Dr. Phillips has the following paragraph :—" Malgaigne and Betz found the use of very small doses (about $\frac{3}{4}$ of a grain in twenty-four hours) to be exceedingly valuable for dysentery, especially in young persons—an apparently paradoxical fact, but established on good evidence ; and, after all, not more strange than the completely opposite action of small and large doses of strychnia, and of many other drugs."

Dr. Hilbers gives the 2nd dilution.

The medicine we have next to discuss is one of the most valuable of the American contributions to the Materia Medica. It is the yellow jasmine,

Gelsemium

(for it seems that we have been wrong hitherto in calling it Gelseminum). The tincture of the root is the preparation used in our practice ; and Dr. Bartholow, who has devoted much attention to this drug, recommends the fresh root to be employed, as the alkaloid gelsemia, on which so much of its activity depends, is lost during desiccation. We should, therefore, prescribe by preference the tincture made in America, where the plant is indigenous.

Gelsemium was first introduced into homœopathic practice by Dr. E. M. Hale, who, in concert with Dr. Douglass, made a number of experiments with it, and published, in 1862, a monograph on its properties. Since then it has acquired an ever-growing reputation among us, and has been proved and tested in a variety of ways. Of late years, it has attracted attention in the old school ; and Berger in Germany,* Bartholow in America,† and Ringer and Murrell in England,‡ have experimented largely with it,—the last-named having proved it, *more Hahnemanniano*, on six persons, in doses sufficient to produce decided effects. Dr. Allen is thus able to give us a pathogenesis containing 682 symptoms, obtained by upwards of 80 observers. In referring you to this article for the physiological effects of the plant, I would add a commendation of Dr. Hale's fourth edition, as supplying the best *résumé* we possess of its therapeutic virtues.

The effects on the healthy human subject of full doses of Gelsemium are almost identical with those we have lately studied as resulting from the action of Conium. The first symptom is heaviness of the eyelids, so that the eyes can hardly be kept open : with this there is giddiness on standing. Then ensues diplopia ; and shortly afterwards the legs, arms and lower jaw become powerless, and the patient cannot stand, move, or speak. At this time there is also ptosis, and sometimes internal strabismus. Here is an illustration of its action :—

" To see what the effects of the drug would be when pushed, I gave to a patient, a sailor, convalescent from periostitis, three doses of twenty minims each—two hours intervening between the first two doses, and one hour between the second and third. About half an hour after the second dose, the usual complaint was made of difficulty of keeping the eyes open from the heaviness of the lids. He saw things double, one image appearing beside the other. During this time the pulse did not appear to be much affected, remaining at 77 ; but after the third dose it became quickened, rising gradually to 96. About two hours after taking the third dose he got out of bed to go to the lavatory, being perfectly conscious. He reached the lavatory, but found himself then

* See *Monthly Hom. Review*, xx., 82.
† *Practitioner*, v., 200.
‡ *Lancet*, 1875-6.

powerless, and quietly sank first on his knees and then at full length. He was quite unable to raise his lids. His lower jaw dropped, and he could not articulate. He was put into bed, and some warm stimulating drink given him, when he soon became better. He told me when I saw him, with the most open-eyed simplicity, that the medicine had done him a great deal of good ; that he could make water very much better since he had had it (I should observe that he previously had suffered from the effects of a troublesome stricture) ; that he knew everything that was going on around him when he sank to the ground, but that he was unable to move, and that his feelings were like those which he had experienced after commencement of intoxication."

We have to enquire in what way Gelsemium produces these effects,—whether it acts upon the nervous centres like Conium, upon the trunks of the motor nerves like Curare, or upon the muscles themselves. The experiments on animals made by Dr. Bartholow point to the cerebro-spinal axis as the seat of the drug's action, and he is sustained in this view by Berger on the one side, and by Ringer and Murrell on the other. The provings of the last-named show that the pathogenetic effects begin to appear within an hour and a half after ingestion, and —unless repeated doses be taken—subside in about the same time. The whole action is therefore what is called functional.

The ocular phenomena occurring under the influence of Gelsemium require somewhat detailed study. They closely resemble, as I have said, those which Conium produces, but ptosis is more marked than defective power of accommodation of vision, and diplopia is far more frequent. This may be either transient or constant, and in either case seems to depend upon loss of power on the part of the sixth nerve, which (as you know) dominates the rectus externus, and is especially affected by the drug. Its paresis probably accounts for the confused vision so often mentioned by the provers, as in S. 152-159 of Allen's pathogenesis. The behaviour of the pupils seems at first sight somewhat contradictory. In poisoning cases they are dilated and insensible to light. Drs. Ringer and Murrell found the same condition set up by dropping the fluid extract or a solution of gelsemia into the eye ; but the internal employment of the drug, in the moderate doses used by them (a drachm of the tincture), caused the pupils to contract. This would at first seem like an opposite action of large and small doses. But the observations of Dr. Tweedy suggest a different explanation.* He found the application of the alkaloid to cause at first ciliary (not conjunctival) injection, with slight contraction of the pupils : then ensued dilatation, whereupon the hyperæmia disappeared. This looks

* *Lancet*, June, 1877, p. 832.

rather as if the contracted pupil were connected with an approach to congestion of the ciliary vessels, and corresponds with that which obtains in iritis and apoplexy. In connection herewith we may note the pain in the brows and eyeballs experienced by several of the provers, and by none more than those of Ringer and Murrell, in one of whom it extended to the occiput, with a sensation as if the crown of the head were being lifted off in two pieces. No such sensations are felt under the influence of Conium ; and, with the weight and oppression of head and limbs so often mentioned, they forcibly suggest that our present drug, besides being a paralyser, is also somewhat of an inflamer, its action not going indeed beyond congestion, but certainly reaching so far.

Such being the physiological effects of Gelsemium,—to those with whom *contraria contrariis* seems an axiom, it at once suggests itself as a remedy for muscular cramp and spasm : and without doubt there are certain ephemeral conditions of this kind in which we may, with advantage, avail ourselves of the antipathic action of the drug. Thus it has effected speedy relaxation of hysterical trismus, of laryngismus stridulus, and of rigidity of the os uteri during parturition. I have myself the highest opinion of its efficacy in simple dysmenorrhœa, and in after-pains, both of which I suppose to be spasmodic in their nature. (I must add, however, that Dr. Guernsey finds it of great value—and in the doses in which he gives it the medicine cannot act otherwise than as a similar—when during labour a cutting pain extends from before backwards and upwards, and is so violent that it impedes the natural pains.) But for spasm of long standing, or of frequent recurrence, we should greatly prefer a homœopathically-acting remedy ; and, on the other hand, should prescribe Gelsemium rather in paralytic conditions. The enuresis of old persons, from weakness of the sphincter vesicæ ; the corresponding state of this and its fellow muscle in debilitated subjects, which shows itself by a tendency to involuntary micturition or defæcation upon emotional impressions ; loss of voice during menstruation, and the post-diphtheritic paralysis of the parts about the throat, and of the eyes and body generally,— all these morbid conditions have yielded to its use.

No less beneficial is its influence in disorders corresponding to its congestive action. The following case of Dr. Madden's illustrates what it can do when the head is thus affected :— " A gentleman had constant, gradually increasing headache for three or four months ; dull, heavy pain, extending to the nape of the neck, frequent throbbing in the temples, and ver-

tigo on rapid movement. I gave Gelsemium, a drop of the
mother-tincture night and morning. For thirty-six hours the
headache markedly increased after each dose; then a sudden
throb like a snap took place in the centre of the head. The
headache at once and entirely ceased, and has not since
returned." Another headache which calls for this medicine is
a sensation as if a band encircled the temples, which goes off
after copious urination. The cerebral congestion of Gelsemium, as also its headache and vertigo, is seen especially in
depressed conditions of system, and causes inability to concentrate the thoughts. It is passive rather than active. In
spinal congestion, I have (as I have mentioned in my *Manual
of Therapeutics*) had results so striking and constant from the
use of Gelsemium, that the medicine and the malady have
become inseparable in my mind.

In affections of the eyes, Gelsemium displays the same
double kind of action which we have seen in the sphere of the
nervous system. Its paralysing influence makes it an apt
remedy for ptosis, and other affections due to loss of power
on the part of the ocular muscles. Among the testimonies
in its favour, I may cite that of Dr. Vilas, of Chicago, who
says* :—" Gelsemium has been of great value in my hospital and private practice in cases of this nature. Morbid
states which failed to respond to other means have been
ameliorated or cured by it ; and electricity has ceased to be
the specific for such troubles." It rivals Conium here, and
exceeds it when affections of deeper parts are the cause of
the loss of power, as in diplopia of central origin.† But
Drs. Allen and Norton have carried the use of the drug a
step farther, viz., to inflammatory affections of the retina and
choroid. Retinitis albuminurica, coming on during pregnancy, chorio-retinitis, in which there seemed to be a bluish
snake before the vision, and serous choroiditis, have been
cured by them with it ; while the latter physician has put on
record several cases of recent detachment of the retina, in
which it seems to have greatly aided in recovery.

In therapeutics, as in pathogenesy, it is the motor nervous
system which is the main sphere of action of Gelsemium. It
must be observed, however, that it is as remedial of toothache
and neuralgia that it has of late found place in the practice of
the old school.‡ It is not easy to understand its action here
upon the antipathic principle, as it is only in toxic doses that

* *American Homœopathist*, i., 5.
† *Brit. Journ. of Hom.*, xxxiii., 569.
‡ *Monthly Hom. Review*, xx., 80.

it affects sensibility. Dr. Ringer found this unimpaired in the subjects of his drachm doses of the tincture, whether generally or in the gums. But, he writes, " one patient, on both occasions on which I experimented on him, complained spontaneously of a numb pain and a little tenderness along the teeth and the edges of the gums of the upper jaw." Dr. Douglass long ago observed the occurrence, under its use, of neuralgic pains. "In my own provings," he says, " I frequently experienced a succession of acute, sudden, darting pains, evidently running along single nerve-branches, in almost every part of the body or limbs, sometimes so sudden and acute as to make me start. At one time, a quick succession of these pains coursed down the outside and front of the tibia for about half an hour, leaving a line of considerable tenderness marking its track." Both he and Dr. J. C. Morgan esteem it very highly in neuralgia, and, while the former speaks of "pretty large doses " as being required, the latter gets excellent results from dilutions like the 5th and 12th. He mentions " indistinct or double periodicity as indicating it."

Another important action of Gelsemium is in the sphere of the circulation. In persons sensitive to its influence Dr. Douglass states that he has repeatedly seen it produce a decided febrile chill with subsequent re-action. It is thus on the homœopathic principle that it prevails as a febrifuge, of which it is one of the most potent. It is not in the acute fever of Aconite, with its agonized restlessness and burning thirst, nor in the delirious heat with dry tongue of Baptisia and Belladonna, that Gelsemium proves beneficial. Its fever is much less active ; the patient's condition is rather torpid and heavy ; the pulse is not very rapid, and inclines to be full and soft ; the tongue has a moist white fur. The main symptoms are those of languor and oppression, with dark crimson face, and dull pains in head, back, and limbs,—the head feeling large and full. Such a fever is no uncommon effect of a chill, and sometimes presents itself in connection with the exanthemata, (especially measles, in which Gelsemium may the more appropriately come in, as it has caused the peculiar rash of this disease). Whenever you meet with it, give Gelsemium in place of Aconite, and you will have every reason to be satisfied with it. From clinical observations, moreover, I am disposed to consider the remittent type of fever as that to which Gelsemium is specially applicable. Whether this would hold good with malarial remittents, I cannot say ; but Gelsemium is one of the many medicines which have repute in the treatment of ague. I have especially in my mind the remittent fever of childhood, for which, on the recommendation of Dr. Ludlam, I have used Gelsemium instead of Aconite for many years past. I know that it is now denied that the "infantile remittent" is a pathological entity. Still, whatever it may be, it is a clinical reality; and it is a great thing to have a remedy which breaks it up as surely as Baptisia does with gastric and Aconite with synochal fever. This Gelsemium effects; and wherever such type of fever manifests itself, having marked exacerbation towards night, and decline of the heat *without perspiration* towards morning, the medicine may be given with sure benefit.

These are the leading forms of disorder in which Gelsemium plays a curative part. Other indications for it may be derived from a study of Dr. Hale's article, which shows it likely to be serviceable (among other things) in nasal and Eustachian catarrh, and in the inflammatory stage of gonorrhœa. Dr. Morgan praises it in sleeplessness from emotional disturbance, as when evening company is too stimulating to the brain.

The nearest analogue of Gelsemium is, as I have said, *Conium.* As an antipyretic it is allied to *Baptisia.*

The 1st dilution is that which I have always given for remittent fever; from the 1st to the 2nd for congestions. The 2nd and higher potencies have been used in paralytic and ocular affections, and for antipathic purposes small doses of the mother-tincture.

Glonoin

is the substance commonly known as nitro-glycerine, and valued for its explosive properties. It is the result of a mixture of glycerine with nitric and sulphuric acids, at an ice-cold temperature. The name Glonoin was formed by its introducer into medical practice, Dr. C. Hering, out of the chemical formula (Gl O NO^5) denoting its composition.

Dr. Hering proved Glonoin on himself and others in 1848, and the experiments were published in the following year. In 1853 Dr. Dudgeon instituted some further provings in this country, the record of which may be read in the eleventh volume of the *British Journal of Homœopathy.* An exhaustive collection of the symptoms thus obtained and of the cures effected by the drug may be found in Hering's *Amerikanische Arzneiprufungen,* and is translated in the *New England*

Medical Gazette for 1874-5. Dr. Allen has few symptoms to add to those herein contained.

The action of Glonoin lies within a very small compass. If any one will touch his tongue with a five-per-cent. solution, he will pretty certainly find in a few minutes that his pulse has increased by twenty, forty, or even sixty beats. He may feel a sense of throbbing all over his body, but will almost always experience it in the head, which will go on beating until a pretty violent bursting headache has developed itself. With this there will probably be some giddiness, a sense of fulness in the head and at the heart, and one of constriction about the throat. If he is sensitive to its action, nausea and vomiting may supervene, faintness may be felt, and even complete insensibility may ensue. Let me read you, in illustration, the record of one of Dr. Dudgeon's provers.

"In good health; pulse 60. At 9 p.m. took one drop of Glonoin, 1st dec., on a piece of sugar. In about half a minute perceived a throbbing of the temporal arteries, soon accompanied by a rather severe throbbing pain in both temples. In a few seconds more the pulse was found increased from 60 to 100, and the heart throbbing most violently and rapidly. In a minute or two a faint, warm, sickening sensation was perceived in the chest and stomach, resembling the threatenings of sea-sickness; also slight giddiness, especially on moving about. The throbbing pain in the temples continued to increase for about ten or fifteen minutes, then gradually diminished, and in about half an hour became considerably easier; the feelings of nausea and giddiness also were lessened; but on returning up stairs very fast, about three-quarters of an hour after taking the medicine, all the symptoms recurred with double force. The temples ached and throbbed excessively, and there was great nausea and giddiness. However, in a few minutes, there was an abatement of these sensations, but leaving slight nausea and throbbing pain in the temples.

"A supper of oysters and stout, at half-past ten, removed the nausea; but the pain in the temples continued, and was very readily aggravated by any exertion of walking, talking, or reading. Went to bed at twelve; had less pain in the recumbent posture, especially when lying on either side; slept well at night. On waking in the morning, felt slight pain, or rather uneasiness, in the temples, with tendency to nausea and giddiness, which have continued all day. Feel fulness of the temples, and very slight nausea, whilst now writing at 8 p.m."

What is the rationale of these striking symptoms? The sudden increase in the frequency of the heart's action may be caused either by direct stimulation of its substance or ganglionic nerves, or by depression of the influence of the vagi. The rapidity with which it supervenes, and the lack of tension in the pulse, lead one to ascribe it to the latter mode of action. That such depression is present is confirmed by Dr. Brunton's experiments on cats, in whom he found the third eyelids drawn half over the eyes "as in division of the vagi." On what, then, depend the head symptoms? At first sight they would seem secondary to the increased action of the heart. But this theory is excluded by the fact that in one of Dr. Dudgeon's provers the head was not affected at all, although the pulse rose very high indeed. We need a special action on the arteries themselves to account for the cerebral phenomena present. And for this we have only to suppose that Glonoin affects the neighbouring vaso-motor centre in the same manner as that of the pneumogastrics. The same sedative influence would then, through the inhibitory fibres of the vagi, set the heart off palpitating, and through the vascular nerves would dilate the arteries. In confirmation of this view, we often find the provers describing the sense of throbbing as felt all over the body, though especially in the head.

All this forcibly reminds us of Amyl nitrite, whose action we lately studied. But a little attention will show that the effects of the two drugs are not identical. Amyl causes a general flushing, without marked sense of throbbing or special localisation in the head; nor is the pulse much affected by it. Glonoin differs from it in all these points. Accordingly, it seems to have been demonstrated that Amyl produces its dilating effects on the arteries by directly paralysing their muscular coats, and acts similarly on other muscular parts ; while Glonoin affects the nervous centres of the circulation, and is limited to this sphere.

It is clear that, if the homœopathic principle is worth anything at all, Glonoin ought to be a remedy for some active disturbances of the cerebral circulation. It would not act, as Belladonna does, upon such congestive states as depend on irritation of the brain substance, and tend to inflammation. With Belladonna the circulation within the cranium is excited because the brain is irritated; with Glonoin the brain is irritated because the circulation is excited. But it would be indicated in such hyperæmiæ as can be produced by excessive heat or cold, by strong emotions, by mechanical jarring, by suppression of the menses or other hæmorrhages and excretions. The first and last of these causes come most frequently before us in connection with the drug, and demand special notice.

1. The cerebral hyperæmia of excessive heat is, in its full development, *sun-stroke*. For this casualty Glonoin has many a time proved a rapid and efficient remedy. It is not a malady often seen in this country; but I have obtained

striking benefit from the drug in its distressing after-effects. In minor degrees of the same trouble, in headaches brought on or aggravated by hot sunshine, and in those which occur in workers by gaslight, Glonoin is very effectual.

2. Perhaps the greatest boon which Dr. Hering has conferred upon patients in introducing Glonoin to medicine is the relief it gives to menstrual disturbance of the cerebral circulation. Every one knows the intense congestion of the brain induced in plethoric constitutions by sudden suppression of the menses. Glonoin is an exquisite *simillimum* here; for in one of Dr. Dudgeon's provers, who took it while the catamenia were present, these immediately ceased, and the headache went on increasing in violence till night. Glonoin is recommended by all under these circumstances, and there are cases on record illustrating its virtues. It is of course no less useful in minor degrees of the same condition. While thus helping the weaker sex during their menstrual life, it becomes especially serviceable as this draws to its close. It does not act, like Lachesis or Amyl nitrite, on the general flushings of the climacteric epoch; but it is most valuable when these are localised in the head. It was from a suggestion of Dr. Kidd's that I first began to use Glonoin for this common trouble, and I have since learned to place the utmost confidence in it. It is also very useful in the congestive conditions of the brain incident to pregnancy.

The consideration of the cerebral hyperæmiæ thus caused has illustrated the form of the disorder in which Glonoin is indicated. But we are of course not limited to such or similar origins in our applications of the drug. Whenever we see fulness of the head with throbbing of the arteries present, and are not led to Aconite or Belladonna (or their congeners) by fever or inflammation, we should think of Glonoin. It thus becomes a frequent remedy for headache. It was the statement of its discoverer, Sobrero, that " even a very small quantity placed on the tongue causes a violent headache of several hours' duration," which led Dr. Hering to investigate its action, Here again Dr. Brunton's experiments (which, I should have mentioned, are in the twelfth volume of the S. Bartholomew's Hospital Medical Reports), come in confirmation. " One of the most remarkable effects of nitroglycerine," he says," is the intense headache it produces, even in infinitesimal doses. . . None of the poison was taken by the mouth, and as it is non-volatile the amount taken in by the lungs must have been infinitesimal. It is possible that, as some writers suppose, a little of it was absorbed by the skin,

2 K

but the quantity thus taken must have been excessively minute." In his own case the headache was several times accompanied by vomiting. The kind of headache it produces has been already illustrated. Fulness, tension, throbbing, bursting—these are the phrases used by the provers to describe it; one of them felt as if he were hanging with the head downwards, and as if there was a great rush of blood thereinto in consequence. When headaches so characterised come before us we may look for the best effects from Glonoin. Dr. Coxe, of Philadelphia, has communicated some excellent illustrative cases, which may be read in Dr. Dudgeon's paper. The medicine is seen to act as rapidly in disease as in health, for in from five to twenty minutes all distress had ceased. As regards conditions, the Glonoin headache is increased by shaking the head or moving the body, and relieved by external pressure; but the patient cannot bear the head covered. In those more serious forms of cerebral hyperæmia which we call puerperal convulsions and apoplexy the place of Glonoin has hardly been determined. In the former there is much more than congestion of the head to be thought of: still, Glonoin may be and has been useful in relieving that part of the disorder. For the simple determination of blood to the head which sometimes precedes apoplexy Kafka says it is very effectual, and also for that which often occurs in softening and tumours of the brain.

In what has now come before us we see the main sphere of the action of Glonoin, and the kind and conditions of the same. The only other obvious application to practice of its pathogenetic effects was to use it for some forms of palpitation, which has been done with success. But Glonoin has had two episodes of old-school history. In 1858 its powers became accidentally known to my friend Mr. Field, then practising as a surgeon in Brighton, who communicated it to his brethren in the pages of the *Medical Times and Gazette* Some contradictory experimentation followed; but on the whole the effects of Glonoin were admitted to be identical with those observed by the homœopathic provers. It was not of course to be expected that the drug should be used therapeutically on our principle; it was given rather as a "sedative." In this capacity it manifested in many hands a striking power of relieving paroxsyms of neuralgia; and we have occasionally availed ourselves of its virtues in this direction. Whether it has any specific action in neuralgia I cannot say; but certainly cases have been relieved by the third attenuation, and some permanently cured. More recently, Dr. Murrell, whom I have often mentioned as co-operating with Dr. Ringer in his experiments, has had his attention directed to nitro-glycerine, and in the *Lancet* for January and February, 1879, has communicated some interesting observations of its action. He entirely confirms Mr. Field's experience of the potent effects of the drug, even when taken in a 1 per cent. solution (our first attenuation) ; and noticed in his own person the marked aggravation on movement which we have seen in the narrative of Dr. Dudgeon's prover. The sphygmograph showed considerable dicrotism of the pulse under its influence. Dr. Murrell was of course struck by the analogy between its action and that of nitrite of amyl, noticing this difference, that its full effect on the circulation took longer to establish, but was slower in departing. He tried it as a substitute for the amyl in four cases of angina pectoris, giving it (in doses increasing *guttatim* till ten or fifteen drops were taken at a time) regularly, as well as on the occurrence of the paroxysms. It acted less rapidly in relieving these, but, on the other hand, had a more permanently good effect,—the last report of all the cases speaking of almost, if not quite, entire freedom from their attacks.

Besides *Amyl nitrite, Hamamelis* (q. v.) has once at least acted like Glonoin on the head.

It has proved beneficial in all dilutions from the 3rd decimal to the 12th centesimal. The first and second decimals have been used, but are liable to aggravate.

Graphites

is plumbago, the black-lead of our pencils, in which form Hahnemann proved it, and the British Homœopathic Pharmacopœia directs it to be used. It is understood to be an allotropic form of carbon, with some small admixture of iron and silica. It is prepared by trituration.

A pathogenesis of Graphites appeared in the first edition of the *Chronic Diseases*, containing 590 symptoms. It was then proved by Nenning on several persons, and by Hartlaub. In the second edition of the *Chronic Diseases* Hahnemann incorporated the 200 symptoms thus obtained, and added a few from Rummel and Kretchmar and a number from his own observation, raising the total to 1,144. Dr. Piper subsequently proved it on himself, taking increasing doses of a one-fifth trituration, but his results were exceedingly meagre. You will find them in Allen.

In his preface, Hahnemann tells us that a German physician, Weinhold, when travelling in Italy, found black-lead used by the workmen in a mirror manufactory as an external application for herpes. He himself adopted the practice, giving the substance internally also; and wrote a book to record its success. Hahnemann was led to include Graphites among his " anti-psoric " medicines ; and its use in cutaneous disease, long obsolete in the old school, flourishes among homœopathists to this day. Dr. Hale has reported a remarkable case of eczema impetiginodes, of twenty years' standing, cured by it in the dilutions from the fifth to the 30th ;* and Bähr, who praises it highly in chronic eczema, also gives three cases of that troublesome disease, mentagra, in which it proved radically curative. I mention these, as easily accessible illustrations of its efficacy ; but if you hunt through homœopathic literature you will find numerous testimonies and narrations to the same effect. Dr. Bayes commends it in " psoriasis palmaris," which is, of course, a chronic eczema ; and suggests that the frequent occurrence of this complaint in domestic servants may have something to do with the black-lead used by them for fire-grates.

It is not easy to define the precise place of Graphites in skin disease. The presence of rhagades generally suggests it to me. Dr. Guernsey says that its characteristic symptom here is the exudation of a thin, sticky, glutinous, transparent fluid from raw places or sores. It probably exerts, like Arsenic, a general influence upon the nutrition of the skin, which may lead to varying effects, pathogenetic and curative, according to the subjects of its influence.

Graphites is also very useful in unhealthy states of the appendages and prolongations of the skin. Dr. Guernsey commends it for falling off of the hair and abnormal growth of the nails. He also speaks well of it in tinnitus aurium, with deafness which is improved by external noise : such an affection is probably due to a morbid state of the meatus or membrana tympani. Dr. Cooper uses it successfully in blepharitis ciliaris, where inflammatory symptoms are absent ; also in stillicidium lachrymarum, from obstruction of the nasal duct. Dr. Bayes ranks it with Aurum in crusts about the nostrils in scrofulous children. Dr. Marston has left on record a cure of fissure of the anus by it.

Beyond the cutaneous region, the best-established action of Graphites is on the ovaries and testes. Hahnemann himself recommended it for delayed menstruation, especially when

* *Brit. Journ. of Hom.*, xxviii., 353.

accompanied with great costiveness. I should mention, by the way, that for constipation itself Graphites is one of our main remedies : the stools are large and knotty, requiring much straining for their expulsion. The use of the drug in catamenial deficiency has become established among homœopathists. Dr. C. Wesselhœft has recorded* a series of cases showing its efficacy in this complaint and for its accompanying disorders. He thinks it especially suitable when the patient is on the wrong side of thirty, saying that Graphites is to the climacteric period what Pulsatilla is in youth. It is, perhaps, better when the menses are infrequent, scanty, and pale, than when they are altogether absent.

Dr. Dudgeon has lately given us an interesting account of the disappearance of an indurated enlargement of the ovaries themselves under its employment ;† and in their male analogues, the testes, Graphites has more than once proved curative of hydrocele. It is highly esteemed in indurations and cicatrisations of the mammæ consequent upon inflammation and abscess.‡

Graphites has lately been selected as the subject for the prize-essay of the Central Homœopathic Society of Germany, —the source from which we have had Reil on Aconite, Bähr on Digitalis, and Sorge on Phosphorus. The successful essayist on this occasion is Dr. H. Goullon. I have not yet been able to get access to his work ; but from some extracts from it translated in the *North American Journal of Homœopathy* it appears to be so complete a collection of clinical experience with the drug, that it can hardly fail to enlarge our knowledge of its use.

Graphites may be compared in its respective spheres with *Pulsatilla ;* with *Arsenic ;* and with *Alumina* and *Plumbum.*

It appears to act almost equally well in substance and dilution,—from Weinhold's twelve-grain doses to the lower triturations employed by Bähr, Cooper, and Marston, and thence to the twelfth dilution of Dudgeon, Hale, and homœopathists generally.

I have now to speak of

Gratiola.

This is the Gratiola officinalis, the common "hedge-hyssop."

* *N. Engl. Med. Gazette*, xi., 459.
† *Brit. Journ. of Hom.*, xxxi. 183.
‡ *N. Engl. Med. Gazette*, xi., 334; and Guernsey's *Obstetrics* 3rd ed., p. 475.

The homœopathic tincture is prepared from the whole plant in the usual manner.

A pathogenesis of Gratiola appears in the *Arzneimittellehre* of Hartlaub and Trinks. Of its 604 symptoms, 72 are warranted by Trinks himself, and 10 are taken from authors: the remainder are from the copious " Ng." But, in addition to this, we have some excellent provings of the drug in full doses, which have been translated from the *Archiv* (xvii, 165) by Dr. de Moor in the third volume of the *Révue de la Matière Médicale Spécifique ;* where also will be found the history of its previous uses. Dr. Allen adds some symptoms from Lembke.

The general knowledge about the physiological action of Gratiola is summed up by Pereira in saying that it " is cathartic, emetic, and diuretic, acting in large doses as an acrid poison." Its dynamic action appears limited and uncertain. Some provers took gtt. xx—l of the tincture, and gr. x—xx of the dried plant, without appreciable disturbance of health. The few genuine and frequently recurring effects of the drug seem worth noting here, as so little is known about it. They are—

1. Determination of blood to the head, with heat and somnolence.

2. Sense of coldness on the vertex, changing to heat.

3. Pain in the occiput on early waking, relieved by rising or lying prone.

4. Sensation in the face as if it were swollen.

5. Objects, even green ones, appear white (after S. 1.).

6. Every morning for weeks swelling of the upper lip, disappearing after a few hours.

7. Teeth ache from cold.

8. Great distension of the stomach after meals.

9. Great somnolence and lassitude after meals.

10. " Pressure at the pit of the stomach, as from a stone rolling from side to side, with cramp-like drawing which mounts into the chest ; at the same time frequent urgings to vomit and eructations ; this condition lasts several days, and is always worse after taking food [four days after] " (*Trinks*).

11. Diarrhœa, greenish yellow and watery.

12. Constriction of and itching at anus.

13. Great rectal and anal irritation, with passage of fœtid mucus.*

* In animals poisoned by Gratiola, Orfila occasionally found the rectum inflamed, even when the drug had not been introduced into the alimentary canal.

14. Burning in urethra after urinating.

I may add a quotation from Taylor (p. 515). "A series of cases observed by M. Bouvier are reported by Orfila, in four of which the plant was used, under the form of a decoction, as an enema. The result was that in one instance violent vomiting and purging, with syncope, was induced, and in all a strong attack of nymphomania. In other cases there was constriction of the throat, with hydrophobic symptoms and convulsions."*

Gratiola, employed in the past to remove " visceral obstructions," and so relieve mental diseases, dropsies, &c., has fallen into disuse in the common practice ; nor has it yet found any defined place in homœopathic therapeutics. It is unmentioned by Hempel, Bayes, Guernsey, and Espanet. Teste only seems to have some practical acquaintance with it. He says—" Gratiola will be found particularly useful in cases bordering upon such as would, by their symptoms, unequivocally point to Chamomilla. Gratiola would seem to be to chronic affections what Chamomilla is to acute. In nervous diseases for example (such as mania, nymphomania, delirium tremens, &c.), and in neuralgic affections caused by the prolonged abuse of coffee, Gratiola often renders good service. I have often given it after Causticum : this seems to be its antidote."

As to dose, it can only be said that less than twenty drops of the tincture failed ordinarily to affect the healthy system.

My last medicine to-day is one not unfamiliar to you,

Guaiacum.

Our tincture is a solution of the gum-resin.

The proving of Guaiacum appeared in the fourth volume of the *Reine Arzneimittellehre*, where it has 29 symptoms from Hahnemann, 113 from three fellow-observers, and 3 from authors. Guaiacum appears also as an antipsoric in the second edition of the *Chronic Diseases ;* but only 15 additional symptoms are credited to it.

I can but refer you to the list of symptoms given by Hahnemann in these records. There is little in them of a

* Referring to the original, I find that in one of the cases the nymphomania was permanent. The last sentence is (not very correctly) based on the following of Orfila:—" In a fifth case, there was added to the *fureur utérine* a spasmodic constriction of the throat, with hydrophobia, convulsions, and death in two days."

significant character.   So far as they go, however, they make
it probable that Guaiacum is homœopathic to some of those
rheumatic and gouty pains for which it has so long been
employed.   Dr. Phillips likewise (though I know not on what
authority), summing up the effect of large doses, says—" Stiffness, of a rheumatic character, is felt in the nape of the neck
and the small of the back, with pains in the bones of the legs,
the limbs feeling as if swelled ; darting pains, apparently of a
rheumatic neuralgic character, extend also from the feet to the
knees."   Hahnemann recommends it in " gouty lancinating
pains in the limbs, especially in contractions produced by
tearing, shooting pains in the limbs, the pains being excited
by the slightest motion and accompanied by heat in the
affected parts, especially when the patient had been injured
by the abuse of Mercury."

We are here reminded of the *quondam* repute of the decoction of the Guaiacum wood in syphilis, which gave it the
name of "lignum vitæ."   It is quite discredited now ; and
probably Hahnemann hit the nail on the head when he cited
the ancient saying, " *Luis venereæ mercurius antidotum, mer-
curii guaiacum.*"

The only observation Dr. Allen has added to those of
Hahnemann is one in which a decoction of six ounces of the
wood in half a quart of water was drunk, and produced
" violent spasmodic inflammatory affection of the air-passages,
especially the larynx, with such violent palpitation of the
heart that suffocation seemed imminent."

Of late there has appeared some evidence that Guaiacum
specifically affects the throat.   It has been recommended by
some writers as abortive of quinsy ; and one of our American
colleagues speaks highly of it in diphtheria.   It is esteemed by
some also in dysmenorrhœa, I presume of rheumatic origin.
It is a medicine deserving, I think, of further investigation.

The mother-tincture, which Hahnemann recommends, will
probably have to be given in most cases.   In diphtheria it is
best administered in warm milk.

HAMAMELIS, HELLEBORUS, HELONIAS, HEPAR SULPHURIS.

Our first medicine to-day is another precious contribution from America to our remedial store, the witch-hazel,

Hamamelis Virginica.

We prepare a tincture from the bark.

A proving of Hamamelis conducted by fourteen persons, mainly with the attenuations, was presented to the American Institute of Homœopathy at its meeting in 1874 by Dr. Wallace McGeorge, and is published in its Transactions for that year. All other knowledge of the pathogenetic and curative effects of the drug is collated by Dr. Hale in the article upon it in his *New Remedies*. You will also find the results of Dr. McGeorge's experiments in Allen, with those of ten other provings or observations.

Hamamelis has long had a popular reputation in America, and is the basis of a patent medicine known as " Pond's Extract," which is largely used as an anodyne application to injuries. Dr. Hering, being in attendance on the proprietor of this preparation, was led to test its real virtues. Dr. Okie did the same, and reported his results in a letter to Dr. Hering published in 1853. Dr. H. C. Preston had already, in 1851, proved the drug on himself, and found it cause marked determination of blood to the head and chest, with epistaxis. The latter symptom was observed upon another, and metrorrhagia in two female subjects.

Dr. Preston was naturally led to use Hamamelis as a remedy for hæmorrhages. But he found it to be no less efficacious in affections of the vessels from which the blood proceeded. It had already been commended for piles : he now used it, internally and externally, for varicosis of the legs. Its next application was to phlebitis, and here also it succeeded excellently well. He was thus led to consider the drug as acting specifically upon the venous system, and, in a series of papers in the *North American Journal of Homœopathy* (1853), developed and illustrated this doctrine. Dr. Ringer, who vouches for the remedy, does well in putting Dr. Preston's name forward as the chief authority for its virtues.

The three leading forms of venous disorder are phlebitis, varicosis, and hæmorrhage.

1. In simple phlebitis you can hardly put too much confidence in Hamamelis. It acts even better than Pulsatilla, which has great virtue here. Dr. Preston commends it for phlegmasia alba dolens ; but I think that it will often cause disappointment there. The lymphatics are, I take it, more frequently at fault than the veins in that disease.

2. In the various forms of varicosis Hamamelis is the prince of remedies. In varicose veins of the leg you will be delighted with the way in which the first or second dilution will ease the pain, while the external application of the diluted tincture will cause the dilated vessels to shrink up. Varicose ulcer of the leg may be healed by similar treatment ; to which also varicocele and circocele have often yielded. It is good for varicosis of the throat, where the parts look bluish from distended veins, and there is more or less discomfort, with pain on swallowing, and hawking of mucus with blood. Such a throat is often seen in gouty subjects. But it is in this same condition at the other end of the digestive tube, viz., in hæmorrhoids, that Hamamelis has won its greatest triumphs. I have cured case after case of "bleeding piles" by the internal use of this medicine ; and indeed can safely say that in an experience of it dating some seventeen years back, I have never failed with it. Numerous testimonies to the same effect are to be found in Dr. Hale's article ; and we can now add to them that of Dr. Ringer, who says that he has found it singularly successful and prompt in arresting bleeding from this source, even when excessive and amounting to half-a-pint a day, repeated almost daily for months or years. It not only checks the bleeding, which by itself might not always seem beneficial; but does so in the only way in which a homœopathic remedy can act, namely, by removing the proximate cause. Even where there is not much bleeding Hamamelis will cure piles, if they are a local manifestation of a general tendency to varicosis.

3. We are thus led to the use of Hamamelis in hæmorrhages generally, for which mischance it is perhaps more frequently indicated than any other remedy. The general

evidence of those who have used it agrees with that of Dr. Preston, that it is in venous hæmorrhages, where the blood flows steadily and without expulsive effort, that Hamamelis is likely to cure. I have myself also suggested* that it is more suitable when the state of the vessels leads to the hæmorrhage than where this is dependent upon altered composition of the blood itself. If this canon be true, it defines the place of Hamamelis in purpura. There are many cases on record showing its efficacy. I have myself seen more than one ; but I think that in all the vessels and not the blood itself were at fault. Dr. Ringer speaks of being disappointed with it in epistaxis occurring in a lad with the hæmorrhagic diathesis ; where, perhaps, the same explanation will hold good. Otherwise, this form of bleeding is remarkably under its control, as also are hæmatemesis, melæna, and hæmoptysis of passive and venous type. Dr. Ringer has known it arrest hæmaturia in four cases which had resisted many other remedies, and to check the oozing of blood which sometimes goes on for weeks after delivery. Dr. Dyce Brown finds it very successful in uterine hæmorrhage generally.† It has also cured vicarious menstruation, and helped much in the treatment of dysentery. I have myself used it in most of these affections, and have so much confidence in its power that I would never be without it in my pocket-case.

If you ask me what is the rationale of this hæmostatic power of Hamamelis and other medicines of ours, I can only answer that it is but an instance of the general homœopathic principle. They cure hæmorrhages because they cause them. Hamamelis certainly does not owe its virtues to the tannin which, like many other barks, it contains ; for it acts well as high as the second and third dilutions, whose very infinitesimal proportion of tannin could hardly prove astringent.

The only other sphere of action in which we know Hamamelis to be capable of vigorous work is that of the generative organs. . Its potent pathogenetic influence on these, in the male subject, was first brought to light by that indefatigable prover, Dr. Burt. He experimented on himself with the drug in 1864 (as you may read in the twenty-third volume of the *British Journal of Homœopathy*), and suffered severely from neuralgic pains in the testicles, which—when strong doses were taken—were so intense as to compel him to discontinue

---

* *Brit. Journ. of Hom.*, xxiii., 256. I have there related a case where, in a sensitive subject, the administration of Hamamelis for epistaxis caused much dilatation and throbbing of the cerebral vessels.

† *Monthly Hom. Review*, xiv., 473.

the proving. Sometimes the pains migrated suddenly to the stomach, causing nausea and faintness. They were accompanied by frequent emissions, and much hypochondriacal depression and irritability. The latter symptom was very marked in Dr. McGeorge's provers.

Dr. Okie had already used it successfully in ovaritis; and Dr. Burt gives three cases of what he calls "ovarian neuralgia" cured by it. The first was probably of a subinflammatory nature: the second and third may have been pure neuroses. But the most important testimony to the value of the medicine in ovarian affections is that of Dr. Ludlam. I quote from his excellent *Lectures, clinical and didactic, on the Diseases of Women* (p. 138). "During the summer term of lectures for the year 1864, I called attention to the efficacy of the hamamelis virginica in ovaritis. The remarkable effects of this remedy, locally and internally, in orchitis led me to infer that it would also be useful in some forms of ovaritis. I have prescribed it in numerous cases with remarkable results. It seems appropriate to the subacute attacks of this disease which are incident to pregnancy and menstruation. In the former case, I have no question of its power, in some instances, to prevent abortion, where such a mishap threatens in consequence of ovarian irritation and inflammation. In the latter, it allays the pain and averts the menstrual derangement which is so liable to follow. It is also useful in gonorrhœal ovaritis, in which variety the suffering is sometimes extreme. This affection bears a close analogy to the gonorrhœal orchitis of the male, in which Hamamelis is also specific." In this last affection Dr. Franklin also, in his *Science and Art of Surgery*, commends it. It probably has a similar action on the whole genito-urinary apparatus. Dr. Payne, an "eclectic" practitioner in America, states that in large doses it causes in women violent contractions of the vagina, and a smarting, burning sensation, followed by pruritus : in men he has known it produce irritation of the urethra, and a discharge, with ardor urinæ. With apparently unconscious homœopathicity he recommends it for the cure of these very conditions. It ought to be useful for gonorrhœa occurring in the female. Dr. McGeorge, in the clinical observations he adds to his provings, speaks warmly of its power, when applied locally, to give permanent relief to vaginismus. It is also attaining a good deal of reputation in dysmenorrhœa (especially, Dr. Pattison says, in the form of hamamelin) : it is probably where this trouble depends upon ovarian irritation that it is beneficial.

There are several points about the action of Hamamelis which lead me to think it likely to prove a useful remedy in gout ; but I must reserve this part of the subject until I have been able to develope and test it further.

The only true analogue to Hamamelis is *Pulsatilla.*

I have generally used the 1st decimal in acute hæmorrhage ; the 1st and 2nd centesimal in other cases.

Our next medicine to-day is the Christmas rose,

Helleborus niger,

of which we prepare a tincture from the fresh root.

The proving is in the third volume of the *Reine Arzneimittellehre*, and contains 92 symptoms from Hahnemann, 162 from eight fellow-observers, and 34 from authors. The latter describe mainly the drastic properties of the plant. The provings do not seem to have been very heroic, judging from a letter of Hahnemann's to Stapf, cited by Dudgeon (*Lectures,* p. 189), in which an eighth of a drop of the tincture is ordered to be taken every hour or two until some violent effects are experienced. Dr. Allen adds a thorough proving by Lembke, and several other observations and experiments.

The black Hellebore seems to have been occasionally used (as an adjunct to or substitute for the Veratrum album) by the Greek physicians in the treatment of mental disorders.* They supposed it to act by its evacuant properties ; but it is probable that it had some specific influence. Hahnemann makes the following remark in point : " I infer from various observations that stupor, an obtusion of the inner sense (*sensorium commune*)—imperfect and heedless sight, although the eyes are perfectly good, imperfect hearing, although the organ of hearing is perfectly sound, imperfect or no taste, although the organ of taste is in good condition, constant or frequent absence of thought, want of recollection of the things which have just taken place, indifference, light slumber without the sleep being refreshing, desire to work without having the power or attention necessary to do anything—is a primary effect of Hellebore." Knorre has reported a cure of melancholia following typhus by it, and recommends it in the same condition occurring in girls at puberty.† I should mention that the condition of brain found *post mortem* in the subject

* So Hahnemann says ; but Dr. Hamilton *(Flora Homœopathica)* considers that it was the H. officinalis they employed.

† *Brit. Journ. of Hom.*, xii., 478.

of S. 80 among Hahnemann's "Observations of others" must not be supposed to have been caused by Hellebore, as the man was a melancholic.

But the chief use of Hellebore is in the various forms of dropsy. Hahnemann gives, as one of his own observations (S. 66), " sudden dropsical swelling of the skin ;" and remarks upon it—" This symptom, with others belonging to the kidneys, appears to show that Hellebore will be a great remedy in certain dropsical affections." The renal symptoms referred to are among those of his fellow-observers,—

S. 104. Abundant urination, without much urging (*Langhammer*).

S. 105. Frequent urging to micturate, and scanty emission (*Ibid*).

S. 106. Emission of a quantity of watery urine (*Stapf*).

The opposite character of the first two, though occurring in the same prover, is explained by the fact that the scanty urine with urging was observed within the first four hours after the dose, the abundant and free passage of the secretion twenty-four hours after it. This precisely corresponds with later observations, which show that one of the glucosides of Helleborus—helleborein—is a diuretic to animals, but causes hyperæmia of the kidneys. Thus the primary effect of Hellebore would be to congest the renal organs and diminish their secretion ; while, as the effect was passing off, an opposite condition would obtain. Now this is just what we have in post-scarlatinal dropsy, where the drug has gained its chief laurels. There is a general *consensus* of testimony to its value here, Dr. Bayes being the only one who speaks of disappointment.

Hellebore is also occasionally used with benefit in other dropsies, as in that left behind by intermittents, and in the ascites of scrofulous children.* But the question of main interest is as to what it can do in hydrocephalus. It produced marked congestion of the brain in Lembke and another ; and its other glucoside—helleborin—causes paralysis in animals, the cerebral meninges being found after death congested, and the substance diminished in consistence and showing extravasation. It would thus be homœopathic to the second stage of encephalitis ; while its power over serous dropsies elsewhere might well extend to the cranial arachnoid, making it useful in such cerebral effusions as occur from

* See *Brit. Journ. of Hom.*, x., 124.

insolation, after typhus, or from the retrocession of mumps or the exanthemata. In chronic hydrocephalus it might well aid the constitutional remedies—Sulphur, Calcarea, and such like—on which we mainly rely. All these are well-attested uses of the drug; but whether it can help in true tubercular meningitis is another question. It is recommended for it, in the stage of effusion, by all the older homœopathic writers; but those of later date seem to have less confidence in it. I have tried it several times myself, in varying dilutions, but never with any benefit.

In all these dropsical affections, very scanty and dark-coloured urine, depositing a sediment like coffee-grounds, is given by Dr. Guernsey as "characteristic" for Helleborus.

The only other sphere of action of Hellebore is the ovario-uterine. Pereira says that it stimulates the pelvic circulation like Aloes, and is an emmenagogue. In the female animals poisoned by helleborein the mucous membrane of the uterus was always found congested. It has some repute among homœopathists in amenorrhœa.

The medicines most allied to Helleborus are *Apis, Apocynum, Cantharis,* and *Kali bromatum.*

The medium and higher dilutions have been those most frequently used; but Dr. Phillips states that he gets excellent results in post-scarlatinal dropsy with ten or fifteen-drop doses of the tincture. I should say that I am indebted to his book for the facts about the glucosides of the plant.

We have now once more to turn to America, which sends us a medicine whose importance is growing upon us of late, the

Helonias dioica.

A tincture is prepared from the root; and the concentrated preparation, helonin, is triturated for our use.

A full account of Helonias is given by Dr. Hale in his *New Remedies.* You will do well to supplement his remarks by reading the excellent article on the drug by Dr. Samuel Jones in the twenty-second volume of the *North American Journal of Homœopathy,* who presents us also with a full schema of its pathogenetic effects, to which Dr. Allen has little to add.

Dr. Jones is one of the two chief provers of Helonias. He took three ounces of the mother tincture and a scruple of helonin in the course of a week, and noted the results at the time and subsequently. It had been reported as beneficial in diabetes and Bright's disease ; and he was desirous to ascertain whether it would cause sugar or albumen to appear in the urine. He found neither ; but he did get an excess of urea, to the extent of a sixth part of the normal amount. At the same time his urine, which was apt to be alkaline, and to deposit amorphous phosphates, became acid, even after a meal; and the phosphatic deposition ceased to be anything more than an exceptional occurrence. During the time, and for twelve days afterwards, he was weak and irritable, and full of aches and pains. Then all these left him, and for a week he felt unusually well. But, he writes, "on the nineteenth day after the last dose had been taken a profound depression of spirits supervened. I was filled with the most abject despair." This condition continued nearly two weeks ; and then, three weeks later, he "became ' bilious,' sleepy during the day, head dull and stupid, poor appetite, food had no taste." He thinks that at this time an examination of the urine would ·have shown a *minus* of urea ; but, strangely enough, he omitted to make it.*

I have dwelt fully on these phenomena, as Helonias has gained a considerable reputation as a "tonic," and it is interesting and important to ascertain its action in health. I cannot think that the "bilious" condition occurring seven weeks after omitting the drug had anything to do with it ; but the depression of the fourth and fifth week seems fairly traceable to its influence. Dr. Burr, the other chief prover of Helonias, who took smaller doses, experienced the same feelings from the fifth day of his proving. He says little of debility, but nothing of increased strength ; and Dr. Jones was decidedly weakened by the drug, so that the healthy reaction subsequently was keenly enjoyed. The changes in the urine have hardly yet received their interpretation.

Helonias, accordingly, may fairly have its "tonic" action explained upon the principle of similarity ; and, judging from the cases Dr. Hale relates, it need not be given in large doses. Its action is compared by all who have used it to that of iron. It possibly acts on the blood-making processes, and may be useful in chlorosis and anæmia where iron disagrees. I once cured an exquisite case of chlorosis with it with considerable rapidity. Dr. Jones (and also Dr. Carroll Dunham) speaks well of it in such mental depression as follows over-dosing

* I have received a letter from Dr. Jones, acknowledging the justice of my rejection of this last group of symptoms, and explaining the omission of testing at the time.

with bromide of potassium ; and no less so in post-diphtheritic debility.

The local actions of Helonias are on the kidneys and the uterus. In the former pain and weight are experienced, and a sensation of burning, as if the kidneys were two bags of hot water; there is also increased urination. The drug has not been proved npon women ; but Dr. Clark, of Portland, states that in six or eight female patients to whom Helonias had been given in the first decimal dilution there occurred " pain in the lower part of the back, through to the uterus, like inflammation, piercing, drawing." The breasts also swelled, and the nipples became sensitive and tender. Finally uterine hæmorrhage set in, and continued till the medicine was given up. Upon the male subject it has acted as an aphrodisiac.

Correspondingly, the chief use of Helonias has been in renal and uterine affections. It is reported curative in phosphatic urine, urinary irritation with impotence, diabetes, and albuminuria : it reminds one here of Phosphoric acid. From its power over affections of the womb it has obtained the appellation of " uterine tonic." In prolapsus, menorrhagia, leucorrhœa, and other atonic states of this organ—even when causing sterility or tendency to miscarriage—it seems really possessed of very great curative virtues. I can hardly claim these uses of the medicine for homœopathy, as it is a stimulant rather than a depressant to both urinary and sexual organs. Dr. Hale would bring in his " secondary homœopathicity " here, arguing that all stimulation is followed by subsequent relaxation ; so that Helonias is primarily homœopathic to renal or uterine irritation, and secondarily to atonic conditions of the same organs. But I must maintain (as I have done in my fifth lecture) that such " secondary homœopathic " action is essentially antipathic; and, if really curative, only shows that *contraria contrariis* as well as *similia similibus* plays a part in specific medication.

Dr. Jones thinks that the key-note of the subjective symptoms of Helonias is " amelioration while doing something." " The headache," he says, " disappears when the attention is engaged. The pains vanish when one is busied. The sense of profound debility is lost when exercising. When one turns from the book and goes into a half reverie then comes the headache. When one sits purposeless then come the burning-aching pains. When one feels as if he could scarcely drag one foot after the other he is astonished to find that the sense of rest is gotten, not by lying on the couch, but by walking."

I have already mentioned the analogy between the virtues of Helonias and some of the effects of *Phosphoric acid* and *Ferrum.*   As a uterine remedy, it most resembles *Stannum.*

The mother tincture of Helonias, and the 1st decimal trituration of helonin, have generally been used.

My last medicine to-day is one of the old Hahnemannian stock, the calcic sulphide,

Hepar sulpnuris.

It is prepared for homœopathic use by " mixing equal parts of finely-powdered clean oyster-shell and quite pure flowers of sulphur, and keeping the mixture for ten minutes heated to a white heat in a crucible hermetically closed." These are Hahnemann's own directions ; and the resulting compound is plainly a sulphide of calcium.   The potencies are made by trituration.

A pathogenesis of Hepar appears in the fourth volume of the *Reine Arzneimittellehre,* containing 282 symptoms from Hahnemann, 16 from two fellow-observers, and 10 from authors— of which 8 are effects of the sulphuretted waters of Neundorf and Aachen.   In the *Chronic Diseases* another pathogenesis appears, in which the last-named symptoms are omitted, but others are added by Hahnemann himself, raising the number to 661.

The term Hepar sulphuris—" liver of sulphur "—appears to have been given in old time especially to the sulphide of potassium.   The virtues ascribed to this drug, however, so closely correspond as far as they go with those of our own calcareous compound, that we may fairly use them in connection with it.   Again, since sulphuretted hydrogen is unmistakably evolved when Hepar is brought into a state of solution, it must share in the pathogenetic properties of that gas and inherit its repute as a remedy.   Lastly, being a compound of the two great constitutional medicines, Sulphur and Calcarea, itself becomes an agent of the same character, having points of resemblance to each of its elements.   Like Sulphur it affects the skin, and like Calcarea the glands.   It is, however, far more like the Sulphur than the Calcarea it contains.   That the other alkaline sulphides act much in the same manner, and that in the *Materia Medica Pura* Hahnemann treats of Sulphur and Hepar together (though giving their pathogeneses separately), is sufficient to indicate this.

But, like many other compounds, Hepar is something over and above its constituent parts; and strikes out (so to speak) an action of its own. I think that Hahnemann pretty closely defined the nature of this action when he recommended the drug as an antidote to the effects of Mercury. In the first instance, indeed, he used it to neutralise mercurial influence chemically, as converting the metal into an insoluble sulphide; and gave largish doses accordingly,—in one bad case three grains every hour.* Later, however, he seems to have recognised a dynamic antidotal virtue in it; and his indications in this direction have been so frequently acted upon with success that there seems little doubt of their being well founded. They have lately received some valuable illustrations from Dr. Bryce, of Edinburgh.† He finds Hepar (which he gives mainly in the sixth trituration) of great use in the treatment of non-patent forms of mercurial poisoning, i.e., in the sufferings of those who have used blue-pill, calomel, and such-like medicines largely or frequently without actual mercurialisation having been induced. The congested livers and follicular throats, as well as the general ill-health, of such patients he shows to be greatly benefited by a course of Hepar. Now for a drug to be a dynamic antidote, in minute doses, to a chronic medicinal disease, it must act upon the principle of similarity; and the symptoms induced by Hepar sufficiently resemble those of Mercury to support the inference drawn from therapeutics. Hepar accordingly has affinities with Mercury, as well as with Sulphur and Calcarea; and its range of influence is consequently a wide one.

Before proceeding to special therapeutics, let me say a word about the general characteristics of the drug. These are well put forward by Dr. A. K. Hills, in a paper which you will find in the Transactions of the American Institute for 1872. Depressed and irritable frame of mind (Dr. Bryce always found this present in the mercurial hepatic disorder cured by it); pains of a bruised and sore feeling, the part affected being very sensitive to touch; craving for sour and strong-tasting articles; difficult expulsion of stools and urine; the patient very chilly, and very sensitive to cold air, which will (e.g.) bring on his cough immediately—these are the principal points he specifies. Dr. Bryce found his patients much affected by change of the weather to damp.

The most important application of Hepar resulting from its analogy to Mercury is its use in *suppuration*. The power

* See *Lesser Writings*, p. 156, 186.
† See *Brit. Journ. of Hom.*, xxxiv., 489.

of the latter to induce suppurative inflammation is well
known ; and its employment in inflammatory states of the
organs it influences when matter threatens to form is as
obvious as it is successful.   Hepar acts similarly (Hahnemann
has observed it to cause suppuration of the axillary and inguinal glands), but it goes farther.   It will often check suppuration when impending :* but, when it is inevitable, it has
wonderful power in promoting it, and conducting it to a
speedy termination. "Drs. Allen and Norton think the result
dependent on the potencies employed ; the higher check suppuration, the lower promote it." This has been the doctrine
and practice of the homœopathic school for many years ; and
testimony to its soundness has now been given by Dr. Ringer.
The later editions of his *Handbook* reiterate the statements
made by him on the subject in the *Lancet* for February, 1874.
He recommends the use of the sulphides to prevent or mature
suppuration generally, for unhealthy ulcerations, for boils and
carbuncles, for those indolent subcutaneous swellings which
may be called scrofulous nodes, and for suppurating scrofulous
glands. He prefers the sulphide of calcium to the others, and
finds the eightieth of a grain generally sufficient as a dose,
though sometimes giving the tenth.

You will not hesitate, moreover, to act on these principles
when more important organs are involved. Dr. Bähr speaks
of " brilliant cures " of pneumonia with Hepar, when the
exudation had become purulent; and cites one which bears
out his commendations.   Twenty weeks after the commencement of a pneumonia, treated allopathically, his advice was
sought for the patient, a boy of six.   " The child was exceedingly emaciated, had a slight hectic fever, was constantly
troubled by a sometimes spasmodic cough, with purulent and
fœtid expectoration, diarrhœa, and loss of appetite.   The
right side of the thorax had become considerably hollowed, the
left was abnormally bulging; on the right side the percussion-
sound was perfectly empty, with intense bronchial respiration
and slight râles   We diagnosed pleuro-pneumonia of the
right side, with absorption of the pleuritic exudation, but
continued presence of the pneumonic infiltration in a state of
purulent dissolution.   After various ineffectual remedies, the
child was finally put upon Hepar, third trituration, with such
excellent results that in eight days already the hollowing of
the chest was considerably less.   In about four weeks the
right lung had almost been restored to its normal condition,
and the curvature of the thorax had entirely disappeared, so

* See *Brit. Journ. Hom.*, vi., 233.

that the child now looks perfectly straight and thoroughly sound and healthy." He recommends the drug also in empyema, which was possibly present in the foregoing case. The use of Hepar in pleurisy, however, has mainly lain on the other side of suppuration, viz., in copious plastic exudation into the sac of some long standing. Wurmb praised it highly here, and Dr. H. Gross has put on record a striking case of cure by it after some months' interval, which you may read in the eighteenth volume of the *British Journal of Homœopathy*.

2. Hepar next follows Mercury in acting on the *liver*. Of its value here we have the fullest account from Dr. Bayes. "Those chronic states of engorgement of the liver," he writes, "inducing great abdominal distress from their interference with the return of blood through the vena portæ, are greatly benefited by a course of Hepar sulphuris. . . . Hæmorrhoids arising from this source are readily cured by this medicine. The obstruction to the abdominal venous circulation often gives great distress to the patient, preventing the abdominal respiration, and hence inducing oppression of breathing. In other cases it induces obstinate constipation, from a congested condition of the veins in the rectum." He gives from the third decimal to the sixth centesimal attenuation. I know that other practical physicians have the same confidence in the power of Hepar to relieve engorgement of the liver and portal system; though Dr. Bryce thinks this to hold good only when the hepatic derangement is traceable to mercurial influence. Hæmorrhoids were among the affections for which sulphuretted hydrogen was given of old; and the pathogenesis has some icteric symptoms.

3. We now follow the line of the Sulphur which enters into the composition of our medicine, and find it influencing the *skin*. Like Sulphur itself, it can cure scabies by its lethal influence on the acarus when locally applied*; but Hahnemann points out that it is also homœopathic to the eruption. " Others besides myself," he writes, " have observed an eruption produced very similar in character to the itch ;" and again, " baths impregnated with sulphuretted hydrogen excite the same itch-like eruption, in the flexures of the joints especially, which itches most at night." Hepar thus becomes suitable for several other eruptions of papular or vesicular character, and Dr. Guernsey thinks this location in the flexures of the joints, as in those of the elbow and knee, a special indication for it. He also recommends it in crusta lactea and intertrigo, when " the eruption spreads by new pimples appearing

* See *Brit. Journ. of Hom.*, xxvi., 46.

just beyond the main disease, which finally become incorporated with it." Dr. Hills thinks it indicated when the skin is unhealthy, so that it chaps and becomes sore at the least provocation. In the old school it is coming much into vogue as an internal remedy for acne. My chief experience with it has been in the local eczemas incidental to certain employments, as the "grocer's itch," and the "psoriasis palmaris" of those who have to handle much mineral matter. It is often beneficial in the treatment of ulcers, especially when of scrofulous origin, and having the characteristic sensitiveness of the drug.

4. But, next to its power over suppuration, the most important action of Hepar is that which it exerts upon the *respiratory mucous membrane.* The conjunctiva is, as we have often had occasion to remember, an offset of the commencement of this tract : and in its affections Hepar plays an important part. It is very useful in blepharitis, especially when the meibomian glands are much involved, and in acute phlegmonous inflammation of the lids. Its influence seems to penetrate to the cornea. Dr. Peters, in a *Treatise on Diseases of the Eyes,* has collected many recorded instances of its value where this membrane was affected; and you may there see how often it has cured cases where onyx, hypopyon and prolapsus iridis were present, and also what power it has over recurring ulceration of the cornea in ophthalmia scrofulosa. Drs. Allen and Norton fully confirm its value in every form of keratitis save the syphilitic, mentioning great photophobia and relief of pain by warmth as characteristic of it. Then it acts upon the ethmoid cells at the root of the nose, where Hahnemann's recommendation of it when boring headache is present has often been verified : the pain comes on, he says, every morning, and lasts from 7 to 12 o'clock. It has less influence on the nasal mucous membrane itself, but acts powerfully on that of the larynx and trachea. Hahnemann pointed out that pathogenesy indicated Hepar and Spongia as the cardinal remedies for croup ; and they remain so to the present day among most homœopathists. There is a general agreement in the canon laid down for its employment by the late Dr. Elb, and excellently illustrated by Dr. Hale,* that it is after resolution has been initiated by Aconite or Spongia, so that the breathing has a rattling rather than a sawing sound, that Hepar is useful. The same principles, *mutatis mutandis,* apply to less formidable affections of the larynx. Dr. Guernsey speaks of its cough as a choking

* See his *Lectures on Diseases of the Chest.*

one,—the patient, he says, " coughs into a choke." Dr. Bayes says that the " sensation as of a clot of mucus or of internal swelling when swallowing " (which is one of Hahnemann's original symptoms) is characteristic for it here ; and Dr. Hills says the same thing of the symptom, " sticking in the throat, as from a splinter, on swallowing, and extending to the ear on yawning." Swallowing ice, he says, will sometimes cause this feeling. Bähr recommends it also in croupous and Hempel in capillary bronchitis.

5. In a recent discussion on diphtheria at the British Homœopathic Society,* Drs. Drury and Leadam agreed in placing Hepar in the front rank of its remedies. The experience of these excellent physicians, and the tendency of the diphtheritic exudation to invade the larynx, would justify its full trial in the disease.

Dr. Guernsey agrees that whenever Hepar is indicated there will be found great sensitiveness to touch, draught of air, or other impressions on the senses. The presence of this symptom may often guide to its employment, as in whitlow when the patient dreads the least approach to the finger, in rheumatic headache when the pressure of the hat is intolerable, and so forth. Herein it resembles Silica, which is its analogue in relation to the suppurative process.

Besides *Sulphur*, *Calcarea*, and *Mercurius*, Hepar has a close analogue—especially in the respiratory sphere—in *Kali bichromicum*.

Dr. Ringer's experience bears out that of many of our own practitioners in indicating the lower triturations of Hepar as containing all its curative virtues. Dr. Bryce is the only one who prefers the 6th.

* See *Brit. Journ. of Hom.*, xxviii., 740.

LECTURE XXXIV.

HYDRASTIS, HYDROCOTYLE, HYOSCYAMUS, HYPERICUM, INDIGO.

We will begin this lecture, as the last, with one from among the American contributions to our Materia Medica, the golden seal,

Hydrastis Canadensis.

The tincture of the fresh and the triturations of the dried root are used in our practice.

Dr. Hale's article in his second edition contains two excellent provings of Hydrastis in substance by medical men (one of which—that of Dr. Burt—is omitted by Allen), and some experiments with the dilutions by a class of students. His fourth edition fairly summarises its curative powers.

It seems that the golden seal has long been in repute among the American Indians as an application to sore eyes and legs. It then came to be considered a "tonic;" and when taken up by the "botanic" practitioners of the country, was used largely by them as a "detergent" in chronic catarrh of the mucous membranes. It has not made its way into ordinary practice, being unnoticed by Stillé and the elder Wood; and the same silence regarding it prevails in the later treatises of the younger Wood and of our own Ringer. But it had long been in use among homœopathists even before their first public notices of it appeared, which were those of Dr. Hastings in the *British Journal* in 1860, and of Dr. Hale in the *North American* in 1858. Dr. Phillips' article contains a full account of the reputation it has gained in the school of Hahnemann, save as to its employment in cancer; and he endorses our estimate of its activity.

Hydrastis has been found to contain two alkaloids, on which most if not all of its efficacy depends. One, hydrastin, is of yellow colour, and is believed to be identical with berberin;

like it, it is " tonic " and " anti-periodic," resembling quinine also in causing ringing of the ears. The other, hydrastia, occurring in white crystals, seems to be that element of the plant which affects the mucous membranes. It is commonly used as a muriate ; and this—in the proportion of a grain to an ounce of water—seems the best form of the drug for local application.

1. Used thus, or as a weak infusion of the dried root, Hydrastis has a marvellous control over chronic catarrh of mucous membrane wherever situated. Dr. Hale and Dr. Phillips give each a long list of local disorders of this nature, in which they or others have found it curative. Their lists include syphilitic coryza ; all forms of sore mouth ; chronic angina ; leucorrhœa, both uterine and vaginal ; chronic conjunctivitis, otorrhœa, and ozæna. Both ecommend the coincident internal administration of the tincture ; and agree that in catarrh of parts which cannot be locally reached the latter alone is sufficient. Thus jaundice from catarrh of the bile-ducts has often yielded to it. Dr. Yeldham praises it as an injection in gleet ; and Mr. Clifton has excellently described* a form of dyspepsia calling for it, whose sodden-looking face, yellow slimy tongue, sour or putrid eructations and combined feeling of distension and empty " goneness " after meals unmistakably point to mucous flux of the stomach. In chronic nasal catarrhs Dr. Lucius Morse (who has written a useful little book on this disorder) esteems it very highly when there is accompanying atony of the digestive organs. Symptomatically, he finds it indicated by the frequent dropping down of mucus from the posterior nares into the throat—a hint of which I have more than once availed myself with advantage.

What is the rationale of this influence ? The provings suggests its being of homœopathic nature. Catarrh of the eyes and nose, with profuse thick white secretion, was Dr. Burt's most prominent symptom ; another had sticky mucus about the fauces, with a broad yellow stripe down his tongue. Dr. Hale writes :—" its action on all mucous surfaces is of a similar character. The natural secretion is at first increased ; then it becomes abnormal in quantity and quality. At first clear, white, transparent, and tenacious, it becomes yellow or thick, green, and even bloody, and nearly always *tenacious ;* so that the discharge may be drawn out in strings, as with Kali bichromicum."

The power which Hydrastis displays over catarrh and even

* *Monthly Hom. Review,* xvii., 157.

erosion of mucous membrane attends it also in the treatment of ulceration of the skin. In most forms of chronic ulcer its application is beneficial; and as a glycerole it is very healing to excoriations—as of the nipple, to fissures, and to intertrigo. Dr. Phillips has cured two cases of rodent ulcer with it, and Dr. Maclimont three of lupus,—by both the internal being recommended together with the external use. Dr. Jousset confirms this favourable experience with Hydrastis in lupus exedens, saying that it has procured him several cures even in advanced cases. He prefers it now to Arsenic. He also speaks of having obtained a "brilliant success" with it in a case of genuine leprosy, in the second (ulcerative) stage. He gave the mother-tincture internally, and applied locally a lotion of one part of the same to five or ten of water. His mode of using it in lupus is very similar. We have only the analogy of its action on mucous membrane to suggest that the curative influence here is specific and homœopathic.

2. The next great sphere of operation for Hydrastis is that weakened and congestive state of the lower bowel whose chief expression is *constipation*. The earlier writers on the drug in this country—Drs. Hastings, Rogerson, Bradshaw, and Bayes —all praise it here ; and I myself know no remedy so constantly efficacious. I agree with Dr. Rogerson in finding it most useful when the constipation is the fruit of sedentary habits, and of the frequent resort to aperient medicines. I have tried various dilutions and modes of administration ; but have found the best to consist in giving a drop of the mother-tincture in water before breakfast, at first every day, and then at increasing intervals. Dr. Phillips praises it in prolapsus ani and in hæmorrhoids,—Dr. Yeldham also in the latter trouble.

3. But by far the most interesting aspect of Hydrastis is its relation to *cancer*. It was first introduced—without name— in 1854, as a new remedy for this disease, by the late Dr. Pattison, who used it as an ingredient in the caustic paste with which he enucleated scirrhous tumours. Its internal use was taken up by homœopathic practitioners—ever foremost in seizing on any fresh means of aid to their patients, and in 1860 and 1861 Drs. Hastings and Bradshaw reported their experience with it, which was hardly favourable. But in the latter year Dr. Bayes, and in 1863 Drs. Marston and Macli-mont, were able to speak of much better results. The latter found relief of pain and improvement in general health nearly always following its administration ; and in some instances its conjoined external application as a lotion so improved or even

removed the symptoms that a contemplated operation was abandoned.

Here is one of their cases :—

" Mrs. F— had suffered for six months from a swelling in her left breast, for which she sought relief. The pain, which was compared to knives being thrust into the part, had become almost unbearable, and the patient was already beginning to assume that worn appearance so characteristic of the cancerous diathesis. The tumour, which had attained a considerable size, was hard, heavy, and adherent to the skin, which was dark, mottled, and very much puckered, the nipple being also retracted. The patient was at once advised to come into town in order to the enucleation of the tumour. This, however, her circumstances prevented; and without any expectation of affording much relief, a lotion of Hydrastis was ordered, with the internal use of the same medicine. The pain almost immediately ceased, and the tumour so speedily decreased in size that at the end of two months it had altogether disappeared, leaving but the puckered skin, which had otherwise regained its natural appearance. When we last heard of this patient she continued perfectly well. It is needful to state that her health rapidly improved during the treatment, and that her countenance regained the aspect of health."

Dr. Marston, writing a year and a half later,* says that this patient " has not again come under notice, though I have no doubt that she would have put in an appearance had anything occurred which would have called for our assistance."

To Dr. Bayes, however, we owe the best knowledge we possess of the power of Hydrastis over cancer. In papers in the nineteenth and twentieth volumes of the *British Journal of Homœopathy*, and in the third volume of the *Annals* of the British Homœopathic Society, he gives a number of cases treated by the drug both internally and externally. His final conclusion is that it has no influence over the cancerous dyscrasia as such, and is of little use in epithelial or uterine carcinoma; but that in scirrhous tumours developed in glandular structure—as in that of the breast—it is often of great value, through a specific influence upon the gland itself. When it fails in mammary scirrhus, it is generally found that the gland has become absorbed or deeply involved in the cancerous mass, so that there is little healthy tissue to act upon. Dr. Marston also assents to this theory ; and what makes it more probable is that Hydrastis has great power of dispersing simple glandular tumours of the breast. But however this may be, I think that these physicians express the general experience of the homœopathic body in this country; and that in suspected mammary scirrhus we are

* *Brit. Journ. of Hom.*, xxiii., 196.

well justified in withholding the knife or the caustic, and first
giving our patients the benefit of the local and internal use
of Hydrastis.

The present state of opinion among British homœopathic
practitioners as to the virtues of Hydrastis in cancer may be
gathered from two papers read within the last three years
before the British Homœopathic Society, with the discussions
following,—the report of which you will find in the eighth
volume of the *Annals*. One is " On the treatment of intractable forms of disease," by Dr. Gutteridge ; the other " On the
antecedent symptoms to local cancerous deposit," by Mr.
Clifton. You will see there that whilst some of our colleagues
have been disappointed in the remedy, several testify unequivocal confidence in it. Dr. Gutteridge says :—" I should
contend, led by my own experience, that the Hydrastis
treatment is the very best yet known for this dire disease.
. . It improves the appetite and condition of the patient
generally ; under its use the complexion alters, the state of
the blood improves. . . It marvellously allays the pain of
cancer, in this respect altogether surpassing opium, morphia,
or any so-called anodyne. It retards the growth of cancer."
Mr. Clifton calls attention to a group of symptoms which he
has often met with in patients who have afterwards developed
cancerous growths. They are those of "atonic dyspepsia"—
obstinate constipation, flatulence, pains in the bowels, kidneys,
and liver, &c., but without the altered tongue and the pain
after food generally seen in such cases. The complexion, too,
was not "bilious," but brownish or earthy ; and the skin was
generally dry or harsh. He has found the "dyspeptic" symptoms in these subjects quite unamenable to the usual remedies
of homœopathy, as to those of the ordinary practice ; but
since he has recognized their significance, and treated them
with more positively anti-cancerous medicines, he has had
very beneficial results. "I may say," he adds, "that Hydrastis
Canadensis has been found more beneficial than any other
drug ;" and I need hardly point out to you its appropriateness
to the condition he describes.

Another important testimony to the (at least) occasional
value of Hydrastis in cancer has been given by Dr. Kidd, in
the appendix to his recently-published *Laws of Therapeutics*.
" In an extensive practice during thirty years," he writes, " I
have been three times encouraged as to the possibility of
curing cancer." In two of the cases he refers to—incipient
scirrhus of the breast, of undoubted malignancy—complete
recovery took place under our present medicine.

Judging from Dr. Hale's book, our American *confrères* do not seem to have followed us in this application of the remedy we have derived from them. But a case is cited there from a Belgian source, in which an apparently hopeless scirrhus of the stomach occurring in an old man was so greatly influenced for the better by Hydrastis, that the patient enjoyed the rest of his life in tolerable comfort.

I have said nothing as to the rationale of the two latter uses of Hydrastis, for they cannot as yet be explained, either on antipathic or on homœopathic principles. We must know more about the physiological action of the drug, on various subjects and under prolonged use, ere we can theorise on the point.

The analogues of Hydrastis in its action on mucous membrane are *Pulsatilla, Kali bichromicum, Ammonium muriaticum,* and *Antimonium crudum.* On the lower bowel it acts like *Collinsonia, Aloes, Sepia,* and *Sulphur ;* and on the mammary gland like *Phytolacca* and *Conium.*

The dose, as has been seen, and as is evident from the quarters from which the praises come, need not be a very minute one ; though unquestionably the drug acts well in at least the lower dilutions.

A favourite indigenous Hindoo medicine now comes before us, which has become the property of homœopathy by being proved. I speak of the

Hydrocotyle Asiatica.

A tincture is prepared from the entire plant.

An article by Dr. Audouit, of Paris, containing a pathogenesis of the drug chiefly obtained from provings on his own person and observations on patients, appeared in the *Journal de la Société Gallicane* in 1856, and was (in substance) translated in the sixteenth volume of the *British Journal of Homœopathy.* This monograph—which, as reprinted separately,* I lay befcre you—constitutes my chief source of information regarding the drug.

Hydrocotyle. came to France from the east, recommended from both East and West Indies as a remedy for leprosy. The first to use it was a Dr. Boileau, of the island of St. Maurice, who has reported as the final result of his experience

* *Etudes pathogénétiques et thérapeutiques sur l'Hydrocotyle Asiatica.* Bailliere, 1857. ·

that in fifty-seven cases of this dire disease* treated by him with the plant, in all, without an exception, its progress was arrested. It is a curious comment upon his statement that he himself subsequently died of this very malady. Other Eastern practitioners, however, found good results from it; and it was tried in the Paris hospitals by Cazenave and Devergie. They could not say much of its power over the few cases of leprosy they had to treat; but they found it very efficacious in some chronic eczemas. Dr. Audouit himself reports cases in which it proved curative of lepra tuberculosa, lupus exedens, and chronic eczema impetiginodes. Altogether, there can be no question of the influence of Hydrocotyle upon the skin; and further provings and more extensive experience may define it.

The pathogenetic symptoms hitherto elicited are not striking. The drug evidently stimulates the cutaneous surface, causing redness, erythema, itching, and much perspiration; also there appears under its use increased secretion of urine, often with deposit. The nerves of sight and hearing, and the trigeminus, become hyperæsthetic; and there is decided irritation of the uterus, even to visible redness of the cervix. Acting on this last hint, Dr. Audouit has given Hydrocotyle with much success in granular ulceration of the neck of the womb, and in pruritus vaginæ. It ought to find a place in the treatment of facial neuralgia.

Dr. Salzer, of Calcutta, states that the repute of Hydrocotyle in elephantiasis led him to try it in a less obstinate thickening of the skin—acne rosacea, and with good effect. I have lately cleared a lady's face of a troublesome eruption of this kind with the drug, being led to it by the evident connexion of the acne with uterine disorder, which had now ceased.

Hydrocotyle reminds me somewhat of the *crude* action of *Silica* and *Lycopodium*, and of that of *Dulcamara*.

Dr. Audouit's usual dilution was the sixth; and this I myself used in the case I have mentioned.

My next medicine is the familiar henbane,

Hyoscyamus.

The homœopathic tincture is made from the herbaceous part of the fresh plant of the H. niger.

* Dr. Helmuth, in his *Surgery* (p. 136) says " lupus ; " but this is a mistake.

The proving of Hyoscyamus is in the fourth volume of the *Reine Arzneimittellehre.* It contains 104 symptoms from Hahnemann, 123 from six fellow observers, and 355 from forty-four authors. Most of these last are recording cases of poisoning; but Greding's observations were made on epileptics, melancholics, and maniacs, and hence—especially when the symptoms belong to the nervous system—must be used with caution. Hyoscyamus has also been proved by the Vienna Society, of whose experiments you may read an account in the sixth volume of the *British Journal of Homœopathy;* and by Dr. John Harley, as recorded in his *Old Vegetable Neurotics.* Dr. Allen, incorporating the above, adds some more poisonings and provings. Besides these sources of information, I may refer you to an exhaustive monograph on Hyoscyamus by Dr. Laurent, constituting one of the theses for the doctorate of the University of Paris (An. 1870, tome 7), and to some recent experimentation with the alkaloid hyoscyamine, carried out by Dr. Lawson, and recorded by him chiefly in the West Riding Medical Reports for 1875-6.

Toxicologists were wont to tell us that the virtues of Belladonna, Hyoscyamus, and Stramonium depend upon a common "active principle," and that their action is therefore essentially identical. I say "were wont," for they seem receding from the position of late. But when we turned to writers on therapeutics, we heard nothing more about the relation of henbane to these "deliriafacients;" but found it classified as a substitute for Opium in cases where the cerebral or intestinal influence of the latter drug is undesirable. If "contraria contrariis" be the rule by which it acts, one of these views must have been wrong. But as they are both founded on indubitable facts, the influence can only be that the "calming, soothing, and tranquillising effect" for which the drug is ordinarily administered is a homœopathic action. It is especially observed, Pereira goes on to say, "in persons suffering from great nervous irritability, and from a too active condition of the sensorial functions." He would have been more correct had he said that it is, in these only that it is observed.

Hyoscyamus has indeed nearly all the actions we have seen in Belladonna, though in a milder degree. It irritates the nervous centres, the mucous membranes, and the skin; but the functional excitement is only moderate, and the circulatory disturbance never goes on to inflammation. Indeed, when the drug is pushed, the phenomena are rather those of congestion with oppression of function. Hence the somnolence so often noted as resulting from it. It requires full doses to produce it—two ounces of the succus (according to Harley) or an equivalent quantity of hyoscyamine; and is accompanied with giddiness and weight across the forehead, flushed cheeks, and injected eyes. It is full of dreams, and is often broken by mutterings and slight jerkings of the limbs. Such a condition is totally different from natural sleep, with its cerebral anæmia. In cases of poisoning, the peculiar condition known as "coma vigil" or "typhomania" is sometimes induced; or a complete apoplectic coma may supervene.

When functional excitement predominates over vascular engorgement, delirium is induced. This is rarely furious; it is either a vivacious talkativeness with hallucinations of the senses, or a spiteful, quarrelsome moodiness. Dr. Lawson describes it as "a mental condition which partakes of all the leading symptoms of simple mania" in a "subdued form." There is no hyperæmia with it. "Muscular twitchings," says Dr. Harley, "and restlessness of the eyeballs are more frequently seen during the action of Hyoscyamus than with that of Belladonna." With this condition insomnia is always present.

The differential diagnosis of the three mydriatics in the treatment of head affections as recognised in the old school (at least as regards henbane) is fairly stated by Dr. Phillips; and precisely corresponds with what we have now seen as the physiological action of the drug. "In cases of cerebral hyperæmia the severer forms are removed by belladonna, while hyoscyamus proves its value when there is little or no congestion, but much excitement. So in the case of delirium; the forms of this disorder for which hyoscyamus is adapted are the milder and less inflammatory ones, whereas the severer cases are better dealt with by belladonna and stramonium. Hyoscyamus is specially useful again in those cases of delirium with hallucinations which are accompanied by little or no cerebral congestion, but where there is great excitability of the nervous system, and where there is reason to fear that the operation of opium would prove injurious."

The two types of cerebral disorder, accordingly, in which Hyoscyamus is useful are those occurring in fever and in delirium tremens.

1. Hahnemann himself, in relating his treatment of the fever—typhus and relapsing—which ravaged Germany after the campaign of 1813, speaks of Hyoscyamus as the suitable medicine when head symptoms became prominent; and it has ever since been the favourite remedy for this condition among

his disciples. It is exquisitely homœopathic thereto, as may be seen from this picture of Dr. Harley's :—" after one hour, pulse increased four beats ; sclerotic and conjunctiva a little injected ; the face—chiefly the cheeks—hot and flushed ; tongue dry and brown down the centre, the rest of the mouth very clammy ; much somnolency and giddiness." The urine always manifests an increase of urea, and of the phosphates and sulphates, just as during the action of Belladonna. Stillé also compares the somnolence with incoherent mutterings produced by Hyoscyamus to that which is so common in typhoid fever. It is the form of typhus which used to be called " febris nervosa versatilis " in which Hyoscyamus has proved most useful, with coma vigil and muttering delirium. It is also very helpful in the typhoid form of puerperal fever. Painless, and it may be involuntary, diarrhœa calls for it in the latter (and indeed in the puerperal state generally); and in both a key-note for the drug is that the patient will not remain covered.

2. The delirium of Hyoscyamus corresponds most nearly with that seen in delirium tremens. " The connexion," says Dr. Harley—and Dioscorides had noted the same thing before him—" between alcoholic intoxication and the effects of henbane on the cerebrum and motor centres is undoubtedly very close." The experiments of the Vienna provers show that the drug has the power also of producing the gastric mucous derangement so often present in this disease. It is an excellent remedy for it, calming the whole system and promoting sleep. It is also of use in nymphomania, in which the tendency to uncover the person is so strong ; and in puerperal mania. Dr. Phillips says that " in hypochondriacal monomania, when the patient suffers from such mental symptoms as syphilophobia, when really he has no reason to think himself the subject of any venereal taint, hyoscyamus will relieve the distressing despondency, and in many instances remove the hallucination." Hahnemann thinks that the delirium of Hyoscyamus closely resembles that of hydrophobia, to which it is undoubtedly homœopathic along the whole line ; but Belladonna and Stramonium, which act so similarly, have been hitherto selected in its stead. It is never curative in chronic insomnia, to which it acts as a mere palliative ; but it is useful where sleep is restless or too dreamful from cerebral excitement or feverishness.

Dr. Lawson has considerably added to our knowledge of the value of Hyoscyamus in cerebral derangements. He finds it of great value in " simple mania, characterised from the first

2 M

more by agitation than excitement, and due to the existence of obscure delusions and hallucinations ;" also in recent cases of chronic mania, and in the recurrent form of the disease, where the paroxysms present as their main features bodily restlessness, " an amiable but troublesome officiousness," and a destructive tendency. It is hardly less useful in the excitement of general paralysis, and in the incessant incoherent talking occurring in some forms of mania. The homœopathicity of the remedy to these morbid conditions is obvious ; and Dr. Lawson admits it in other words. " The succussion," he says, " produced in the mind already muddled with delusions and hallucinations by the antagonism of new forms of mental aberration, together with the subsequent deep and prolonged sleep produced, may tend to leave the mental state more composed after the artificially produced delusions and hallucinations have passed away." This is, like Trousseau's " substitution " and Dr. Harley's mutual interference of circles of water, merely homœopathy in other words. Dr. Hayward has lately shown us that such large and paralysing doses as Dr. Lawson employs are not always necessary,* and Drs. Ringer and Bury have found atropia and daturia—the alkaloids of Belladonna and Stramonium—to have quite as calming an effect in mania as hyoscyamine itself.†

I have mentioned, on Dr. Harley's authority, the frequent occurrence of muscular twitchings during the action of Hyoscyamus. Dr. Oulmont, of Paris, has lately published‡ some interesting observations upon its use in mercurial and senile tremors, and even paralysis agitans. Dr. Hammond, and also Dr. Lawson, praises it in the tremors of sclerosis of the nervous centres. We have long known its value in what might be termed "local chorea" in children, as squinting, stammering, twitching of the face, &c.; but this is an extension of its field of action which, being thoroughly homœopathic, we shall do well to follow up. Dr. Guernsey seems to consider jerking and twitching of the muscles, including those of the face and eyes, an actual " key-note " for the remedy.

The only other recognised use of Hyoscyamus in the homœopathic school is in the relief of cough. Hahnemann observed it cause dry cough at night, constant while lying down, but relieved on sitting up ; and such a cough is daily being eased by the drug, even in infinitesimal doses. Dr.

* Brit. Journ. of Hom., xxxv., 162.
† Practitioner. March, 1877.
‡ Ibid, x., 1.

Phillips transfers this use of it to his pages, and leaves it to be understood that it is as a " sedative " that it acts. But, if so, why this precision as to the kind of cough it relieves ? A sedative merely deadens nervous susceptibility, and would do so as readily were a cough nocturnal or diurnal.

Hyoscyamus may yet receive wider applications. Hahnemann says that it causes epistaxis and frequent catamenia, and refers to its repute in chronic hæmorrhages. He describes, moreover, a form of toothache in which it is remedial.* " It occurs," he says, " only from cold air, mostly in the morning, with rush of blood to the interior of the head, that makes the tooth loose with a formicating pain in it, and on chewing there occurs a sensation as if it would fall out, whilst at the same time there is a tearing pain in the gum." It is also worth noting that Wepfer, in a case of poisoning observed by him, records severe pains in the iliac region and in all the joints as having occurred ; while Schneller, one of the Vienna provers, experienced similar sensations. He speaks of drawing and tearing pain in the joints, especially in the wrists and knees. Stillé says that while general sensibility is, in most cases, very much impaired, there may at the same time be some neuralgic pains in the course of the principal nervous trunks.

In *Belladonna* and *Stramonium* I have named the only true analogues of Hyoscyamus.

As regards dose, Hahnemann recommended the 12th dilution, and those from the 1st to the 4th decimal have been much employed in later times. But Dr. Harley's experiments would indicate that the juice of henbane is not always a very active poison, as much as three ounces of the succus of the Pharmacopœia being necessary to develop its full physiological effects. I, however, have seen its dryness of mouth and throat supervene under the use of drop doses of the first dilution. There is probably a good deal of variability in the activity of the plant ; and it might be well to follow Dr. Oulmont's recommendation, and try whether the substitution of the alkaloid would give us as good results. Dr. Allen gives a separate pathogenesis of it. One eighth of a grain of hyoscyamine, according to Dr. Harley, has the same potency as three ounces of the succus ; and Dr. Oulmont gives it in granules each containing a milligramme (gr. $\frac{1}{65}$). Dr. Lawson's dose in mania is three-quarters of a grain, given once, and rarely repeated.

* *Lesser Writings*, p. 642.

I have next to speak of the S. John's wort,

Hypericum perforatum.

A tincture is prepared from the entire fresh plant.

A proving of Hypericum is recorded in the fifth and sixth volumes of the *Hygea*. Three women took each one dose of four drops of the mother tincture, and the effects lasted for some weeks. Several other persons have tested it, as you will see in Allen's *Encyclopædia*.

The S. John's wort was of some ancient renown in medicine. Dioscorides praised it for sciatica and agues. The following extract from Johnson's edition of Gerarde's *Herball* will show the account that was made of it in 1633. " S. John's wort with his floures and seed boyled and drunken, provoketh urine, and is right good against the stone in the bladder, and stoppeth the laske," whatever that may be. " The leaves stamped are good to be layd upon burnings, scalds, and all wounds ; and also for rotten and filthy ulcers. The leaves, floures, and seeds stamped, and put into a glass with oyle olive, and set in the hot sunne for certaine weeks together, and then strained from those herbes, and the like quantity of new put in, and sunned in like manner, doth make an oyle of the colour of blood, which is a most precious remedy for deep wounds, and those that are thorow the body, for sinewes that are pricked, or any wound made with a venomed weapon." He then describes a " compound oyle," prepared with Hypericum, white wine, and oil of olives and turpentine, which he says is the finest balsam in the world.

This repute of Hypericum as a vulnerary, after slumbering for some time, has awakened again in the homœopathic school. Its action on the nervous system, as inferred from the provings, led Dr. Franklin to use it in injuries involving the nerves ; and, in the large opportunities he enjoyed during the American war, he learned to place the utmost confidence in its use. You will find his recommendations in his *Science and Art of Surgery*. " Injuries of parts rich in nerves, particularly the fingers and toes, and the matrix of the nails;" open *painful* wounds, with general prostration from loss of blood, and great nervous depression ; and lacerated wounds— these, he says, are the special spheres of its action. He considers that it stands in the same relation to laceration as Arnica to contusion of the tissues. He recommends the higher dilutions internally, and locally one part of the tincture to twenty of warm water. Dr. Ludlam had previously published* two good cases of injury to the spinal cord benefited by Hypericum, and had suggested that it might prove to be the Arnica of the nervous centres.

My friend Dr. Edward Madden has made a short proving of Hypericum for me, taking at length as much as 260 drops of the mother tincture in the day. It had little effect save the diuretic one noted in the old herbal, and a few neuralgic shoots in the eye-balls and the right ulnar nerve. Dr. Brinckner experienced this last pain (but in the left arm) while proving the dilutions.

Time will not allow of my beginning upon Ignatia to-day, so I will in conclusion say the few words that are necessary about

Indigo.

The dye of commerce is triturated for homœopathic use.

Indigo has been well proved, in substance and the lower triturations, first by Professor Martin and his pupils, and then by Lembke. Their results, with a few other observations, make up nearly 590 symptons in Allen's *Encyclopædia*.

A feeling as if the brain were distending at the centre; epistaxis; toothache, of a rheumatic character; bloating of the stomach; and a good deal of irritation of the bladder, with mucus in the urine—these are the only noteworthy effects I can discover in the pathogenesis of Indigo. As a remedy, it has been used in the old school with occasional success in epilepsy and chorea. Teste states that he has cured with it some worm-fevers in children, and has found it of service in chronic catarrh of the bladder, and in urethral stricture threatening after gonorrhœa. It is a drug I have never myself used; nor has Espanet or Bayes anything to say about it. Dr. Guernsey mentions it once only, as indicated by burning in the mammæ during the menses.

* See *Brit. Journ. of Hom,* xvii., 523.

LECTURE XXXV.

IGNATIA, IODINE AND THE IODIDES.

We begin to-day with a medicine which owes its fame almost entirely to Hahnemann and his disciples, the seed of the Strychnos S. Ignatii, S. Ignatius bean,

Ignatia.

It is ordinarily treated with alcohol to form a tincture; but the results of Jörg's provings seem to show that a trituration of the bean would better preserve the virtues of the drug.

Ignatia was fully proved by Hahnemann himself, and 620 of the 795 symptoms ascribed to it in the third edition of the second volume of the *Reine Arzneimittellehre* are his. 121 of the remainder are from Jörg; they are marked " Hartlaub and Trinks," being taken from their compendium. They were obtained by the Professor himself and twelve of his pupils, who took doses of from 10 to 200 drops of the tincture, and from one to four grains of the powdered bean.

Ignatia contains a considerable amount of strychnia, more indeed in proportion than Nux vomica itself. It is doubtless to this alkaloid that it owes much of its energy. Yet strychnia could not take the place of either, nor could Ignatia and Nux vomica be given interchangeably. The study of the effects of our present medicine will show its own distinctive individuality, and this study could nowhere better be carried out than in Hahnemann's pathogenesis. He has bestowed special pains upon it, enriching it with notes and references between the symptoms; and his preface is full of important observations.

In poisonous quantities Ignatia simply produces tetanic spasms, and death by dyspnœa. But these phenomena are resolved into their elements by the symptoms resulting from smaller doses. Ignatia *exalts the impressionability of the incident nerves all over the body.* We have hence pains and other morbid sensations well-nigh everywhere; increased susceptibility of the special senses; emotional sensitiveness; and—probably from reflex excitation—twitchings, constrictions, and spasms. This action of the drug, however, is not deep and lasting. An alternating series of symptoms—numbness, torpor, depression —soon appear, which are themselves as superficial as their predecessors. The febrile symptoms which the drug causes have the same characteristics. Its chill is readily removed by external warmth; and its heat is unaccompanied by thirst. So is it with the mental and moral phenomena which occur. The sense of being in a hurry; the ready starting, irritability, impatience and querulousness which mark its first effect, often alternate with undue hilarity or silent melancholy.

These symptoms have naturally led to the use of Ignatia in the treatment of *hysteria.* Comparing the moral state it suits with that which indicates Nux vomica, Hahnemann says:— " it is not where anger, urgency, violence predominate, but where there prevail rapid alternations between hilarity and desire to weep." I do not say that Ignatia will follow hysteria into all its ramifications ; but it will remove many of its painful, spasmodic, and convulsive phenomena (some of which will come before us directly), and by its continued use will greatly improve the fundamental perversion of the nervous functions, especially the emotional instability. It is also of frequent service in other neurotic affections. Before Hahnemann's time it was in use for epilepsy, when brought on by violent emotions. He agrees that in a first attack so caused, when assuming a threatening aspect either on account of its duration or rapid recurrence, it may even be permanently cured by a single small dose : this his own experience confirms. He says, moreover, that epileptic fits which only occur after chagrin or grief about a moral wrong, and never appear from any other cause, may be prevented by the drug. But he cannot allow that chronic and settled epilepsies are ever curable by it. This " chagrin " (that is, sense of offence) is a *causa mali* to which he thinks Ignatia specially adapted, when it affects persons who are not in the habit of breaking out into vehemence or of seeking revenge, but who keep it concealed and dwell upon it in their recollections. But when fright or grief are the exciting emotions Ignatia has been found hardly less useful. It is often of service in the eclampsia of children* or of puerperal women, when thus caused or from reflex irritation, where the phenomena are spinal rather

* See Dr. Hirsch in *Brit. Journ. of Hom..* xxvi., 221.

than cerebral.   In neuralgia, also, it has found a place.   This
is excellently characterised by Gerson in his article on the
therapeutics of prosopalgia, which you will find translated in
the twentieth volume of the *British Journal of Homœopathy*.
Its neuralgia is that of hyperæsthetic patients, which nevertheless is borne patiently, or at most with quiet weeping ; it is
not deeply rooted, and often alternates with pain of the same
kind elsewhere.   Dr. Nankivell has communicated a striking
cure of sciatica with it.*

Ignatia also causes, and has cured, several local affections,
though probably acting always on the nervous elements of the
part.   It readily excites headache, especially a pressive aching
in limited spots, shifting from one to the other.   Sometimes
the concentrated pressure is described as if from a pointed
body, and resembles the "clavus hystericus," in which the
medicine has often been found useful.   In the fifteenth volume
of the *Monthly Homœopathic Review* you will find a graphic
picture of the headache of Ignatia, by Dr. Shuldham :   it is
of course accompanied with great impressionability of the
senses, and frequently passes off with the evacuation of a
large quantity of pale limpid urine.   At its height it is often
agonising ; there is restlessness then and chilliness throughout.
Then there occurs a peculiar disturbance of vision which
Hahnemann compares to the "spurious vertigo" of Herz : "a
circle of white, shining, flickering zig-zags when looking out
of the line of vision ; the letters at which one looks becoming
invisible, and those which are close by becoming so much
more bright."   In the throat Ignatia causes a sensation as if a
lump were there ; there is a sore pain when swallowing, but
between the acts of deglutition the lump is felt most, and
there is then (and then only, Hahnemann says) a sense of
sticking.   Nervous sore throats so characterised are readily
cured by the medicine ; the "lump" is no real swelling.   A
peculiar feeling of weakness at the pit of the stomach was
complained of by more than one of the provers ; and this is
said by Hahnemann to be a characteristic symptom of Ignatia.
The great formation of flatulence which is noted is a frequent
hysterical symptom.   Then we observe in several of the
provers a remarkable tendency to prolapse of the rectum at
stool.   This trouble when occurring in children, and also proc-
talgia in sensitive adults, has often been removed by Ignatia.
Dr. Hirsch finds it no less useful in constipation from weakness of the lower bowel ; and confirms the general impression
of its usefulness when ascarides infest this part.   The menses

* *Monthly Hom. Review*, xv., 30.

are premature and profuse. There is itching of the skin, of which Hahnemann observes that it is characterised by ready disappearance after scratching. Sleep is absent, or very light, or prevented by startings.

Besides the epilepsy I have mentioned, Hahnemann found Ignatia in use for intermittents. His own observations led him to lay down that " only those forms of ague can be cured by it which are characterised by thirst during the cold, and absence cf thirst during the hot stage."

Chamomilla, Coffea, Nux vomica and *Stramonium* are the general analogues of Ignatia. It is, like the first-named, pre-eminently a women and children's remedy.

The medicine seems in favour alike with those who use infinitesimals and those who prefer more substantial doses.

We shall be engaged during the rest of our time to-day (and perhaps longer) with Iodine and the iodides.

Iodum

(as it is now called) is prepared for homœopathic practice in a saturated alcoholic solution, which contains about one tenth part of the drug, and is reckoned as 1x in making the subsequent attenuations. These should be freshly prepared whenever the drug is to be employed in acute disease.

The extensive use into which Iodine soon came after its discovery in 1812 led to a rapid accumulation of observations as to its physiological effects. It was soon selected for proving by Jörg, who, with five of his pupils, took it in doses of from half a grain to two grains. The symptoms thus obtained were collated by Hartlaub and Trinks in the second volume of their *Arzneimittellehre*, and a few added as observed by themselves and Schreter. Hahnemann had already published in the first edition of his *Chronic Diseases* 153 symptoms of his own as caused by the drug ; and in the second edition he incorporated these with the collection of Hartlaub and Trinks, and some new observations from Gross and von Gersdorff, making 724 in all. Of this total 348 are from authors. Some of Hartlaub and Trinks' citations are effects of iodide of potassium—Kali iodatum ; and of these Hahnemann has not availed himself. We must therefore go back to their work for them ; and we shall also find there a separate pathogenesis of the compound, apparently from provings, but without name or other indication of origin. It contains 383 symptoms.   Dr. Allen, in accordance with his usual practice, gives separate pathogeneses of Iodum and Kali iodatum, under these headings respectively.   He omits from the former all Hahnemann's citations from authors, on the advice of Dr. Hering, strengthened by the investigations regarding them with which I have been able to supply him.   On the other hand, he supplies numerous fresh observations of undoubted validity.   His pathogenesis of Kali iodatum is chiefly made up of collections from periodical medical literature, and so far is excellent; but it is, in my judgment, marred by the admission of the more than dubious symptoms furnished by Dr. Houat, in his *Nouvelles Données.*   I must warn you against accepting as genuine any effects of the drug warranted by this writer only.

For the general literature of Iodine, I would refer you, besides the articles in Stillé and Ringer, to Dr. Cogswell's *Essay on Iodine and its compounds;* to a collection of "Observations on the curative and noxious effects of Iodine," by Dr. Wilcox, in the first volume of the *Annals;* and to a "Study of Iodine," by Dr. Madden and myself, in the twenty-first volume of the *British Journal of Homœopathy.*   In this last you will find references to authorities for any unsupported statements I shall make on the present occasion.

You will notice that I have spoken of Iodine and of its compound with potassium in the same paragraph.   I have done so advisedly.   I am quite unable to see any difference *in kind* between the physiological effects of the two substances; although the presence of the alkali undoubtedly modifies these as regards force and frequency of appearance, and makes a considerable difference in practical use.   Chemistry points in the same direction.   M. Sée* justly argues that Iodine must necessarily unite with sodium in the stomach and potassium in- the blood, and circulate so compounded throughout the frame; so that to give Iodine is virtually to give an alkaline iodide.   On the other hand Professor Binz† has shown that when iodide of potassium reaches the tissues it is decomposed, and free Iodine liberated.   The presence of protoplasm and of carbonic acid is all that is necessary to effect this change, as he has demonstrated by experiment.‡   Kämmerer

* *London Medical Record*, i., 757.
† *Practitioner*, xii., 15.
‡ No such decomposition takes place when bromide of potassium is similarly treated, and we have already seen that the compounds of Bromine with the alkalies have an action entirely different from that of the pure substance, and requiring separate discussion.

had been previously led to the same conclusion; but Stillé justly points out that only a small proportion of the iodide undergoes this decomposition, the greater part escaping unchanged by the urine, and therefore—unless it has destructive work to do, of which more anon—being literally wasted. Thus the ultimate effect of giving iodide of potassium is to supply free Iodine to act on the living matter of the body; and we may speak of the effects of either as belonging to the action of Iodine. The chief difference is that the local irritant influence of the metalloid is greatly diminished by its union with the alkali, so that large doses can ordinarily be introduced through the stomach without resentment on the part of that organ. A good many of the noxious effects of Iodine noted by the older observers arose from its being given in simple alcoholic solution. Such a tincture, unless largely diluted, would precipitate the drug on entering the stomach, and leave it there in substance to irritate the mucous membrane as we all know it does the skin. Hence the violent gastro-enteric irritation, the vomiting, colic and diarrhœa, which Hahnemann cites from many authors. Those who, like Coindet and Gairdner, used the drug more carefully had no such accidents; and since iodide of potassium has been the form of administration they have been rarely seen. The "iodism" observed by such therapeutists belongs either to the nervous system or to the distant tissues, as we shall see presently : it is set up subsequent to absorption.

What, then, are the remote effects of Iodine when introduced into the circulation and diffused through the frame?

1. They are, first of all, *irritative* in nature. The peculiar form which iodic irritation takes is best studied in its most frequent seat—the upper portion of the respiratory mucous membrane. "There is first noticed," says Dr. Ringer, "some slight running at the nose, with occasional sneezing, and a little frontal headache; these symptoms become more marked, when the conjunctiva of the eyes is injected, and the tears abundantly flow.* The loose tissues about the orbit become swollen, reddened, and œdematous, while occasionally a peculiar rash appears on the skin of the face. . . . The nose is sometimes reddened, especially at the tip, and is at the same time rather swollen. The rash has not always the same look. It is often very much like acne, and is always hard, shotty, and indurated, but the papules may be broad and large, and covered with what looks like a half-developed vesicle or pus-

---

* This conjunctival irritation may go on to acute œdematous inflammation with chemosis, as observed by Ricord.

tule." Some instances of the occurrence of this coryza—always from Kali iodatum—are collected in the twenty-third volume of the *British Journal of Homœopathy ;* where you will find it noted of the watery nasal discharge that it feels cool, and causes no excoriation, herein differing from that of Arsenic.

Erythema, with œdema, of skin and mucous membrane are the phenomena here presented to us ; and we see it going on to infarction of glandular structure in the acne of the former, and to copious flux in the latter. Similar effects may at times be seen from the drug over the whole cutaneous surface, and in nearly every part of the mucous tracts. There is a stomatitis incident to its use, accompanied with desquamation and ptyalism. Angina is a characteristic symptom of saturation of the system with it. Besides the gastritis and enteritis of its local influence, there is a gastric—and also an enteric—catarrh occasionally resulting from small doses, and seen after introduction of the drug into the circulation otherwise than by the stomach.* It seems under these circumstances largely eliminated by the peptic glands, and may cause their degeneration in the process, as in a case of Rose's cited by Boehm (Ziemssen, xvii., 296). The lower portions of the respiratory tract exhibit signs of the same irritation that we have seen in the upper. In the larynx and trachea we may have hoarseness, aphonia, and chronic inflammation, even simulating laryngeal phthisis ; and while the bronchi are but moderately affected, the lungs show the influence of the drug by congestive oppression, hæmoptysis, and even pneumonia. The genito-urinary tract is the only part which seems to resist its action. The skin manifests it sometimes in such inte.ise erythema as that described by Dr. Inman,[†] or, more commonly, in eruptions of acne or of pustules, and, more rarely, of bullæ.[‡]

Nor does the iodic irritation limit itself to skin and mucous membrane. Serous membrane also feels it, if the effusion into pleura and peritoneum found in autopsy means anything ;—Wallace also noting that, among his patients who took full doses of iodide of potassium for syphilis, several had acute pain over the left false ribs, with cough, dyspnœa, and fever.[§] Glandular structure also is very frequently affected. The first result is stimulation to increased action, whence we have the salivation and diuresis‖ often noted, and the increase

* See Stillé, ii., 850.
† *New Theory and Practice of Medicine,* p. 270.
‡ Stillé, ii., 853.
§ *Lancet,* 1835-6, i., 9.
‖ In children albuminuria has more than once been produced by its external application.

of the biliary and pancreatic secretions, as observed (among others) by Jörg's provers and by Gairdner. The testes feel its influence in increase of sexual appetite, and the ovaries show it in menorrhagia. The ultimate effect is either chronic inflammation, as recorded by Christison of the liver and by Sée of the kidneys, or atrophy, of which the mammæ and testicles are the subjects. The last result of the action of Iodine has been much doubted by recent writers; but their scepticism only arises from ignorance of the older observations. Hahnemann cites some of these; and to every one he mentions I could add two others. Diminution in the functional energy of the ovaries makes it probable that these organs are similarly affected,—barrenness having occurred from the use of the drug in young females previously prolific, and the menses being often suppressed.

Whether the lymphatic glands are similarly influenced by Iodine is a question of much interest in its bearing on therapeutics. Hahnemann cites Röchling as having observed "induration of the axillary glands" from its use. But when we examine the original, we find that the author is reporting the treatment by Iodine of glands already enlarged, which it caused to suppurate readily; and that his "Vereiterung" has been transcribed "Verhärtung." The mistake is Hartlaub and Trinks', from whom Hahnemann has copied. Dr. Cartwright, however, has put on record two cases in which the glands of the neck enlarged under the action of the drug given for other complaints.* This has also been observed (in three instances) as a pathogenetic effect of the waters of Hall, in Upper Austria, whose power over goitre shows that the Iodine they contain is one at least of their active ingredients.

For the effects I have now ascribed to Iodine abundant evidence is given in the works I have mentioned at the outset. And as we study them the interesting fact comes out that all these irritations belong to the class of medicinal actions which Dr. Drysdale has distinguished as "contingent." They are not "absolute" effects of the drug, requiring only its administration in certain quantity, and their absence being the exception to the rule. It is rather the other way. Iodine locally applied, whether to skin or mucous membrane, will certainly irritate. But introduce it into the circulation, and this result cannot be predicted. Often enough it produces no obvious physiological effect at all, even when given in large

* *Monthly Hom. Review*, xii., 411.

doses.* When it does irritate, in one person its influence will
fall on the Schneiderian mucous membrane, in another on the
mouth or stomach, in another on the pleura, in another on the
skin. And of all these actions that is true which Dr. Imbert-
Gourbeyre has noted and formulised, that with *contingenter*
goes *omni dosi.* It is frequently remarked by Dr. Ringer,
when speaking of the various phenomena of what *he* calls
iodism, that "even minute medicinal doses will sometimes
produce" this or that effect. He explains in one place that
he means a grain of iodide of potassium or even less. We
shall see this even more strikingly exhibited when we come to
the phenomena of iodism as described by the older observers.

2. Of these I now proceed to speak as the *neurotic* effects
of the drug. I suspect that they are really irritative in nature,
peculiar only in the seat being the various portions of the
nervous substance. But, phenomenally, they are best classed
separately.

It was early noted by the introducer of Iodine into practice
—Coindet of Geneva—that when the system became saturated with the drug a peculiar train of symptoms manifested
themselves. These were insomnia, palpitation, tremors, and
anxietas ; and therewith rapid emaciation, often associated
with bulimia. The obviously nervous symptoms first mentioned were largely seen and recorded during the Iodine-
mania which set in on the publication of Coindet's results.
Gairdner† has fully described the tremors, which resemble
those of Mercury. Manson and Cooper have seen these go on
to twitchings and other convulsive movements, and Brodie has
known them end in paralysis. The action on the brain manifested in the insomnia has shown itself in various other ways.
Determination of blood to the head is frequent, causing headache with sense of fulness, giddiness, drowsiness, epistaxis,
and even a sort of intoxication. One of the subjects of
Wallace's large doses of iodide of potassium was seized while
taking it with violent headache, and had dilated pupils and an
incessant motion of the eyes like that of a child with con-
genital cataract. Muscular tremors then supervened, and
lastly hemiplegia; from which he recovered but slowly.

* This fact is universally known as regards iodide of potassium, and
Gairdner says of Iodine itself—"Some persons take it in large doses for
a length of time with perfect impunity." "Others," he adds, "from
that peculiar, undescribed, and unintelligible state of constitution called
by physicians an idiosyncrasy, are speedily and violently affected by
very small doses."

† *Essay on the effects of Iodine on the human constitution.*
London, 1824.

Gairdner has observed and described the *anxietas* characteristic of the drug. It differs, he says, from hypochondriasis in this respect, that the patients occupy themselves with the present rather than with the future.* They describe it commonly as a feeling of (psychical) sinking and faintness which is particularly depressing; and they have been heard to complain of this even when suffering violent pain.† The sensory centres are also affected, as by obscuration of vision, partial deafness, and illusions of the sense of touch. The first of these may depend on irritation of the retina. Hempel cites a case in which the symptoms suggest retinitis (the patient, however, was an hysteric); and Ricord states that he has seen iodide of potassium produce transitory amaurosis, like that of Bright's disease, and dependent on sub-retinal œdema.

But the most complete observations of this form of iodism are those of Rilliet, of Geneva. A memoir presented by him to the French Academy of Medicine was referred to Trousseau, and his report thereon may be read in the twenty-fifth volume of its *Bulletin*.‡ It seems that Geneva is singular in the entire absence of Iodine—so universally diffused elsewhere—from its air and waters; so that its inhabitants offer a virgin soil in which the drug can bear fruit. Hence, says M. Chatin, the frequency of goitre there; but hence pretty certainly the remarkable susceptibility displayed to the influence of the substance when administered medicinally. The Genevan bronchoceles are cured with doses of iodide of potassium of less than a milligramme in amount; and it is while taking such "nearly infinitesimal quantities," as Trousseau calls them, that the "grave accidents" he cites from Rilliet occur. They have been seen in these sensitive subjects from taking a tenthousandth part of the iodide in their table salt; and even from staying at the sea-side, where it is calculated that they inhale from the fiftieth to the tenth of a milligramme in a day.

The first symptom of iodism which manifests itself is the emaciation. It sets in suddenly and proceeds with startling rapidity. The goitre (if there is one), the mammæ, and the

* Dr. Allen (S. 16) gives this observation in the converse sense, but he is in error. Gairdner's statement, as extracted above, may be read at p. 12 of his Essay. [Dr. Allen has corrected himself in his supplement.]

† Ringer also has observed that "iodide of potassium sometimes produces distressing depression of mind and body. The patient becomes irritable, dejected, listless, and wretched. Exercise soon produces fatigue and even fainting."

‡ See also Rilliet's own *Memoire sur l'iodisme* (Paris, 1860).

testicles go first ; then the face falls in ; then the whole body wastes. There is no gastro-enteritis ; but exaggerated appetite is present, going on to bulimia : there is also much nervous palpitation. Then supervenes a condition of hypochondriasis or hysteria with weakness, sadness, insomnia, and nervous susceptibility. The younger Coindet is quoted as characterising this state as "a very troublesome condition of the nervous system, which the subjects can hardly describe ; it is an internal agitation, similar to that caused by hearing bad news, or by remorseful feelings after a quarrel ; together with inability to fix the attention when reading or drawing, weeping, and intolerance of the slightest opposition." There are painful sensations in the stomach, especially at its greater curvature ; and the face is pale, green, or yellow.

I cite these observations especially for the light they throw on the *emaciation* of Iodine. This phenomenon has early and constantly attracted attention ; and it has been noted that it is commonly accompanied by profuse sweats and accelerated pulse, thus making it resemble closely the wasting of tuberculosis. There are three ways in which it has been accounted for. The first and most common is to say that Iodine is a stimulant to the absorbents ; and that thus, absorption being rendered over-active, atrophy follows upon its use. I shall show reason for objecting to this explanation even of the local effects of the drug ; and I think that it quite fails when applied to the emaciation of the system at large. The absorbents are set for the nutrition, not for the wasting, of the body as a whole. The lacteals take up the chyle from the intestines, and the lymphatics absorb the not altogether effete products of the disintegration of the tissues, and the residue (if any) of the liquor sanguinis which has been poured forth from the capillaries for their nutrition. Chyle and lymph, thus selected and taken up by the absorbent vessels, are passed through the chain of absorbent glands, in which they undergo that progressive elaboration which fits them to be discharged, as blood, into the torrent of the circulation. It is evident, therefore, that a drug which has the property of stimulating the absorbent system must promote rather than lower the nutrition of the frame.* A second view would account for the atrophy of Iodine by the gastro-enteritis which it is undoubtedly liable to occasion, attributing it to

* The notion here combated is identical with the Hunterian theory of ulceration, which supposed this process to depend upon an over-active state of the absorbents. Long given up in this sphere, it still holds its place in speculation on the *modus operandi* of drugs.

the impairment of digestion which must result from this state of the *primæ viæ*. But a larger survey of the facts will at once show this view to be untenable, as there is no constant connexion between the gastro-enteric symptoms and the emaciation ; while Arsenic, which affects the alimentary canal far more certainly and severely, causes by no means so rapid and intense a wasting. Lastly, Iodine has been styled a "liquefacient" of the tissues, and is supposed to promote their disintegration with such rapidity that the waste is in excess of the supply, and hence atrophy. We may have to call up some such action when we come to consider the power of the drug over syphilitic and other neoplasms ; but we cannot, I think, use it to explain the general wasting which is induced. To begin with, the quantity which needs to be introduced is quite insufficient to effect such a process. We have, moreover, called to mind that the very function of the lymphatic absorbents is to take up such tissue-substance, disintegrated but not altogether effete, and, having elaborated it into blood, to pour it back into the circulation. Thus, supposing the absorbent system to continue healthy, the result of such increased rapidity in the disintegration of tissue would only be an increase in the purity of the substance and the energy of the functions of the entire organism.

In this "supposing" I have indicated what I believe to be the true direction in which to look for an explanation of the atrophy of Iodine. Its sphere is the great absorbent system, especially in its lacteal portion ; but its action there—probably by irritation of the active protoplasm—is depressant * rather than stimulant. Given a sluggish taking up of the chyle by the lacteals, and an insufficient elaboration of their contents by the mesenteric glands, and we have at once a most important channel of nutrition choked up and rendered useless. The fatty aliments being those which the lacteals chiefly select, the emaciation becomes more rapidly apparent than if it had been the albuminous elements whose supply was cut off. But you will remember how Hughes Bennett, following Ascherson of Berlin, has shown that the presence of oil is essential to the assimilation of albumen ; and infers that if the fatty elements of food be insufficiently supplied, the albumen remaining unassimilated in the blood will be deposited in the tissues as tubercle. If it is still tenable to explain in this way the occurrence of primary tuberculosis,

---

* Dr. H. Goullon says that the mesenteric glands are found reduced in size after poisoning by Iodine ; but I know not his authority for the statement.

2 N

it may account for the occasional development of phthisis pulmonalis in iodised patients in whom no previous tendency thereto had existed.

3. One word yet upon the possible *hæmatic* influence of Iodine. It can hardly be imagined that so universal an irritant of the living matter should circulate in the blood without affecting its corpuscles. But whether this be the rationale or not, it is certain that iodide of potassium every now and then causes petechiæ and purpura, and that under the long-continued influence of Iodine the blood and the secretions become thin and watery.

I may here also note the evident influence on the heart which the drug has displayed. The palpitations of the iodism of Coindet and Rilliet, the faintness noted by Gairdner and Ringer, the death by syncope of Rose's patient (who was poisoned by an Iodine injection into an ovarian cyst)—all these, combined with the dilatation of the right ventricle of which we shall presently hear from Goullon, point unmistakeably to a lethal influence on the substance of the organ like that we have seen exerted by Arsenic. The importance of this fact will appear as we proceed.

We have now completed our survey of the physiological action of Iodine : its therapeutic applications we must reserve for our next lecture.

LECTURE XXXVI.

IODINE AND THE IODIDES (*continued*)—IRIS.

In our last lecture we reviewed at some length the physiological effects of Iodine. We have now to consider its recognised uses as a medicine, and see what relation they bear to its action as a poison; subsequently reviewing the further applications of it which have been made, derived from the latter according to the principle of similarity.

I. The earliest and the prerogative application of Iodine is its use in *bronchocele*. "From time immemorial," as Stillé says, "sponges and other marine products containing Iodine have been recognised as popular remedies for goitre." When this substance was discovered in one of such products, the *fucus vesiculosus* (as well as the sponge itself), it was the happy thought of Coindet to see if it would not prove to be the active ingredient of the weed. He found it to be so; and from that time to this the curative action of Iodine in bronchocele has been one of the few certainties (with rare exceptions) of ordinary medicine.

What is the rationale of its action? Let me read you a short narrative : it is from the pen of one of the veterans of Homœopathy, Dr. Goullon, sen.*

"A man, 62 years of age, very bilious, and from his youth affected with gout, got from an allopathic doctor for sciatica two scruples of Kali iodatum in four ounces of water, with directions to take morning and night a tablespoonful. After about eight days there came on *a rapidly growing swelling of the thyroid gland*, with some sensitiveness to the touch, and a feeling of oppression. He was, however, ordered to continue the medicine, and in the second week he got all the signs of endocarditis—oppression, weakness almost amounting to fainting, tumultuous throbbing, intermitting and unequal beats of heart and pulse, tensive pain across the chest. The right ventricle gradually became dilated." The medicine was

---

* Translated fron *Allg. hom. Zeit.*, xlv., 63, in *Brit. Journ. of Hom.*, xi., 335.

omitted, and Mercurius, Arsenicum and Sepia in succession removed the symptoms.

I give you this for what it is worth. Let no one say, however, in derogation of homœopathic doctrine, that Iodine has never produced goitre ; and do not let the singularity of the occurrence weigh too much with you, having regard to the peculiarly contingent and idiosyncratic nature of all the effects of the drug. But let us consider what bronchocele is, and what are the phenomena of its disappearance under Iodine.

The thyroid body, whose enlargement constitutes the disease, is one of those ductless glands whose operation is doubtless concerned with the composition of the blood itself. It may be (as Mr. Simon thinks) a *diverticulum* for the cerebral circulation, as the spleen is for that of the stomach ; but its structure forbids the supposition that this is its only function any more than that is of the spleen. The albuminous matter it separates from its large supply of blood is contained in the interstices of its honeycomb-like structure ; and is probably taken up from thence by its no less abundant lymphatics. Simple bronchocele (with which alone we are at present concerned) seems to be a failure on the part of the lymphatics to undertake this absorption, so that the secretion accumulates ; and this, and not any increase in its fibrous or connective tissue, constitutes (at first, at least) the hypertrophy of the gland. It may come on rapidly, like the splenic enlargement of ague ; and, like that, may rapidly subside. In old and hard goitres, of course, the stroma itself must have become thickened, and the fluid possibly absorbed. These are permanent.

Now the conclusions at which we have already arrived as to the action of Iodine on the lymphatic system, and the case of Dr. Goullon's just related, suggest forcibly that Iodine acts homœopathically in the cure of the simple, recent and soft goitre which depends upon unabsorbed secretion. Another fact pointing in the same direction is the frequent occurrence, noted by all observers, of increase of the tumour, with hardness, pain, and tenderness, when needlessly large doses are given. But still more convincing is the minute quantity which often suffices for the cure. I have already mentioned the experience of the Genevese practitioners. But in regions whose inhabitants are less susceptible to the drug we have observations of the same kind. Dr. Kidd records a case in which a large but soft goitre, of many months' standing, entirely disappeared in two months under the hundredth of a grain of

Iodine night and morning.* A still more striking instance is related in the *Revue homœopathique Belge* for August, 1874.† The enlargement was of fifteen years' standing, and had reached the size of a child's head; but was soft. Iodine 6 was given on August 3rd, 1873, and repeated every few days up to the end of the year. Improvement was felt after the second dose, and on January 1st, 1874, the tumour was found to have completely disappeared. Mr. Cameron has even had a case in which the 30th dilution effected the purpose; but it took a twelvemonth in doing it.‡

It is otherwise, I think, with the old hard goitres we sometimes meet. Mr. Cameron treated two such cases with his 30th dilution, but effected little more than relief of distressful sensations,—that is, of irritation of the tumour such as large doses cause. Dr. Kidd, in the valuable paper on the subject to which I have already referred, mentions a hard goitre in which he could get no effect from Iodine till he gave half a grain three times a day; but with these doses he did cure it, and with still larger quantities the most indurated bronchoceles have been known to be melted down. I think that we must here suppose a destructive action of the drug to be exerted, such as we shall have to invoke to account for its power over syphilitic gummata; and that we shall often do well to use its local instead of internal exhibition. The success of the application of ointment of biniodide of mercury in India is, I understand, very constant and gratifying.

When goitre is cystic, Iodine must be still more locally applied. It must be injected into the cavity; though even there, as we shall see with hydrocele, it may act after a specific manner. But it may find place as a homœopathic remedy in yet another form of the disease, the exophthalmic. The coincident affection of the heart in Dr. Goullon's case rather suggests that the thyroid enlargement was vascular; and Trousseau, commenting on the iodism described by Rilliet, says he has seen the same condition in cases of Graves' disease. Dr. Horatio Wood says of Iodine, that "experience has demonstrated its value" in exophthalmic goitre also; but I know of no record thereof.

II. The transition from bronchocele to *scrofula* is natural. Enlargement of the thyroid was supposed to be so intimately connected with the scrofulous diathesis that the name "struma"

---

* *Brit. Journ. of Hom.*, xxv., 180. Dr. Kidd's first decimal is evidently our present first centesimal.

† See *ibid.*, xxxii., 720.

‡ *Ibid.*, iii., 469.

was applied to it; and when Dr. Stillé says that the marine products containing Iodine have long been recognised as popular remedies for goitre, he adds, "and for scrofula." Accordingly, when this substance was discovered to be their active ingredient, and was found powerfully curative of bronchocele, it was at once applied to the treatment of scrofula. The names of Manson* and Lugol† stand foremost among those who have tested and written upon it; and their testimony to its virtues is very earnest.

What is scrofula, and what is Iodine calculated to do in its treatment in the light of the physiological action of the drug?

According to the doctrine of Niemeyer, now generally received, scrofula is that vulnerability of constitution which we call "delicacy" *plus* a tendency on the part of the lymphatic glands in the neighbourhood of any disordered part to take on hyperplasia and become enlarged. The other so-called "strumous" affections are in no way specifically distinct from the same diseases in non-strumous subjects, though they are more readily induced and more difficult to cure. But this doctrine, though it well connects the facts, does not explain why the lymphatic glands are so apt to take on the morbid action specified. It leaves out of sight, moreover, what I think cannot be gainsaid, that these glands may be and often are primarily affected. I must agree with Dr. H. Goullon, in his excellent treatise on *Scrofulous Affections*, that scrofula is essentially a morbid condition of the lymphatic and lacteal system, whereby the lymph and chyle are supplied in an imperfect or vitiated state to the blood, and the nutritive processes thereby impaired.

If this be so, we can well understand that Iodine may change for the better the whole scrofulous diathesis, owing to the profound action we have seen it to possess upon the lacteo-lymphatic system; and that we are quite within the range of homœopathy when we so use it. It must be especially suitable to the sanguine form of the scrofulous constitution, and where the tendency is to emaciation rather than to the flabby plumpness indicating Calcarea. As regards the several local disorders, it must depend upon the elective affinity of the drug for the part affected whether it shall have any specific influence over its morbid conditions. Of these we shall speak farther on But we must consider here the action of Iodine upon the

* *On the effects of Iodine.* London, 1825.
† *On Iodine in Scrofula*, translated by O'Shaughnessy. London 1831.

absorbent glands themselves when affected by scrofula. I have shown its power of engorging them ; and I have no doubt that here, as with goitre, the recent affection is fully under the homœopathic action of the drug, and may be dispersed by small doses. My colleague Dr. Belcher has the utmost confidence in it when the glands of the neck are the part affected : he gives grain doses of the first decimal trituration of Kali iodatum, and applies a weak solution locally. Dr. Goullon relates two cases of laryngismus stridulus obviously dependent on enlarged bronchial glands, where Iodine in small doses was curative. Dr. Dunham mentions another, saying that he was guided to the choice of Iodine by the fact of the child having previously suffered from marasmus. I have myself great confidence in it in this marasmus itself, the "tabes mesenterica" of childhood. Under its use the hectic first subsides ; and the remaining symptoms, if proper diet and hygiene can be secured, steadily disappear. I give the third decimal dilution.

Here also, however, I suspect that any power which Iodine may have over old indurations and suppurations of the cervical glands is due to its destructive action, and requires substantial doses. It was early noted that it promoted the formation of matter in these adenopathies.

III. I have next to speak of the action of Iodine in *syphilis*. Why it should have been tried in this disease, unless it were from the analogy between its effects and those of Mercury, I cannot say. But it was so tried ; and the results—especially when it was given freely by Wallace of Dublin * as iodide of potassium—were highly satisfactory. It is now the accepted remedy for tertiary, as Mercury is for secondary syphilis. That it is as Iodine that it cures, though given in combination with potassium, appears from Dr. Guillemin's experience, who finds the simple tincture do all that can be done by the iodide.†

I think that there is no reason for doubting that Iodine, like Mercury, finds much in constitutional syphilis to which it is homœopathic. As regards the general state, it is unquestionably an impoverisher of the blood and a waster of the tissues as the syphilitic virus is.‡ "I would remark," says Trousseau,

---

* *Lancet*, 1835-36, vol. i.

† *Gaz. Hebd. de Méd et de Chir.*, 1865, p. 134, et seq.

‡ "By the syphilographers it is held that the iodides promote constructive metamorphosis ; and that a gain in body-weight is a result of their use. . . In the physiological state the iodides increase waste and the elimination of the products of waste, and emaciation with a general depression of the vital functions ensues, when they are administered for lengthened periods." (Bartholow).

" that in some circumstances certain cachexiæ, *and the syphilitic among them,* take a form identical with that ascribed by M. Rilliet to iodism." He then relates a case of the kind : it was cured by iodide of potassium. Skin and mucous membrane, moreover, are very similarly affected by drug and by disease— the former especially. Iodide of potassium has even been observed (by Ricord) to cause a cachectic-looking rupia on the legs in a non-syphilitic person. The evidence of dose, moreover, is in the same direction, especially when Iodine itself is given. Dr. Guillemin's doses are very small compared with the corresponding quantities of the iodides ordinarily administered, and Zeissl speaks of obtaining excellent effects from two minims of the compound tincture twice a day ; while from our own school we have the testimony of Dr. Jousset, who (following Tessier) has " obtained very rapid results from Iodine in the 30th, and even the 500th dilution." Here, therefore, I think that it is reasonable to suppose that it cures, as Mercury does, in virtue of its power to affect the same parts and in a similar manner. But the benefits of largely increased dosage in the tertiary gummatous deposits on bones and in viscera are so great and indubitable that I think we must look now to a different *modus operandi.* What this is has been discussed by Dr. Madden in a very interesting paper which you will find in the twenty-sixth volume of the *British Journal of Homœopathy.* He points out that these affections are of the nature of organized new growths, which are therefore quasiparasitical to the body, and require parasiticides to destroy the 1. The strong antiseptic power of Iodine suggests, he thinks, that it may have such an action ; or, as seems to me more probable, it deals with these foreign deposits as it does with the lead or mercury it is so successful in eliminating from the system.* Either way, it must be given for such purpose in full doses, and the indications for its use must not be looked for in its pathogenesis.

IV. The same explanation probably applies to the virtues of Iodine in chronic rheumatism, gout, and rheumatoid arthritis. They are undoubted ; and in the latter obstinate affection Iodine really seems the most hopeful remedy we have. This is the testimony of Laségue,† of Trousseau,† of

---

* Stillé seems to take the same view, for he thinks that the iodide should be used in preference to iodine itself " whenever the elimination of some effete, imperfectly organised, or abnormal material is the object to be accomplished," the latter being chosen " whenever it is intended to modify the living and normal elements of the economy."

† See Trousseau's *Clinical Lectures* (New Syd. Soc.), iv., 430.

Fuller,* and of Horatio Wood. Full doses and local application are ordinarily required.

V. We have now passed in review the diathetic relations of Iodine. It only remains to consider the disorders of those parts to which it is a specific irritant, and note how far it has proved useful in their treatment. The homœopathicity of the action here needs no argument.

1. Iodine is not a leading remedy in affections of the mucous membrane of the alimentary canal, though it will often control these—as the diarrhœa of phthisis and marasmus—when given for the diseases of which they are an accompaniment. Some references to its occasional uses here may be found in the study of the drug (by Dr. Madden and myself) which I mentioned when I began. I may add to these the vomiting of pregnancy, and perhaps some chronic alterations of the glandular system of the stomach characterised by the same symptom. But while thus inferior to Arsenic as a remedy for affections of the alimentary mucous membrane, it just as far excels the latter drug in those of the respiratory tract. It is very useful in severe local coryza, where the nose is red and swollen. Kali iodatum may be given internally, or Iodine applied by olfaction.† The latter mode of treatment is commended by Ringer in the daily attacks of coryza from which some people suffer, and, conjoined with the internal administration of the drug, has proved highly beneficial in strumous ozæna. A case of recovery of the sense of smell, lost for three years, under the use of Iodine, is cited by Wilcox : the patient was taking the drug for a chronic ophthalmia. In a case of my own of profuse dark discharge from the nose, without constitutional symptoms, occurring in a child after exposure to the contagion of diphtheria, when other apparently well-indicated remedies had failed the first dilution of Kali iodatum effected a rapid cure. Over the extension of this mucous tract to the eye Iodine has little influence, though its constitutional action may make it helpful in strumous ophthalmia. But on that which penetrates the Eustachian tubes it exerts much power, and has often proved curative in catarrhal deafness.‡ In affections of the larynx and trachea Iodine takes the highest rank § Before its discovery in the ashes of burnt sponge Hahnemann had proved that substance, and discerned its

* On Gout, Rheumatic Gout, &c.
† See Brit. Journ. of Hom., xxiv., 168.
‡ See a case of mine in Monthly Hom. Review, xii., 538.
§ See case of syphilitic laryngitis treated by it in Brit. Journ. of Hom., vi., 68.

specific laryngeal action; so that as a remedy for catarrhal
and inflammatory affections of the part, and even for croup
itself, Spongia has long been in high repute in the homœopathic school. It has been with croup as with goitre : Iodine
has been suspected to have the chief credit of the curative
power of the sponge, and experiment has confirmed the suggestion. Koch was the Coindet of this revolution; and since
his communication to the *Hygea* in 1841. Iodine has taken in
most hands the place of Spongia in membranous croup, the
other being given only in the catarrhal form. Dr. Elb's
excellent essay on the disease, which you will find translated
in the tenth volume of the *British Journal of Homœopathy*,
will tell you all that is necessary about this piece of therapeutics. As soon as he has satisfied himself as to the existence
of true croup, he gives a dose of Iodine, from the 2nd to the
6th decimal dilution. " Like the sudden subsidence of a
storm," he writes, " so wonderfully quick is its action. The
anxiety and imminent suffocation and whistling cough cease
as if by magic, and the dyspnœa becomes so much diminished
that we may safely wait an hour before giving a dose of
Aconite, which speedily procures remission of the fever, with
perspiration." He then continues the two every hour alternately as long as there is need. Drs. Arnold and Dake have
added the recommendation—supported by their experience—
of giving inhalations of the drug in rebellious cases.

You will ask, remembering that I have spoken in similar
terms of the action of Bromine, how we are to differentiate
between them. I can only repeat Dr. Meyhoffer's suggestion,
that constitutional prostration is the characteristic indication
for the preference of Bromine, which is thus suited to diphtheritic croup, while Iodine suits the sporadic and more sthenic
form. If, however, you should agree with those who think
that true croup is always connected with diphtheria, I may
mention that Dr. Kidd regards Iodine as the most important
remedy we have for the latter disease.

Dr. Kafka would have us esteem Iodine as highly in
pneumonia as in laryngitis membranacea. The term " croupous " applied by the German pathologists to acute primary
inflammation of the lungs implies for him the pathological
identity of the two processes, and he treats them accordingly.
He maintains, on the strength of a prolonged experience, that
if Iodine be administered when the physical signs first appear
it will arrest the progress of localisation, and abort the whole
disease. He gives a drop of the 1st, 2nd, or 3rd decimal
dilution every hour or even half-hour, and says that improve-

ment may generally be looked for after the fifth or sixth dose, and that within twenty-four hours the disease will be evidently conquered. He does not consider Aconite necessary, but says that the stronger the fever the smaller should be the dose of Iodine, lest aggravation should ensue.

These doctrines about the treatment of pneumonia have lately been the subject of an interesting controversy in the pages of the *Revue homœopathique Belge*,—the Belgian physicians mostly adhering to Jahr's prescription of Aconite followed by Sulphur, and Dr. Jousset joining in the discussion to maintain the sufficiency of Tessier's Bryonia and Phosphorus. As, however, neither class of Dr. Kafka's opponents claim his aborting results, it seems reasonable that his recommendations should be tested.

Before leaving the respiratory sphere, I must speak of the use of Iodine in pulmonary phthisis. Its potent action on the lungs, its modifying influence over scrofula, and the hectic character of its emaciation and fever would make it from a homœopathic point of view the most hopeful of remedies for this disease. My own experience is that of Bähr, that " more than any other remedy it effects curative results, especially if tuberculosis is the result of scrofulosis, in the case of young and robust individuals." This means, I take it, when phthisis is scrofulous pneumonia rather than primary tuberculosis of the lung. Nevertheless, in a case where the severity of the constitutional symptoms and the deficiency of physical signs gave me every reason to dread the presence of tubercle, Iodine alone effected a speedy and most satisfactory cure. I am firmly persuaded that, so far as medicines go, our best hope of future success in phthisis lies in our knowing better how to use Iodine for it. Tessier and Jousset recommend a course of Sulphur and Iodine, in high attenuation, as the best ordinary medication for the disease.

As regards the genito-urinary mucous membrane, I have only to say that Dr. Bumstead finds Kali iodatum in ordinary doses increase urethal discharge in gleet, and that Dr. Franklin esteems it, in the 3rd decimal dilution, highly conducive to its cure.*

2. The action of Iodine on the serous membranes has been little utilised in the homœopathic school; but to it belongs, I think, the occasional curative power of iodide of potassium in hydrocephalus and hydrothorax. To it, also, I am inclined to

---

* *Science and Art of Surgery*, i., 400.—" Discharges from the urethra or vagina which have recently been cured are very prone to recur under the influence of this medicine " (Stillé).

refer the usefulness of Iodine when locally applied or injected to remove effusions into serous or synovial cavities. It is commonly supposed to act here by setting up adhesive inflammation of the walls of the sac. But Dr. Jousset has disproved this hypothesis in the case of hydrocele, and shewn that inflammation is not essential, or even favourable, to the curative process.* Iodine is found in the serous effusions of hydrocele and hydrarthrosis when it is taken internally : to apply or inject it is merely to intensify its influence by concentration, and, when the disorder is local, seems the most rational practice.

3. I can hardly say anything definite of the power of Iodine in cutaneous affections apart from syphilides and scrofulides. Dr. Neligan thinks the iodide of potassium superior to any other drug in these cases, and Mr. Hunt extols cod-liver oil as the only medicine to be compared with Arsenic in its power over skin disease. We shall have to inquire directly how far the power of this oil is to be ascribed to the Iodine it contains. I think that the acne-like character of some of the iodic eruptions hints at an action on its part upon the sebaceous glands, and suggests it as a leading remedy in seborrhœa, molluscum, wens, and the several forms of acne itself. In the two last-named affections it has actually been found curative. Dr. Thin, indeed, examining microscopically specimens of skin the seat of bullæ induced by Kali iodatum, found no alteration in the sebaceous glands, and that the lesion had occurred at points in the coats of the blood-vessels. He thinks that to extravasation thus caused the acne, the bullæ and pustules, and the purpura, which characterise the progressive degrees of the iodic skin affection, are due.†

4. And now as to the glands. Iodine has cured mercurial salivation, and that of pregnancy. Pereira and Watson rank it next to Mercury in chronic disease of the liver, and Dr. Dudgeon once cured with it an obstinate case of jaundice in which he suspected organic disease.‡ Iodine is the leading remedy for diseases of the pancreas in the organology of Rademacher ; and several cases of acute and chronic disease of this gland are cited by Dr. Wilcox in which it effected a cure. You will think of it if you ever encounter the diarrhœa adiposa ; and perhaps Dr. Herbert Nankivell's observation, that Iodine enables fatty food to be digested which otherwise

See *Brit. Journ. of Hom.*, xvi., 259.

† *Lancet*, 1878, ii., 696.

‡ *Brit. Journ. of Hom.*, xxii., 357. See a similar case in vol. xxxiv., p. 381.

could not be given, belongs to this action of the drug. If, too, it can improve the functional action of the pancreas, it is the better fitted to aid in phthisis.

The specific influence of Iodine upon the glands of the generative system would suggest its frequent employment in morbid states of these glands, especially when occurring in scrofulous and tubercular subjects. In such patients prostatitis in the male, and amenorrhœa, galactorrhœa and leucorrhœa in the female subject have been cured by it. I speak with more diffidence when I suggest that to such an influence .is due the dispersion of mammary, ovarian, and uterine tumours which has sometimes been accomplished by Iodine. It is worth noting, however, that the tumours of the uterus which have—in Dr. Ashwell's words*—"melted down" under the action of Iodine appear invariably to have originated in the cervix, i. e. in the glandular and secreting portion of the organ. In inflammation and induration of this part, moreover, Iodine is a remedy of tried value. Here, probably, what has been said about strumous glands holds good (Trousseau and Pidoux speak of its having caused metritis, with discharge) ; and the ovary seems to bear to Iodine just the same relation as the thyroid. Ovarian dropsy (at least of the unilocular kind) is analogous to cystic bronchocele, and, like it, is far more amenable to the injection than to the administration of the drug. Iodine should be borne in mind, I think, in cases of sterility where the strumous diathesis exists.

5. The group of symptoms I have described as constituting the iodism of Coindet and Rilliet point to the action of the drug on the nervous and circulatory systems, and on the blood itself. Trousseau compares them to false chlorosis, simulating phthisis. The tremors suggest mercurial palsy and paralysis agitans, and perhaps chorea, in which affection, and in some cases of paralysis, Manson has found it very useful. I often give it with advantage in the chronic congestive vertigo of old people. It ought to be (perhaps in high dilution) beneficial in insomnia, and in hypochondriasis of the kind it causes. It may be useful in palpitation ;† and its power over the muscular substance of the heart perhaps explains the undoubted good done by iodide of potassium in internal aneurism,

---

* See Guy's Hospital Reports, vol. i.

† "In a case altogether exceptional," Trousseau writes, "M. Rilliet has seen palpitation cease, instead of appearing or increasing, under iodism ; *the patient was one habitually subject to it.*" Dr. Guernsey praises it in cases of debility where at every exertion all the arteries throb painfully.

which does not always require the large doses of it now in vogue. I have had one of the innominata under care, in which great relief has been obtained by the persistent use of this remedy, in grain doses twice a day ; and it is worth noting that Dr. Neligan speaks highly of the biniodide of mercury in the treatment of organic—especially valvular—disease of the heart. The Iodine is surely the prepotent agent in this preparation. I shall also have to speak of Spongia as a cardiac remedy.

I have now done with Iodine—this drug which M. Sée, reechoing Hahnemann, calls an " heroic but dangerous medicine, requiring the greatest prudence on the part of the physician." Here again *magis venenum, magis remedium.* Iodine, so recently discovered, already stands in the front rank of therapeutic agents; and I know of none which promise so much in the future.

A word before closing on the iodides. The compound Iodine forms with potassium has already come before us, and the substitution of sodium or ammonium makes little difference in the result ; though Dr. Bartholow finds small doses of iodide of ammonium specially effective in affections of the respiratory mucous membrane, where he admits that the drug acts "substitutively." With the alkaline earths—as barium and calcium ; with the metals—as iron, mercury, and lead ; and with sulphur, Iodine forms compounds which owe their energy mainly to their bases, though its presence gives them a somewhat distinctive character and special direction. The iodide of carbon forms a substance quite unique, save as it corresponds with the sulphide of the same element, which has already come before us. It is unknown to medicine. "Iodoform " (a teriodide of formyl), taken internally, acts both pathogenetically and curatively like Iodine ; but it is—as its name suggests—an analogue of chloroform, and has anæsthetic properties, of which much use has been made by way of local application. But of all iodic compounds the most important is cod-liver oil—

Oleum jecoris aselli. When this potent therapeutic agent was first introduced into practice, it was a common opinion that its peculiar virtues were due to the Iodine it contained. To the homœopathic physician, the infinitesimal proportion (one part in 40,000) in which the drug existed occasioned no difficulty; and he could point triumphantly to the perfect homœopathicity of Iodine to most of the maladies in which cod-liver oil was found beneficial. Of late years, however, so much evidence has accumulated as to the importance of oily matters in the nutritive operations, that it has become usual among ourselves as well as in the old school to regard cod oil as a purely dietetic agent. I cannot myself subscribe to this conclusion. Without questioning for a moment the great value of an easily digested animal oil as an article of diet in badly nourished frames, I do strongly doubt whether the whole virtues of cod-liver oil can be ascribed to this mode of action. When we remember that in a teaspoonful of this oil we are adminstering a dose of Iodine equal to a drop and a half of its third decimal dilution, and that we are generally giving it in cases to which the drug is thoroughly homœo-pathic, can we doubt that it exerts a curative action? If we disbelieve this, we have no reason for believing in the action of infinitesimals anywhere. Moreover, were it the oleaginous matter *per se* which cures, why should all attempts to find a substitute for the oil of fishes be so unsuccessful? and how was it that the first disease in which cod oil won its laurels was not scrofula or phthisis, but chronic rheumatism? I conclude, then, that the virtues of cod-liver oil are due, in a great measure, to the Iodine it contains; and that the pathogenesy of this drug should always be borne in mind in our prescription of the oil. Iodine will obviously be given best in the form of cod-liver oil where there is much wasting; as we then introduce at one and the same time both the specific to cure the pathological tendency, and the most suitable pabulum wherewith to repair the organism after the ravages of disease.

I must again pass by the strict alphabetical order, as it will be impossible to discuss Ipecacuanha to-day. I will, in its stead, bring before you a plant which, though not peculiar to the American continent, has been made known as a medicine by American practitioners. It is the common blue-flag,

Iris versicolor.

A tincture is prepared from the root.

Iris has been well proved, both in substance and in the attenuations. Dr. Allen gives symptoms from seventeen experimenters. Some of these provings are recorded in detail in the second edition of Dr. Hale's *New Remedies*, and in the fourth edition you can read a full account of the extensive clinical experience which has been obtained with it.

Iris has long had a reputation among those who employ the indigenous plants of America as a very active emetic and purgative, and as an excitant of the salivary and biliary secretions. Our provings, while they agree with this description, both enlarge and precisionise it. Enlarge,—for they show that the pancreas is irritated as much as or more than the salivary glands and liver. This is shown by the continual burning felt in this region by one of the provers, who at the same time was passing frequent watery evacuations ; and by the highly congested state of the organ in animals poisoned by Iris. And precisionise,—for they indicate the vomiting and diarrhœa of Iris to be the result of hypersecretion along the alimentary tract, and that the morbid condition set up has little tendency to run on to inflammation. The vomiting is often acid ; and the purging is accompanied by severe colic and burning in the rectum, suggesting that the stools also have this acid quality. With the salivation there is a thick and flat, or even greasy, taste in the whole mouth, but no fœtor.

These gastro-intestinal symptoms of Iris were the first to be turned to account in homœopathic practice. Dr. Kitchen called attention to them in the *North American Journal of Homœopathy* in 1851. He stated that he found the drug of eminent value in many forms of vomiting and diarrhœa, several of which he instanced and illustrated from practice. The two definite maladies in which, consequent upon his statements, Iris has achieved a reputation are cholera nostras and sick headache. To the first the drug is completely homœopathic, and many testimonies from America coincide with those of Dr. Lade and myself in this country in warrant of its striking efficacy. About cholera infantum the evidence is more conflicting. I have myself been disappointed with it in this disorder : the vomiting is often checked by the Iris, but the purging rarely. Cholera infantum is not so characteristically bilious as is the autumnal attack to which adults are liable.

As regards the so-called sick-headache, there is more to be said. It was the vomiting which accompanies the malady by which Dr. Kitchen was led to prescribe it, and he found it very effectual in relieving both this feature of the paroxysms and the pain itself. Iris thus found a place among the remedies for sick-headache ; but it was natural to suppose, from all we knew of its physiological action, that it was the gastro-hepatic variety of the disease to which it was applicable, and not true nervous migraine. In the *North American Journal of Homœopathy* for February, 1875, however, I came across an observation by Dr. Bigler, of Rochester, U.S., that " Iris

hardly ever fails to cure a case of sick-headache when preceded by a blur before the eyes." Now just at that time
migraine, under the impetus given by Dr. Anstie, was being
studied in its neurotic aspect, and Liveing especially had
brought out the frequency with which the preliminary phenomenon was a disturbance of vision on the affected side very
like the "blur" mentioned by Dr. Bigler. I had hitherto
given Iris in sick-headache only when I supposed it to be of
gastro-hepatic origin ; and had every reason to be pleased
with it. I now, however, began to give it in true migraine,
when ushered in by the characteristic blur, and have obtained
at least one decisive result in the treatment of this very
obstinate malady.

I am the more confirmed in the validity of this application
of the drug by a variety of facts which indicate a true action
on the nervous system, especially in relation to neuralgia, as
exerted by it. Drs. Kitchen and Holcombe have each reported success in the treatment of facial neuralgia by it ; and
the latter caused a pretty severe attack of the same in his
own person by taking two or three drops of a strong tincture
four times daily for a few days. It was on the right side,
involved all the divisions of the trigeminus, and was accompanied with copious diuresis. Again, Dr. Conrad Wesselhœft,
also proving the drug on himself, found it induce a genuine
sciatica of the left leg, which was a trouble quite unknown to
him previously.

It is interesting to notice that this last result followed the
taking of the fifth dilution,—the drug in substance having had
but little effect on the prover. It is thus suggested that, in an
attenuated form, Iris may develope properties unknown to
those who (as the practitioners mentioned above, including
myself) have used it only in a comparatively crude state. A
striking series of experiences in point have lately been communicated by Dr. Claude, of Paris.* He was led, by a
German recommendation, to try the drug in high dilution as
a remedy for constipation, and got results which surprised
him. He relates nine cases in which Iris, in the dilutions
from the 12th to the 30th, acted—often with marvellous rapidity
—as what would be called an aperient, relaxing the most
obstinately constipated bowels. It does not seem to cure the
evil radically, but is always effective as a temporary remedy.
Below the 12th dilution, its effect in this direction is *nil*. I
may mention that several of the subjects of Dr. Claude's
treatment were *migraineuses*, and one laboured under chronic

* *L'Art Médical,* vol. xlv.

ptyalism : the last was cured, and the others were much benefited. This is a very valuable contribution to our knowledge of the drug.

Iris has in other cases cured salivation, mercurial and idiopathic ; also some cutaneous affections (especially, Dr. Hale says, when connected with acid secretions in children), and sthenic seminal emissions. It should be thought of in acute affections of the pancreas.

The analogues of Iris are *Antimonium tartaricum, Colchicum, Iodum, Ipecacuanha, Mercurius,* and *Podophyllum.* The neurotic properties it is now displaying give it other allies. Of its dosage I have already spoken.

LECTURE XXXVII.

IPECACUANHA, JABORANDI, KALI BICHROMICUM.

I have to-day to bring first before you the famous medicine

Ipecacuanha.

From the powdered bark of the root a tincture is made by percolation; or (which I think better) we triturate it.

There is a pathogenesis of Ipecacuanha in the third volume of the *Reine Arzneimittellehre*. It contains 146 symptoms from Hahnemann; 46 from 3 fellow-observers; and 41 from 11 authors. Of the last, those of Geoffroy, Scott and Murray are alone to be depended on; the rest are too impure. Dr. Allen adds several other experiments and observations. But the most complete collection of the effects, physiological and therapeutical, of the drug is that of Dr. Imbert-Gourbeyre. It has been reprinted in a separate form (Paris: Baillière and Son) from *L'Art Médical* for 1868, where it first appeared; it is also translated in vols. xxvi—xxviii of the *British Journal of Homœopathy*. In one of these shapes it should be before you in your study of the medicine; and my remarks here will to a large extent be a summary of and commentary on its contents.

1. I must first speak of the relation of Ipecacuanha to vomiting. It has long been known as a certain, though tardy and mild, emetic; and has been used accordingly. An interesting paper was furnished a century ago to the *Medical Observations and Inquiries* (vol. vi.), showing how small were the doses needed to effect this purpose, from two to four grains nearly always proving sufficient. Physiological investigation has since proved that this action is specific, that is, it is set up when the drug is introduced into the system otherwise than through the stomach. But it has also proved that—unlike Tartar emetic and Apomorphia—Ipecacuanha always, however introduced, excites vomiting through the stomach.

Divide the pneumogastrics so that their gastric extremities shall not be impressionable and no vomiting can be set up by Ipecacuan, while the two other emetics act as usual. This explains why Ipecacuan operates so much more freely and quickly when introduced into the stomach than when injected subcutaneously while exactly the opposite is true of the others.

Other investigations have shown what is the nature of the action of the drug on the stomach. An increased production (of gastric mucus is the usual effect in man but the catarrhal nature of this is shown by experiments on animals in whom the hypodermic injection of emetia (the alkaloid of Ipecacuan) causes a slight inflammation of the gastro-intestinal mucous membrane.

The emetic action of Ipecacuanha was naturally seized upon as a *point d'appui* for the application of *similia similibus* and from Hahnemanns time onwards it has been the main remedy in the Homoeopathic school here vomiting had to be checked. But it was a curious thing to see the practice adopted small dose and all by the practitioners of traditional medicine. When Dr. Ringer in the first edition of his *Handbook of Therapeutics*, stated that several forms of vomiting could be cured by drop doses of Ipecacuanha wine and when subsequently his experience was echoed from all parts of the country it seems to me that the small end of the wedge made an effective entrance. If this were true there was no reason why any other piece of homoeopathic medication might not be true; and the *tuto, cito it jucunde* of the practice was obvious. A feeble attempt was made to evade the inference by ascribing to Ipecacuan a "tonic effect on the sympathetic system generally." Under the cover of this shield cases illustrative of the practice were for a time admitted into the pages of the *Practitioner* even from Homeeopathic sources. But when it appeared to be successful in doses too small for even "increase frequency of administration" (by no means always present) to bring them up to an orthodox amount; and when Tartar emetic to which no ingenuity could ascribe a tonic action) was shown to have a similar effect the ground became dangerous and the subject was abruptly dropped. *De mortuis nil nisi bonum* would never be my wish more strongly than in the case of Anstie; but I must regretfully feel that in this instance prejudice was too much for his cadour.

Practitioner, xiii, 252; see also St. Barth, Hosp. Reports, v, and vii.

While, therefore, the older treaties on Materia Medica spoke of Ipecacuanha only as a means of causing vomiting, their successors all devote some space to showing how it may check it. To Dr. Ringers catalogue of the forms of the trouble in which it is useful or useless we can mainly subscribe. The former embraces the vomiting of pregnancy, suckling, and menstruation, that of acute catarrh and cancer of the stomach, of whooping cough, of chronic alcoholism and of simple debility, the latter consists of the vomiting of infants from intolerance of milk, and that of hysterias. But I cannot at all agree with Dr. Phillips that it is almost solely when the vomiting is sympathetic that Ipecacuanha is useful. That of chronic alcoholism, which he himself specifies, is surely as much gastric as nervous On the contrary, I should say, the more purely sympathetic the vomiting is, the more effected by an impression on the nervous centre of the action which does not take the route of the stomach, the less valuable Ipecacuanha becomes. Thus it is of no avail in vomiting from cerebral disease. In pregnancy, where it is so useful the stomach itself is always more or less affected: and even here, I find that Nux vomica, which meets the reflex nervous irritation, materially assists it action. Hahnemann recommended it where there is chronic disposition to vomit without bringing anything away, and Dr. Guernsey thinks constant nausea characteristic of it.

Nor, it for the vomiting only of gastric irritation that Ipecacuanha helps us; it goes a long way in curing the disorder itself. In acute catarrh of the stomach, especially in children, it wins the applause of the both schools; and in many dyspepsia depending on chronic catarrh of the same organ it is highly beneficial. Upon the intestines it acts in the same manner. In moderate doses it causes mucous diarrhoea, with much griping, the stools being often green or greenish yellow; and when emetia is injected subcutaneously the intestinal lining is always found inflamed. Correspondingly, it has been used largely in the school of Hahnemann in the mucous diarrhoea of children, even when inflammatory symptoms appear. Dr. Ringer's experience is no less favourable. "The dysenteric diarrhoea of children," he writes, "whether acute or chronic, will generally yield to hourly drop doses of Ipecacuanha wine. The especial indication for this remedy are slimy stools, green or not, and with or without blood." Vomiting, he says, if present, is an additional reason for giving it." It has often been found useful in cholera nostras, and even in the cholerine which prevails during the epidemics of the Asiatic form of the disease. Our excellent Hindoo colleague, Dr. Mahendra La'l Sircar, has just put on record a case of poisoning by 35 grains of the powder,* in which the symptoms (save for the greenish tinge of the stools) presented, as he says, " a complete picture of cholera at the onset." Cramps, abdominal and general, were very marked.

This leads us to the use of Ipecacuanha in dysentery. It was in the treatment of this disease, so prevalent at the end of the seventeenth century, that it first won its spurs ; so that it became known as the "radix anti-dysenterica." But the practice ere long fell into neglect and disuse, and Hahnemann could speak of it in his day as abandoned. It has been revived in our own by means of a different mode of administration. Formerly an infusion was used ; but now the drug is given in powder, in a single dose of twenty or thirty grains. By rest and a little laudanum this is prevailed upon to keep down ; and then the most beneficial results appear. " The tormina and tenesmus," writes Dr. Maclean,† " subside ; the motions quickly become feculent ; blood and slime disappear ; and often after a profuse action of the skin the patient falls into a natural sleep and awakes refreshed." A second dose is sometimes required ; but rarely a third. This Ipecacuanha treatment of dysentery is now prevalent throughout India ; and is most highly esteemed.

Is it homœopathy ? Hahnemann argued that Ipecacuanha was incapable of curing the essential symptoms of dysentery, since it was incapable of producing similar ones in healthy persons. "Incapable" is a perilous word to use in pathogenesy ; and subsequent experiment has shown that Ipecacuanha can inflame the intestines, so that its relation to dysentery might fairly be argued to be that of similarity.‡ But I am not sure whether we can claim the present practice for our method. The large dose required, and the advantage gained by giving it in substance, point to a local action of the drug, which indeed (as Dr. Noel de Mussy has pointed out)§

drug in the dysenteric diarrhœa of children, endeavours to connect its *modus operandi* here with that which obtains in epidemic dysentery. But though he speaks of giving from two to five grains for a dose, when we come to his actual prescription we find that he orders one only, though to adults he gives from twenty to sixty. Dr. Ringer's dropdoses of the wine still more completely decide the question.

* *Calcutta Journal of Medicine*, vii., 447.
† Reynolds' *System of Medicine*, vol. i., art. Dysentery.
‡ See *London Medical Record*, iii., 59.
§ *Brit. Journ. of Hom.*, xxxiii., 752.

is often given with advantage in injection. It seems to cause a transpiration of the intestinal mucous membrane analogous to that seen on the skin, and so to promote the resolution of the disease. Homœopathic practitioners have not found it very efficacious in their small doses, save as an adjunct to other remedies. Hahnemann admits that it may diminish the quantity of blood, and relieve the tormina, of the affection; as to these symptoms it is quite homœopathic. But there is another feature of dysentery which Ipecacuanha, though it has never caused it, may well relieve. I mean the tenesmus. This is an action very analogous to the vomiting we have seen and the cough we shall soon see caused by the drug ; and like these it may be quieted by it, as Teste has affirmed.

2. We come now to the action of Ipecacuanha on the respiratory organs. When these receive it by inhalation as those by ingestion a similar train of phenomena is wont to appear. Irritation of the mucous membrane is set up—increased secretion going on to catarrhal inflammation. But more marked than this, and often out of all proportion to it, is the involvement of the extremities of the incident nerves. Continual sneezing, spasmodic cough, and especially dyspnœa of asthmatic kind, are the sufferings of those who have the misfortune to be susceptible to Ipecacuanha whenever they are exposed to its emanations.

Dr. Imbert-Gourbeyre has collected numerous instances of this effect of the drug. It is of the contingent order, only appearing in certain persons. But with them it results *omni dosi*. They may be at the top of the house, while Ipecacuanha is being powdered on the basement; yet ere long they will feel the influence of their enemy. Sometimes their conjunctival and Schneiderian membranes are most affected; the eyes are reddened, smart, and water, and there is a copious defluxion from the nose, with incessant sneezing. More commonly the influence is felt lower down, in dyspnœa, wheezing, and cough, ending in profuse mucous expectoration. They suffer like the subjects of hay-fever and -asthma : only the irritant is different.

This being so, Ipecacuanha should play an important part in the disorders of the respiratory apparatus ; and it does so in both schools of medicine. In coryza it should be given where sneezing is very troublesome. In hay-fever it does all that a palliative can do, though nothing seems really curative save destruction of the living matter which, in the form of pollen, Dr. Blackley has demonstrated to be its cause. It is of great service in croup and in pertussis. Its repute as an

emetic in these disorders is probably due to its dynamic properties. For croup M. Teste strongly recommends the
alternation of Ipecacuanha with Bryonia. There is certainly
a spasmodic as well as an inflammatory element in most cases
of croup ; and as Bryonia, which we have seen to have the
power of setting up membranous inflammation of the air-
passages, controls the latter, Ipecacuanha may well help by
its influence on the former. In whooping-cough I have the
utmost confidence in it as long. as, or whenever, catarrhal
symptoms are present. When the cough is pure spasm
Drosera, Corallium, or Cuprum is preferable. It is thus (often
in alternation with Aconite) the usual remedy for the malady in
its first two or three weeks, and gives unequivocal relief. In
simple spasmodic coughs resembling pertussis, with much
retching and mucous expectoration, Ipecacuanha is often
rapidly curative. Dr. Guernsey praises it also for incessant
and most violent cough with every breath, such as sometimes
occurs in children with measles. It relieves, he says, " like a
charm." It is hardly suited to pure spasmodic asthma, where,
if it relieves the paroxysm, it must do so as any other
nauseant would, by inducing general relaxation. Nor has it
power over acute bronchitis. But in bronchitic asthma its use
is most beneficial, in small frequent doses during the attack,
and at longer intervals subsequently. And there are cases of
bronchitis which are half asthma, neuroses as much as phlo-
goses ; and here Ipecacuanha acts beautifully. I have put
one such case on record in the fifth volume of the *Annals* of
the British Homœopathic Society (p. 199).

Dr Ringer has lately extended the influence of Ipecacuan
over the disorders of respiration, by introducing the wine
into the chest in fine spray. By this means he is able greatly
to relieve and even cure chronic cases of winter-cough,
where the bronchial membrane is always engorged, and the
incident nerves in continual excitement. The success he has
obtained should encourage us to repeat the experiment, and
perhaps to use the drug in this form in hay-fever and in the
asthmatic paroxysm. It is the more rational so to do, as the
power of Ipecacuan to cause respiratory troubles through the
stomach is less than it has when inhaled, in which case it does
so (as we have seen) in the minutest dose. That the action,
however, is specific, and not merely local, is certain. In
poisoning by impure emetia the mucous membrane of the
bronchiæ is found inflamed ; and Stillé relates an interesting
case in which a person susceptible to it had a violent paroxysm
of asthma from a dose of the wine. " After the paroxysm,

and when expectoration became free again, a large quantity of sputa was ejected, which any person at first sight would have pronounced to be a mass of small, nearly transparent worms. These bodies were no doubt formed of concrete mucus moulded in the smaller air-tubes," and shew that the action of Ipecacuanha reaches even to these. Dr. Jousset esteems it highly in alternation with Bryonia (both in the 12th dilùtion) in the treatment of acute capillary bronchitis.

I think that, both in the digestive apparatus and in the respiratory organs, the condition indicating Ipecacuanha may be defined as "a moderate inflammatory irritation of the mucous surface, resulting, through a reflex excitation conveyed by the incident nerves of the part, in vigorous expulsive muscular movements."

3. I have now to speak of the use of Ipecacuanha in hæmorrhages. Dr. Imbert-Gourbeyre has collected various testimonies to its value here, and has convincingly shown it to be homœopathic in its *modus operandi*. Several authors have seen it produce epistaxis and hæmoptysis in connection with its respiratory troubles ; and in an observation of asthma caused by its emanations, and lasting some days, it is noted that menstruation appeared prematurely, and not only the sputa, but also the stools and urine, were sometimes tinged with blood. It is now forgotten in ordinary practice, save when, as by Higginbotham and Peter, it is recommended as hæmostatic by producing vomiting; but among homœopathists, and in their non-perturbative doses, it holds high rank as a remedy in intestinal hæmorrhage, in hæmoptysis, menorrhagia and metrorrhagia, and hæmatemesis. The presence also of blood in the *ejecta* is always held to strengthen the indications for it in vomiting, dysentery, and pertussis.

4. What amount of direct action Ipecacuan exerts on the nervous system in health is uncertain. But it has found an occasional place in the treatment of neurotic affections in both schools of medicine, as may be seen from Dr. Imbert-Gourbeyre's collection. I can speak only of cerebro-spinal meningitis and of intermittent fever. In an epidemic of the former disease occurring at Avignon in 1846-7, Dr. Bechet was led to Ipecacuan as the medicine most similar to the symptoms present; and he gave it (in the mother tincture) in every case with such great relative success that it was appropriated (of course without acknowledgment) by the practitioners of the old school in the place, and vaunted as a specific.* In ague it has long been in esteem as an emetic ; but Sauret at least

* See *Brit. Journ. of Hom.*, xi., 305.

has published an obstinate case in which it cured without causing nausea and vomiting.   Roux observed, in the same journal, that such facts were long since known in the school of Hahnemann.   The presence of much gastric derangement, and vomiting during the paroxysms, have always been held to indicate it, also supervention of the fit in the evening or night; but Jahr says that he always commences with it in the treatment of ague unless some other remedy is distinctly indicated, and that by pursuing this course he has cured many cases by the first prescription.   Bähr thinks its place to be in intermittents when epidemic in a district ordinarily non-malarious.   If in any of these visitations it cures the first case, it will cure all the rest.

Our contention that it is by its specific action that Ipeca-cuanha checks intermittents, as it does hæmorrhages, has been powerfully sustained by a recent treatise from the pen of an old-school practitioner—Dr. Woodhull, of the United States Army.   It is entitled " The non-emetic uses of Ipecacuanha" (Philadelphia, 1876).   Besides the other applications of the drug I have mentioned above, he relates as his experience in ague that he has treated with it fifty cases, giving one or two grains at intervals of from three to six hours.   In no uncomplicated case did it fail; and in one half of those treated no chill appeared after its administration.

Among the miscellaneous facts adduced by Dr. Imbert-Gourbeyre in his exhaustive collection is one where intense pain, with profuse lachrymation, congestion of the eyes, photo-phobia going on to blindness in one eye, and appearance of iridescent rings of fire before the other, occurred four times from exposure to the dust of Ipecacuanha.   He gives also a case of choroiditis (by which name I think we must designate this attack), where coloured haloes surrounded all bright objects, rapidly removed by the medicine in medium dilutions.

Dr. Guernsey, besides the constant nausea I have already mentioned, considers a pain about the umbilicus passing off into the uterus, and a continual flow of bright red blood, to be infallible indications for its use in uterine hæmorrhage.   Teste considers that its symptoms generally, and not only its fever, are wont to supervene during the night; and Dr. Chargé warns us against giving it to sensitive children in the evening, for fear of producing nocturnal exacerbations.

Hahnemann esteemed Ipecacuanha an antidote to opium-poisoning; and it has been found of great value in weaning the system from the opium-habit.

The analogues of Ipecacuanha are *Antimonium tartaricum* and *Arsenicum*.

The first and second decimal triturations, and the first decimal dilution, answer well for all the homœopathic applications of Ipecacuanha. The drop doses of the wine made so fashionable by Dr. Ringer are about equal to a drop and a half of our Ix.

I have next to make some remarks upon a South American plant which has recently been introduced into general medicine—the pilocarpus pinnatus, or

Jaborandi.

The leaves are the medicinal portion of the plant, and appear to owe most if not all of their activity to an alkaloid contained in them, which has been called pilocarpia. An alcoholic solution of this last, and triturations of the dried leaves as imported, will probably be the officinal homœopathic preparations.

The physiological effects of full doses of Jaborandi have been so thoroughly ascertained by physicians of the old school—among whom I may especially name Gubler, Robin, and Ringer—that they have left nothing for us to do in this direction. Provings of smaller doses, however, are required, and have been supplied by two members of our own body—Drs. Watkins and Thayer, both of the United States. The pathogenesis in Allen's *Encyclopædia* comprises a full view of the results thus obtained.

Jaborandi was introduced into practice at Paris in 1874 by Dr. Coutinho, of Pernambuco, who showed that in the form of an infusion of the leaves it displayed uncommon activity as a diaphoretic and sialogogue. I cannot better display its operation than by reading you (from Allen) the description given by Robin of the general effects of its administration.

"Very soon," he writes, "the face becomes red; the temporal arteries throb more strongly; then there is a peculiar feeling of heat in the mouth and on the face, and the flow of saliva begins. In a little while the forehead becomes moist, and the face more red; then beads of perspiration appear on the forehead, cheeks, and temples. The flow of saliva increases, all the salivary glands successively contributing to this effect; the mouth is filled with immense quantities of fluid, and expectoration is incessant; at the same time perspiration

JABORANDI.

covers the face and neck; then the whole body becomes red
and moist, and a pleasant warmth is experienced; in a few
minutes perspiration breaks out over the whole surface, and
soon runs down on all sides. Meantime other symptoms have
supervened. The eyelids first become moist, then the
lachrymal secretion gradually augments, and, after collecting
in the canthi, rolls slowly over the cheeks; at the same time
there is a copious discharge from the Schneiderian membrane,
increased by the tears which escape through the nasal canal ;
moreover, there is increased activity of the mucous glands of
the pharynx, trachea, and bronchi. All these effects reach
their maximum of intensity in about three-quarters of an
hour after taking the drug, continuing thus for thirty or forty
minutes. Lying on one side, that the saliva may run more
freely, the patient spits ten or fifteen times a minute ; the flow
is so rapid that he can hardly speak ; the salivary glands are
enlarged, and the mouth becomes hotter. The body is bathed
in perspiration ; a shirt is wet through in a few moments. Now
a feeling of comfort, or of weakness, as the case may be, is
experienced. Thirst is intense. The pupils are slightly contracted. By degrees the excessive activity of the secretory
processes is diminished ; in an hour and a quarter, or an hour
and three quarters, the lachrymation, the nasal discharge, the
bronchial expectoration, and finally the flow of saliva and the
perspiration, are sensibly lessened, and the parts involved
gradually return to their normal condition. When the perspiration and flow of saliva have ceased, the subject is prostrated
and drowsy. The parts which secreted so copiously are now
very dry, especially the mouth and the pharynx. There is
also much thirst." These are the effects of six grammes of
the powdered leaves, given in infusion ; but similar results may
be obtained from the subcutaneous injection of minute quantities of pilocarpia.

Later experimentation has filled in the outline of this
picture. It has been ascertained that the rapidity of the circulation is notably increased by Jaborandi, but the arterial
tension and the temperature lowered. The secretion of the
kidneys is ordinarily unaffected. The medicine acts strongly
upon the eye, contracting the pupil, and causing tension of
the accommodative apparatus, so as to induce a temporary
myopia.

Jaborandi is thus a medicine analogous on the one hand to
Amyl nitrite, on the other to Physostigma and Muscaria, and
in both spheres of action precisely antagonistic to Atropia—a
minute dose of which will accordingly arrest the whole group

of symptoms caused by it. It goes beyond Amyl nitrite in that perspiration succeeds its flush. Its diaphoretic effect may be regarded as neurotic in origin ; though the same can hardly be said of its ptyalism, as this occurs even when the nerves—cerebro-spinal and sympathetic—of a salivary gland are divided. It becomes, accordingly, in our hands a remedy for excessive perspirations connected with nervous depression. When the flushes of the menopausia are accompanied with sweating, Jaborandi or its alkaloid should be their best aid, and I have recently had a case at the hospital where it has reduced their recurrence from half-hourly intervals to two or three a-day. In the hands of Dr. Chase, of Cambridge, U.S., it has proved curative of the sweatings of convalescence from acute disease and palliative of those of phthisis. In all these cases Jaborandi itself was given, in the first trituration. Dr. Ringer has obtained similar results with small doses of pilocarpia in perspirations, including those curious unilateral sweatings which sometimes occur in connection with disease—functional or organic—of the nervous centres.* The drug should be tried in the salivation of pregnancy and in that which sometimes results from cold ; although the former, being a reflex phenomenon, is hardly likely to yield to it. I have myself tried it in one case without result. Allopathically, it would seem a possible help in uræmia, especially as the urea of the perspiration is found greatly increased by its use.

An application of Jaborandi to morbid perspirations has recently been made on a larger scale by Dr. Murrell, whom association with Dr. Ringer has naturally predisposed in favour of similarly-acting medicines. Giving either the twentieth of a grain of a salt of pilocarpia, or about fifteen minims of a tincture of Jaborandi, he treated thirty-three cases, mostly phthisical. "In every case the drug did some good, and in most cases it was a great success." It acts somewhat slowly, producing little effect the first night ; but when once the sweating has been checked by it "there is, as a rule, no return for many weeks."†

I have nothing further to say of the analogues or of the dose of Jaborandi.

Our third and last medicine to-day is a salt which, known only as a caustic in the old school, has through physiological

* *Practitioner*, Dec., 1876.
† *Ibid*, Dec., 1879.

proving become among homœopathists a widely used and most valued remedy.   It is the bichromate of potash,

Kali bichromicum.

It is prepared by trituration or aqueous solution up to the third potency; above that with alcohol.

This substance was first proved in England, under the superintendence of Dr. Drysdale, on 11 men and 5 women. The results, with experiments on animals and observations on the workmen engaged in its manufacture, were published by him in the *British Journal of Homœopathy* for 1846.   In 1845 the Austrian Society selected the drug for proving, which they carried out on 12 men and 2 women, publishing the results in their journal for 1847.   Dr. Arneth, who conducted the proving and undertook the publication, has embodied in his article all that was known upon the subject up to that date.   These ample materials form the pathogenesis of Kali bichromicum given by Allen, and from them Dr. Drysdale has constructed the arrangement of the drug which appears in the first part of the *Hahnemann Materia Medica.*   Numerous clinical cases are appended there; and a series of others has been furnished by the same physician to the fifteenth volume of the *British Journal.*

We have thus in Kali bichromicum a fully proved and largely tried medicine.   As it may be quite strange to some of my hearers, I must expound it *ab initio.*

Dr. Drysdale well characterises it as "a pure irritant to the organic tissues."   Comparing it with Arsenic, we observe that neurotic, hæmatic and myotic influences are altogether wanting; but its sphere of tissue-irritation is wider, omitting indeed the serous membranes, but extending beyond the mucous membranes and the skin to the fibrous tissues on the one hand, and to some of the glands on the other.   I will endeavour to describe its physiological effects under these headings.

1. The action of Kali bichromicum on the mucous membranes is as marked as that of Arsenic and of Tartar emetic.   It causes a morbid increase in the quantity of mucus formed, which mucus sometimes is tough and stringy, and sometimes degenerates into pus.   Higher grades of the inflammatory process are seen in the respiratory mucous membrane, and (when the poison has been swallowed) along the alimentary tract.   In the former region, false membranes have

been formed ; in the latter, the tendency is towards ulceration. The portions of the mucous tracts chiefly affected are the mouth, throat, cardiac portion of the stomach, duodenum and jejunum, and rectum ; and the whole respiratory membrane, including the conjunctiva. These toxicological actions are pictured in the physiological provings. The provers have sore and injected fauces ; sour eructations and heartburn, slow digestion, bitter taste, nausea and vomiting, with thickly coated tongue ; dysenteric purging ; coryza, hoarseness, and cough.

2. The action of Kali bichromicum on the skin, like that of Croton and Tartar emetic, is most fully displayed as the result of its external application ; although, as also with them, the effect is specific, and may appear under other circumstances. In the account of the English proving given in the *British Journal* you will find some coloured engravings of the effects of the poison upon the skin. Papules, pustules and ulcers are the most characteristic forms : the ulcers have hard bases and overhanging edges, are deep and generally dry.

3. The glands chiefly affected by Kali bichromicum are the liver and the kidneys. On the former its action is very marked. Here is a group of symptoms occurring in one prover :—" aching for some days in the right hypochondrium ; scanty, pale, clay-coloured stools, sometimes twice a day ; metallic taste, fœtid breath, and confusion in the head." In animals poisoned by it, the liver is found congested, enlarged, friable, of a dark reddish-brown colour, but presenting on its surface whitish-yellow spots extending into its substance, of soft consistence, and slightly depressed. The kidneys are also found intensely congested, the tubular portion softened and undistinguishable from the rest, and the urine either purulent or altogether suppressed.

4. The fibrous tissues are much irritated, as shown by the marked tearing pains experienced by the provers, especially about the joints. Still more striking is the effect upon the periosteum, which manifests not only pain at certain spots, but its characteristic hard swellings. These symptoms are observed especially in the parietal, malar, and maxillary bones, and in the tibia. I see no evidence that Kali bichromicum influences the bones themselves ; but its curious effects upon the nasal septum show a decided power of destroying the cartilages. Dr. Drysdale thus describes what happens to the workers in chrome. " For the first days there is discharge of clear water from the nose, with sneezing, chiefly on going into the open air ; then soreness and redness of the nose.

with sensation of a fœtid smell. Then they have great pain and tenderness, most at the junction of the cartilage, and the septum ulcerates quite through, while the nose becomes obstructed by the repeated formation of hard elastic plugs (called by the workmen clinkers). Finally, the membrane loses its sensibility and remains dry, with the septum gone, and frequently loss of smell for years."

The pathogenetic effects I have now described are faithfully represented in the clinical use of the drug. Kali bichromicum is of no service in idiopathic nervous affections, or in toxæmic fevers. The apparent exception of supra-orbital neuralgia, which it has often cured (especially when occurring on the left side), is probably not a real one; as this is the neuralgia most frequently induced by gastric derangement. Two leading forms of cachexia, however, are prominently pictured in its pathogenesis, viz., syphilis and chronic rheumatism.

I. Of syphilis Dr. Drysdale writes:—"the resemblance in many respects between the action of this medicine and that of the syphilitic virus, and also its analogy to Mercury, would lead us to hope that we may find in it another remedy for that disease. Though we would not place any weight on such a merely superficial resemblance, yet we cannot refrain from noticing the likeness that the chrome ulcer when healed presents to the indurated chancre. A more correct way of judging of the resemblance is in the further development of the constitutional symptoms. We have in this remedy the rash on the skin; then the sore throat, which has been mistaken for syphilitic; then the periosteal pains; then the rheumatism; and lastly the diseases of the skin, chiefly of the pustular character, which have the hard dark scab, and leave the depressed cicatrix." Experience has confirmed the hope here expressed, as will be seen in the remarks I shall make upon its curative power over affections of the throat, eye, skin and periosteum.

II. The rheumatoid pains induced by Kali bichromicum are so numerous and characteristic, that it can hardly fail to take its place as a remedy for rheumatic affections. Experience has here also confirmed the indications of pathogenesy. It is especially on the middle ground between rheumatism and syphilis—in periosteal and syphilitic rheumatism—that Kali bichromicum plays so distinguished a part. It will be seen, however, that its action is by no means limited to cases such as this. The rheumatism calling for Kali bichromicum is chronic, and of the "cold" variety.

Let us now follow the curative action of the drug along

the road we have already traversed in describing its pathogenetic effects.

1. In chronic catarrh and ulcerations of the alimentary
mucous membrane Kali bichromicum is often our very best
medicine. The common chronic ulcer of the pharynx rapidly
heals under its action. I agree also with Drs. Watzke and
Russell in rating it very highly as a remedy for syphilitic sore
throat. It will not, I believe, arrest the destructive ulceration sometimes set up (requiring Mercury or Iodine); but
will subdue chronic inflammation and heal up superficial
ulcers very effectually. Then it is very useful in dyspepsia
and vomiting from chronic gastric catarrh, where the tongue
has a thick yellowish coat, differing herein from the white coat
of Antimonium crudum. Mr. Clifton has contributed some
valuable indications for the medicine here.* He agrees with
Dr. Lippe (of whose remarks I shall speak hereafter) that it
is especially useful in the dyspepsia of beer-drinkers, and
where *weight* (not pain) is complained of after food. He
notes that under the rough yellow fur of the tongue the
surface of the organ is red; and he confirms the general
experience of alternation of gastric sufferings with rheumatism
being characteristic of the drug. Kali bichromicum is hardly
less useful in helping to heal the round ulcer of the stomach,
and those of the duodenum resulting from burns; and in
chronic diarrhœa from intestinal ulceration it vies with Mercurius corrosivus, and has effected some brilliant cures.

Still more striking is the power of this remedy in affections
of the respiratory mucous membrane. In acute coryza, and
in catarrh of larynx, trachea, and bronchi, such as occurs in
influenza, it is often rapidly curative; especially (I think)
when the digestive mucous membrane is simultaneously involved. There is also a large accumulation of evidence
tending to show that it is a potent remedy for true membranous croup, whether diphtheritic or apparently primary.
I cannot yet compare it with Iodine and Bromine here, save
that thickness and tenacity of the false membrane will always
be an indication for it. It seems gaining in reputation as an
anti-diphtheritic medicine among our American *confrères*, who
see more of the disease now-a-days than we do. I have
myself seen it act exceedingly well when the deposit invaded
the nares. It is, however, more especially in the chronic
affections of the respiratory tract that Kali bichromicum is
efficacious. The great indication for it in these is the tough,
tenacious, glutinous character of the expectoration, which

* *Monthly Hom. Review*, xvii., 154.

may often be drawn out in long strings. Dr. Meyhoffer esteems it highly in chronic laryngeal catarrh, and when bronchitis lingers long in a sub-acute condition. He administers it by inhalation as well as internally. It might be useful in ulceration of the larynx, syphilitic or simple.

The lining membrane of the nose, and its offset to the eyes, is therapeutically as well as physiologically a special seat of the action of Kali bichromicum. It is very good for chronic coryza, where the discharge is thick, yellow, and glutinous, and the nose tender. Used locally as well, it has cured polypus narium in many instances.* It is worthy of trial in ozæna after the same manner. The internal use of the drug alone I have never seen curative of this disease; though Mr. Lord found it very successful in horses, with whom it is a frequent occurrence. In acute glanders affecting these subjects Mr. Moore has found it curative; and the suppurating nostrils and pustular skin of the disease plainly indicate it, at any rate in alternation with the Arsenicum or Lachesis required by the constitutional condition. In the sphere of the eyes Kali bichromicum stands high among the remedies for catarrhal and strumous ophthalmia; and its action on the fibrous structures has enabled it to cure even rheumatic† and syphilitic inflammations of the ball. It is especially useful in catarrho-rheumatic ophthalmia. Drs. Allen and Norton mention a case of pannus from granular lids, in which the eyes cleared up wonderfully under the medicine. They have found it useful also to remove opacities of the cornea.

The other uses of the drug may be more briefly passed over.

2. It has often been used with great advantage in pustular eruptions; and is a valuable remedy, externally as well as internally used, for ulcers on the legs. Dr. Edward Blake has lately‡ communicated some interesting experience with it in lupus non-exedens, which he has several times succeeded

---

* See one in *Brit. Journ. of Hom.*, xxviii., 356. Dr. Ransford has communicated (*Ibid.*, xxiv., 304) a case which he calls "malignant ulceration of the nose," cured by the internal use of the bichromate. I should rather have called it polypus, possibly malignant. Dr. Ransford has found fault with this criticism (*Ibid.*, xxxii., 651); but his only reply is to repeat testimonies as to the malignancy of the affection. This I do not question: I only submit that it was a polypoid growth rather than an ulcerative process.

† One of the Austrian provers, who took the second trituration, had "several bright red spots and streaks on the white of the left eye," which looks like sclerotic injection.

‡ *Brit. Journ. of Hom.*, xxxii., 643.

in curing with the 5th decimal attenuation. I have had a similar result in one case of my own.

3. Kali bichromicum is a decided hepatic medicine, much resembling Mercurius. Dull pain in the right hypochondrium, especially when limited to a small spot, and whitish stools, are indications for its use. Its action on the kidneys has led to its use in the suppression of urine which sometimes follows upon Asiatic cholera; and so far with apparent success.

4. The action of Kali bichromicum upon fibrous tissue has led to its successful use in a number of local rheumatisms, and such-like maladies. In Dr. Drysdale's article you will find cases of rheumatic headache, of lumbago and sciatica, and of periostitis, which have been very satisfactorily cured by it.

Two of our American colleagues, Drs. Lippe and Kitchen, have within the last few years written upon Kali bichromicum. The concurrence of their experience is interesting, as the former uses the higher infinitesimals while the latter gives semi-material doses. Dr. Lippe compares its eruption to that of measles, and says that in this disease the cough and expectoration are often such as to indicate the drug. Dr. Kitchen mainly confirms our experience with it in chronic affections of the respiratory tract, where he thinks yellow expectoration a great indication for it.

Hepar sulphuris, Kali iodatum and the mercurial preparations are the medicines which have most analogy to the general action of Kali bichromicum. In its effects on the mucous membranes and skin it resembles also *Arsenic* and *Tartar emetic. Spongia, Iodine* and *Bromine* act like it upon the larynx and trachea; *Mercurius* on the liver; and *Mezereum* and *Phytolacca* on the periosteum.

I recommend by way of dose the first six dilutions. The 3rd is most commonly used, except in syphilis, where the lowest potencies of this salt and of the neutral chromate have been employed with most benefit. In acute affections, however, I nearly always prefer the 6th, unless I give the 12th. For external use, as to ulcers, one grain of the pure salt to eight ounces of water will be found quite strong enough.

KALI CARBONICUM, CHLORICUM, NITRICUM, AND PERMAN-
GANICUM; KALMIA, KREOSOTE, LACTUCA.

OF the compounds of potassium we have already studied
the iodide, the bromide, and the bichromate—all of which
belong less to it than to the other element entering into their
composition; and free potash itself has come before us under
the name of Causticum. We have now to consider the remaining drugs of this order which we use in homœopathic
practice.

The first of these is the carbonate,

Kali carbonicum.

It is prepared by solution in distilled water, or by trituration.

Hahnemann published a proving of Kali carbonicum in
the first edition of the *Chronic Diseases*, containing 938
symptoms, a good many of which were contributed by Rummel
and von Gersdorff. In the second edition the list has swollen
to 1,650, a few of the additions being Hartlaub's and Goullon's,
but most of them coming from Nenning. Dr. Allen's additions are few and unimportant.

The carbonate of potash is not credited with any specific
action of its own in old-school therapeutics; but is classed
with the acetate, citrate, and other vegetable salts of the alkali.
The only exception is whooping-cough, where it has some
reputation. This—as with cochineal—has been sustained
in homœopathic practice: von Bönninghausen thought it
specially indicated where there was much puffiness of the
upper eyelids present. Dr. Drury recommends it also in
cough from relaxed uvula.* It is in affections of the respiratory organs that it has found its chief use. Dr. Bayes com-

* *Annals*, iv., 543.

mends it in ulceration of the nostrils ; and in a series of cases of ozæna—or, rather, chronic nasal catarrh—published by Dr. S. C. Jones in the *American Journal of Homœopathic Materia Medica*,* Kali carbonicum was the remedy most frequently successful. He thinks the presence of ulceration within the nose the special indication for its use. Hahnemann says— " it is rarely that ulcerative pulmonary phthisis can be cured without this antipsoric," and the suggestion has been generally carried out and substantiated by his disciples. It seems agreed that the chief indication for it is—as with Stannum— profuse purulent expectoration, but also—which is peculiar to it—much pain in the walls of the chest. It will so often remove these pains, and the pains themselves are so frequently pleuritic in nature, that it has come to be thought that Kali carbonicum is a true remedy for pleurisy, and not only when occurring in connection with phthisis. I suspect that it is only when the pleuræ are affected by extension from the lungs that it proves useful, and that the "phthisis" in which it has been beneficial is pneumonic rather than tubercular.

Another specific action of Kali carbonicum is that which it exerts upon the ovario-uterine system. Hahnemann commends it in suppression of the menses, or when these delay in making their first appearance at the time of puberty ; and to such negative conditions of the periodic function it has generally been considered applicable. But Dr. H. Goullon has of late commended it to us as no less valuable in menorrhagia.† It is spoken of very highly in Noack and Trinks' *Handbuch* for aching in the back, with sense of weakness there, in pregnant women (an experience I have often confirmed), and for the effects of want of care after miscarriage and childbirth.

Besides these more defined uses of Kali carbonicum, it is a medicine which not unfrequently comes into play in the treatment of complex cases of chronic disease. When the symptoms present are, on consulting our repertories, found in its pathogenesis, we may generally use it—preferably in the higher dilutions—with good hope of benefit. A good many such cases have been at various times contributed to the *Allgemeine homöopathische Zeitung* by Dr. Schelling, who is an enthusiast for the medicine. Dr. Guernsey considers the sharp, stitching, jerking pains we have seen it removing from the walls of the chest an indication for its employment generally, and Hahnemann himself had remarked that "stitching is the most characteristic pain of Kali."

* Oct. and Nov., 1875.
† See *Brit. Journ. of Hom.*, xxv., 515.

It will be seen from this that Causticum is not so close an analogue of Kali carbonicum as their chemical relationship would suggest. *Natrum muriaticum* and *Stannum* are perhaps the medicines which most resemble it.

As Kali carbonicum was used by the earlier Hahnemannians much more than it is now, I should have supposed that the higher dilutions were the most efficacious. Dr. Clotar Müller, however, writes :—"as long as I employed this medicine in 6 or 30, I saw little or no benefit. But since I have for many years, by Dr. Gruber's advice, given it in 1 and 2, I have seen better results, especially in some cases of pulmonary tuberculosis." Dr. Bayes, also, seems quite satisfied with the third and lower potencies.

Before passing to other salts of potash which have an individuality of their own, I would mention that the presence of this substance as a natural constituent of the body has given it a place among Dr. Schüssler's "tissue-remedies." He uses the chloride, phosphate, and sulphate (Kali muriaticum, phosphoricum, sulphuricum) ; and thinks the first of great value in croupous inflammations of mucous membrane and severe affections of the skin ; the third in catarrhs and superficial disorders of the same parts ; and the second in nervous debility and septic conditions of the blood. I mention these points, though Dr. Schüssler's structure seems to me much founded on guess-work. The large proportion of potash normally present in muscle is the only fact of the kind which I should regard as practically significant.

We come now to the chlorate of potash,

Kali chloricum,

which also is prepared by trituration or aqueous solution.

A proving of Kali chloricum was published in the sixteenth volume of Stapf's *Archiv*, by Professor Martin of Jena. Eleven persons took part in it, using the crude drug. Dr. Allen giving Martin's results, adds several other observations.

The chlorate of potash was found by Stevens, when taken internally, to give the venous blood an arterial hue ; and the same result was obtained by O'Shaughnessy when he injected it into the vessels of animals. Taking this in connection with the large amount of oxygen it contains, and the readiness with which it parts with it, the salt was supposed to be a means of conveying oxygen to the blood and tissues; and was given accordingly in scorbutic conditions, in scarlet and other adynamic fevers, and in diphtheria. This theory is now considered invalid, as the salt is found unchanged in the urine, and other alkaline salts (as nitre) produce a similar effect on the blood. But practical men seem no less to believe in its power of improving cachectic states of the system; and give it accordingly in such diseases as syphilis, cancer* and phthisis, where the general condition is of this nature. Dr. Charles Drysdale and Mr. Allingham treat infantile syphilis with this medicine alone, and with excellent results;† Drs. Cotton and Chambers find it very beneficial in phthisis occurring in patients of broken-down constitutions. I venture to suggest that the agent of these effects is not the oxygen of the drug, but the chlorine. The liberation of this gas when hydrochloric acid is applied to the salt is well known, and it finds plenty of this acid in the stomach. Chlorine water, prepared by mixing the two in aqueous solution before administration, is in the same repute as chlorate of potash in acute disease, and might have like effects in chronic. This view is further supported by the deodorising influence of the chlorate when applied in solution, which is well known, but nowhere better illustrated than in a paper by Mr. Evan Fraser in the eighteenth volume of the *British Journal of Homœopathy*. It is far more likely that chlorine is at work here than oxygen, for the foul surfaces are already freely exposed to the latter element. The small quantity required for this purpose, moreover—Mr. Fraser finds ten grains to a pint of sufficient strength—quite corresponds with the fact that the larger part of the doses ordinarily given passes out unchanged in the urine (sometimes, I may mention, causing nephritis on its way). The decomposition of a very small quantity would liberate chlorine enough to do plenty of work.

However, whether it be chlorine or oxygen by which the salt influences cachectic conditions, the practice seems to belong to iatro-chemistry rather than to dynamism and homœopathy. But we can justly claim for the latter a still better established use of chlorate of potash—its power over *stomatitis*. I will state this in the words of Dr. Ringer. "It is of signal service in mercurial and simple salivation, in ulcerative stomatitis and aphthæ. It is particularly useful in ulceration of the edges of the gums. The influence of the chlorate on this form of ulceration is almost magical: in one or two days it

---

* See *Brit. Journ. of Hom.*, xxv., 518.
† *Treatment of Syphilis without Mercury* (1st ed.), pp. 130—132.

cleans the dirty-looking sores, and heals them in a day or two more. It is said to cure follicular and phagedenic ulceration like a charm." Let me now read you a case reported in the *Medical Times and Gazette* for May 22nd, 1858. A child had been taking from March 16th to May 18th, three times daily, at first ten and then five grains of the salt for strumous ophthalmia. "On May 18th she came with a very sore mouth. The saliva dripped from her lips, there were numerous follicular ulcers on the tongue and inside of lips, and one large one occupied a surface the size of a shilling on the back part of the dorsum of the tongue. The salivary glands were enlarged and tender, and the mouth full of saliva, although the ptyalism was not extreme nor were the gums sore. In this latter respect and in the existence of the larger ulcers on the tongue, the stomatitis differed from that caused by mercury." Nor is this an isolated occurrence. Mr. Hutchinson reports three other cases, and Mr. Traill a fourth,—the former describing the form of stomatitis it causes as exactly resembling that over which it exerts curative powers ; and salivation is ascribed to it by Isambert and other writers. It is eliminated by this secretion as freely as by the urine.

I hardly know whether Kali chloricum is as much used in the homœopathic treatment of affections in the mouth as it deserves to be. I never require any other medicine for simple stomatitis—that exudative inflammation of the buccal mucous membrane which the French call "muguet." I have lately found it very beneficial in one of those rare cases of epithelial degeneration of the mucous membrane of the mouth which Paget has described as often forerunning cancer, and an instance of which Dr. Cooper has mentioned as cured by him with Muriatic acid. In my case I gave that medicine with little effect. Mr. Fraser thinks that Kali chloricum has a specific power over ulceration in this region, and gives a good case where the process in the throat of a syphilitic patient was arrested by it. Dr. Joslin found it of eminent service in an epidemic of gangrenous stomatitis occurring in a Children's Home.

The pathogenesis may possibly guide us to further uses of the salt. Dr. Drysdale has recorded* a case of facial paralysis, beginning with face-ache, in which a rapid cure was effected by the first decimal trituration of Kali chloricum after the failure of Belladonna and Rhus. He was led to the medicine, not by the paralysis, but by the presence of tenderness on touch or pressure of the affected side, which is prominent

* *Brit. Journ.*, xxv., 316.

among its symptoms. It produced, however, in a person who took fifteen grammes a sensation as if half the head, face, and nose were paralysed.

In its action on the mouth Kali chloricum has for analogues *Mercury, Iodine, Nitric* and *Muriatic acids,* and *Iris.*

The 1st decimal trituration has been that which I have always used.

The third salt of potash which comes before us to-day is the nitrate,—the saltpetre or nitre of common parlance,

Kali nitricum.

The nitre of the shops, dissolved in hot water and deposited in crystals as it cools, is triturated for our use.

Nitre is one of the best-proved medicines we have. The pathogenesis in the second edition of the *Chronic Diseases* contains 588 symptoms from Schreter, Tietze, and Nenning (very few being from Hahnemann), and 122 from authors. A second pathogenesis, obtained by ten persons chiefly from good-sized doses of the first trituration, was published in the *Archiv,* and is translated in the first volume of the *Révue de la Matière Médicale specifique.* Jörg and eight pupils have also contributed to its proving,* besides Alexander of old ; and numerous cases of poisoning with the salt are related in the *Révue* (p. 336) and by Hempel. Dr. Allen embodies all these materials, giving 1,119 symptoms to the drug.

Before I practised homœopathically, nitre was a very favourite remedy of mine in the febrile affections of childhood. I supposed it to act chemically on the hot and hyperinotic blood, and dynamically on the excited circulation. I see no reason for supposing that I was wrong. Hahnemann says that " inasmuch as the production of cold in the system is the primary effect of Nitrum, its action in inflammatory fevers must be palliative only." It is so ; but in these ephemeral affections a palliative answers much the same purposes as a curative, as Hahnemann himself has said in reference to Opium. I have better remedies now ; but I remember with affection my formerly used nitre.

I confess, moreover, that I have not found a place for it in

---

* In my last edition, I spoke also of Löffler (and four associates) as having joined in the proving of nitre. In this I was mistaken, having been misled by Hempel. It was the nitrate of soda (Natrum nitricum) which Löffler proved, as Dr. Allen shows.

my new therapeutics; nor, it would seem, have others in our school. There is little trace of its use in homœopathic literature : Bayes and Teste omit it altogether, and Hempel and Espanet give but theoretical indications for its employment. All I can do, therefore, is to tell you what has been ascertained as to its physiological action.

Nitre shows the general properties which are now recognised as belonging to the salts of potash : it paralyses the spinal cord and the heart, arresting the action of the latter in diastole. This effect—seen best in experiments on animals— is pretty obvious in the poisonings and provings. It further acts like the alkalies generally on the blood, exerting there a spoliative and antiplastic influence. It is, moreover, an undoubted diuretic, and the solid constituents of the urine seem increased *pari passu* with the liquid. Sugar was found in it in one case of poisoning. The irritant influence on the kidneys suggested herein is also manifested elsewhere,—in poisonings by g stro-enteritis, and in provings by irritation of the respiratory mucous membrane (including the conjunctiva), the testicle and epididymis, the joints, and (in one instance) the salivary glands. There was often much pyrexia. In one case of poisoning there was acute œdema of the whole body : in another, after recovery from the first effects, chorea and great irritability of temper.

From these facts therapeutic indications may yet be drawn. Some hints, moreover, for dynamic uses of the salt may be got from its reputation in old-school therapeutics. Its action in acute rheumatism is hardly that of a mere alkali; and Alexander and Frank, among its provers, have experienced great pains in joints and muscles. The value of nitre-paper in relieving asthma is undoubted, and is not traceable to any known action of the drug ; Hahnemann mentions asthma as a morbid state especially calling for it. It has been praised in enuresis, to which, if that affection be paretic in nature, it is surely homœopathic.

I hope that thus we may some day find a place for nitre among our remedies, and that its extensive provings may not always remain barren. At present I can say nothing about allied medicines or dose.

The permanganate of potash,

Kali permanganicum,

is the last of its salts which I have to mention. It has been best known hitherto in the solution of it sold as "Condy's Fluid," where it disinfects and deodorises by means of the large proportion of oxygen it contains, and yields to organic matters. It has now received a most heroic proving from Dr. H. C. Allen, of Cleveland, which you may read in the twenty-fifth volume of the *British Journal of Homœopathy*. Its power is shown herein to set up acute inflammation of the throat, extending to the nares (whence the discharge was sanious), larynx, and salivary glands, and along the Eustachian tubes. With these symptoms there were diuresis and obstinate constipation, and much weakness. Putting together this elective affinity for the throat and its neighbourhood (for its action is not local,—as Stillé says, "upon mucous surfaces it causes neither pain nor irritation"), and the chemical power of the drug in dissolving the false membrane and destroying the offensive emanations of diphtheria, Dr. Allen tried it in a desperate case of the malignant form of this disease, with the most rapid and brilliant results. The usual remedies had been given without effect: the odour of the breath had become almost unbearable; a dark-coloured offensive diarrhœa had set in, while, " with vomiting, fluids taken by the mouth were returned by the nose, and a general prostration seemed to be the precursor of a fatal termination. At this stage," says Dr. Allen, "I dissolved three grains of the permanganate in one half-glass of water, and gave her a teaspoonful at 9 p.m., to be repeated every hour until I saw her. Called at 12 p.m., found her much improved, breathing easier, and a warm perspiration had made its appearance. Continued the medicine. The next morning I found her sitting up in her bed, and her whole appearance changed. On examining the throat, to my astonishment I found the membrane hitherto so extensive almost gone, a small patch on the left tonsil only being visible. The offensive character of the breath was completely changed; in fact, I could discover no odour at all. Continued the medicine every three hours while awake, and she went on to a speedy convalescence."

Dr. Allen adds : " This is only one of a number I could relate treated with the permanganate, all with equally good results." To my mind it recalls many a case in which I would have given anything for such a medicine, but which went down to the grave, untouched by the ordinary means. I have only had one good opportunity since of trying it ; and though the effect was *nil*, the case was hardly a fair one to be the test of any remedy, as paralysis of the velum palati occurred early, and allowed fluids to return through the nose. The tender mucous membrane, thus irritated, broke out in hæmorrhage, and the poor little fellow sank exhausted. I have also failed to meet with more than one* communication of its use, successful or otherwise, at the hands of others.

Drs. Drummond and Woodgates speak highly of a gargle of the permanganate (grs. iv. to ʒviij) in ulcerated sore-throat.†

My next medicine, the mountain-laurel,

Kalmia latifolia,

is another of those which have been proved by Dr. Constantine Hering. His pathogenesis, obtained by several persons with the dilutions from the 1st to the 30th, is contained in the *Materia Medica of American Provings.* Dr. Allen adds provings, made with substantial doses, by five other persons.

Kalmia sometimes proves poisonous to animals eating it, and even to human beings partaking of the honey of bees which have ransacked its blossoms or of pheasants who have lived upon it. From instances of the latter kind (confirmed by the more heroic provings given by Allen) it has been ascertained to act like Digitalis, diminishing the force and frequency of the heart's action in a very marked manner, and causing nausea and dimness of sight. Much pain is complained of in the region of the cervical vertebræ, which suggests that like its analogue it acts through the medulla oblongata. It has been comparatively little used in disease. Dr. Hering thinks it shares the relation of Ledum and Rhododendron to rheumatism—certainly few medicines cause so many rheumatoid pains ; and that it will be found useful in rheumatic affections of the heart. Dr. Bayes says he has found it curative in face-pains of this character, worse at night, and seemingly situated in the periosteum. Mr. Clifton reports a still fuller experience ; he has frequently used it with beneficial results in rheumatism, in organic heart-affections, and in neuralgia. The rheumatism in which it is indicated is acute, but non-febrile ; it shifts much, especially from above to below ; the pains are worse on the least motion and towards midnight. It gives relief when the pains seem suddenly to leave the extremities and go to the heart, without actual inflammation of the organ being set

---

* See *Brit. Journ. of Hom.*, xxxiv., 386.
† *Monthly Hom. Review,* vols. xi. and xii.

up. In organic disease of the heart, with pain and slow weak pulse, he has often seen benefit from it. He argues that the neuralgia in which it is useful is "rheumatic," *i.e.*, excited by cold in otherwise tolerably healthy subjects. It is nearly always, he says, on the right side, and often goes down the arm. The pain is generally succeeded by numbness, and may be associated (as in a case of brachialgia he records) with the characteristic slow pulse of the medicine. I would advise you to read Mr. Clifton's remarks in full : you will find them in the twenty-first volume of the *Monthly Homœopathic Review* (p. 423).

In the twenty-second volume of the same journal you will find an interesting study of Allen's pathogenesis of Kalmia, by Dr. Dyce Brown. He analyses especially the symptoms which point to its action on the cerebro-spinal system, the muscles, and the joints, and points out its homœopathic appropriateness to many morbid conditions of neurotic and rheumatic nature. Dr. Dunham, in his *Lectures* (I. 194), relates a case of rheumatic endocarditis so completely cured by it, that no valvular murmur remained.

The tincture is made from the leaves. Dr. Bayes gave the third decimal attenuation.

Let us now consider the place occupied in specific therapeutics by that product of the distillation of wood tar called

Kreosotum,

of which we make alcoholic attenuations for use.

A proving of Kreosote was carried out on seven persons (five of whom were females) by the late Dr. Wahle of Rome, and published in the sixteenth volume of the *Archiv*. Small doses only were employed, none taking over a drop. Dr. Syrbius also has proved it (rather more boldly) on himself and seven others. The results of these and other observations are given by Allen. Much interesting matter is contained in Dr. Cormack's monograph on the drug ; and Teste's article should by all means be consulted.

The results of Dr. Cormack's experiments on animals seem to me negative as respects the medicinal value of Kreosote. It appears to suspend the functions of the first organ through whose capillaries it passes, causing vertigo and stupor if introduced into the carotids, asphyxia if injected into the veins. These effects are probably due to the coagulation of the albumen of the blood, since Kreosote exerts an influence of this kind under all circumstances. Upon this influence, indeed, the remedial powers of the drug when applied locally seem to depend. If your experience leads you to think favourably of these uses, pray do not abandon them till you get something better. The point is quite outside the domain of homœopathy ; she says neither yea nor nay to the practice.

When we come to the dynamic effects of Kreosote, however, the aspect of things is changed. Pereira is never more homœopathic in his unconscious honesty than in treating of the properties of this drug. " Swallowed in large doses," he writes, " it causes *vomiting* and purging;" and again, " when the dose has been considerably augmented, *diarrhœa*, or even *dysentery*, has been produced." And then he goes on to tell us that " as an internal remedy, Kreosote has been principally celebrated, in this country, as a medicine possessing extraordinary powers of arresting *vomiting ;*" that in Sweden it was found very useful in a wide-spread epidemic of *dysentery ;* and that Mr. Spinks and Dr. Kesteven have published cases of its successful employment in common *diarrhœa.* While to crown all, we have this sentence :—" occasionally it increases the quantity of the urinary secretion ; but in diabetes it sometimes has an opposite effect."

The power of Kreosote over vomiting is the only one of these actions upon which I need dwell. It is recognised by us with our small doses as heartily as by the old school with their large. We agree, moreover, that it is in *sympathetic* vomiting that Kreosote proves specific—where the irritation starts from some other organ than the stomach. Thus the vomiting of phthisis, of hepatic and uterine cancer, and of chronic kidney disease, is often checked by it. I must say, however, that I once had a chronic case of suspected cancer of the stomach under treatment, the vomiting of which was always arrested by Kreosote when it became troublesome. I believe that some esteem it very highly in hysterical vomiting.

Dr. Hilbers considers that Kreosote has great power of sustaining the strength in some of these exhausting diseases, as well as of checking the vomiting; and relies much upon it in the treatment of phthisis. Like the other antiseptics, moreover (as Arsenic and Carbo), Kreosote has a dynamic influence over foul discharges and putrescent processes. I once made a very pretty cure with it of persistent lochial discharge, which had become brown and offensive. Wahle's provings, indeed, show that it has a very decided action on the uterus, vagina, and vulva, causing much leucorrhœa—yellow, offensive, and acrid, with itching, biting, smarting, and burning in the pudenda, and between the labia and the thighs; also menorrhagia, generally of dark colour and acrid character. These symptoms have naturally led to its use when uterine discharges have assumed morbid features of this kind, and frequently with success. You will find its indications very clearly given in Dr. Guernsey's *Obstetrics*. Besides those already mentioned, he notes two other among its pathogenetic effects as guiding symptoms for its choice—viz., a paroxysmal, intermitting character of the menstrual flow, and sharp stitches darting from the abdomen into the vagina. The morbid nature of the uterine discharges of Kreosote have, naturally enough, led to its trial in cancer and gangrene of the womb; but I am unable to speak of any success.

But we owe to the fertile and original mind of M. Teste a remarkable development of the uses of Kreosote. He calls attention to the effects of the continued use of smoked meat— "a sort of scurvy carrying off the teeth, foul breath, costiveness, a general malaise, and a real cacohymia." He then suggests that the power of Kreosote when locally applied, not merely to relieve temporarily the pain of toothache, but to arrest the progress of caries, is of a dynamic nature. Putting these facts together, he justifies by them the following statement drawn from his experience :

1. Kreosote is in children of all ages, as well as in adults, the chief remedy for *odontalgia*, when it is caused by caries of the teeth.

2. When *dentition* is so badly performed as to become a disease, comprising general irritation and cachexia with degeneration of the teeth themselves, especially when the child is constipated, Kreosote is the specific remedy.

These statements I can confirm from repeated trials in my own practice, which have yielded me almost uniform success. Dr. Madden also writes :—" I like Kreosote in dentition very much. My first case was our own baby. She had been extremely fretful and irritable and sleepless for three or four days, and Chamomilla had done no good. I gave Kreosote 24, and in a quarter of an hour she was asleep, and slept eleven hours right off, and woke cheerful. The nurse was almost frightened, thinking I must have given an opiate." Dr. Guernsey also speaks of Kreosote as " an invaluable remedy in difficult dentition," giving similar indications to those of Teste ; and adding that the symptoms are usually worst from 6 p.m. to 6 a.m., so that the child (and nurse) gets little sleep.

I cannot follow M. Teste, however, when he goes on to extol Kreosote as " the specific for syphilis in nursing children." If he limits it, as he seems to do subsequently, to cases " where the disease manifests itself under the exanthematous form," I shall not disagree. But I have failed to see any effect from Kreosote upon the profound cacohymia which this sad disease so often manifests.

M. Teste further adds that Kreosote is most suitable to delicate cachectic children : and, when given to those of a lively, vigorous, and sanguine constitution, makes them feel so uncomfortable that the exhibition of Ferrum metallicum as an antidote becomes necessary.

It may be well to remember, when we are studying the constitutional action of Kreosote, the virtues ascribed of old to tar water, as by Bishop Berkeley in his *Siris*. Dr. Sharp has called attention to these, characterising the condition of body in which it was so commended as a " dyscrasia where there is a strong tendency in the fluids to decomposition, and in the solids to disorganization." Kreosote, which is one of the most important constituents of tar, may possibly inherit its renown.

You will see from what I have now said that I cannot accept the present identification of Kreosote with *Carbolic acid* as a remedy. The two have similar chemical properties, and coincide at some points of their spheres of action ; but these are quite distinct. Closer analogues of Kreosote are *Carbo animalis* and *vegetabilis ; Mercurius ;* and *Petroleum*.

I have used from the second to the sixth dilution for vomiting and uterine discharges ; but have followed M. Teste in giving the 12th in toothache, and the 24th in morbid dentition and infantile syphilis.

I conclude this lecture with a short account of the virtues of the wild lettuce,

Lactuca virosa.

The milky juice of this plant and of the milder Lactuca sativa has long been in use as lactucarium. In homœopathic practice a tincture prepared from the entire plant is employed.

The general knowledge about the action of lactucarium is well epitomised by Pereira. There is a proving of Lactuca virosa in the fifth volume of the *Hygea ;* and a summary of the experiments, with remarks and observations from authors, is given by Dr. Seidel in the second volume of the *Journal für Arzneimittellehre*, and translated in the first volume of the *Révue de la Matière Médicale specifique.* All the provers (fifteen in number) took considerable doses of the tincture or extract. Dr. Allen gives a few additional symptoms.

As very little is known about this drug (it is not mentioned by Hempel or Teste) I will read you in full the summary of its effects furnished by Dr. Seidel.

"The general character of the action of Lactuca virosa can be traced from the preceding experiments as follows :—

"Immediately after taking it, there was a sensation of heat in the stomach, accompanied by an uneasiness which mounted into the throat, and an insipid taste. After a quarter of an hour, this sensation gave place to an icy coldness in the stomach and throat. At the same time, the prover experienced a contraction at the pit of the stomach, which was followed by real præcordial anguish ; the thorax seemed compressed and narrowed, especially while sitting with the body bent. He felt a desire to breathe deeply, an ardent longing for the open air ; and had frequent yawnings. It was not till after this that the head became confused and giddy, without, however, the judgment being obscured. He had a sensation (a physical one) of wavering in the brain, which rendered every posture of the body uncertain, and was accompanied with buzzings in the depth of the ears. After from fifteen to thirty minutes there supervened, in the midst of eructations which gave but slight relief, gurglings in the abdomen with emission of flatulence, which last did good. The præcordial anguish diminished, and alternated with heats, flying shootings, and sensations of cold in the chest. Deglutition became difficult, not because of any obstacle in the throat, but because the muscles of the pharynx refused their office. There were also constant sighings. Keeping himself seated with the body bent relieved the stomach ; and sitting upright did good to the chest. The thorax could not bear any pressure ; there was cloudiness of the head, but the veil which covered the sight disappeared when he fixedly regarded an object. At the end of an hour mucosity had accumulated in the throat, which with some was at the same time rough ; and a cough was set up whose short paroxysms grievously pained the chest and the head. This cough became more violent afterwards, and the headache grew worse. This last was characterised at one time by confusion merely, at another by painful pressings. In some subjects, there was at this time a 'clavus hystericus.' With these there were fulness in the abdomen, obscuration of sight, and difficulty of breathing. The above symptoms increased

2 Q

up to the third or fourth hour, and then diminished little by little. Those of the chest, especially the oppression and desire to breathe deeply, continued several days. Those of the abdomen went off most frequently with emissions of flatulence or with a scanty stool, pappy or loose, which took place the first day, and was followed by a long constipation. During the first few hours, the secretion of urine was restrained, but later it increased considerably. There was shuddering, with great prostration and lassitude, for the first days; and in the nights deep sleep, quiet, sometimes lethargic; but afterwards the sleep was agitated and interrupted. The pulse was somewhat less frequent during the first days. The disposition manifested itself in sadness, anxiety, and causeless chagrin."

Besides these symptoms, I note the hepatic sufferings of many of the provers : with one " the liver was swollen, hard, the pressure of the hand under the false ribs could not be borne, with a rather pressive pain."

The facts here given warrant Dr. Seidel in further saying that " the pure milky juice of the lettuce, as it is contained in 'lactucarium,' seems to act principally on the brain and nervous system, and to exert less sensible effects in the vegetative sphere than preparations in which the juice of the whole plant is employed." The observations summarized by Pereira embrace the neurotic properties only of the drug. It is regarded as a " sedative," diminishing the force and frequency of the pulse, and disposing to sleep. Hence its name of " lettuce-opium." It differs, however, from Opium in causing no excitement either of brain or circulation.

In ordinary practice, lactucarium has been employed as an " anodyne, hypnotic, antispasmodic, and sedative ;" but its operation is considered uncertain. In the school of Hahnemann Lactuca has hitherto found little if any employment; the only symptom indicated by Allen as having been frequently verified is " incessant spasmodic cough, which threatens to burst the chest : it is always caused by a peculiar tickling in the fauces, which in turn seems to be produced by a sensation of suffocation in the throat." It seems indicated however, in some forms of hepatic and pulmonary congestion, of clavus, and of cerebral weakness with somnolence. At any rate, should a repertory ever direct us to it, we may prescribe it with confidence that the symptoms are genuine effects of the drug.

The dilution best suited to obtain the homœopathic action has not yet been ascertained.

LECTURE XXXIX.

LACHESIS AND THE SERPENT-POISONS.

I shall devote to-day's lecture to the medicine we call Lachesis, taking occasion thereby to discourse upon the medicinal use of serpent-venom generally, and upon the other members of the family which, as Crotalus, Naja, Elaps, and Vipera respectively, have place in the Materia Medica of Homœopathy.

We prepare such substances by triturating the virus, or dissolving it in glycerine. Alcohol is not considered a suitable menstruum for the lower attenuations; but it seems to make no difference when we get into the region of infinitesimals.

Of our sources of information as to the physiological effects of snake-venom we must place first in order the *Wirkungen des Schlangengiftes* of Dr. Constantine Hering. A copy of this rare book I am able to lay before you. Published in 1837, it contains a full collection of the phenomena of snake-bites, as observed and recorded by authors before that time. These are arranged in the Hahnemannian schema, and incorporated with them are numerous symptoms obtained by the author and seventeen fellow-observers on both healthy and sick persons. This collection contains symptoms obtained from the lance-headed viper, *Lachesis trigonocephalus;* the rattlesnake, *Crotalus horridus;* the cobra, *Naja tripudians;* and from the Italian and German species of viper—*Vipera Redi* and *torva*. The provings of Lachesis venom were all made with the thirtieth dilution; but some of the symptoms recorded appeared in Dr. Hering himself while triturating it, and from taking the first and second attenuations so prepared. Crotalus was proved in these last-named potencies, and among the effects referred to are some obtained from swallowing the poison-bag made into pills with cheese.

The next great contribution to our knowledge on this subject was made by Dr. Rutherfurd Russell, who—in conjunction with Dr. Stokes—proved the poison of the cobra on ten male and three female subjects, using the first, third, and sixth attenuations. An account of these excellent experiments is given in detail in the eleventh and twelfth volumes of the *British Journal of Homœopathy.*

Dr. Allen, as is his wont (and in this case I think with ample warrant), separates the pathogeneses of the various snake-poisons. Those of Lachesis, Crotalus, and Naja, while containing the material specified above, add fresh observations,— of the effects of bites with the two latter, of symptoms observed in patients taking the drug with the former. He gives us, for the first time, a complete pathogenesis of *Elaps corallinus,* the Brazilian coral-snake, made of three provings instituted by Drs. Mure and Lippe—the 3rd and 4th attenuations being used.

Dr. Russell prefixes to his proving several fresh narratives of poisoning by cobra-bites. But this branch of the subject has received special attention of late. Sir Joseph Fayrer's great work on *The Thanatophidia of India* is known to all ; but, as it is too much of a *livre de luxe* to be generally accessible, I will make my references to the narratives of poisoning extracted from it which Dr. Pyburn has collected in the sixteenth volume of the *Monthly Homœopathic Review.* I would also commend to your notice the essay of Dr. Weir Mitchell, " On the Venom of the Rattlesnake," contained in the twelfth volume of the *Smithsonian Contributions to Knowledge* (Washington, 1860) ; and also an account of a series of inoculations of the same virus, practised with the hope that they would prove prophylactic of yellow fever, given by Dr. Neidhard in his treatise *On Crotalus horridus in Yellow Fever* (second edition, New York, 1868). Finally, I would refer you to a useful account of some recent experimentation on animals as to the effect of serpent-bites, contributed to the thirty-fourth volume of the *British Journal* by Dr. Bayes, under the title of " The Differential Symptomatology of Naja tripudians and Crotalus poisons."

I must repeat here what I said under the head of Apis, that it is no longer necessary to apologize for our use of serpent-venom as a medicine introduced through the ordinary channel. It is now fully admitted, by those most qualified to judge, that such virus does act however admitted into the circulation, though most certain and rapid in its influence when it enters the blood direct.

I think that the results of serpent-bites, or of the inoculation of their venom, will be found to fall into three groups, corresponding to three leading forms of disease.

I. In the first group the symptoms are those of direct

poisoning of the nervous centres without local inflammation or blood changes. From the experiments of Dr. Brunton and Sir J. Fayrer on animals, it would appear that "the great shock of the poison is first felt in the nervous centres of the cord, gradually involving those of the medulla oblongata and of the ganglia of the mesocephale, and lastly implicating the functional integrity of the hemispheres of the brain." The sympathetic system (at any rate in its cardiac portion) they think the last to suffer; as though paralysis of the vagus is indicated by augmented pulsation of the heart as well as cessation of the respiration, by inducing the latter process artificially the heart can be kept going and life prolonged for a considerable period. I am inclined to think that—at any rate with Naja—the medulla and mesocephale are sometimes affected even earlier than the cord. Mr. F. Buckland, in his interesting *Curiosities of Natural History*, relates how, having skinned a rat which had been killed by a cobra-bite, he omitted to notice that on one of his fingers, near the nail, there was a small raw place. Shortly afterwards, however, while walking, "*all of a sudden I felt*," he writes, "*just as if somebody had come behind me, and struck me a severe blow on the head and neck*, and at the same time I experienced a most acute pain and sense of oppression at the chest, as though a hot iron had been run in and a hundredweight put on top of it." Sometimes the symptoms are those of epilepsy, as in the second case in Dr. Pyburn's paper; sometimes they are tetaniform, as in the fourth; most frequently there is nothing but profound prostration with speedily supervening unconsciousness. From the sense of being heated all over experienced in the third and fourth cases, we may infer paresis of the vaso-motor system. A bitten person who recovered speaks of a "violent throbbing headache" soon coming on (case 6). Inoculation of the rattlesnake virus produced at the moment vertigo, which soon passed away; more rarely a nervous trembling of longer duration. Other neurotic effects of the inoculation were headache, generally occupying the frontal and orbital region, and lasting on an average twenty-one hours; and neuralgic pains in the head and neck.

The outline thus given us in the effects of direct introduction of snake-venom is filled in by the experiments which have been made with the diluted virus taken internally. These must be studied in the records I have mentioned. The main effects here also are seen in the parts supplied from the nerves arising at the base of the brain, especially the pneumogastric. The throat and laryngeal symptoms of Lachesis are very numerous and distinctive. Beyond hawking of mucus they are purely subjective; but they include well-nigh every form of distress from which the parts can suffer. Dryness, pain, burning, rawness, swelling is complained of, also a sense as if a morsel of food had remained after eating; swallowing is difficult and painful, but more so when "empty" than when ingesting food, and more for liquids than for solids. The larynx is painful and sensitive; there is hoarseness, with continual tickling cough, and a constant desire to draw a deep breath. All the symptoms are aggravated by external pressure, and the contact and weight of mere covering are resented.

The headache produced by Naja (its seat being chiefly in one or other temporal region) was often very severe, and accompanied with profound depression. The headache of Lachesis was especially marked by a tendency to extend into the root of the nose.

II. The second form of serpent poisoning which seems to obtain is the *purpuric* or *hæmorrhagic*. Dr. Pyburn refers to some instances of this,* but a fuller account of it is given by Dr. Neidhard and by Dr. Mitchell.

Dr. Neidhard shows the inoculations to have produced, in from eighteen to twenty-four hours, the hæmorrhagic condition of the gums which authors regard as a characteristic symptom of yellow fever, and pathologically identical with its black vomit. With this there were febrile heat, thirst and anorexia, red countenance, and injected conjunctiva; then jaundice and swelling of the face, with angina tonsillaris.

Dr. Mitchell found, when death was not caused by the ordinary nervous shock, decomposition of the blood set up, resulting in its complete diffluence and non-coagulability. Ecchymoses and hæmorrhages were constant in the animals poisoned by him. He thinks the fibrin affected rather than the corpuscles, but Sir J. Fayrer found the latter altered in form and non-adherent.

In a later contribution to the *Medical Times and Gazette*,† Dr. Mitchell speaks again of the striking power of snake venom to cause hæmorrhages. You have only, he says, to moisten the intestinal peritoneum with it, and blood will be forthwith effused at the spot.

He concludes his account of the action of the rattlesnake venom by "calling attention to the singular likeness between the symptoms and lesions of Crotalus poisoning and those of certain maladies, such as yellow fever." He points out that

* Pp. 676, 677.
† Feb. 6, 1869.

in either there is " a class of cases in which death seems to occur suddenly and inexplicably, as though caused by an overwhelming dose of the poison." This holds good also of scarlatina. " A second class of cases survive the first shock of the malady, and then begin to exhibit the train of symptoms which terminate in more or less complete degradation of the blood. All these maladies, varying among themselves, exhibiting, as it were, preferences for this or that organ, agree in the destruction of the fibrin of the blood which their fatal cases frequently exhibit. In yellow fever the likeness to the venom-poisoning is most distinctly preserved, as we trace the symptoms of both diseases to the point where the diffluent blood leaks out into the mucous and serous cavities." The effects of inoculation, as I have cited them, quite sustain Dr. Mitchell's comparison; and the angina tonsillaris noted there again adds scarlatina to the similar diseases.

The *jaundice* of snake-bites is one element in the resemblance of their phenomena to those of yellow fever. Frerichs* mentions several cases of its occurrence. It is not caused by obstruction to the flow of bile; and it depends either upon disordered innervation, or upon changes in the blood hindering the due metamorphosis of the reabsorbed secretion. Of jaundice from the former cause we have an instance in that form of it which has followed (often suddenly) from mental emotions. The rapidity with which yellowness sometimes supervenes upon bites, especially of the viper (" in less than an hour" Mead says he has seen it†), suggests this explanation of it. But there is a jaundice which appears later on in the course of snake poisoning, which rather denotes that which is characteristic of yellow fever, and which not unfrequently complicates pyæmia, typhus, and other acute blood infections. In these maladies there is no change in the secreting structure of the liver, and hardly enough in its circulation, to account for the deep and lasting jaundice observed. Moreover, " it is worthy of notice," writes Frerichs, " that when the diseases just alluded to are complicated with jaundice, a group of severe symptoms, such as *hæmorrhages from the gastro-intestinal mucous membrane, ecchymoses of the surface*, albuminuria, *hæmaturia*, suppression of urine, &c., manifest themselves." Such symptoms plainly point to an extensive disorganization of the blood, and have already come before us as effects of serpent poisoning. I have in another

* *Diseases of the Liver* (New Syd. Soc.), vol. i, p. 160.
† *Ibid.*

place gone into the theory of their causation,* and will only here suggest that they depend upon some destructive agent which may either be furnished by the liver itself, as in acute atrophy of that organ, or formed independently of it as in these fevers. In the former case they find their *simile* in Phosphorus; in the latter in snake-venom.

You will observe that it is almost entirely from the poison of the rattlesnake that we obtain the hæmatic effects of serpent venom. The comparative experiments of Dr. Brunton and Sir J. Fayrer led them to the conclusion that "there is a greater tendency to both local and general hæmorrhage and extravasation of blood and of the colouring-matter of the blood" in poisoning by the rattlesnake than in that of either the cobra or the viper. So in Hering's pathogenesis of Crotalus we have (as from bites) "hæmorrhage from all the organs of the body, eyes, ears, nose, mouth, and urethra," to which there is nothing corresponding under Lachesis and Naja.

III. In the third place we have those symptoms which result from the local affection induced by the bite. The inflammation set up is always of an asthenic character. In form it is a cellulitis or an erysipelas. Its sanies is absorbed either by the lymphatics, causing angioleucitis, abscess of the lymphatic glands, and inflammation of the areolar tissue higher up; or by the veins, resulting in pyæmia. The local inflammation often goes on to gangrene; and with this, and the other secondary consequences described, there is constitutional disorder of a typhoid type.

These phenomena at once open a wide range of action for serpent venom, when administered as a remedy according to the principle *similia similibus.* Whenever a local affection assumes a malignant character, and from thence proceed poisoning of the blood and prostration of the nervous energies, its use is indicated. Traumatic gangrene, carbuncle, malignant pustule, malignant erysipelas, putrid sore throat, are instances of such a pathological state. The effects of dissection wounds, and pyæmia in general, come within the same category; and the second stage of malignant scarlatina often belongs to it, where, as Watson puts it, "the system is reinoculated from" the ulcerated and gangrenous throat.

We have now to inquire how far these indications have been carried out in practice. The materials for such an inquiry are scattered throughout our literature; but there are three records of especial fulness to which I shall make re-

* *Brit. Journ. of Hom.,* xxii., 127.

ference. The first is an article on Lachesis by its introducer, Dr. C. Hering, in the second volume of the *British Journal of Homœopathy.* The second is a series of cases of severe disease, illustrating the action of the same remedy, by Dr. Carroll Dunham, in the fourth volume of the *American Homœopathic Review.*[*] The third is a paper on the snake-poisons, by Dr. Bradshaw, of Nottingham, which you will find in the first volume of the *Annals of the British Homœopathic Society.*

I. In the *neurotic* sphere of these poisons they have proved most valuable remedies. They heal, as they hurt, especially when the nerves having their centres in the medulla oblongata are disordered. Hence their usefulness in affections of the throat and larynx, the bronchi, and the heart.

Lachesis is a great medicine for what may be called a "nervous sore throat." In its acute form the sense of aching is out of all proportion to the visible mischief. When chronic, it is the "irritable throat," always uneasy, and causing choking, hawking, and coughing. The feeling as of a dry spot in the throat, or of general dryness of the part, especially on waking from sleep, also of a lump in the throat on empty deglutition, is characteristic of it. Several of Dr. Hering's cases are of this kind ; and there is a striking one in the twenty-second volume of the *British Journal of Homœopathy* (p. 488). It is thought by some that Lachesis even controls inflammations of the throat, as tonsillitis[†] and syphilitic angina.[‡] Naja certainly effected, in Dr. Russell's hands, a rapid cure of an acute pharyngo-laryngitis.[§] He considered it indicated when the fauces had a dark-red colour.

The affection of the larynx in which Lachesis has been found curative is a catarrh with little secretion and much sensitiveness. The cough is dry, coming as it were from a sense of tickling in the larynx, provoked by deep inspiration, by speaking, and especially by external pressure, which cannot be borne, and aggravates the whole trouble. "There is moreover a sense of fulness in the trachea and a very painful aching in the os hyoides." I quote from Dr. Carroll Dunham, whose comparison of Lachesis with Belladonna, Phosphorus, Causticum and Rumex crispus is a masterly piece of work.[||]

[*] See also the article on the drug in the second volume of his *Lectures on Materia Medica.*
[†] *Amer. Journ. of Hom. Mat. Med.*, i, 126.
[‡] Hering, Case 4. *Amer. Hom. Rev.*, iv, 410. *Brit. Journ of Hom.*, xxxi, 127.
[§] *Brit. Journ. of Hom.*, xii, 213.
[||] See *Hom. the Science of Therapeutics*, p. 417.

Naja has proved in my hands very useful in cough. laryngismus, and even spasmodic stricture of the œsophagus, when
these are the result of spinal irritation affecting the nucha.

Lachesis has no power over bronchitis, as such ; but it has
rendered great service in this affection as a neurotic ally. It
is indicated when the cough is spasmodic and suffocative ; and,
though abundance of fluid mucus is heard in the chest, it is
not expectorated,* or only after long effort.† Such coughs
occur especially in the subjects of cyanosis and cardiac disease ;
and in their bronchial attacks Lachesis should always be
thought of.

Both Lachesis and Naja are of great value in cardiac
affections ; not, I think, by direct action on the substance
of the organ, but by influencing its innervation. In the
"tremulous irritability of the heart" left behind after
scarlatina‡ and such-like fevers, and in the sympathetic
cough of cardiac affections, Lachesis is highly praised. Dr.
Hale has lately recorded a case of rapid heart's action (the
pulse was 160) from paresis of the vagus in which it was
rapidly curative.§ Naja was Dr. Russell's favourite remedy
for chronic nervous palpitation, for the restoration of a heart
damaged by acute inflammation, and for assuaging the sufferings of chronic hypertrophy and valvular disease. ‖ Its power
of removing valvular murmurs (apparently from fibrinous deposition) remaining in young persons after acute rheumatism
is really very striking ; and I have lately seen it do the same
thing in a man of fifty. Dr. Bradshaw reports a case of angina
pectoris cured with it (Case 1).

Besides these pneumogastric disorders, we have *headache* as a
trouble in which both Lachesis and Naja have done good
service. The headaches of Lachesis are fully discussed and
illustrated in Dr. Black's papers in the fifth volume of the
British Journal of Homœopathy (pp. 403, 424—435).¶ The
"nervous" and the "sick" headache are its spheres ; the pain
is unilateral and the face pale. It is also good for the burning
vertex headaches of the menopausia. The headache of Naja
is a dull but severe pain in the temporo-frontal region, with
much depression of spirits.** Dr. Russell also speaks well of

* *Amer. Hom. Review*, iv, 415.
† Bayes, *Applied Homœopathy*, p. 109.
‡ *Annals*, iv, 167.
§ *American Homœopathist*, ii.
‖ *Brit. Journ. of Hom.*, xii, 372, 549 ; *Annals*, i, 297
¶ See also *Brit. Journ of Hom.*, xxii, 482.
** *Brit. Journ.*, xii, 214.

it in weight and pressure at the vertex, with cold feet and flushes of the face.

I have no knowledge of the application to practice of the epileptic and tetanic phenomena occasionally induced by snake venom, though it would seem specially homœopathic to traumatic tetanus, and no less so to hydrophobia.*   But one of the most valuable uses of Lachesis hangs on the paresis of the sympathetic which we have seen induced in sufferers from the bite.   It is in that *vaso-motor ataxy*, or ganglionic nervousness, which is exhibited chiefly in the "flushings" of the climacteric period, but which has other manifestations.   It constitutes or complicates most affections occurring at this time of life, and Lachesis is helpful in all of them.   This is the general testimony of those who have used it.†   The eighth case of Dr. Hering's series is one of nervous dyspepsia, which reads like a neurosis of the solar plexus.

In these nervous affections "characteristic" symptoms of drugs, however trivial, are often useful guides.   One of these, as regards Lachesis, is that symptoms especially appear, or are aggravated, on waking from sleep; another, that external pressure, even of the clothes, is intolerable to the patient; another that (where the organ affected is bilateral) the symptoms begin on the left side and tend to pass over to the right.   I should have said that in graver maladies such *nugæ* would be out of place, but they seem to influence our transatlantic colleagues in the most serious cases—the commencement on the left side in diphtheria and scarlatina anginosa, the aggravation after sleeping in croup.   A sense of mental depression and uneasiness on waking is often noted by Dr. Guernsey as characteristic of Lachesis.

II. Next, what use has been made of the *hæmatic* action of serpent venom?

Of purpura I find two cases in which Lachesis was given.‡ In both it rapidly dissipated the symptoms.   The hæmorrhage was subcutaneous only.   The constant oozing of blood from an ulcer remaining after post-scarlatinal abscess led to its use in one instance,§ and with the best results.   Dr. Liebold and also Drs. Allen and Norton consider the snake-poisons, and

* The symptoms induced in dogs by the bite of the cobra often shadowed out, and in one case strikingly imitated, even to the rage, the phenomena of hydrophobia (*Brit. Journ. of Hom.*, xi, 82—84).

† *Monthly Hom. Review*, ix, 763; *Brit. Journ. of Hom.*, xxxi, 127—131.

‡ *Amer. Journ. of Hom. Mat. Med.*, iv, 66; *Brit. Journ. of Hom.*, xxii, 489.

§ *Amer. Hom. Rev.*, iv., 362.

particularly Lachesis, the best remedies for retinitis apoplectica.
Our information regarding its employment in yellow fever
comes from Drs. Holcombe* and Neidhard.† The former at
first used Lachesis in alternation with Arsenicum, so that his
experience was of doubtful value. But in a second epidemic,
having come to the just conclusion that the serpent-poisons
were the most truly homœopathic remedies for the disease
which we possess, he gave them in every case,—choosing
Crotalus in preference to Lachesis when blood-poisoning was
predominant. On both occasions he got excellent results.
Dr. Neidhard, in an epidemic occurring in Philadelphia in
1853, was led to rely more and more exclusively on Crotalus
in its treatment. He found the dilutions from the third downwards far superior to the higher. In 1858 some more cases
occurred, and again Crotalus served him well. He was thus
led to give it in cognate forms of disease (as he considers them)
—the "bilious remittents" of his neighbourhood, which often
assume a malignant form, and then closely resemble the true
"typhus icterodes." Here, also, he found the remedy of signal
value.

Serpent venom (and especially Crotalus) should be borne in
mind as a remedy :—

First, whenever jaundice, primary or secondary, is accompanied with ecchymoses or hæmorrhages. Here it compares
with Phosphorus, which would supplant it when the liver
was intimately affected, as in acute atrophy of that organ.
Jaundice from mental emotion would also suggest snake
venom, and here rather that of the viper, as its remedy.

Secondly, whenever a purpuric condition supervenes upon
other diseases, as typhus and variola, constituting their hæmorrhagic forms. These are very fatal, and a powerful remedy
for them is much needed. Arsenic is tolerably homœopathic,
but is hardly rapid enough in its action.

Thirdly, when the epidemic cerebro-spinal meningitis appears
in the form known as "malignant purpuric" or "spotted
fever."‡ Here the prostration is early and intense ; the
febrile reaction slight ; and the appearance of petechiæ constant, with sometimes hæmorrhages.

III. Malignant local inflammations, with secondary blood
infection and nervous prostration, have proved pre-eminently
the sphere of action of Lachesis. A typical instance is traumatic gangrene. Of this disease Dr. D. M. Dake has pub-

* *North Amer. Journ. of Hom.*, iii.
† Op. cit.
‡ *Brit. Journ. of Hom.*, xxiii, 394-5.

lished three cases, which are so decisive as to overcome even Dr. Hempel's scepticism as to the virtue of the remedy. They are given at length in the second edition of his *Materia Medica ;* and in the fourth volume of the *American Homœo-pathic Review* Dr. Searle, of Brooklyn, has recorded two others.   To these I would add the testimony of Dr. Franklin, who, as army-surgeon in the late civil war in America, had abundant opportunity of seeing the disease.   " I have used this remedy," he writes in his *Science and Art of Surgery,* " in a number of cases of gangrene following wounds, and have never been disappointed in its results.   In a case of compound com-minuted leg-fracture, terminating in gangrene and threaten-ing speedy destruction of the limb, the gangrene was quickly checked by the internal and external use of Lachesis, the inflammation subsiding, and the healing process moving on to a complete cure.   In another case of compound dislocation of the ankle-joint, with fracture of malleolus externus, followed by gangrene, Lachesis effected a speedy cure, the patient making a good recovery under the surgical treatment em-ployed.   I cannot recommend too highly the use of this agent for gangrene, and am confident that the observations of all who have employed or may employ it will bear me out in the assertion that it is eminently curative of gangrenous affections."

It is affections of this kind, moreover, which form the bulk of the paper of Dr. Carroll Dunham to which I have referred. He begins with a case of septicæmia occurring in his own person, as the result of a wound incurred during the post-mortem examination of a case of puerperal peritonitis.   Both the local and general symptoms were severe, but they rapidly yielded to Lachesis 12, three times a day.   Next he relates an epidemic of malignant pustule, in which he treated eight cases with Lachesis alone.   " It relieved the pain within a few hours after the first dose was given, and the patients all recovered very speedily."   Then he speaks of three cases of phlebitis supervening upon ulcers (probably syphilitic) of the lower extremities.   There was a great and sudden prostration of strength, low muttering delirium, and general typhoid symp-toms, indicating pyæmic infection.   The effect of Lachesis was all that could be desired, the patients rallying promptly, and all symptoms of phlebitis speedily disappearing.   Last, he narrates one case, and refers to others, of carbuncle, in which the constitutional symptoms denoted very great prostration, *not* preceded or attended by the nervous and vascular erethism which is sometimes observed in similar cases.   The absence of this condition is, he thinks, in all these disorders the indication for Lachesis as against Arsenicum, when the asthenia is not so complete as to call for Carbo vegetabilis.

Dr. Dunham finally refers to the usefulness of Lachesis in certain cases of diphtheria. In these the tumefaction of the throat was slight, and the redness of the mucous membrane hardly noticeable, the diphtheritic deposits consisting merely of two or three patches hardly larger than a pin's head. But the prostration of strength was quite alarming;* the pulse became, in a very short time, slow, feeble, and compressed; a cold, clammy sweat frequently covered the forehead and extremities; the breath was foetid; the appetite entirely destroyed. "In such cases," he writes, "in all in which the constitutional symptoms thus predominated over the local, Lachesis produced prompt and lasting improvement, so much so that very rarely was any other remedy given subsequently." To the same effect is the testimony of Dr. Tietze, of Philadelphia, in the fourth volume of the *United States Medical and Surgical Journal.* He mentions a purple, livid colour of the affected parts, with dull, dry appearance and little swelling, also pain out of all proportion to the amount of inflammation, as local characteristics of the remedy. He places it as third to Belladonna and Apis in throat affections, in the descent from sthenic to asthenic conditions. Dr. E. M. Hale also contributes to the *American Journal of Homœopathic Materia Medica*† three similar cases of diphtheria in children, which made a rapid recovery under Lachesis, while the rest of the family (altogether eight in number) under old-school treatment succumbed to the disease.

Cognate to diphtheria is scarlatina. We have already seen how Dr. Mitchell suggests the similarity between the phenomena of snake-poisoning in its most *foudroyant* form, and those of the invasion of malignant scarlet, as well as yellow, fever. Dr. P P. Wells sustains the comparison from the homœopathic point of view.‡ But there is another stage of scarlatina in which the power of Lachesis comes into play. It is when the throat symptoms assume a virulent character, and therewith signs of blood poisoning and prostration show

---

* "In acute cases" (of snake-poisoning) "the symptoms of depression are most marked, and the heart and nerve centres are suddenly and fearfully enfeebled, so that the irritability is lessened, and is finally lost earlier than occurs in other forms of death" (Mitchell, *loc. cit*). "The principal constitutional effect of the venom is a general prostration of the most appalling character" (*Ibid*).

† Vol. i., p. 184.

‡ *Amer. Hom. Review*, IV, 335; see also p. 556.

themselves. I am reminded as I speak of a case of this kind where Lachesis rapidly removed the patient from the sphere of gravest foreboding into that of happy convalescence.

I have already suggested malignant erysipelas, and pyæmic infection in general, as morbid states of this kind, and thus indicative of snake venom in their treatment. Severe symptoms resulting from insect stings would also call for it in preference to Apis or Ledum : there is on record a case of the bite of the tarantula in which it proved very efficacious.* The following narrative, moreover, suggests the homœopathicity of Crotalus to glanders. " On the Rio Grande, in October, 1857, two horses were bitten by the same rattlesnake while grazing. A few hours afterwards the sub-maxillary, parotid, and all glands situated about the head and neck were greatly enlarged ; from the nostrils and gums a clear mucous discharge ran down ; the eyes were glairy, with the pupils greatly dilated ; and the coat was rough and staring." After antidotes, " both horses recovered ; one, although reduced in flesh and thrown out of condition, was fit for work in a week, but the other only just escaped with his life, became a perfect skeleton, and only commenced to mend at the end of three weeks."†

There are other uses of snake-venom, to which I cannot do more than refer. Both Lachesis and Naja have a decided ovarian action, and have proved useful in chronic affections of this organ.‡ I am inclined to think that Lachesis acts most on the right, Naja on the left ovary. As regards Lachesis I am here in accord with Dr. Guernsey, but at variance with Dr. Lippe.§ The ovarian action of Naja was first observed by Dr. Holcombe in a patient to whom he was giving the medicine for cardiac disease, and it was the left ovary in which the " violent crampy pain" was developed. Lachesis has cured inflammation of the cæcum ;‖ and I have often seen it arrest threatened ulceration about the ancle in cases of varicosis of the leg. It is also of great value in ulcers themselves, when of the " irritable" kind. Naja was of use in Dr. Bradshaw's hands (as also in Dr. Russell's) in spinal irritation, and in the cough of pulmonary and laryngeal phthisis. Dr. Hilbers also esteems Crotalus highly for phthisical cough. But the

---

* *Amer. Journ. of Hom. Mat. Med.*, iv., 106.
† *Monthly Hom. Review*, xiv., 442.
‡ *Amer. Journ. of Hom. Mat. Med.*, i., 44 ; *United States Med. and Surg. Journ.*, ii., 85.
§ *Cincinnati Medical Advance*, Sept., 1876, p. 216.
‖ *Brit. Journ. of Hom.*, v., 40.

three spheres of action in which we have seen the poison of serpents at work are its main field of operation. It is here an exquisite instance of the operation of the law of similars. The circles of its poisonous and curative action exactly coincide. Not only is it true here that *quantum venenum, tantum remedium*, but also *quale venenum, tale remedium.*

In all this I have been speaking of the three great examples of snake-venom, Lachesis, Naja, and Crotalus. Of the poison of the viper I can say little, save that Dr. Jousset esteems it in the treatment of chronic hepatic congestion, relating an instance of its efficacy in his *Leçons Cliniques* (p. 269). Elaps, in its proving, manifested most influence upon the eyes and ears, causing partial amaurosis in the former, and deafness, noises, and even discharge of matter and blood from the latter. It has been found useful in some forms of amblyopia, deafness and tinnitus, and otorrhœa,* and Mr. Clifton has recorded several cases of chronic inflammation of the nasal and pharyngeal lining in which it was curative. Mr. Hitchman esteems it highly in the cough of phthisis.

The analogues of serpent venom are *Apis* of course, and *Arsenicum.*

The observations of the curative action of Lachesis at least, if worth anything at all, prove the validity, not only of our therapeutic rule, but also of the infinitesimal dose. The results gained with it are all due to the sixth or higher attenuations, for we have never had lower ones in our hands. Dr. Hayward, whose energy has recently provided us with a fresh supply of rattlesnake and cobra poison, is endeavouring also to replenish our stock of that of the lance-headed viper. It will then be interesting to ascertain if Lachesis will do more in the lower than it has done in the higher potencies. Crotalus and Naja have usually been given in the first three attenuations : Elaps in the 6th and 12th.

* See *Brit. Journ. of Hom.*, xxxiv., 466.

LECTURE XL.

LEDUM, LEPTANDRA, LILIUM, LITHIUM, LOBELIA, LYCO-PODIUM, LYCOPUS.

I have to-day to bring before you a series of minor medicines, with one only—Lycopodium—of primary importance.

We will begin with the marsh tea, or wild rosemary—

Ledum palustre.

The tincture is prepared from the small twigs and leaves.

The proving of Ledum is in the fourth volume of the *Reine Arzneimittellehre*. It contains 186 symptoms from Hahnemann, 148 from six others, and four from authors. Lembke also has proved it (in the mother tincture) : his results are incorporated with Hahnemann's by Allen.

In his " Essay on a new principle for ascertaining the curative power of Drugs," published in *Hufeland's Journal* in 1796, Hahnemann speaks of having ascertained that Ledum caused difficult and painful respiration, a painful shooting sensation in all parts of the throat, and troublesome itching of the skin. Hence, he thought, upon the principle *similia similibus* then just dawning upon him, were explained its virtues in whooping-cough and asthma, in inflammatory and even maligant sore-throat, and in chronic cutaneous diseases. In his *Fragmenta de viribus* (1805) he published his first pathogenesis of the plant, whose 75 symptoms have now swelled to the fuller list in the *Materia Medica Pura*. Besides the symptoms already mentioned, its most noteworthy effects seem to be a determination of blood to the head and chest, causing a sort of intoxication in the one, and cough with bright sanguineous expectoration in the other ; pain and swelling in the joints, including that of the great toe ; and boring pains in the bones. These pains are worst in the evening, but easy while the patient is in bed. They shift about much. The articular pains are relieved by movement.

2 R

In his preface to the pathogenesis, Hahnemann says that Ledum will prove suitable only in chronic maladies characterised by coldness and deficiency of animal heat. Its chief use in the homœopathic school has been in non-inflammatory articular affections; of which you may read two excellent illustrations in the ninth volume of the *British Journal of Homœopathy.* Dr. Drury has several times expressed his high appreciation of it in hæmoptysis, in which Dr. Jousset also commends it; and Dr. Drysdale has recorded a case in which it immediately removed a nocturnal itching of the feet.* But I think that for our best knowledge of how to use Ledum we are indebted to M. Teste. He thinks that it acts specially on parts of the body where the cellular tissue is wanting, as the fingers and toes; and hence affects the small joints rather than the large. He recommends it accordingly for traumatic whitlow, and for true gout of a sub-acute nature, seated in the hands or feet, and causing little swelling. Ledum produces several of the symptoms of gout, including the distension of the veins of the extremities in the evening. He goes on to affirm that Ledum is to punctured wounds what Arnica is to contusions. Besides some obvious applications of this property of the drug, he mentions that it gives almost immediate relief to the itching caused by mosquito-bites; and this even when given internally in the fifteenth dilution. In the stings of bees and wasps, he says, the result is less prompt, but still very satisfactory.

There is a general agreement as to the efficacy of this last application of Ledum, though the tincture is commonly used in a less diluted form, and applied locally also.† As a remedy for punctured wounds it supplies the gap left by Arnica, Calendula, and Hypericum, which correspond to contused, incised, and lacerated wounds respectively. M. Teste notes the intense coldness which sometimes accompanies these injuries as corroborating the choice of Ledum for them; and one of our Belgian confrères has just communicated a case in which daily epileptiform attacks supervened in a child after a wound in the head from scissors, which almost immediately yielded to the remedy.‡

On the skin, M. Teste says, Ledum causes "an eczematous eruption, with a tingling itching, that spreads over the whole

---

* *Brit. Journ. of Hom.,* xxix., 166.

† See *Monthly Hom. Rev.,* xiii., 203; *Brit. Journ. of Hom,* xxxiv., 353.

‡ *Revue Hom. Belge,* Oct., 1875, and *Brit. Journ. of Hom.,* xxxiv., 337.

body, penetrates into the mouth, probably also into the air-passages, and occasions a spasmodic cough, which is sometimes very violent." A similar condition is sometimes met with idiopathically in gouty subjects.

M. Teste compares Ledum with *Rhus, Arnica,* and *Croton ;* to which may be added *Pulsatilla* and *Ruta.*

His recommendations are best carried out with his dilutions, viz. about the sixth or twelth.

My next is an American medicine, the "black root,"

Leptandra Virginica.

The tincture of the root, and triturations of leptandrin, are the officinal preparations.

A proving of this medicine by Dr. Burt and another is given by Dr. Hale in the second edition of his *New Remedies ;* and in the fourth edition you may read all that is known of its curative effects.

The action of Leptandra is upon the *liver* and *bowels.* Dr. Burt suffered from dull aching distress in the region of the liver and gall-bladder, extending to the spine. With this there were such sympathetic symptoms as frontal headache, soreness of the eyeballs, and pain in the left shoulder. A student who took the drug for two weeks reports that it gave him actual jaundice. The intestinal evacuations are much affected by Leptandra. Its most frequent and characteristic effect is seen in stools frequent, profuse, *black, fœtid,* and papescent : they are difficult to retain. Under the prolonged use of the drug the stools become watery, and later have quantities of mucus in them.

Leptandra has not been much used as a remedy ; but such applications as it has received have been in precise accordance with the pathogenetic effects I have now described. In certain cases of " bilious headache " and " liver-complaint," especially when the characteristic blackish stools are present, it has been found very useful ; and it has occasionally proved curative in chronic diarrhœa and dysentery.

It most resembles *Bryonia, Iris,* and *Podophyllum.*

The lower potencies only have been used.

I have now to bring before you another American contri-bution to the Materia Medica, which, though only of recent introduction, bids fair to take an important place, especially in uterine therapeutics. I refer to the tiger lily,

Lilium tigrinum.

The tincture is prepared from the flowers.

We owe this remedy to the late Dr. W. E. Payne, of Bath, Maine, U.S. Provings of it carried out at his instigation—by fourteen persons in all, of whom nine were women—have been appearing from time to time in America; and they are gathered up by him into one view in the Transactions of the American Institute for 1867 and 1870. A *résumé* of the symptoms produced, with an account of what has been done with the medicine clinically, may be read in the fourth edition of Dr. Hale's *New Remedies;* and the pathogenetic effects in full are in Allen.

Dr. Payne was led to prove Lilium from the reported death of a child in convulsions from eating the pollen. Nothing further of this kind was manifested; but in the female provers a series of symptoms occurred in the sexual organs which showed a most potent influence of the plant. "The symptoms," says Dr. Payne, "connected with the female reproductive organs, and the consecutive moral conditions, are very pronounced and peculiar." The ovaries were the seat of peculiar sharp and burning pains. "In the uterine region there was severe pressing, bearing-down sensation, with the feeling as if the whole internal parts would be forced through the vagina, making the desire irresistible to press the hands firmly against the vulva to prevent the parts from escaping; the whole genital organs felt as if swollen, with smarting and irritation of the labia, great tenderness to touch, and acrid brownish leucorrhœa. In three of the provers the uterus was found, on examination, to be prolapsed and anteverted." Two women described the bearing-down sensation as not confined to the pelvis, but causing a sense of dragging in the thorax even to the shoulders. With it there was tenesmus of the bladder and rectum, diarrhœa (especially on first rising in the morning), and frequent micturition : also a mental state of conjoined irritability of temper and depression of spirits, with inability for mental exertion. The uterine symptoms began to get worse about 5 p.m., and increased up to midnight. In the male provers the sexual organs were much less affected; but there was considerable oppression and palpitation of the heart. When taken in moderate doses the effects were not immediate, but were very persistent; and tended to recur at longer or shorter intervals, and in groups which preserved a definite order.

Lilium has been too recently proved for any extensive experience with it to have accumulated; and my impression is that on the whole it has disappointed expectation. One reason of this may be, as Dr. Hale suggests, that its slowness of action has not been borne in mind. But it can hardly fail to find some place in the treatment of some of the congestive and even inflammatory state of the ovaries, uterus, vagina and vulva which we encounter, especially when the moral symptoms are those of the drug. Dr. Payne found much benefit from it in sub-involution after childbirth, and Dr. Hale in ovarian neuralgia.

Of Lilium Dr. Dyce Brown has given us one of his best "Studies in the Materia Medica," in which I advise you to read up the symptomatology of the drug. You will find it in the *Monthly Homœopathic Review* for August, 1877. He makes a good point when he recommends the medicine to be given in mental and moral disturbances connected with uterine disorder, and those which occasionally manifest themselves in pregnancy, childbed, and the climacteric age,—those, in fact, for which Actæa has hitherto been our main remedy. Dr. Woodyatt, of Chicago, thinks very highly of Lilium in cases of ciliary spasm, where the nervo-muscular derangement of the eye has caused a certain degree of astigmatism. He has recorded several cases in which such conditions disappeared under its use.*

Dr. Dunham, who was specially great in comparisons, has left us some between Lilium on the one side, and Podophyllum, Sepia, Pulsatilla, Platina, and Helonias on the other. You will find them at p. 344 of the first volume of his collected writings. *Platina* and *Helonias* seems best to correspond,—the former to the mental symptoms and the latter to the uterine condition induced by Lilium; and each proved antidotal to it in these spheres respectively.

And now a few words upon the carbonate of lithia,

Lithium carbonicum,

which we prepare by trituration.

A proving of this salt—made almost entirely with the lower attenuations—is given by Dr. Hering in the third and fourth

---

* See *Monthly Hom. Review*, xxii., 143; *Medical Counselor*, Oct., 1879; and Transactions of Amer. Ophthalmological and Otological Society, 1878, p. 61; 1879, p. 99.

volumes of the *American Homœopathic Review*. The schema of symptoms has been transferred to the first volume of the fourth edition of the *New Remedies*, and to Allen.

Dr. Hering considers that the symptoms of the eyes, heart and kidneys induced by Lithium are most significant; and in these regions its curative powers seem to have found what little scope they have, as you may see from Dr. Hale's therapeutic article on the drug. Dr. Carroll Dunham has reported a case of hemiopia from excessive use of the eyes—only the lateral half of objects being visible—which was soon cured by it.* This symptom is marked in its pathogenesis. The same physician found great and lasting benefit from it in his own case, when his heart was seriously damaged by acute rheumatism.†

In the case of hemiopia the 30th dilution was given ; but Dr. Dunham's own recovery ensued upon inhaling the emanations from the third trituration, as he was raising it to a higher potency.

I have now to speak of the Indian tobacco,

Lobelia inflata.

From the powder as imported a tincture or triturations are made for homœopathic practice.

Of the pathogenetic effects of Lobelia we have much information, from the frequent over-dosing with it which occurs in the hands of "botanic" practitioners. It was first proved after the Hahnemannian manner by Dr. Alphonse Noack on himself and five others, all using substantial doses. A treatise on the drug, embodying the results of his experiments, appeared in the fifteenth volume of the *Hygea* (1843), and has been translated into English in the appendix to the first volume of the *British Journal of Homœopathy*. There are articles on the drug, containing and adding to Noack's materials, by Dr. Jeanes in the *Materia Medica of American Provings*, and by Dr. Hale in the fourth edition of his *New Remedies*. Dr. Allen gives also the results of a proving recently made in the old school, by Dr. Barrallier, of Toulon, in which eleven persons co-operated.

The name "Indian tobacco," commonly given to Lobelia, fairly expresses its poisonous action. Like its namesake, it is

---

* See *Brit. Journ. of Hom.*, xxvi., 489.
† See *Monthly Hom. Review*, Feb., 1876.

nauseant, depressant, relaxant; and is used for these purposes as an enema in strangulated hernia or rigid os uteri.
But its main sphere of action is the pneumogastric nerve; as Dr.
Bartholow says—"Lobelia . . affects especially the medulla
oblongata and its respiratory centre (nucleus of pneumogastric)." The symptoms of Noack's provers decisively point to
this; and they have led to its successful use in many nervous
affections of the stomach and respiratory organs. The dyspepsia in which Dr. Jeanes has often found it curative is
characterised by a sense of weakness and oppression at the
epigastrium, and at the same time some oppression at the
chest. There is often acidity, with heart-burn and lateritious
urine, and a sensation as of a lump in the throat-pit, impeding
respiration and deglutition. Dr. Noack gives two cases of
cardialgia in which small doses of the mother tincture were
very effectual. The pain was pressive in character. It has
also been found beneficial in "stomach-cough," and in the
cough of phthisis. "When a tormenting dry cough and an
nsufferable tickling in the throat rob the patient of rest," it is,
says Neumann, "in the highest degree beneficial."

This brings us to the respiratory section of the pneumogastric tract, and to the use of Lobelia in *asthma*. The
testimony to its value here is abundant and unexceptionable.
It is true that asthma, so capricious in its behaviour under
climatic conditions, is hardly less so in relation to medicines.
It is difficult to say beforehand when Lobelia will do good ;
but when it does, the relief in the paroxysm is rapid, and even
a permanent cure is occasionally obtained. What is the
rationale of its action here? Dr. Hyde Salter * supposed
that it relaxed the bronchial spasm in virtue of its nauseating
property, as Tartar emetic would do it ; saying that it rarely
relieves the paroxysm before it induces its physiological
effects. But he has not shown us that Tartar emetic could be
substituted for it with similar results. Elliotson,† Pereira
and Ringer, on the other hand, recommend the use of small
doses ($\mathbb{m}$ v) at the commencement, gradually increased up to
the point of physiological effect, and then suspended. The
first-named physician has found too large a dose aggravate
the dyspnœa. Then Darwin tells how

        " fell Lobelia's *suffocating* breath
      Loads the dank pinions of the gale with death."

One of Jeanes' provers who took the tincture in tea-spoon-

* *On Asthma*, 2nd ed. (1868).
† *Lancet*, Jan. 23, 1833, April 15, 1837.

ful doses every fifteen minutes until nearly an ounce had been ingested, without exciting vomiting, complained of a general tightness of the chest, with short and somewhat laborious breathing. In the other provers the influence of the drug seemed mainly expended on the stomach ; but where the respiration was affected, it was always with embarrassment. Dr. Phillips also speaks of "extreme spasmodic difficulty of breathing," as attending the distressing condition induced by over-dosing with Lobelia ; and Dr. Barrallier experienced, from forty drops of the tincture, "extremely difficult breathing caused by a very strong constriction at the middle of the chest, which impedes the respiratory movements." I am inclined, therefore, to think that it acts homœopathically in asthma. It is a confirmation of this view that it often gives relief when administered in minute and infinitesimal doses—from the second to the sixth dilution, as I myself can testify.

Dr. Jeanes speaks highly of Lobelia in asthma ; but when he comes to narrate a case, and to give characteristics, it seems to be the paroxysmal dyspnœa of emphysema which he has in mind. "The symptoms," he writes, "which I have found most strongly to indicate the lobelia are," besides the gastric phenomena already enumerated, "constant dyspnœa, which is increased by slight exertion, and aggravated so much by slight exposures to cold as to form a kind of asthmatic paroxysm." Bähr also says that "Lobelia inflata is more adapted to emphysema than to asthma." I have seen it decidedly beneficial so far as the sensations are concerned in this affection.

These have been the practical applications of Lobelia. There are, however, certain residuary phenomena in its pathogenesis which require noting. They are these :—

1 Heat, fulness, and sometimes aching in the head.

2. Much dreaming, generally distressing.

3. Hemiopia.

4. Scratching, burning, and dryness in the throat.

5. Pain as if a nail were driven through the pit of the stomach to the spine, spreading right and left, with twisting sensation.

6. Circumscribed burning pain at the edge of the right false ribs, extending across the epigastrium and round to the left scapula. The spot originally affected subsequently became the seat of a violent boring pain, and felt as if paralysed.

7. Distension of abdomen, disordering respiration.

8. Diuresis.

9. Urine deposits a pink sediment, in which is a small

brown crystal resembling—under the microscope—a goose-berry (probably uric acid).

10. Distressing heaviness of the male genitals.

11. Prickling sensation through the whole body, extending even to the fingers and toes.

Most of these are individual symptoms ; but the fourth was experienced by all the provers, and more from small than from large doses. One of them could not go on with the experiment on account of it : he says it "far exceeded in severity that of Mezereum, Ledum, Polygonum, and Euphorbia."

There is also in Teste a catalogue of symptoms which his experience has furnished as those to which Lobelia is particularly adapted.

The analogies of Lobelia are *Antimonium tartaricum*, *Digitalis, Ipecacuanha,* and *Tabacum.*

I have already indicated the dilutions in which Lobelia has done most service.

I now come to one of those curious medicines whose virtues we owe almost entirely to the Hahnemannian process of trituration. It is the club-moss,

Lycopodium.

The well-known unmoistenable powder, prepared from the spores of the plant, is triturated for our use. The value of this mode of preparation has been peculiarly demonstrated in the case of Lycopodium by some microscopical researches carried on by Mr. Isaac Thompson, of Liverpool. He found, on examination of the powder, that it was made up of a number of little particles, each about the $\frac{1}{800}$th of an inch in diameter, and in shape like a nut. On pounding a small quantity in an agate mortar, these nuts were found to be fractured, and their contents dispersed. These the addition of a drop of water showed to be oil-globules. It seems most probable that the medicinal virtues of Lycopodium reside in this peculiar oleaginous matter with which its sporules are filled ; and hence the comparative inertness of all preparations of the drug which do not involve complete fracture* or solution of the investing envelope. No tincture but an ethereal one is found to effect solution ; and for fracture even trituration with milk-sugar must be prolonged—in the case of the first decimal—for at least two hours.

* Rau had made the same statement many years ago (*Hygea*, xiii., 284).

The earliest record of pathogenetic effects due to Lycopodium is contained in the first edition of the *Chronic Diseases*, where the drug has 891 symptoms. In the second edition the number has swelled to 1608. Some of the additions are from the fellow-observers Hahnemann acknowledges; but the majority of them are his own. It has since been proved on several occasions in Germany by individual experimenters, and twice in the collective manner—viz : by Huber and nine others in 1856 and by Professor Martin and ten of his pupils in 1859. The record of the last-named testing may be read in the eighteenth volume of the *British Journal of Homœopathy*. Dr. Allen combines the whole series of observations into one splendid pathogenesis, comprising over 3000 symptoms. He has still further contributed to our knowledge of the drug, by giving us, in the *North American Journal of Homœopathy* for August, 1877, a *catalogue raisonnée* of its " clinical symptoms " so far as recorded. There is an admirable study of Hahnemann's pathogenesis of the drug, by Dr. Pope, in the seventeenth volume of the *British Journal*.

Martin's provings were conducted with the crude drug, and sometimes the first trituration. The general symptoms were those of excitement,—quickened circulation, headache, increased appetite, more frequent evacuations, stronger sexual desire. The chief local affinity manifested was for the urinary organs. There was frequent and sometimes painful micturition ; and the urine was cloudy and sedimentous, occasionally charged with mucus and even blood.

This may be called the crude action of Lycopodium ; and therewith correspond its traditional uses. These were confined to urinary affections. In the spasmodic retention of urine of children, and in catarrh of the bladder in adults, it had considerable repute as a remedy even before Hahnemann's trituration developed its more extensive powers.

When we turn to the proving in the *Chronic Diseases*, a very different scene is manifested. Instead of acute disorder, we are looking upon gradually advancing chronic disease : instead of excitement we have depression and decay. Whether we regard the phenomena as genuine pathogenetic effects of the drug, or (which seems to me more probable) as symptoms of the patients to whom it was proving beneficial, in either case they picture its sphere and kind of action. Mental, nervous, and bodily weakness ; sallow or grayish-yellow complexion, and cold extremities ; anorexia, slow and depressed digestion, flatulence and constipation ; a passive catarrh of the air-passages ; and an unhealthy state of the skin—are the morbid conditions presented to us. This is the general character of the profounder action of Lycopodium. Let us pass on to fix its sphere as a remedy from clinical experience.

We may lay it down that Lycopodium has no direct neurotic or hæmatic influence. It is a purely vegetative remedy, affecting the three great tracts of mucous membrane with their cutaneous continuation.

1. The digestive canal, with the liver, is the most important seat of the action of Lycopodium. There is a form of dyspepsia in which it is quite specific. A typical case of this is related by Dr. Hutchinson in the twenty-fifth volume of the *British Journal of Homœopathy*. It is so illustrative of the medicine that I will read you the patient's description of her sufferings. She complained of " pain under the ribs and all round the waist, with shooting pains up the shoulder-blades ; pain across the stomach and straight down on each side of it, sometimes very severe ; nausea ; the food often thrown up, with a sour and then a bitter taste ; water-brash ; obstinate constipation ; very painful hæmorrhoids, with great loss of blood ; coldness in the extremities ; cramp in the legs and thighs ; the action of the kidneys is undue and most disturbing at night. The last two nights I have not closed my eyes, and the pain has been increasing. My complexion is deadly pale, with a mixture of ash and yellow combined." This condition had lasted two months or more. Lycopodium 12 was prescribed twice a day, and the diet regulated. In a week the pain had subsided, and the other symptoms were disappearing ; and she was soon restored to health.

The constituent elements of such dyspepsia occasionally appear separately, and often require this remedy. In water-brash it will frequently prove curative. For flatulence the choice generally lies between Lycopodium and Carbo vegetabilis. I think the former most suitable when the distension takes place in the intestines, the latter when the wind accumulates in the stomach, oppressing the breathing. Dr. Bayes has lately noted some additional features of the flatulence of Lycopodium.[*] It is incarcerated, causing bloating and distension ; the pain is referred to the right hypochondrium and intestines ; and palpitation during digestion is often complained of. I may add that constipation is nearly always an accompanying symptom. For this trouble itself Lycopodium stands very high as a remedy. Teste commends it strongly in the constipation—sometimes so obstinate—of young children. He also praises it in a very different condition of

* *Brit. Journ. of Hom.*, xxx., 153.

the bowels, viz., that most dangerous enteritis which is set up in infants by the ingestion of food which they cannot digest.   I have more than once verified this recommendation. I should mention that this physician thinks Lycopodium to correspond best to the indigestions caused by heavy farinaceous and fermentable food.

Dr. Guernsey finds most of the characteristic symptoms of Lycopodium in the sphere of the digestive organs.   They are— that the smallest quantity of food produces either satiety, or a sense of fulness even up to the throat ; much fermentation of the food, causing a feeling of "working" in the stomach, and audible borborygmi, which are most noticeable in the left hypochondrium ; and pains shooting across from the right to the left side of the abdomen.   He does not lay so much stress on distension of the abdomen ; but both in the provings, and in Dr. Allen's collection of symptoms removed by the medicine, you will find it a very prominent feature.   Bähr describes the pathological condition calling for it as chronic gastric and intestinal catarrh (though the tongue is not much coated), and lays stress on hopeless depression of the mind and "jaundiced, yellowish-gray, or dingy-sallow hue " of the complexion as especially indicative of it.

Besides the above-named affections, acidity and heartburn are prominent features of Lycopodium, indicating its appropriateness to acid dyspepsia ; and it has as a marked symptom unconquerable sleep after dinner, followed by great exhaustion. It is probable that some of its digestive disturbance is due to its influence upon the liver.   In Professor Martin's provings, this organ occasionally gave signals of distress ; and Dr. Pope says that in old hepatic congestions he has found Lycopodium more useful than any other medicine, Sulphur perhaps excepted.   Jahr and Bayes state a similar experience.

2. In the respiratory sphere Lycopodium manifests great power in what may be called " chronic influenza : " i. e. where catarrh becomes persistent, with much general weakness. Some forms of chronic bronchitis and even of pneumonia come within this category.   Teste commends it highly for " chronic pneumonia, with purulent, foul-smelling expectoration, even when one of the lungs (especially the left) has become partially hepatised."   Dr. Pope adds that few medicines are so valuable in pulmonary phthisis as this, when perseveringly used.   " The cough," he says, " the gastric irritation, the exhaustion, and the intercurrent attacks of pleurisy, are wonderfully mitigated by it."   It is probable that the phthisis of this writer and the chronic pneumonia of the former are the same

disease. Dr. Meyhoffer, whose opinion on respiratory affections is so weighty, says that he had no opinion of Lycopodium until he was led to try it in chronic pneumonia; but since then he has had for it in this disease and in chronic passive bronchitis characterised by copious muco-serous or muco-purulent expectoration the utmost respect. I am myself very fond of the drug in cases of suspected phthisis in young men, where yet there is no evidence of tubercular deposition.

Mr. David Wilson has lately called our attention to the fan-like movement of the alæ nasi noted in the pathogenesis of Lycopodium, which he believes to be a pathognomonic indication for the choice of this drug in diseases of children and young people. Much controversy was excited by the manner in which Mr. Wilson put forward this statement; but I cannot in this instance join my good friends his assailants. There is nothing à priori improbable in his statement. " When this symptom is clearly marked," he writes, " no matter through what organ or tissue the symptoms of any attack of illness may manifest themselves in children and young people, I venture to submit that the whole group of the phenomena in such attacks will be found under Lycopodium." This is a pure matter of experience; and a good many cases have since been published which go to confirm Mr. Wilson's statement. It is of course in respiratory affections that this symptom is most frequently present.

3. Of the action of Lycopodium on the urinary organs I have already spoken. Dr. Arnold says that he has seen in several cases an increase in the secretion of urine on the administration of Lycopodium, especially when any dropsical affection was present. He has likewise observed diminution of the quantity of urine in cases where it was morbidly increased. I find it the very best medicine where the patient is suffering from an excess of lithic acid gravel; and look upon copious sediments of this nature as one of the most unerring indications for its choice in dyspepsia. Dr. Guernsey also adopts this symptom—under the title of " red sand in the urine " —as one of his chief general key-notes for the drug. He says that, connected with its presence, there is frequently pain before passing water, shown in young children by crying and screaming at the time, and by adults referred to the renal region.

4. Lycopodium is very good for the intertrigo of children and for dry porrigo capitis. It is said to be curative in that scourge of Poland, the plica polonica; and in pruritus ani.

With three additional observations I will conclude. First, I would mention that the 2nd trituration has caused an inflammatory rheumatism of the right fore-arm, wrist, hand, and fingers.* Secondly, that Dr. Bayes recommends it for syphilitic ulcerations of the fauces, superficial but spreading ; and that among the high dilutionists in America it is much thought of in diphtheria when the deposit first invades the right tonsil (in this distinguished from Lachesis). The third point is more curious. Lycopodium has occasionally been suggested for aneurism, but I had thought little of it, though in a case treated by Dr. Madden and myself what *seemed* an aortic aneurism ceased to be discoverable while we were giving the medicine for the general health. But I have since seen most striking results from it in an unmistakeable carotid aneurism in an old lady, for whose dyspeptic symptoms the remedy had often proved serviceable. The shooting pains which accompanied the swelling disappeared in the first three days of taking the Lycopodium ; and in a fortnight the enlargement of the artery was reduced one half, at which point it has since continued stationary, giving her no pain or inconvenience.

You will do well also to consider the list of symptoms prefixed by Hahnemann to his pathogenesis, as indications for the choice of Lycopodium in disease. They may yet yield fresh therapeutic applications of this valuable drug.

The analogues of Lycopodium in the digestive sphere are *Bryonia* and *Nux vomica*. I know no medicines really resembling it as a whole.

The higher attenuations are those most used in practice. I nearly always employ the twelfth.

I have finally another wolf's foot to bring before you, but botany has saved us from confusion by slightly varying the nomenclature. It is the bugle-weed,

Lycopus Virginicus.

The tincture is prepared from the whole plant.

Dr. Morrisson has enriched pathogenesy by a thorough proving of Lycopus upon his own person, the account of which you will find in the sixteenth volume of the *Monthly Homœopathic Review*. It is rendered especially valuable by pulse-tracings having been obtained from the sphygmograph to show the action of the drug upon the heart. There is also in

* *Brit. Journ. of Hom.*, ii, 285.

the second edition of Dr. Hale's *New Remedies* a short proving of the drug by Dr. G. E. Chandler, and Allen gives results from yet another experimenter.

Lycopus has long had, among the "eclectic" practitioners of America, the reputation of being an arterial sedative, somewhat like Digitalis. Drs. Chandler and Morrisson both found it exert an indubitable action upon the heart. In the former, whose health was perfect, the strangeness of his cardiac sensations, and the slowness of his pulse (which at one time was only 48), led him to seek an examination ; when the first sound was found to be absent, and replaced by the blowing sound of mitral regurgitation. Dr. Morrisson's heart was somewhat feeble, and its action inclined to intermit, ere he commenced his proving ; but the pulse-tracing taken then was of very healthy character compared with those which subsequently appeared. The organ was first oppressed and then depressed by the drug :* the sphygmographic signs of debility increased day by day until the proving was suspended, and irregularity—not mere intermission—of pulse became the rule instead of the exception.

Dr. Hale says that Lycopus has become one of his most favoured and trusted remedies in functional diseases of the heart, especially when there is cardiac irritability with depressed force. Dr. Morrisson has recorded two cases of the same kind in which the drug was very useful : in one of these there was a great tendency to exophthalmos, showing the cardiac symptoms to be those belonging to Graves' disease. In the *British Journal of Homœopathy* for April, 1876 (vol. xxxiv., p. 388) is a case reported from Honolulu, in which double valvular disease of the heart, with all its associated symptoms, was so greatly relieved by the continued use of the medicine, that the patient was able to return to work ; and, though some abnormal sound continued audible, he considered himself in perfect health. All this is very promising ; and the drug should be fairly tested.

The dilutions from the first to the third decimal have been those used—the provings having been conducted with full doses of the mother-tincture.

Omitting for the present the four medicines next on our list, I shall pass on when we meet again to speak of Mercurius.

* Dr. Morrisson explains that by cardiac "depression" he means feeble and excitable action, by "oppression" heavy and laboured action, as if the heart were obliged to make great efforts to do its work.

LECTURE XLI.

MERCURIUS.

I shall begin to-day to speak of the various mercurial preparations. Under the common name of

Mercurius

—by which, and not by that of hydrargyrum, the metal has always been known to homœopathic therapeutics—I shall include all those salts and compounds of it which produce pure mercurial effects, as distinguished from such as—like the cyanides, the iodides, and the sulphides—have peculiar properties of their own. These I shall discuss in a subsequent lecture.

Homœopathic pharmacy embraces all the ordinary mercurials, triturating those that are insoluble, and dissolving the perchloride—Mercurius corrosivus, as we call it—in rectified spirit. But besides these we have two peculiar preparations of the drug. One, known as Mercurius vivus, is a trituration of the metal with milk-sugar. It answers to the blue pill and grey powder of ordinary practice, for which it is a substitute in our hands. The other—Mercurius solubilis—is a preparation of Hahnemann's own, and is known in Germany to this day by his name (Merc. sol. Hahnemanni). It is made by dissolving metallic quicksilver in nitric acid, and then precipitating it from solution by caustic ammonia. The result is an impure oxide, of doubtful and varying composition. Therapeutically it is effective enough; but from the chemical side the Pharmacopœia seems justified in recommending its displacement by Mercurius vivus, according (as it truly says) to Hahnemann's own later practice. Its solubility is only comparative; and it is prepared by trituration.

We have pathogeneses of most of the mercurial preparations. Hahnemann experimented mainly with his own black oxide,—in substantial doses, Noack and Trinks say. In the last edition of the first volume of the *Reine Arzneimittellehre*, 1,264 symptoms are credited to it, of which nearly half are his own, the rest being furnished by eight associates.* Dr. Allen does little more than reproduce this proving; but he gives an entirely new and most valuable one of Mercurius vivus, chiefly made up of observations on workmen and others exposed to the emanations of the metal, and containing 840 symptoms. He also presents or completes Hahnemann's provings of the acetate (M. aceticus) and the chloride (calomel, M. dulcis). These constitute the mercurial preparations whose action, physiological and therapeutical, I am now about to discuss.

As regards other sources of information, I have availed myself of the treatises on the ill effects of mercury by Dietrich, Mathias, and Habershon, and of the later studies of its action by Overbeck, Kussmaul, and Hallopeau.†

I have now to describe, on the basis afforded by these materials, the pathogenetic effects of Mercury. The field is such a wide one that you will pardon me if I traverse it somewhat rapidly. It is only at controverted points that I can stay to adduce evidence and discuss arguments; but I will ask you to believe that I make no statement without having gone through these processes on my own account beforehand. Even as it is, I find that any satisfactory treatment of the subject will occupy an entire lecture, so that I must ask you to wait for the therapeutics of Mercury until our next meeting.

I. When an unirritating preparation of Mercury is gradually introduced into the system, before any local manifestation of its influence occurs a profound change is being wrought in the blood. Its full hæmatic effect is thus stated by the late Dr. Headland, in his well-known treatise *On the Action of Medicines :*—" By some inscrutable chemical power, of whose agency we know nothing, it is able to decompose the blood : by some destructive agency it deprives it of one third of its fibrin, one seventh of its albumen, one third or more of its globules ; and at the same time loads it with a fetid fatty matter, the product of decomposition." Trousseau and Pidoux well describe the cachexia which results from this action. The

---

* I must express some doubt as to the validity of the contributions to this pathogenesis of Hahnemann's son Friedrich. They are twice as numerous as those of his seven fellow-provers put together; and many of them are of such severity that, though not impossible effects of mercurial *poisoning*, they are extremely unlikely to have been developed in provings, as they purport to have been. I strongly suspect that the list has been filled in from his imagination.

† *Du Mercure action physiologique et therapeutique,* 1878.

blood loses colour and consistence; pallor of the surface occurs,
followed by œdema and anasarca. All the symptoms of
anæmia are present, such as palpitation, sighing, breathlessness; and in young females the menses are suppressed, and
chlorosis sets in. In other cases ecchymoses and passive
hæmorrhages appear.

The diminished number of the red corpuscles of the blood
under the influence of Mercury, indicated by these symptoms
and affirmed by Headland, has been substantiated by recent
researches, in which the new method of counting their number
has been employed. A condition of " hypoglobulia " is always
found to exist when the drug has been given in sufficient
quantity to induce its characteristic effects.[*]

With the early stage of this affection of the blood there is
slight pyrexia. Hahnemann, who in his treatise *On Venereal
Diseases* taught that the cure of syphilis depended on the
supervention of this " mercurial fever," thus describes it in his
own graphic and detailed manner :—

" The patient gets a metallic taste in the mouth, a disagreeable smell in the nose, a painless audible rumbling in the
bowels, an earthy complexion, a pinched nose, blue rings
round the eyes, pale leaden-coloured lips, an uninterrupted or
frequently recurring shuddering (always getting stronger) that
thrills deeply even into the interior of the body. His pulse
becomes small, hard, and very rapid ; there is an inclination
to vomit, or at least nausea at everything, especially at animal
diet, but chiefly a very violent headache of a tearing and pressive character, which sometimes rages without intermission in
the occiput or over the root of the nose. The nose, ears,
hands, and feet are cold. The thirst is inconsiderable, the
bowels constipated, great sleeplessness, the short dreams of a
fearful character, accompanied by frequent slight perspirations. The weakness is extreme, as also the listlessness and
anxious oppression, which the patient thinks he never before
felt anything like. The eyes become sparkling as if full of
water, the nose is as if stuffed with catarrh : the muscles of the
neck are somewhat stiff, as from rheumatism ; the back of the
tongue is whitish. At this period the patient experiences, if
all goes on well, some discomfort in swallowing, a shooting
pain in the root of the tongue, on both sides of the mouth a
looseness or setting on edge of the teeth (the gums recede a
little towards the roots of the teeth, become somewhat spongy,
red, painful, swollen); there is a moderate swelling of the
tonsils and submaxillary glands, and a peculiar rancid odour

* See Hallopeau, *op. cit.*, p. 90.

from the mouth, without the occurrence, however, of a notable increase in the secretion of saliva, and without diarrhœa or immoderate perspiration."

All this, you will observe, is prior to the full development of the first local effects—the stomatitis and salivation. When the gums grow tender, the saturation of the system is complete. This is shown by the effects which ensue in certain morbid products and conditions when present. Indurations are resolved, and exudations of lymph absorbed ; on the other hand, old cicatrices grow tender and may even reopen. All the secretions at the same time tend to increase in quantity and greater fluidity in consistence.

II. If now the drug is continued, or if the patient be unhealthy or expose himself to cold, certain inflammations are apt to arise. I think we must distinguish these from the inflammations which the corrosive sublimate of Mercury is capable of producing. It acts, like Arsenic and Iodine, by its essentially irritant properties, selecting tissues and organs for this influence by elective affinity. The blander preparations of Mercury have no such property ; yet it is well known that stomatitis is much more readily induced by them than by the perchloride, and the same is true of certain other affections. I shall, therefore, here describe the inflammations, ulcerations, and other effects specifically induced by Mercury as such ; and later on shall mention the modifications and additions which ensue when the perchloride is given.

In the light of this view, let us consider the phenomena presented by mercurial poisoning in the several parts of the body it affects. We will begin by studying its action on the alimentary canal and its associated glands.

1. I think that the general action of Mercury on the alimentary canal may be stated as follows. The mildest degree of its influence is shown in an increased secretion from the whole mucous tract, and from the salivary and pancreatic glands which open into it. The full constitutional action is manifested in irritation with diminished secretion — often amounting to congestion or actual inflammation—along the whole tract, but in some regions attacking chiefly the mucous surface, in others the glandular involutions. Thus in the mouth we have intense stomatitis, while the salivary glands secrete vigorously. In the small intestine, on the other hand, the mucous membrane shows little sign of disturbance, while the liver often becomes congested, and its secretion diminished.

Let us see how far these principles hold good in the several portions of the tract.

a. The mercurial stomatitis I trust that you have never seen in any severe form; but it is necessary that we should have it before us. I will describe it in the graphic language of Dr. George Wood. He thus pictures the onset of the affection: " The first phenomenon presented is often a whitish appearance of the lower gums, probably owing to opacity of the epithelium. Soon afterwards the gums are seen to be somewhat swollen, rising up between the teeth, and reddened at their edges. At the same time they are somewhat tender to the touch, and not unfrequently pain is produced at the roots of the teeth by firmly closing the jaws. A metallic taste, as of copper in the mouth, is also among the first symptoms; and I have repeatedly been able to detect the approach of salivation by the peculiar fetor of the breath, before any other sign had presented itself. It not unfrequently happens that the above symptoms have existed for some time before any increase of saliva appears; and occasionally there is at first seen a dryish condition of the tongue." The second stage he thus depicts: " The gums, tongue, cheeks and fauces, one or all, swell and become painful; deglutition is painful; the teeth, if carious, begin to ache; the tongue is somewhat furred, and indented by the teeth at its edges; the saliva is discharged copiously; the salivary glands swell, together with the neighbouring areolar tissue, and the breath is very offensive, having a peculiar fetor which distinguishes the mercurial sore-mouth from all other analogous affections." If the disease run on, it reaches a third stage, which Dr. Wood describes in this manner: " The swelling, internal and external, increases; the tongue sometimes projects from the mouth, in consequence of its greatly increased bulk, and is covered with a very thick, soft, yellowish white fur, extremely offensive to the smell; the parotid and submaxillary glands become much enlarged and painful; the patient cannot open his jaws, swallows with great difficulty and pain, and is wholly unable to articulate; the saliva streams from the mouth; the odour of the breath is insupportably fetid, and sometimes scents the whole apartment; ulceration of the gums, cheeks, and tongue takes place, with occasionally copious and exhausting hæmorrhage; the teeth loosen and fall out; and even gangrene of the soft parts, and necrosis of the alveolar processes, sometimes occurs." This gangrene may extend to the face and neck; and, though most commonly spreading from the mouth or throat, sometimes begins at once on the external surface.

Sir Thomas Watson calls attention to the special character of this mercurial inflammation. "It is," he says, "superficial, spreading, erysipelatous: it leads to ulceration without any distinct occurrence of suppuration; the ulcers enlarge." Ulcers, I should say, are apt to occur in the mouth under mercurial influences without actual stomatitis, as in those professionally engaged in the venereal wards of hospitals (see Allen's S. 47 of M. vivus). I would notice also the peculiar fœtor of the breath, as connected with the fatty matter of the same character we have seen formed in the blood; and the tendency to hæmorrhage. Observe, moreover, that while the drug is thus raging on the mucous surface, the salivary glands are simply stimulated, and pour out their secretion profusely. Orfila—and he is followed by Trousseau and Pidoux—states that in mercurial salivation there is no true inflammation of the glands, but only effusion into the cellular tissue around them. But there is evidence that (in its ordinary forms) the drug can cause hyperæmia of these organs; and in one case, when under the poisonous influence of the perchloride they enlarged and became tender, the salivary secretion was diminished.

A word as to the contents of the mouth. The tongue is affected like the cavity generally, so far as its mucous membrane is concerned. The submucous tissue is also involved in the inflammation, as shown by the great enlargement of the organ; but I do not know that the muscular substance is affected. As to the teeth, there is much need of a thorough and unprejudiced study of the influence of Mercury upon them. Does it attack them immediately, setting up true caries? or do they loosen and fall out as a consequence of the degenerated state of the gums, themselves remaining entire? The latter alternative seems at present to be that best supported by evidence, *as the rule;* but the observations made on the workers in the metal show the teeth frequently becoming discoloured and carious. The mercurial stomatitis begins in the alveolo-dental periosteum (as the early tenderness there indicates); and it is curious that it is difficult, if not impossible, to induce it in infants prior to dentition or in persons who have lost their teeth.

b. The throat may be either acutely or chronically affected by Mercury. The acute affection is identical with the mercurial stomatitis, which it commonly accompanies: there is much swelling always, ulceration often, gangrene sometimes. Hahnemann reports, from M. solubilis—" suppuration of the tonsils, with sharp, sticking pain in the fauces when swallowing." The chronic angina of Mercury is graphically described by Dietrich. It is characterised by a dark or bluish redness; great sense of dryness, with hawking of tenacious, glassy mucus; and enlargement of the mucous follicles.

c. The stomach is, so far as I know, affected by the per-chloride only of all the mercurial preparations ; so I will say nothing of it here.

d. The small intestines are very rarely inflamed by Mercury ; but the two great glands which pour their secretions into this part of the bowel suffer from the drug in a very considerable degree.

(1.) The physiological similarity between the salivary glands and the pancreas makes it probable that—as with Iodine and Iris—a drug which powerfully influences the one will affect the other also. That it is so in the case of Mercury is argued by Dietrich on the ground of the symptoms occasionally occurring during life ; while Hughes Bennett in experiments on animals, and Wibmer in examination of the bodies of those who have been long treated by mercurial frictions, have found the gland reddened and hypertrophied. The most striking case, however, is one cited by Dr. H. Wood. " A woman after excessive salivation experienced deep-seated epigastric pain and heat, with nausea, thirst and fever, and voided thin stools containing liquid resembling salivary fluid. At the post-mortem the pancreas was found weighing eight ounces, red, congested, and with its duct dilated."

(2.) That Mercury acts upon the liver, and is a cholagogue, would have been thought till lately too obvious to need de-monstration. But the experiments conducted by Drs. Scott and Handfield Jones, and those carried out by a committee of the British Medical Association under the presidency of Dr. Hughes Bennett, ascertained the fact that in the lower animals at least Mercury rather diminishes the secretion of bile than increases it. Dr. Rutherford, also, whose experiments have rehabilitated most of the vegetable cholagogues, found calomel without effect on the biliary secretion in the dog,—though, as we shall see, a very different result was obtained when corrosive sublimate was administered. There is of course no proof that the same thing happens in the human subject ; but we seem to have a strong probability that it is so. Nor is it any evidence to the contrary that an increased quantity of bile is found in the stools after the administration of mercurials. It must be remembered that this secretion is ordinarily reabsorbed after being poured into the duodenum, so that its presence is hardly to be traced in the stools. To find it there may thus simply mean that the bowels have from some cause been unable to take it up. But it is not shown hereby that Mercury has no action on the liver. On the contrary, the diminished secretion sometimes observed under its use may well be a sign of the congestion of the gland which post-mortem examination shows to be present in acute mercurial poisoning. This may be accompanied by jaundice, of the occurrence of which there are several cases on record,* and in continued exposure to the malign influence it may go on to chronic hepatitis, with enlargment or atrophy and induration.†

e. While Mercury has little influence upon the small intestines, the large—cæcum, colon, and rectum—are a special seat of its influence. Diarrhœa not unfrequently accompanies or replaces salivation ; and the tendency to tenesmus shows that its seat is the lower portion of the bowel. In poisoning by corrosive sublimate, as we shall see, the whole tract exhibits marks of intense inflammation.

This is the place in which to speak of the effect of Mercury upon the intestinal evacuations. The stools produced by it are of various characters. When given as a purgative in the form of calomel or blue-pill, it causes copious fluid evacuations, of a dark brown or yellowish colour—sometimes, especially in children, of a green hue. I suppose these evacuations to consist of an increased quantity of the biliary and other intestinal secretions. The green " calomel stools " of children are generally supposed to consist of bile, altered in tint by superabundant acid in the intestines. Others, however, consider them to be due simply to the presence of the subsulphide of Mercury in the fæces, their colour being a phenomenon analogous to the blackness of the stools in those who are taking iron. The objection to this view is that they have been induced by doses of calomel far too small to cause any general coloration of the fæces.—The purging caused by mercurials always tends, if severe, to assume the dysenteric character ; i.e. to consist of slimy and bloody stools, with tormina and tenesmus.

2. The respiratory mucous membrane is not a special seat of the influence of Mercury. Conjunctivitis, however, is no uncommon manifestation of its action : it occurred in Overbeck's experiments on animals, and in Hahnemann's proving

* Taylor, On Poisons, 1st ed., p. 396. Johnson, Cheyne, and Chapman, quoted by Black, in Introduction to the Study of Homœopathy, p. 119. Budd, On Diseases of the Liver, 3rd ed., p. 478. Hempel, p. 61,
† Taylor, op. cit., p. 397. Graves, cited in Med. Times and Gazette, xix, 452. Overbeck, in Ibid., Jan. 18, 1862. Wibmer, cited by Hempel, p. 506. Allen, S. 390 and 400 of M. vivus.

of M. solubilis and Hering's of the biniodide. Coryza sometimes occurs in mercurialisation and among the workmen;
and one of the dogs poisoned by corrosive sublimate in Dr.
Hughes Bennett's experiments had constant muco-purulent
discharge from the nose. Epistaxis was not an uncommon
effect of M. solubilis. Pneumonia generally complicates the
febrile mercurial eruptions of which we shall speak presently.

These phenomena, however, appear far less frequently from
Mercury than from Arsenic and Iodine.

3. The reverse of the comparison obtains in the genito-
urinary tract, which, according to Christison, suffers more
from corrosive sublimate than from Arsenic. Of this I shall
speak subsequently; but from Mercurius solubilis two of Hahnemann's provers had balanitis and balanorrhœa; and another
(Hornburg) reports the following symptom :—" A number of
small red vesicles at the termination of the glans penis under
the prepuce, which become converted four days later into
ulcers, which break open and pour forth a yellowish white,
staining, strong-smelling matter; afterwards the larger ulcers
bled, and, when touching them, a pain was felt in them which
affected the whole body; they were round; their edges, which
looked like raw flesh, overhung the ulcers, the base of which was
covered with a cheesy lining."* A similar symptom was experienced by one of the provers of Cinnabar.

These phenomena are of much interest with reference to
the relation of Mercury to chancre. Other facts are mentioned by Trousseau and Pidoux which bear on the same
point. They allow that Mercury may cause serious ulceration at the side of the penis or in the vulva. They relate how
a dog whom Bretonneau had mercurialised, copulating with
one of his kind, had his penis swelled, inflamed, ulcerated, and
finally gangrenous. And they state that women labouring
under puerperal fever, and treated with mercurial frictions,
were liable to get membranous inflammation of the vulva
followed by sphacelus.

4. I have now to speak of the action of Mercury on the skin.
I have already mentioned its diaphoresis; and will only add
that the secretion is often vitiated as well as increased, being
sometimes sour, sometimes fœtid. It is especially marked
at night. But whenever Mercury has been given to any large
extent in disease, there have been seen occasional instances of
its power of causing cutaneous eruptions. These have been
noticed by several writers, and especially by Pearson, whose
"eczema mercuriale"—a form of eczema rubrum—is classical.

* S. 657 in the R.A.M.L., S. 1056 in Allen.

But the fullest account of them is given by Alley, in his *Observations on the Hydrargyria* (London, 1810). By this name he denotes the vesicular disease arising from the exhibition of Mercury. He describes it as occurring in three forms, and Bazin confirms his observations. The first is a roseolous efflorescence, with minute vesiculation, and without constitutional symptoms. The second form is distinctly febrile; and in this, in its appearance, and in its catarrhal complications closely resembles measles. In the third variety the fever is more intense, the fauces are much involved, actual pneumonia is present, and the appearance of the surface is like that of vesicular erysipelas. The cuticle, and often the hair and nails, exfoliate subsequently. Other observers have seen pustulation, and others ulceration, occur.

5. Dietrich states that periostitis is a not uncommon effect of the long-continued use of Mercury. Pereira considers that this affection is rather to be ascribed to the venereal disease for which the drug had been administered. But Graves affirms that periostitis attacked patients who had taken a great deal of Mercury, even if they had never been affected with syphilis, as often as they took cold; and almost all later observers admit this action of the poison. Trousseau and Pidoux mention a case of a worker in quicksilver who suffered as severely from nocturnal bone-pains as if he were syphilitic, which he was not. We have already seen that the primitive effect of the drug on the mouth is an alveolo-dental periostitis.

These workmen in Mercury give us many opportunities of observing the profounder and more lasting effects of the mineral on the frame. Thus it has been noted of those who labour in the quicksilver mines of Idria that they are liable to congestion, followed by enlargement or atrophy of the liver; inflammation and abscess of the lymphatic glands; neuralgia of the fifth pair; various eruptions and ulcers of the skin; and swellings of the salivary glands, periosteum, and bones.* Kussmaul, indeed, found no hepatic or osseous affections among the Erlangen workmen whom he observed. But the most striking effects seen here are neurotic in seat and nature; and of these I have yet to speak.

III. The neurotic effects of Mercury are manifest chiefly in the musculo-motor, and in the ideational and emotional spheres.

1. The "mercurial tremor" is as characteristic an action of the drug as its salivation. It is chiefly seen in workmen at quicksilver mines, or in trades—as water-gilding—where

* Stillé, *Mat. Med.*, in loc.

the metal is much used. Mérat's account of the affection is
followed by most writers.* The disease, he states, may begin
suddenly ; but in general it makes its approaches by slow
steps. The first symptom is unsteadiness of the arms, then
quivering, finally tremors, the several movements of which
become more and more extensive until they resemble convulsions, and render it difficult or impossible for the patient
to walk, to speak, or even to chew. All voluntary motions,
such as carrying a morsel to the mouth, are effected by
several violent starts. The arms are generally attacked first,
and also most. severely. The tremors have been compared
to those of chorea, of delirium tremens, and of paralysis
agitans. Of the last Watson says : " The mercurial tremor
consists in a sort of convulsive agitation of the voluntary
muscles, which is most violent when efforts are made to move
the limbs by the help of those muscles ; whenever, in fact,
volition is brought to bear upon them. It differs, therefore,
from the shaking palsy, inasmuch as the tremor ceases when
the muscles are supported, or are not brought into action."
In other respects it closely resembles this disorder, far more
so than multiple sclerosis, to which it has been compared
by Hallopeau. The concomitant symptoms of the trembling
are a peculiar brown tint of the whole body, dry skin, constipation and flatus, but no colic. The pulse is always slow.
In severe or advanced forms of the disease, the tremor is
accompanied or replaced by paralysis.

2. The milder effects of Mercury in the ideational and
emotional sphere are thus described by Dr. G. Wood :—
" The most prominent nervous phenomenon of mercurialisation
is an increased susceptibility to impressions ; slight causes
producing a disturbance of the mental equanimity, and unpleasant influences of all kinds having more than their
ordinary effect. A fretful, peevish state of mind, and irritable condition of temper, are not uncommon ; and restlessness, wakefulness, and general uneasiness are frequently added
to the other sufferings." Naunyn describes (after Kussmaul)
a similar condition (under the title of " mercurial erethism ")
as preceding the development of tremor in the workmen.
" Every unexpected or perplexing event," he writes, " excites
the patient in the highest degree. The visit and conversation of the physician put him into a state of complete
bewilderment, even to syncope : he grows pale, and stammers
in answering the simplest questions. To perform his allotted
task requires the greatest effort, or is even impossible if he

* Appendix to his *Traité de la colique métallique.*

sees or thinks that he is being watched. There is also great solicitude and feeling of anxiety without any reason for it. There is sleeplessness, or sleep which is restless, frequently broken and disturbed by frightful dreams, headache, and palpitation. In the severer forms there are frequently hallucinations, usually of a frightful nature." The graver cerebral symptoms are chiefly seen in those in whom tremor has long existed : they are mental weakness, loss of memory, delirium (often like that of alcoholism), apathy. The sufferers may die comatose and hemiplegic ; and the cerebral hemispheres are found after death the seat of softening, with effusion into the ventricles.

There can be no doubt, I think, that these phenomena imply inflammatory irritation of the gray matter of the brain and perhaps the cord. Accordingly, a mercurial neurosis may sometimes assume other forms. Dr. Anstie relates a terrible case of neuralgia of the limbs induced by it,* and Dr. Bartholow " has seen a well-marked case of locomotor ataxia, characterised by pains, ocular disorders, spermatorrhœa, plantar anæsthesia, and incoordination of muscular acts, result from the inhalation of mercurial fumes."†

Such are, as fully as I can present them to you, the pathogenetic effects of Mercury, as such. I have endeavoured to be just to this much-abused drug,—nothing to extenuate, indeed, but nought to set down in malice. The tendency at the present day—perhaps in reaction from the extremes of the non-mercurialist syphilographers of thirty years ago — is to minimise its noxious effects. That men can believe it a comparatively harmless drug only shows that they are using it in a comparatively harmless way ; it does not negative the observations made in days when it was given in injurious excess or under circumstances where its influence is long-continued and penetrating. We at least can use such observations as contributing to that pathogenetic knowledge of the metal which, upon the principle of similarity, shall enable us to employ it beneficially as a medicine.

* *On Neuralgia*, p. 24.

† Hallopeau, also, relates several forms of cerebro-spinal disease resulting from mercurial influence.

LECTURE XLII.

MERCURIUS (*continued*).

At our last meeting we considered in some detail the pathogenetic action of Mercury. We may classify its effects in three divisions.

In the first, we have the results of administering a single evacuant dose—results manifesting themselves, as you know, almost entirely in the sphere of the liver and the intestines.

Secondly, we have the phenomena following its gradual but *rapid* introduction into the system,—in what we may call acute mercurialisation. It here shows no direct irritant action on the living tissue, and exerts its primary influence upon the blood. It sets up therein a series of changes involving spoliation, liquefaction, and decomposition; and thereupon follow certain local affections, mainly of the mucous membranes and the skin. These are of a low and diffuse inflammatory character, and readily pass into suppuration, ulceration, and gangrene.

Thirdly come the effects of gradual and *slow* impregnation of the organism with the metal—chronic hydrargyrosis. These include a profound disturbance of the nutritive functions, but chiefly consist of neurotic disorders—manifested by tremor, erethism, and neuralgic pain, and going on to imbecility and paralysis.

Now the aim of homœopathy must be to take up all these forms of its physiological action, and fit them to the corresponding morbid conditions of idiopathic origin which occur in practice. That it has done so you may see by the essays upon it by Dr. Quin in the second volume of the *Annals*, and by Dr. Leadam in the twelfth volume of the *British Journal of Homœopathy ;* by the section devoted to it in the first volume of Hartmann's *Practical Observations ;* or, perhaps, the best way of appreciating the place and value assigned to it in our practice is to look through Bähr's *Therapeutics*, and see what and how numerous are the diseases for which he indicates it, and where it may be applied with best advantage. You will find reproduced in such a list the whole series of pathogenetic effects which on the last occasion of our meeting passed before us. But we shall not be able to limit our considerations to such applications of the medicine. The first and second of the forms under which we have classified its physiological action actually represent the traditional uses of the drug; and we shall have to estimate these, and to weigh their advantages and disadvantages in an impartial scale.

I. First, then, let us speak of the effects of the single evacuant dose of a mercurial. To the practitioners of the old school they indicate the usefulness of the drug when the portal system needs depletion; and, had we no more excellent way of accomplishing such a purpose, we might be obliged to avail ourselves of it. Dr. Kidd has shown how a judicious use may be made of this property of the drug, where consti-pation and portal obstruction hinder the development of the specific action of Digitalis in cardiac dropsy.* But the evil that is done by the habitual use of blue-pill and other mercu-rial purgatives for what is called "biliousness" is incalculable. They promote the recurrence of the very attacks they at first seem to relieve; and they gradually induce—as Dr. Bryce has shown—a chronic poisoning by the metal, an hydrargyrosis which, though slight, is real, and makes the patient's life a very miserable one.

On the other hand, homœopathic experience has taught us that the British use of the drug in disorders of the liver (I say the *British* use, for in French and German treatises this medication is always spoken of as foreign to their practice) is largely based on the principle of similarity, and obtainable by small doses. I have already shown that experimentation, while opposing the notion that Mercury directly stimulates the secreting function of the liver, shows it to cause conges-tion of the organ and jaundice. In both these hepatic affec-tions the medicine ranks *facile princeps* among homœopathic practitioners; and it acts well in quite minute doses, as the third, sixth, and twelfth attenuations. It is an admirable remedy for what is called a "torpid" liver, where deficient secretion of bile is indicated by pale, costive, and offensive motions, loss of appetite, and depression of spirits. That there is congestion present in these cases seems indicated by the dull pain in the right hypochondrium, of which the patients usually complain. So in simple jaundice as it occurs in children (where probably the same congestion is present), Mercury will generally do all that is required. For acute

* *Laws of Therapeutics*, ch. x.

parenchymatous inflammation of the liver, Dr. Gerson speaks of calomel in our doses as highly as do the Indian practitioners of the old school.

Dr. Ringer has some excellent remarks on this subject, which might have been written by any homœopathist. Admitting the full force of the experiments which have been made, he yet argues that they must not neutralise the experience of generations; and that "it is not difficult to conceive that Mercury in disease may set aside some condition hindering the formation of bile, and thus act as a cholagogue, while yet in health it may even check this secretion." He advises minute doses—from the sixth to the half of a grain of grey powder twice or three times a day; and says that were those who decry mercurial preparations to use the drug in this way, they would obtain the desired effect without the bad results they fear.*

II. But it is the second of our three actions of the drug—acute mercurialisation—upon which I am desirous of fixing your special attention; as it is that whereby it has played so great a part in the history of medicine, and coincidently has wrought so great ruin and destruction among mankind. With the exception (if it be an exception) of blood-letting, I know of no more mischievous treatment ever devised than the induction of the constitutional influence of this drug, as shown by stomatitis and ptyalism. It was bad enough to rob a man of a large proportion of his vital fluid; but it was intensifying the injury indeed to poison the remainder. Hundreds of deaths, and hundreds of thousands of ruined healths—to say nothing of temporary suffering and disease—have attested its influence all over Europe. It is little wonder that the wiser practice of the present day tends more and more to abandon its use. The change is indicated in the two editions of Sir Thomas Watson's classical *Lectures* which appeared in 1857 and in 1871 respectively. In the former Mercury takes rank after venesection in the treatment of most inflammations; in the latter it has followed its principal into the limbo of doubt-

---

* My *Monthly Homœopathic* reviewer objects to this explanation of mine of the action of Mercury in torpid liver, and thinks that in endorsing Dr. Ringer's suggestion as to its *modus operandi*, I am passing by the principle of similarity. But this I am not doing; for I mean that the condition it removes is that which it causes, viz. :— congestion, and such an explanation seems to me as good homœopathy (and better pharmacology) as to say that it stimulates the secreting cells of the liver in small doses while depressing them in large. My critic cites Dr. Rutherford's recent experiments as supporting this position; but I cannot find any such statement made by him.

ful and perilous means of practice. The same abandonment
had at one time largely, though not universa'ly, taken place
in the treatment of syphilis.

What is the reason of this pernicious effect of a drug
supposed to be given as a medicine—an effect unique in its
instance ? Arsenic and Iodine are far more potent as poisons;
yet they have not wrought this mischief. Any injurious
effects they have had have been (so to speak) extraneous and
incidental : by proper dosage and mode of administration
they have readily been avoided. But the ill-doing of Mercury
has been an essential part of its use, and so inherent therein
that because of it that use itself has been dropped. The fact
is that when Mercury has been employed (as it most largely
has been) in the treatment of syphilitic and of inflammatory
affections, it has been its physiological action that has been
used for the purpose. The cure has been sought, not directly,
but through the medium of "salivation"—that is, by the
full constitutional influence of the drug as implied by that
phenomenon. "When we fail to induce some affection of the
mouth," writes Pereira, "we do not obtain the beneficial effects
of mercury." Thus, instead of the poison being transformed
into a medicine, it has been used as a poison ; and hence its
prejudicial effects. When it is now employed in this way, the
nature of its action is recognised, and it is pushed to as slight
an extent as possible. To "touch the gums" now is just to
excite the mercurial fever which we described in Hahnemann's
words, and which he, at the time he wrote, conceived to be
necessary (and as much as was necessary) for the cure of all
syphilitic manifestations. This is to lessen the mischief,
indeed ; yet mischief it still is. It is still doing evil that good
may come ; and though such a proceeding is not so rigidly
proscribed in medicine as in morals, yet it is only to be
adopted to avert greater evils, and with full knowledge and
circumspect discreetness in its application. In our hands who
aim at specific indications—who seek to absorb all physiological into therapeutical action, such an employment of a drug
must be, if ever resorted to, a rare and regretted exception to
our general practice. We should rather turn the bane into
the antidote, and use Mercury to cure instead of to cause the
morbid conditions it is capable of setting up, when, as not
unfrequently happens, they come before us from other causation.

That we have succeeded in doing this appears from the
different estimation in which the medicine is held in the two
schools of practice. It had become, as I have said, quite a

badge of the more advanced section of the old practice to renounce the use of Mercury in disease. It was declared to have no influence on the liver; to be of doubtful necessity in syphilis; and to act perniciously in most acute inflammations. On the other hand, the applications of it which are made according to our law and in our doses are continually affording us satisfaction. Few medicines are so frequently in our hands; and in none have we more thorough confidence. This looks a little as if we had found the clue to the right use of this and other poisons.

It was, as I have said, mainly for the treatment of syphilitic and inflammatory affections that the induction of acute mercurialisation was practised. The most celebrated use of the drug, and that which has best held its ground in the present day, has been as a remedy against *syphilis*. Let us enquire into its relation to this disease, and its sphere of action therein.

I assume the correctness of the modern doctrine regarding syphilis, in so far as it refuses the name to the soft chancre with its suppurating bubo, and allows it only to the indurated sore and its sequelæ. I also range myself with those who follow Hahnemann in believing the appearance of the induration to be evidence that the system—that is, the blood—is already contaminated with the venereal poison. I have discussed this question in an article " On Hahnemann's Doctrine of Syphilis " in the twenty-seventh volume of the *British Journal of Homœopathy*, and need not detain you with the evidence and arguments here.

Syphilis, then, is a poisoning of the blood analogous to the exanthemata—let us say, to inoculated smallpox. It has a stage of incubation, which is yet (as Lancereaux has pointed out) not without signs of impaired health. Slight feverishness, lassitude, aching of the bones and headache are often present; and careful observation finds chloro-anæmia to have already set in. Hahnemann shows from earlier authors that of old time this stage of incubation was more prolonged, and the evidences (debility and fatigue, dulness of the sensorium, depression of spirits, earthy complexion with blue borders round the eyes, &c.) of ill health during its existence more obvious. Then ensues the lesion which marks the point of entrance of the virus. It is essentially an induration, whatever may be present on its superficial aspect; and it is soon followed by a similar condition of some of the inguinal glands, doubtless the result of absorption. This is analogous to the pustule of variolous inoculation; and now, after a time, follows the specific fever of the disease, with its rash and sore-throat. The rash is macular or papular, less frequently squamous. The sore-throat is ulcerative, generally indolently so. Iritis, and sometimes laryngitis and periostitis, may occur at this time. Lastly, we have *sequelæ* of the syphilitic as of other blood infections ; and these are in its case the infiltrations of the viscera and the periosteum which are known as gummata or nodes.

It is, I think, very helpful thus (with Mr. Hutchinson) to regard primary, secondary, and tertiary syphilis as stages of a chronic exanthema, differing only in its prolonged course from the acute affections which bear the same name. It is certain, again, that Mercury has some influence over this malady, and that of a specific kind. Few would maintain now-a-days that it antidotes the venereal poison as an alkali neutralises an acid ; and none, I think, would suppose that it eliminates the *materies morbi* by its ptyalism or other evacuation. We must look, therefore, to its physiological effects to see what it is capable of doing as a therapeutic agent, and how it does it.

Now it would be easy to make capital out of the admissions of writers on the subject, and argue that Mercury does all it can do in syphilis in virtue of its homœopathicity thereto. "It is singular," says Dr. Ringer, "how similar the phenomena produced by Mercury are to those which result from syphilis ;" and in so speaking he does but echo the expressions of many who have gone before him.* But as our object is truth, and not the support of a theory, we must not be content with these testimonies ; but, remembering that Kussmaul, after an exhaustive enquiry into the effects of Mercury on the workers in it, comes (as Trousseau and Pidoux had done) to the opposite conclusion, must examine for ourselves to see how it is.

I think that the result of such an enquiry must be that the physiological effects of Mercury present a nearly perfect parallel to one stage of the syphilitic history, but diverge widely from it before and afterwards. This stage is not that of the primary incubation. A slightly febrile chloro-anæmia is indeed the original constitutional effect of both poisons. But that induced by syphilis eventuates in plastic deposits— the indurated sore and glands ; while the local symptoms of Mercury are those of liquefaction of tissue, — any glands

---

* Thus Stillé : "Alterative medicines act to a great degree in the same direction as the diseases which they cure ; mercury, for example, tends to produce lesions which bear a close resemblance to, if they are not identical with, those caused by syphilis."

affected by it swelling from irritation approaching to inflam,
mation, and tending to suppurate. The condition of blood
from which such opposite results proceed can hardly be really,
though it may be phenomenally, the same. Again, there is
nothing in the effects, actual or possible, of Mercury to correspond with the gummy infiltrations of the tertiary period. So
that, although the drug may affect every part which is invaded
by the disease, though a mere "organopathy" may regard
it as a *simile* thereto, true homœopathy cannot allow that it
acts in all these parts after a like manner, and must hence (I
submit) refuse it the name. If Mercury can do anything to
resolve the primary indurations and tertiary infiltrations of
syphilis, it must do it by its physiological action ; and we
must not think that we are homœopathising in so using it.

It is otherwise with the secondary stage of the disease.
Again we have a febrile chloro-anæmia, of still more marked
character, to which, with its rheumatoid pains (aggravated by
rest and the warmth of bed) in the head and face, behind the
sternum, and around the joints, and its termination in falling
of the hair, Mercury is obviously and strikingly homœopathic.
And here it is hardly less so to the resulting local manifestations,
which may be described as low inflammatory processes in
skin, mucous membrane, and periosteum. We are strictly
within the lines of our method when we treat with small doses
of the drug the syphilitic pyrexia, and the exanthemata, the
ulcers of mouth and throat, and the subacute periostitis, of
the secondary period. As regards the chloro-anæmia, it has
been recently ascertained that Mercury, when given in syphilis,
increases the number of the red globules of the blood. We
have already seen that it diminishes them in health ; and
here also it is noted that, if the drug be pushed too far, it
reduces their number again.

These seem the necessary deductions from the facts of the
case. Let us see how they agree with experience.

We have in the case of syphilis an excellent opportunity of
estimating the real effects of treatment ; for we have abundant
material for the natural history of the disease. Expectant
treatment has been carried out on a large scale by the opponents of the use of Mercury. The results may be read in the
excellent treatise of Dr. Charles Drysdale, *On the treatment
of Syphilis and other diseases without Mercury.* Syphilis,
say the non-mercurialists, when allowed to run its course
under hygienic measures and local applications, is rarely other
than a mild and indolent disease, wearing itself out with little
injury to the frame. In the words of one of them—the late

Mr. Syme—" the case may be tedious, and the skin, throat, or periosteum may be slightly affected; but none of the serious effects which used to be so much dreaded ever appear, and even the trivial ones just noticed comparatively seldom present themselves." This is perhaps too broad a statement, and more exceptions should have been allowed; but it goes little beyond the conclusions arrived at after the non-mercurial treatment of thousands of cases in the great military hospitals of France.

Can Mercury do better? In endeavouring to answer this question we are much hindered by the confusion which has existed till within the last few years between the soft chancre and the indurated sore. Since Mercury is perfectly homœopathic to the former, as we have seen, it may well promote its healing if given in moderate doses. And since this chancre is far more frequent than the other, and is never followed by constitutional symptoms, it may easily be supposed by one who lumps all his cases together that the Mercury he gives prevents the occurrence of secondaries. This is the statement of Hahnemann,* and of two of his followers, Schneider† and Jahr‡—all these speaking from prolonged or extensive experience. On the other hand, Dr. Yeldham in his excellent *Homœopathy in Venereal Diseases*, and Bähr in his *System of Therapeutics*, discriminating more scientifically, admit that the indurated chancre is generally followed by secondary symptoms, whatever be the treatment adopted for it. The latter allows nine to fifteen weeks for the continuance of the chancre, which is about the same time it occupies when left to nature. Dr. Yeldham, whose doses approach more nearly to those of the old school, considers that he really shortens the duration of both primary and secondary symptoms.‖ If it be so, it may be that a slight physiological action is produced, though not enough to affect the mouth. But I venture to think that a careful reckoning of his dates will show that his indurated chancres and even his dry syphilides lasted nearly if not quite as long as those of expectant treatment, as the same is related by Dr. Charles Drysdale. The most marked effects were healing of ulcers and improvement in general health, both of which belong to the truly homœopathic action of the drug.

* See *Brit. Journ. of Hom.*, xxvii, 396.

† *Ibid.*, xxii, 620.

‡ *On Venereal Diseases.*

‖ He gives from one to three grains of the first, or from five to ten grains of the second decimal attenuation of Mercurius solubilis (*i.e.*, from $\frac{3}{10}$ to $\frac{1}{20}$ of a grain) three times a day.

The conclusion seems to be that it is only at certain points and stages of the syphilitic process that Mercury can antidote it after a specific manner, that is (again to quote our own Drysdale's definition) by the absorption of its whole physiological into its therapeutical action. But these points and stages are important enough. The blood disorder; the affections of mouth and throat; the sub-acute inflammation of the periosteum; some of the exanthemata, and perhaps the laryngitis, are to be included among them. Again, the whole series of manifestations of hereditary syphilis are within its range, whether they take the form of bullæ, abscesses, and marasmus, or the slower and less fatal variety which consists in snuffles, stomatitis, readily moistening syphilides, pale earthy colour of skin, and epiphyseal periostitis in the long bones. And further uses are suggested by the results of its abuse. When the local manifestations of the disease become *destructive;* when the eruptions take the form of impetigo or rupia, when rapid ulceration affects the mucous membranes, or when caries invades the bones:—here, when the cause is not Mercury itself, its administration is most effective. Thus Dr. Gerson speaks highly of corrosive sublimate in the phagedænic or sloughing chancre; and Dr. Yeldham has known Mercurius solubilis arrest phagedænic ulceration when other remedies, ordinarily recommended for that condition, had failed. Dr. George Wood, moreover, writes of the syphilitic cachexia: "I have seen the lowest condition of shattered health, which for years had resisted various treatment under the idea that it was mercurial disease, get well under a careful administration of blue-pill, as if cured by a charm." Colles makes a similar statement.

We claim all such cures, I say, for the homœopathic action of Mercury. Whether w should ever go beyond it, and use the drug for syphilitic manifestations where some measure of physiological action must be set up, is a question. It seems quite unnecessary to do so for the primary sore and the secondary syphilides, as they only want time for their disappearance; and to disperse the tertiary gummata when they are causing mischief, we can nearly always depend upon the iodide of potassium. The only disease in which the practice has sometimes seemed needful, even in our hands, is syphilitic iritis, in which it every now and then happens that nothing will affect the disease until Mercury is given to touch the mouth. You remember the vivid description of Watson: "The instant that the patient's gums and breath acknowledge the specific influence of Mercury upon his system, a welcome

change becomes apparent : the red zone surrounding the
cornea begins to fade ; the drops of lymph to lessen ; the iris
to resume its proper tint ; and the puckered and irregular
pupil once more to approach to the perfect circle ; till at
length the eye is restored to its original integrity, and beauty,
and usefulness." The eye is so precious an organ that one
would willingly submit to a temporary sacrifice of general
health, if really necessary for its restoration. Should you
ever have to push Mercury to this extent, let me remind you
of the method of Law, who divided a grain of calomel into
twelve parts, giving one every hour till the mouth was touched,
which it usually was ere thirty-six doses had been taken.
Trousseau and Pidoux have carried his plan farther, making
twenty-four doses of the grain, and giving one every two
hours only. In this way, they say, they rarely require as
much as three grains to effect their purpose.

I have said all this from the homœopathic stand-point. In
the old school men seem passing from the entire renunciation
of Mercury in syphilis to a renewed recognition of its power
over the disease. The recent deliverances of Mr. Hutchinson
are very significant on this point. His recommendations to
avoid physiological action are cautious enough ; but when he
speaks of it being "desirable to introduce a considerable
quantity of the drug into the system, and to protract its use
over a very long time," we seem to be beginning the old
career again. To all disposed to enter upon it, I would recommend the perusal of the work of Andrew Mathias, a surgeon to the Queen in 1816, *On the Mercurial Disease.* He
argues, quite in Hahnemannian fashion, that Mercury cures
syphilis by setting up a specific disease of its own which is
incompatible with it. And he shows from numerous observations (as Hahnemann had done before) that if the drug be
given too largely or too long the venereal symptoms will cease
to improve, will take on a retrograde action, and will be complicated with fresh lesions of a similar but distinctive character. It is interesting to observe that, according to him,
when this mercurial disease has subsided, the old venereal
symptoms will reappear, having been suspended only by the
presence of the other. Hahnemann makes such suspension,
instead of extinction, the mark of a different as opposed to a
similar disease ; and so our position is confirmed, that while
Mercury is homœopathic to syphilis at points, it is not so as
whole to whole.

It would seem that Hahnemann himself was once of the
same opinion ; for in his treatise on Venereal Diseases pub-

lished in 1789, he says—"Mercury does not cure syphilis by causing evacuations, but rather by the gradual or sudden *antipathic* irritation of the fibres of a specific nature which it sets up." It is true that in 1796 he argued that the drug was a *simile* to the disease; but let us see how he characterises the latter. "Syphilis depends upon a virus, which, besides other peculiarities that it developes in the human body, has an especial tendency to produce inflammatory and suppurating swellings of the glands (to weaken the tone?); to make the mechanical connexion of the fibres so disposed to separation that numerous spreading ulcers arise, whose incurable character may be known by their round figure; and, lastly, to increase the irritability." It is quite evident that the second only of these features belongs to true syphilis. Hahnemann himself goes on to specify a number of points in which "the mercurial disease is very different from the nature of syphilis."

Fault has been found with me* that I have laid too much stress upon the absence of homœopathic relationship between Mercury and certain manifestations of syphilis, and that I ought to have minimised such points of divergence in the interest of the general similarity it possesses. Now if the fact was only that the homœopathicity of Mercury to syphilis was not perfect, the exception taken to my argument would be well warranted. But my position is that in a considerable range of the manifestation of the disease the drug is not only not homœopathic, but actually antipathic; and that it can only be by inducing its physiological and destructive influence that it can here effect any change. This is an important matter; and, as the general similarity between the effects of the two agents is recognised by all, it seemed to me most useful to you to point out wherein this relation did not hold good, and where accordingly you must not expect to use Mercury with benefit as a homœopathic remedy.

The other great use which has been made of mercurialisation is in the treatment of inflammatory affections. But before entering upon this subject (which indeed I must reserve for our next meeting) I will speak of certain general conditions to which the constitutional effects of the drug shew it to be homœopathically suitable. I will not include among these (though I might do so) scurvy and chlorosis, as the former is so satisfactorily met by dietetic means, and the latter by the judicious administration of iron and similar remedies. But I shall have to say something of scrofula, of rheumatism and of the eruptive fevers.

* *Monthly Homœopathic Review*, xx, 452.

1. I have shown how the very forms of venereal disease which are ordinarily supposed to contra-indicate Mercury to us suggest its choice. Such affections are especially met with in the scrofulous; and it is an accepted canon in old school therapeutics that where this diathesis exists Mercury is strictly forbidden. We on the contrary, and for the converse of the same reason, use it largely in many manifestations of scrofula. It would seem capable even of developing this diathesis, as Alibert and others have shewn that persons exposed to mercurial influence frequently beget scrofulous children. It is useful when the morbid phenomena show themselves in the eye, the ear, the glands, and the bones ; also in weeping eruptions and ulcerations of the surface. In strumous ophthalmia especially you will find it (as I shall have to tell you when we speak of the irritant salts of the metal) an excellent medicine. But for the whole subject of the relation of Mercury to scrofula I would refer you to Dr. H. Goullon's treatise on the disease, here as always the best source of information as to its therapeutics. You will find cases there of scrofulous otorrhœa, eczema, and periostitis in which M. solubilis was strikingly successful.

2. Another constitutional affection in whose treatment Mercury plays a part is rheumatism. The "mercurial rheumatism" is too well-known for any demonstration of its homœopathicity to the disease to be necessary. It is common among the workmen in the metal, as may be seen from S. 555-565 of Allen's pathogenesis of it. When, moreover, Dr. Anstie describes, as frequent premonitory symptoms of an impending rheumatic fever, a "sallow and red tint of the face," with "oily perspiration," we are at once reminded of the pathogenetic effects of the drug. The occurrence of profuse and odorous perspirations, which give no relief, has in all affections been regarded as a "key-note" for Mercury; and it is a well-known and almost pathognomonic symptom of rheumatism. It is in subacute forms of the disease, readily relapsing, where the pains do not shift about much, and are markedly worse at night—the patient being very sensitive to cold—that Mercury is so useful. Some excellent cases illustrative of its virtues are recorded by Dr. Yeldham in the third and fourth volumes of the *Annals*.

3. Again, the description I have given, from Alley, of the febrile eruptions induced by Mercury forcibly suggests the three great eruptive fevers, measles, scarlatina, and small-pox. His severer degrees of "hydrargyria" very fairly correspond to

these in their ascending scale. Mercury suits well the exanthem and the catarrhal symptoms of ordinary measles, and
may, with Aconite for its fever, do àll that is required in its
treatment.   In scarlatina its place is in the anginose form of
the disease ; where the swelling, ulceration, and tendency to
gangrene make it exquisitely homœopathic, and where it is
thoroughly efficacious.   In variola it takes up the treatment
where Tartar emetic has—if it has—to leave it, namely, where
in spite of the former remedy the pocks are going on to suppuration, and the secondary fever is setting in.   It is here
highly praised by all homœopathic writers.

The remainder of the therapeutics of Mercury, and the
action of its special preparations, I must reserve for my next
lecture.

LECTURE XLIII.

MERCURIUS (*continued*).

I have said that it was for inflammation that the induction of the constitutional effects of Mercury was chiefly practised. Now here, too (as well as with syphilis), it would seem that we might convict our antagonists, out of their own mouths, of homœopathising in what they were doing. In the words of Sir Thomas Watson : " When Mercury is gradually introduced into the human body in small quantities, it produces sooner or later very remarkable effects. It *causes* inflammation. Perhaps it may be for that reason that the professors of homœopathy prescribe ' Mercurius ' so often." It is, indeed. But here also we must discriminate, though it be apparently to our own disadvantage. The seat and kind of the phlogosis induced by Mercury is not generally that for which it has been so renowned as a remedy. It is in adhesive inflammations of serous membranes, in membranous croup and exudative iritis, that it has been given : it is its physiological effect that has been desired, and this has been induced accordingly. It has been regarded as contra-indicated in mucous and parenchymatous inflammations, and where the tendency has been to ulceration and suppuration. These *contras*, however, are our *pros*. We cannot claim for homœopathy the ancient antiphlogistic employment of Mercury ; but we find great use for it in the treatment of all inflammations where we desire to check suppuration when impending, and heal ulceration when extending.

1. In affections of the mouth Mercury naturally holds a high place. It is not homœopathic to the true membranous stomatitis of children—the muguet of the French ; but it is so to the stomacace of adults, and to thrush, which always tends to ulceration. It is rarely necessary, however, to give anything but Borax in this last disease, when the morbid process is limited to the mouth. For simple ulceration, as well as syphilitic, of the mucous membrane of the buccal cavity Mercury is specific, especially when followed up by Nitric

acid.　Cancrum oris is another idiopathic disease of this part which closely resembles the pathogenetic effects of Mercury. We of course treat it with this drug ; but it is rather amusing to find a writer of the old school advocating the practice. Hempel cites such an one in the person of Dr. Duncan, of Dublin.

The coexistence with other symptoms of the mercurial mouth will always suggest and often establish its appropriateness to the whole case.

With the mouth we class the salivary glands, the tongue, and the teeth.

a. Mercury has cured idiopathic salivation, as from pregnancy.　Drs. Marcy and Hunt recommend in this affection a wash for the mouth made of two grains of the second trituration of Mercurius corrosivus to a pint of water.　In inflammations of the salivary glands Mercury must always be the leading remedy.　I may specify two—mumps, in which we always give it, though whether it affects the natural course of the disease I cannot say ; and the tenderness and swelling, threatening suppuration, left behind after scarlatina, or appearing during typhus, in which the iodides at any rate act most efficiently.

b. In subacute inflammations of the lingual mucous membrane, and even in acute glossitis, Mercury has acted very well. Dr. Guernsey points out a very heavy, thick, yellow, moist covering of the tongue as indicating the drug, saying that it should rarely be given when the tongue is dry.　Dr. Quin notes sweet taste in the mouth as a characteristic symptom for it.

c. In our present uncertainty as to the action of Mercury on the teeth it would be premature to fix its curative place in their diseases.　If it is true that its abuse can cause them to become carious, the medicine ought to be useful in checking this process.　More certainly it is of value in periostitis of the sockets, a frequent cause of toothache : its steady use here will often supersede extraction.　The feeling as if the teeth were elongated as well as tender is a special indication for it.

2. I have now to speak of Mercury in affections of the throat.　Simple catarrhal angina is a malady in which I think this medicine far too frequently used.　It is recommended in Domestic Guides to homœopathic treatment whenever there is any tendency to ulceration ; and every mucous exudation on the tonsils is taken for an ulcer, and treated accordingly.　But these phenomena, even if truly ulcerative, are

but superficial accidents of an acute sore-throat, where there is much pain and bright redness. Cut away this inflamed base with your Belladonna and (if needful) Aconite; the ulcer will not remain behind. In my own experience, the angina calling for Mercury has been of rare occurrence. It is of a subacute or torpid character, with pale or bluish-red swelling; and ulceration is often present. Its power of checking suppuration makes it often useful in quinsy. Hartmann praises it here; and Dr. Ringer writes: " When in quinsy or scarlatina the tonsils are so enlarged as almost to meet, and when the difficulty of swallowing is nearly insuperable, and it may be there is even danger of suffocation, if at such a time a third of a grain of grey powder be taken every hour, in a few hours the swelling is much reduced, and the danger, discomfort, and distress much removed. The effect of the mercury in such cases is often most signal." Dr. Imbert-Gourbeyre, also, has defined the place and illustrated the virtue of Mercury in quinsy in a memoir on the treatment of angina by mercurials, Belladonna, and Aconite, translated from the *Moniteur des Hôpitaux* in the fourteenth volume of the *British Journal of Homœopathy*.

When anything like the cynanche maligna or putrid sore-throat of the old writers is present, Mercurius is an indispensible remedy. On the other hand, those same characteristics of its action which make it so suitable for the sore-throat of scarlatina unfit it for that of diphtheria. There is so much phenomenal resemblance between the effects of Mercury and the symptoms of diphtheria, that the preparations of this drug were at first extensively used in its treatment. They failed, however, in most hands to show any power of arresting the morbid process. Nor should we expect them to do so. For in diphtheria there is ordinarily neither ulceration nor gangrene, but a false membrane formed upon a comparatively unbroken surface. Until it has been proved that Mercury can cause this pathological formation, there is no evidence that it is truly homœopathic to the diphtheritic process. I reserve the question of the action of the cyanide and iodides, which will come before us presently.

Mercury may occasionally be useful in chronic ulcers of the throat, simple, scrofulous, and syphilitic; and would probably cure such a chronic angina as that described by Dietrich, were we to meet with it as an idiopathic affection. I shall have to speak again of this action in relation to the iodide and to Cinnabar.

3. The only gastric affection in which I can indicate the

ordinary mercurials as specific is the sudden vomiting of milk
in infants, which so often depends upon degenerative change
of the mucous membrane of the stomach. Here Dr. Ringer
highly commends minute doses of grey powder or calomel,
which can hardly act otherwise than homœopathically. Nor
can I say much about them in the substantive affections of
the intestinal mucous membrane, though we shall see corrosive sublimate playing a distinguished part here. The late
Dr. Petroz has published some cases tending to show that the
black sulphide (Ethiops mineral) has considerable control
over the enteric lesion of typhoid fever,* and Dr. von Tunzelmann has more recently written in corroboration.† I have
myself lately had a case in point, where the diarrhœa and
hæmorrhage from the intestinal ulceration was seriously im-
perilling an otherwise happy progress, and where the Ethiops
mineral speedily wrought a change for the better. It is the
lymphatic-glandular apparatus of the intestines which is here
in fault, and Mercury finds its proper sphere of operation.

It is obvious, upon the principle of similarity, that Mercury
should be beneficial in many forms of diarrhœa ; and so it is.
Few medicines are more frequently called for in the diarrhœa
of infants and young children, when the evacuations are vitiated, of various colours, slimy and offensive, sometimes excoriating the anus. Dr. Guernsey adds, as indications for
M. solubilis, much pain before the stool and great relief immediately afterwards ; also much straining.   Calomel ("M.
dulcis" of our nomenclature) is the best form in which to use
it here ; as this preparation of the drug most readily causes
bowel affections in the healthy.

Here again Dr. Ringer supplies welcome corroboration to
our practice, and has contributed most practical descriptions
of the use of the medicine. In children, where " three or four
pale, clayey, pasty, stinking motions are passed in the course
of the day," frequent doses of a third of a grain of grey
powder will soon set matters right. In their dysenteric
diarrhœa, where the motions are "slimy," and often mixed
with blood, the eightieth of a grain of corrosive sublimate will
cure "with remarkable speed and certainty." "The great
indication for the bichloride," he writes, "is the slimy character of the motions." Here he is curiously at one with Dr.
Guernsey, who says, "Mercurius is rarely indicated in diarrhœa
when there is no slime." A sixth of a grain of grey powder
given hourly will soon check cholera infantum and chronic

* See *Brit. Journ. of Hom.*, xxiii., 634.
† *Monthly Hom. Review*, xviii., 77.

diarrhœa with green stools in the same subjects. His whole section on this subject may be commended to ycur study, and affords a most gratifying instance of the progress made by our ideas. If such teachings prevail, Mercury will soon be found a blessing where so long it has been a curse.

4. The mercurial preparations occupy a less important place as remedies for affections of the respiratory mucous membrane. M. solubilis has a high domestic reputation as a remedy for "running colds;" but I confess that I myself prefer Euphrasia and Kali bichromicum. I can confirm, however, Dr. Bayes' statement that "catarrhal cough, with yellow muco-purulent expectoration, often yields very readily" to it in the sixth dilution. Perhaps we in this country undervalue Mercury in bronchitis, for our German brethren seem to estimate it very highly, judging from the testimony of Trinks, Bähr, and Hirschel. Here is what the latter writes about it. " How the allopaths, and much more their patients, are to be pitied, that their school should lack a knowledge of Mercurius as a cough remedy! Where is there a more certain, a more specifically acting remedy for the appropriate kinds of cough of a catarrhal, inflammatory, organic nature, running down from the fauces through the trachea and into the finest bronchi, decisive in acute affections, ameliorating in the chronic, slime-loosening, resolvent, restorative, where there are roughness, burning, feeling of soreness from the fauces down to the sternum, hoarseness of voice, dry cough, raw, concussive, exhaustive ; sputum ropy, watery, spittle-like, nasty, bloody ; catarrhal headache, coryza, diarrhœa, fever, non-ameliorating night-sweats—here is the province of Mercurius. It is the sovereign remedy of inflammatory bronchial catarrh."

5. Coming now to the uro-genital organs, I have already pointed out the homœopathicity of Mercury to the soft chancre, as to any non-syphilitic ulcer forming on the genitals. I will only add that Dr. Yeldham recommends M. solubilis as the best medicine in balanitis. Bähr treats gonorrhœa with Mercury almost throughout, but his results are not striking.

6. The traditional use of Mercury in inflammations of the serous membranes has (as I have said) no relation to its specific influence upon them, and is upon our principles quite inadmissible. We hold it of very questionable advantage to prevent lymphous exudation by a poison which causes a lower form of effusion to take its place. I shall have something to say presently of the specific relation of M. corrosivus to peritonitis.

7. As to cutaneous diseases, I have already spoken of those

of a syphilitic nature. You will always bear in mind excessive perspiration, especially when of a viscid consistence and strong odour, and occurring chiefly at night, as an indication for the drug. When this symptom is itself the disease, as in hidrosis pedum, Hartmann speaks of M. solubilis as not unfrequently curative. The presence of moisture of the skin, moreover, in febrile and inflammatory conditions, favours the choice of Mercurius, as it makes against Aconite and Belladonna. The only non-specific skin affections in which we have any experience with the drug are eczema rubrum and lepra. In the last-named affection, when not of too long standing, I have found it very effective ; and " psoriasis in spots over the whole body " (lepra is psoriasis circinata) has been observed by Kussmaul in the workers. I should say, however, in addition, that Hartmann praises it in intertrigo (to which it is certainly homœopathic), especially when the excoriation developes not merely in the folds of the skin, but also at other spots.

8. As regards affections of the bones and joints, I have spoken of the value of Mercury in scrofulous and rheumatic periostitis. It is recommended by Hartmann in caries developing itself in strumous subjects after variola, or from injury to the bone. He also finds it of great service in the so-called " claudicatio spontanea " of childhood, which he considers dependent upon a greater or less degree of inflammation of the capsular ligament of the hip-joint and of the neighbouring glands. If there is much pain, he preludes with or substitutes Belladonna.

I have yet to speak of certain curative actions of Mercury, for which I have hitherto found no situation. I refer to its place in the therapeutics of eye and ear disease, and of the affections of glands.

9. You will find, if you consult the treatises on diseases of the eyes given us by Dr. Angell and Drs. Allen and Norton respectively, that they are in thorough agreement as to the high place occupied by the mercurial preparations in the treatment of these affections. Of their recommendations as to corrosive sublimate and other irritant salts of Mercury I will speak presently ; but they concur in praising the ordinary forms of the drug in blepharitis, where the lids are red, thick, and swollen ; in superficial keratitis ; and in episcleritis. They also give it in preference in all inflammations of the eye owning a syphilitic origin. Drs. Allen and Norton regard Mercury as the principal remedy for iritis ; though I must say that I think its homœopathicity here has yet to be established.

"No case of iritis of any form," says Kussmaul, "has been noticed among workers in Mercury ;" and this though keratitis and scleritis have not uncommonly been observed. It is more suitable to retinitis, which is suggested by the symptoms of both workers and provers, and seems several times to have been cured by it—the "incipient amaurosis" in which Hartmann commends M. solubilis being presumably of this nature.

The symptomatic indications for Mercurius in these disorders are that the discharges are profuse, burning and acrid, and thin ; and that the pains are all worse at night and for warmth—the heat of a light giving more inconvenience than its luminosity. It is thus especially useful in the affections, both of the mucous and nervous structures of the eyeball, which occur in those much exposed to the glare of a fire, as workers in foundries.

10. "In acute as well as chronic suppurations of the middle ear," writes Dr. Houghton, "Mercurius (vivus or solubilis) is more frequently indicated than any other remedy." The pains here too are aggravated at night, especially in the warmth of bed, abating towards morning. In chronic cases, the pus may be fœtid and even bloody. A good instance is related by Rentsch,* in which otorrhœa of this kind, and very profuse, had existed for a long time (after measles), and a polypus had formed. M. solubilis, internally and locally, cured in four weeks.

11. As regards the glands, I have already spoken of the usefulness of Mercurius in strumous adenitis ; and would only add that Hartmann highly commends it in incipient mastitis during lactation, when the pain has the characteristic feature of increasing from evening till midnight, and after this remitting.

III. Very little use has yet been made homœopathically of the neurotic effects of chronic mercurialisation. The metal ought to find place in the treatment of many chronic inflammations of the gray matter of the brain and cord. Bähr relates a case of acute myelitis cured by it. Hartmann commends it in stammering after apoplexy, and relates the following curious case, in which it was certainly strongly indicated.

"In a man already advanced in years, there appeared slight transient vertigo, which afterwards occurred more frequently, and continued a longer time ; in the periods between the attacks, he laboured under loss of memory, weakness of understanding, and absence of mind, from which he had never suffered previously. Sometimes cardiac anxiety, or again ptyalism, which continued for a whole day, at which

* Goullon on Scrofula, p. 204.

time his mental powers seemed unimpaired, supplied the place of the
vertiginous attacks. He had used many remedies by the advice of
physicians, but none of them had benefited him ; on the contrary, the
morbid state seemed to increase, and finally complete mania was developed, which always disappeared entirely on the supervention of
ptyalism. When the cardiac anxiety occurred, it had always been
conjoined with the settled idea that he would lose his reason.

Mercurius solubilis 2, repeated in three days, effected a rapid and
permanent cure.''

We may thus be encouraged to follow the indication of the
pathogenetic effects of Mercury, and give it where the premonitory symptoms of cerebral disease exist. When Sir
Thomas Watson says—" I have known several obscure but
threatening symptoms of brain disease clear entirely away, when
the gums were made sore by mercury, and kept slightly
tender for some little time," one feels tempted to suppose that
the power of the metal to cause such phenomena had something
to do with the cure, and that the stomatitis induced was at
least unnecessary.—Mercury ought to find place, moreover, in
the therapeutics of paralysis agitans.

The only full analogue of Mercury is *Iodine*. The medicines
resembling it in their action upon special tissues and organs I
have mentioned in their several places.

The range of the dose of Mercury is necessarily extensive.
In syphilitic affections most of us—even those who are otherwise addicted to high dilutions, as Jahr and Hartmann—give
the low triturations ; none however going so far as even to touch
the gums. In most of the other disorders calling for M. vivus
or solubilis the attenuations from the third decimal to the
sixth centesimal will be found suitable ; and Hartmann recommends us. even when we go as high as the twelfth (which
he thinks far enough), to make our potencies by trituration
rather than solution. This seems to have been Hahnemann's
practice ; for in 1822 he recommends M. solubilis to be given
ordinarily in the twelfth trituration.

I proceed now to speak of the more distinctive mercurial
preparations. They are the bichloride, the cyanide, the
iodides, the red oxide, and the sulphide.

Mercurius corrosivus—the bi- or perchloride of chemistry
hitherto, the mercuric chloride of present nomenclature, the
corrosive sublimate of common language—is, as you know
well, a most potent poison, and in our hands is a most valued
medicine. It is prepared by trituration, or solution in rectified spirit. Hahnemann has given a few symptoms as produced by it, and Dr. Buchner has proved it (in fractional doses)

on himself and seven others. To the results thus obtained Dr. Allen adds numerous effects of poisoning, making a pathogenesis of upwards of eleven hundred symptoms, which we may supplement yet further by using the observations made by Lewin in the treatment (on a large scale) of syphilitic disorders by the hypodermic injection of the drug.*

Corrosive sublimate is, of course, a mercurial, and therefore capable of inducing the constitutional effects of the metal ; but these are by no means readily obtained from it, and no mercurialist in the past ever used it to cause salivation. We, in like manner, should be chary of employing it as a remedial agent in conditions answering to those of pure mercurial influence, preferring for such purposes the M. solubilis or vivus. But M. corrosivus has a sphere of its own as a specific irritant to the living tissue, in which for range and intensity it is rivalled only by Arsenic. It affects in this way the stomach and large intestine, the respiratory mucous membrane and the lungs, the kidneys and external uro-genital organs, and the peritoneum. I will speak of each action, and of its therapeutic applications, separately.

1. Upon the alimentary canal the sublimate acts, when swallowed, as a corrosive caustic, chemically destroying the mucous membrane wherever it comes in contact with it. But observation and experiment show that, when otherwise introduced into the system, it still exerts an irritant influence upon certain parts of the digestive tract, which influence must, therefore, be of an elective and dynamic character, and suitable for homœopathic application. The parts so affected are the mouth and throat, the stomach, and the large intestine.

The best observations of these actions are those of Dr. Lewin, as his doses were moderate ($\frac{1}{10}$ to $\frac{3}{8}$ of a grain) and his experiments extensive. He found mouth affections in thirty-five per cent. of his cases. They consisted either of slight stomatitis and moderate ptyalism, with some tenderness and swelling of the salivary glands ; or of stomatitis ulcerosa, the ulcers being covered with a dirty yellow coat, which he compares (hardly justly, I think) to a diphtheritic membrane, without ptyalism; or of pure increase of the flow of saliva, of unchanged quality, and without any evidence of inflammation. If the patients caught cold they had redness and swelling of the tonsils and neighbouring lymphatic glands, hypertrophy-

* The Treatment of Syphilis by subcutaneous sublimate injections. By Dr. George Lewin. Translated by Drs. Proegler and Gale. Philadelphia : Lindsay and Blakiston. 1872.

of the former being no uncommon effect of a prolonged course of injections. Gastro-enteric symptoms were observed only when the maximum dose I have mentioned was overstepped. " In lighter cases, the intoxication is ushered in by gastric disturbances, like anorexia, coated tongue, bad taste, sometimes metallic, yet but seldom does the patient complain of nausea and vomiting. After a little time, pain of a sharp, burning character is experienced, a symptom which manifests itself not only spontaneously, but by pressure on the abdomen, especially in the region of the stomach and right hypochondrium. A little later, diarrhœa commences, tinged with blood only when occurring profusely. The patients present a markedly pale appearance, and complain of great languor. After the injection of relatively larger doses, the symptoms were aggravated, patients generally complaining of a vertiginous feeling, and after walking a few steps they would feel obliged to seize hold of something for support. . . With the already painful affections of the abdomen, vomiting occurred, sometimes with bloody dysenteric stools and tenesmus." I need hardly remind you that similar phenomena are observed in acute poisoning by the sublimate, and post-mortem investigation, while showing all the signs of inflammation (including those of dysentery), finds them limited to the stomach and large intestine, the smaller bowel remaining intact.

Quite in accordance with these facts is the use made of M. corrosivus in homœopathic therapeutics. In affections of the mouth and stomach, indeed, it is not much employed, though Hartmann recommends it (fifteenth dilution) in " very malignant, obstinate stomacace, arising after debilitating, prostrating diseases;" and Dr. Pemberton Dudley esteems it highly, in the second and third decimal triturations, in chronic gastric catarrh, with distension and soreness of the epigastrium and of the transverse colon. But when the large intestines are affected, whether with simple inflammation, with chronic ulceration, or with dysentery, its effects are amongst the most brilliant things in medicine. Hahnemann was the first to recommend it in dysentery, saying (1822) that he had found it almost specific in the common autumnal invasion of the complaint. He gave the fifteenth dilution in single dose; but Dr. Ringer reports correspondingly good results with hourly-repeated doses of a hundredth of a grain. All homœopathists, whether high or low dilutionists, concur to praise it here; and though some would limit its use to a certain variety of the disease, we have Dr. Espanet saying, " In the numerous cases of dysentery which I have treated in Algeria, I have never found the least advantage from substituting for M. corrosivus another remedy which seemed more homœopathic to the febrile phenomena or the abdominal symptoms. Dr. Feuille, of Algiers, has made the same remark."*

2. Corrosive sublimate inflames the respiratory mucous membrane of the eyes, nose, and bronchi, and also the lungs. It is highly esteemed in strumous ophthalmia, as you may see by referring to the cases reported by Dr. Böcker in the third and Dr. Kidd in the twenty-second volume of the *British Journal of Homœopathy*. Predominance of inflammatory and ulcerative symptoms call for it here, with great photophobia and profuse acrid discharges. Drs. Allen and Norton warmly commend it in syphilitic iritis and choroiditis, and in albuminuric retinitis. Dr. Jousset, and with him Dr. Dekeersmaecker, treats purulent ophthalmia by instillations of its third decimal dilution. It should be serviceable in the bronchitis of Bright's disease, and in syphilitic phthisis (*i.e.*, chronic pneumonia in these subjects).

3. The kidneys are very much affected by this poison. Suppression of urine is a very common phenomenon, and post-mortem investigation shows it to be connected with acute congestion or inflammation of the secreting structure of these organs. The urine is albuminous and bloody during life, in one case (cited by Allen) "presenting granular, fatty tubuli in large numbers, showing on their surface epithelial cells of the tubuli uriniferi also in a state of granular degeneration;" and the patients die with all the symptoms of uræmic poisoning. Lower down we have frequent and painful micturition, and sometimes swelling of the penis and scrotum, with blackness of the latter, and intense inflammation—even to sloughing —of the vulva.

M. corrosivus is considered by Dr. Ludlam the best remedy for the albuminous nephritis of pregnancy, and is commended by Bähr in nephritis suppurativa. Dr. Yeldham gives it, in alternation with Aconite, in the first stage of gonorrhœa. I have mentioned its usefulness in phagedænic and sloughing chancre; its homœopathicity thereto is now manifest.

4. Inflammation of the peritoneum and effusion into its sac is a frequent feature in poisoning by corrosive sublimate; and there is reason to suppose that it has a similar influence on other serous membranes. The cerebral arachnoid has been found inflamed by it, and Allen's 883d symptom suggests the spinal arachnoid as in the same state: "Loss of power and stiffness of the extremities, gradually increasing day by day,

* *Bulletin de la Soc. Med. Hom. de France*, xix., 179.

with excessive pain on any attempt to change the position, until the patient becomes entirely paralysed."

I have myself the highest esteem for M. corrosivus in peritonitis. I have used it here more frequently than Bryonia, and with most gratifying results.

Besides these more obvious applications of the peculiar properties of M. corrosivus, it has been used in homœopathic practice in several important disorders, as by Dr. Lawrence Newton in ulceration of the cartilages of the joints,* by Jahr and Hofrichter in syphilitic exostoses,† and in the eczema impetiginodes of scrofulous children. The discovery lately made by Dr. Rutherford, that it alone of the mercurial preparations is a true cholagogue, may possibly lead to further applications of it as an hepatic remedy. For the present, I must say no more of it.

Mercurius cyanatus, the bicyanide of the metal, "mercuric cyanide," we know at present almost entirely from its effects in a few cases of poisoning by it which have occurred, whose symptoms are furnished us by Allen. It does not corrode chemically as the perchloride does, so that its effects on the mouth and throat are of dynamic origin. Among these we find, in one case, " buccal mucous membrane red and injected (third day), a round ulcer, with grayish base and upright edges, and encircled with bright red, on the inside of the right cheek (fourth day), the ulcer in the mouth has spread, and is covered by a large, gray, leathery coating (fifth and sixth days);" and again, " a grayish, diphtheritic-looking deposit around the anus, quite similar to those on the inside of the cheeks;" and again, " a white, opalescent coating on the pillars of the velum palati and on the tonsils." In another case we have " the lips, tongue, and inside of the cheeks covered with a grayish-white pulp (fourth day)." In both instances these local symptoms were accompanied with great prostration.

It is not surprising that such phenomena should have suggested M. cyanatus as a remedy for diphtheria. Dr. Beck, of France, was the first to make the application; and Dr. Villers, of St. Petersburgh, learning it from him, reports that he has had astonishing success with it. Some of his cases are given by Dr. Oehme, in his excellent *Therapeutics of Diphtheritis*. Dr. Villers has lately reported that in ten years' time he has treated over a hundred cases of the disease, of all degrees of severity, without a single death, never giving anything but

* *Monthly Hom. Review*, xiv., 543.
† Jahr's *Venereal Diseases* translated by Hempel, p. 412.

M. cyanatus. He began with the sixth dilution, but now prefers the thirtieth. Its effects are very rapid, the exudation generally clearing away within twenty-four hours, and the general symptoms improving *pari passu.*

Dr. Villers is not without supporters in this experience of his. One of them is an old-school physician of the same city, Erichsen by name, who claims to have been more successful with the cyanide than with any other remedy, giving from one forty-eighth to one ninety-sixth of a grain for a dose. Even when the false membranes extended into the larynx, he found them clear away under the action of the drug. Of twenty-five cases thus treated, he lost three only,—one from cardiac paralysis, one from suppurating parotitis, and one from meningitis ; but even in these cases the local disease was gone.* He of course omits to credit the remedy to his homœopathic colleague. Dr. Jousset esteems it the best medicine in the putrid form of the disease ; and Dr. Burt, of Chicago, has lately stated that for the last three years he has been administering it in diphtheria with such wonderful curative results, that now, as soon as he is certain that he has a case of diphtheria to treat, he "at once puts the patient upon the cyanuret of Mercury, with a feeling of almost absolute certainty of curing him." In two at least of his cases the membrane had invaded the air-passages.† The two last-named practitioners have employed the lower triturations.

Dr. Burt experimented with the poison on a dog, injecting it under the skin. Great prostration, with feebleness of circulation and respiration, were produced ; and on post-mortem examination the larynx was found inflamed, with its mucous membrane and that of the posterior nares loaded with mucus, and the right ventricle contained a white fibrinous clot. In the *Homœopathic Times* for October, 1877, Dr. W. A. Allen writes, " A partial proving of the cyanide gave great prostration and weakness, a low febrile condition, a whitish-gray deposit upon the tonsils and mouth, extending along the right side of the tongue, with slightly swollen tonsils and difficult deglutition. These symptoms are given as communicated to me by the prover. The prostration and other symptoms were so severe that he ceased taking the drug,—the second potency had been used,—and rapidly recovered by the use of Baptisia." I think that such facts should encourage us to a free and trusting use of this remedy when we encounter the disease in question.

* *St. Petersburg Med. Wochenschrift,* 1877.
† *American Homœopathist,* ii., 22.

Mercurius iodatus, ⎫
Mercurius biniodatus. ⎰ By these names we designate the
two compounds which Iodine forms with Mercury,—the green
and red iodides (*fulvus* and *ruber*) of common language, the
mercurous and mercuric iodides of our present chemical nomenclature. They are prepared by trituration. I group them
together, as they have much in common, but shall not fail to
indicate their distinctive places.

The mercurial iodides are prepared by trituration. Both
have been proved in the school of Hahnemann,—the protiodide by Drs. Lord and Blakely, on six persons, the biniodide
by the Philadelphia Provers' Union. The pathogenesis obtained by the latter experimenters is given by Hering in his
Materia Medica ; both may be read in Allen.

They add little to our knowledge of the physiological action
of the compounds, which had been ascertained to behave
mainly like Mercury, though the double equivalent of the
halogen in the biniodide makes it exceedingly irritant. Their
use in the old school has been mainly in the treatment of
syphilis, and Lugol's experience with Iodine in scrofula made
it supposed that they would be especially suitable to patients
having this diathesis. I do not know that the idea has been
confirmed, and it has not prevailed in the homœopathic school.
Here the compounds (and especially the biniodide) have been
reckoned the best mercurials for secondary syphilides ; and
Drs. Yeldham, Clotar Müller and Meyhoffer on the one side,
Drs. Farrington and MacFarlane on the other, concur to commend them, the former giving the lower triturations, the latter
the highest dilutions.

The other chief sphere of action of the mercurial iodides in
homœopathic practice has been affections of the throat, especially when its glandular apparatus is involved. Dr. G. W.
Cook, of New York, introduced the protiodide as a remedy for
follicular pharyngitis, giving it in the first trituration;* and
since Dr. Black communicated his favourable experience with
it in 1857-8,† it has been the favourite remedy for the disorder
in this country.‡ Dr. Cooper praises it in chronic enlargement of the tonsils, when an inflammatory tendency is still
present and superficial ulcerations are seen.§ Dr. Blakely, its
chief prover, considers it indicated in affections of the throat

---

* See Jahr's *Manual*, ed. Snelling, *sub voce.*
† *Brit. Journ. of Hom.*, vols. xv. and xvi.
‡ See *Ibid*, xxxi., 287.
§ *Monthly Hom. Review*, xi., 580.

(and, indeed, of most other parts) where the tongue is coated bright yellow at the base, but is clean in front.*

A more questionable use of these compounds is their application to diphtheria. There is nothing in their pathogenesis to lead to their employment here, yet there is no question of their being in extensive use and high esteem. Dr. Ludlam, indeed, produces† a formidable array of symptoms as produced by the iodide, on the authority of Dr. Cook ; but if the original be consulted, it will be seen that the author is describing the morbid conditions he has *cured* with it. I myself have used them largely, and closely watched their effects, but I have not been able to satisfy myself of their exerting any action upon the morbid process. However, one cannot ignore the favourable results which Drs. Black, Ludlam and Helmuth report from the iodide, and Drs. Madden, Joslin and Dowling from the biniodide. I myself have seen excellent effects from the latter when the scarlatinal throat has assumed a diphtheritic character, with much swelling of the external glands ; and Dr. Russell found it curative in the dangerous parotitis of typhus.‡

Dr. Holcombe praises M. iodatus in chronic catarrh of the posterior nares, when the patient is annoyed by constant dropping of mucus into the pharynx.

Mercurius oxidatus ruber, the old " red precipitate," is also prepared by trituration. Allen gives a short pathogenesis of it, derived from fourteen observers, one of whom was a prover. Hartmann Jahr, and also the later homœopathists of Germany esteem it highly in the severer forms of both primary and secondary syphilis, when M. vivus or solubilis seems ineffective. They all give it in the first trituration, and its *modus operandi* may be inferred from what Hartmann says, that in one case he was compelled to give the sixth of a grain of the pure oxide three times a day before he could check the disease, and that no medicinal symptoms appeared, *save soreness of the gums and some loose teeth*. It removed a chronic blepharitis in the prover I have mentioned, and is esteemed by some in strumous ophthalmia and the other conjunctival affections for which the mercurials are suitable.

Mercurius sulphuratus, the compound of Mercury with Sulphur, appears* in Allen's *Encyclopædia* under its own name of

* *United States Med. Investigator*, iv., 165.
† *Clinical Lectures on Diphtheria*, p. 103.
‡ *Clinical Lectures*, p. 343.

Cinnabar (it is the vermilion of commerce). His pathogenesis of it is mainly made up of a very thorough proving instituted by Dr. Neidhard, and carried out on more than twenty persons, using various potencies of the drug. The record of these experiments may be read in detail in Metcalf's *Homœopathic Provings.*

Cinnabar is prepared, like the other insoluble mercurials, by trituration. Dr. Neidhard was led to prove it by the idea that " substances found in a naturally compound state are probably better calculated to eradicate the many complicated chronic diseases than the simple substances." I hardly think, however, that the results in this instance have supported his supposition. The proving yielded little but the disappearance (under the third trituration) of a chronic sore throat similar to that described by Dietrich as caused by Mercury, and the almost invariable production of sleeplessness by night with sleepiness by day. Therapeutically, Cinnabar is in repute in the transition stage between primary and secondary syphilis, when vegetations and mucous patches are the predominating lesions. Jahr and many others praise it here, as you may see from consulting this writer's treatise on venereal diseases. It is also esteemed in neglected chancres, and in those which have already been treated with mercury, but without the induction of the constitutional effects of the drug.

LECTURE XLIV.

MAGNESIA CARBONICA AND MURIATICA, MANGANUM, MENY-
ANTHES, MEZEREUM, MILLEFOLIUM, MOSCHUS, MUREX,
NATRUM CARBONICUM, MURIATICUM, AND SULPHURICUM,
NUPHAR.

We begin to-day with the magnesian salts, two of which are
used in homœopathic practice. The carbonate,

Magnesia carbonica,

is prepared by trituration.

A pathogenesis of it appeared in the first edition of the
Chronic Diseases, containing 128 symptoms, probably observed
upon patients taking the twelfth dilution. In the second
edition the list has increased to 890. A few of the additions
are from Schreter and Wahle; but the great bulk of them
are taken from a pathogenesis of 801 symptoms in the second
volume of Hartlaub and Trinks' *Arzneimittellehre,*—unnamed,
but supposed to proceed from the fertile manufactory of " Ng."
Dr. Allen inserts all these from the original.

Magnesia, in its simple carbonated form, is known only as
an antacid and mild laxative. Trousseau and Pidoux point
out that the evacuations produced by it are, at first, simple
liquid fæces; but that its continued use sets up sub-acute
inflammation of the intestinal mucous membrane. It may
thus find homœopathic employment in some bowel-affections
of children. Dr. Guernsey says that it is indicated when their
motions are sour-smelling, and resemble the green scum of a
frog-pond : the diarrhœa caused by Magnesia is certainly
generally of this colour. But the chief use to which it has
been put in the school of Hahnemann is in the treatment of
scanty and delaying menses, when, on their appearance, they
are of dark colour and pitchy consistence. It may also, it
seems, find place in the treatment of menorrhagia, when the
flow has the characteristic of being worse at night in bed. Mr.

Clifton relates a case of this kind in which, after the comparative failure of other remedies, it effected a speedy cure, and at the same time removed a greenish diarrhœa to which the patient was subject, and enabled her to take milk, which for years she had not been able to do without causing distress at the stomach and sour risings. He gave the 6th attenuation.

It is recommended by Hahnemann himself for the toothache of pregnancy, where it has often served me well. The pain, Dr. Guernsey says, is characteristically insupportable during repose : the patient must get up and walk about. Dr. Priel, of Riceys, published some time ago a number of cases of cataract in which it had been given with effect, 13 out of 22 patients finding improvement more or less marked from its use.* He also employed the 6th potency.

The chloride of magnesium,

Magnesia muriatica,

is prepared by aqueous solution.

The first edition of the *Chronic Diseases* gives 69 symptoms to this salt. As the sixth dilution is recommended for administration, they were possibly obtained from the third. In the second edition, 749 symptoms are ascribed to it—most of the additions here also proceeding from Nenning, through Hartlaub and Trinks.

Hahnemann thought that the virtues of sea-bathing might be partly due to the large proportion of chloride of magnesium contained in the water ; and considered the salt a powerful antipsoric. It has hardly, however, fulfilled his anticipations ; though experience has sustained his recommendation of it in " knotty, hard, difficult, insufficient and delaying stools," which sometimes (Dr. Guernsey says) crumble to pieces directly they pass the anus. Noack and Trinks commend it in chronic congestion and induration of the liver. Magnesia muriatica also shares with Magnesia carbonica a uterine action. Hahnemann indicates its use in " hysterical uterine and abdominal cramps, which extend even into the thighs and are followed by leucorrhœa ;" and Dr. Bayes speaks of finding it very useful here, and in leucorrhœa generally. He gives the third or sixth dilution.

Here, also, we have some valuable clinical information from Mr. Clifton. He has communicated to the twenty-first volume of the *Monthly Homœopathic Review* a series of eight cases of

* See *Bulletin de la Soc. Med. Hom. de France*, vols. v. and vi.

congestion and enlargement of the liver in which the drug was most beneficial. They all occurred in women whose uterine health was imperfect; and had been connected for months or years with recurring attacks of indigestion, " biliousness," constipation, with large round motions like balls, and inability to lie on the right side (in one case on either side). He gave the 5th dilution.

Dr. Guernsey says that Magnesia muriatica is one of the most important remedies in hysterical conditions. Sleeplessness, the characteristic constipation mentioned above, and frequent fainting attacks which seem to start from the stomach, are his main indications for it.

I have next to speak of the metal Manganesium, or

Manganum.

Triturations, or in the case of the acetate aqueous solutions, are made for homœopathic use.

A pathogenesis of Manganese, obtained from the acetate, appears in the sixth volume of the *Materia Medica Pura*. It contains 89 symptoms from Hahnemann, and 242 from ten fellow-observers. A second pathogenesis was published in the second edition of the *Chronic Diseases*, adding to these the 124 symptoms recorded as obtained from the drug in Hartlaub and Trinks' *Arzneimittellehre*.

Hahnemann's provings led him to think that Manganese would prove indispensable in some of the most troublesome chronic diseases, especially some insupportable pains in the periosteum and joints, some weaknesses of the senses, and some affections of the larynx and trachea. The provings of the native black oxide and the chloride since instituted by Dr. Lembke, of Riga, on his own person—an account of which is given by Hempel and Allen—confirm the first and last of these actions, and show it to affect the head much like Ferrum. The hoarse cough it causes is characterised by being relieved on lying down.

From the statements of Noack and Trinks it would seem that Hahnemann's recommendations of Manganese have been carried out with some success in inflammations of the bones, periosteum, and joints; and in chronic laryngeal disease. In the first named conditions Dr. Guernsey mentions great sensitiveness of the bones as a special indication for it; and Bähr praises it in a form of laryngo-tracheitis chronica which is

very common among persons who use their organs of speech a
good deal. The hoarseness depends upon the presence of
hard and tenacious mucus, so that towards noon, when this
has been cleared away, the voice is tolerably clear. It has also
been used with some benefit in Eustachian deafness and in
chronic cutaneous eruptions. It is a medicine which seems
to deserve more attention than is at present given to it.
From some observations of its pathogenetic effects collected
by Pereira, it appears that in workmen engaged upon it it
produces paralysis of the motor nerves, beginning with paraplegia. This differs from the paralysis of lead in not being
associated with colic or constipation, and from that of mercury
in first affecting the lower extremities, and in not presenting
tremors of the affected part. The sulphate has a decided
action on the liver. This organ was found inflamed in animals
poisoned by it, and both in these and in the human subject it
acts as a vigorous cholagogue. Dr. Leared has published a
number of cases showing the good effects of Manganese in pain
after food occurring in weakly females.

Besides these facts, sundry speculations have been
hazarded as to the value of the preparations of Manganese
in chloro-anæmia. I have read them with attention ; but am
not much impressed with the theoretical reasoning or with its
practical results.

I can say nothing as to this drug also of analogous medicines or dose.

I have now a few remarks to make on the buck-bean, marsh-
trefoil, or

Menyanthes trifoliata.

The tincture is prepared from the entire plant, dried.

There is a pathogenesis of Menyanthes in the fifth volume of
the *Reine Arzneimittellehre*, containing 28 symptoms from
Hahnemann, and 267 from nine others.

There is little in the proving which is characteristic, though
pressure as of a weight on the vertex is emphasised by Dr.
Allen's type ; and Menyanthes has rarely been employed in
medicine. Hahnemann recommends it in some forms of ague
where the chill predominates. Teste remarks, " According to
to my own experience, Menyanthes is most closely analogous
to Drosera, except that the effects of Drosera are more intense
than those of Menyanthes. Obscuration of sight, which is

one of the first symptoms of these drugs, developes itself alike under the influence of one or the other. It is a sort of white mist, or vibrations, which are sometimes so violent that they prevent sight, come on irregularly, of varied duration, especially in the open air, during a walk, and without any other sensation. I experienced this symptom from either drug so violently, while walking on the Boulevard, that I dared not cross lest I should be crushed by the carriages. The pains of Drosera and Menyanthes are likewise alike. In their action on the air-passages they differ only in the degree of intensity. Menyanthes is little used, and never will be used much. I have employed it with success in a case of amaurosis ; but there are few diseases where Menyanthes is indicated which could not be cured much better with Drosera. This opinion, however, is founded on my own impressions, which I am always willing to distrust."

We will now speak of the spurge-olive, Daphne

Mezereum.

We make a tincture of the recent, or triturations of the dried bark.

A proving of Mezereum appeared in the *Fragmenta de viribus*, containing 62 symptoms from Hahnemann, and 34 from authors. The drug did not reappear among his medicines till the second edition of the *Chronic Diseases* was published, where it has a pathogenesis of 610 symptoms, the additions being from ten others. Most of these are taken from a proving published by Stapf in the fourth volume of the *Archiv*, in which eleven persons took part, using the mother-tincture. Several subsequent provings of like kind have been made with Mezereum in the homœopathic school, so that Dr. Allen can give us a pathogenesis of it drawn from 52 observers, and containing 1,566 symptoms.

Mezereum was one of the vegetable substances—as guaiacum and sarsaparilla—with which it was attempted to replace Mercury in the treatment of syphilis. It still holds a place in the compound decoction of sarsaparilla of the British Pharmacopœia, but is quite neglected as a specific agent. Ringer and Wood barely allude to it, and Dr. Phillips (who might have done better) merely summarises Pereira's article on the drug. Yet one of its antisyphilitic applications has stood the test of later practice, and is vouched for by such practitioners as Hufeland and Alexander Russell. I refer to its influence over nodes and nocturnal bone pains—*dolores osteocopi* as they used to be called. Hahnemann's pathogenesis in the *Fragmenta* mentions such pains as caused by it in the cranium, clavicle, and thighs, and several of the later provers report the same experience; in homœopathic practice we use it with much confidence in these affections, and in simple or rheumatic periostitis. Whether it acts upon the bones themselves, I hesitate to say. There is, however, a case on record in which it seemed to check the necrosis of the jaw produced by phosphorus; and Noack and Trinks mention several osseous diseases as benefited by it.

But the homœopathic method has added another valuable application of Mezereum, namely, to cutaneous affections. The plant is a violent acrid, and irritates the skin when applied externally, as it does the throat, stomach, and intestines when swallowed. The former, however, unlike the latter, is a specific action; and is manifested when the drug is otherwise introduced into the circulation. Hahnemann relates* the case of a man who took Mezereum for a long time for the cure of some complaints that he had, and became at length affected with an intolerable itching over the whole body, which did not allow him an hour's sleep. This was removed in twenty-four hours by camphor. Bergius also, cited by him, has observed an itching vesicular eruption over the whole body, caused by the internal use of the drug; and several of the provers had similar symptoms. Mezereum is recommended by Hahnemann, and by Noack and Trinks, for several forms of cutaneous eruption; but Rückert gives no instance of its use. Dr. Robert Cooper, however, has communicated to the thirteenth volume of the *Monthly Homœopathic Review* a chronic case of pityriasis capitis, with loss of hair and great itching, in which Mezereum in the third decimal dilution effected a very satisfactory cure. Bähr, moreover, considers Mezereum about the best medicine for shingles; and not only for the eruption, but also for the consecutive neuralgia. I have tried it in one case, occurring in an old man, with the best results.

A valuable study of the action of Mezereum on the skin was contributed to the World's Convention of 1876 by Dr. Gerstel, of Vienna: you will find it in the Transactions of the meeting. He brings together in one view the cutaneous symptoms of the drug, adding to them a proving on himself, which resulted in a general itching similar to that experienced by Hahnemann's patient. He concludes that this is the

* *Lesser Writings*, p. 381.

mildest form of the Mezereum skin disease, and corresponds with *prurigo ;* that it especially belongs to parts where the panniculus adiposus is deficient ; and that the itching—which may pass on into burning—is characteristically worst in the evening and increased by warmth. He then follows up the effects of the drug into their higher grades, where they are seen manifested in exfoliation and vesiculation. As concomitant symptoms he notes general coldness, which he traces to contraction of the superficial blood-vessels, and twitching of the subcutaneous muscles. The whole action shows the Mezereum atoms irritating the dermic tissue, congesting its blood-vessels, and causing an acrid exudation, while at the same time they fret the associated muscular elements to spasm. He illustrates these facts by citing several interesting cases of cure—including prurigo senilis, pityriasis versicolor, mentagra, and the so-called " herpes crustaceus."

Dr. Dunham some time ago contributed to the *American Homœopathic Review* a number of symptoms of Mezereum as given him by a son of the late Dr. Wahle of Rome. No information is vouchsafed as to their origin, and they read to me far more like clinical than pathogenetic observations. But even taking them in the former sense, they extend the action of the drug to pustulation and ulcers of the skin, and they have been verified in practice. Dr. Dunham himself wrote :— " these symptoms suggest at once the applicability of Mezereum to crusta lactea, to various forms of pure impetigo, and to some of those mercurial or mercurio-syphilitic ulcers on the lower extremities which often prove so difficult to cure. I have frequently had occasion to witness the prompt curative action of Mezereum in these affections, in which I have generally used the 200th potency. This has proved efficacious in cases in which the lower dilutions have been inert. The characteristics of the Mezereum skin diseases are well defined in the above symptoms, viz. : itching occurring in the evening when in bed, aggravated and changed to burning by touch or by scratching; sensitiveness to touch ; ulcers with an areola, sensitive and easily bleeding, painful at night ; the pus tends to form an adherent scab, under which a quantity of pus collects." He also relates an interesting case of deafness cured by the drug. which was chosen on the ground of the affection having resulted from the repercussion of an impetigo of the scalp, closely resembling that described by Wahle. You will find these facts of his about Mezereum in the first volume of his collected writings.

Besides the skin, Mezereum specifically irritates the genito-urinary organs. "The urinary organs," says Pereira, "are sometimes affected by it, an irritation similar to that of cantharides being set up;" and Hahnemann found it produce blennorrhœa of the urethra and vulva. He mentions leucorrhœa of some years' standing as having been cured by it ; and in Dr. Cooper's case " terrible irritation of the vagina " was present, and disappeared under the use of the remedy. There is also a case narrated by Hempel of poisoning by the external application of Mezereum, in which symptoms of cerebral depression supervened like those we have seen produced under similar circumstances by Anacardium. I may add that it is recommended in prosopalgia affecting the left infra-orbital nerve : the pain is apt to extend to the temple.

Altogether, Mezereum is an active and promising medicine; and from what we have seen as to the nature of its provings may be used in accordance with them with all confidence.

Its analogues are *Anacardium, Guaiacum, Phytolacca*, and *Rhus.*

With the exception of the experience reported by Dr. Dunham, the lower potencies have chiefly been used.

I have next to speak of the common yarrow, Achillea

Millefolium.

The tincture is prepared from the entire plant.

Dr. Hering has given us for Millefolium one of his exhaustive collections of observations. It was first published in his *Amerikanische Arzneiprufungen ;* and has been translated, with additions, in the ninth volume of the *New England Medical Gazette.* It contains symptoms from six provers of the plant.

The yarrow has long been in popular repute as a vulnerary and hæmostatic. Its virtues of the latter kind have been sedulously cultivated by homœopathists. Hahnemann wrote of it in 1796: "We should endeavour to find out if the millefoil cannot itself produce hæmorrhage in large doses, as it is so efficacious in moderate doses in chronic hæmorrhages." I cannot discover that it has ever done so when internally administered, but it is noted by the older writers that if a leaf of it is put into the nose it causes blood to flow. Hering indeed cites Hahnemann as stating, in his *Apotheker-lexicon* (1793-9), that it causes nose-bleed and hæmaturia, but he gives no explanations or authorities. However, it is a very good medicine for hæmorrhages in our small doses, which makes it probable that its action is of the homœopathic kind. I have myself seen it act well in hæmoptysis and recurring epistaxis; and Dr. Hering cites several instances of its successful use, among others one of hæmaturia.

This is the only application of Millefolium with which I am acquainted; but you may possibly discover others from a study of Dr. Hering's collection, which contains recommendations of it (from domestic and old-school sources) in numerous forms of disease. It may be useful in " phthisis florida."

Hamamelis and *Ipecacuanha* are allied remedies. The hæmorrhage of Millefolium is not so passive and venous as that of the former, and less connected with expulsive action— cough, vomiting, &c.—than that of the latter.

I use the first decimal dilution. In the case of hæmaturia mentioned, quarter-drop doses of the mother-tincture were employed. I have seen drop doses of it seriously aggravate an hæmoptysis, which supports the homœopathicity of the action.

We come now to that curious animal secretion, musk—

Moschus,

of which we make a tincture or triturations.

There is a pathogenesis of Moschus in the first volume of the *Materia Medica Pura*. It contains 2 symptoms only from Hahnemann, 111 from three fellow-observers, and 39 from authors. The provings seem to have been made with the pure substance or mother-tincture, and we have others from Professor Jörg on himself, six pupils, and two females; so that our knowledge of the physiological action of musk is considerable. Dr. Langheinz, in an article which you will find translated from the *Vierteljahrschrift* in the twenty-second volume of the *British Journal of Homœopathy*, has shown that the symptoms cited by Hahnemann from authors are mostly of doubtful validity. You may read Jörg's experiments in his pages; and in Dr. Allen's collection you will find some curious effects observed in those who have made triturations of the drug.

Musk has long been known as a pretty powerful nervine stimulant. In this way it affected the provers, exciting the circulation and sexual organs, and causing headache with fulness and drowsiness. In this way also it is used in medi-

2 X

cine. I know of no distinctive homœopathic applications of it, though we utilise the virtues it has more largely than do our brethren of the old school. I always carry it in my pocket-case, on account of its great value in two conditions demanding speedy relief. There are the *hysterical paroxysm* and *nervous palpitation.* I know nothing which so rapidly dissipates an hysterical attack, even when it has gone as far as unconsciousness, as Moschus. It is probably homœopathic to this condition, as it was early noted that in hysterical subjects the odour of the drug was liable to bring on their attacks. It is of no less potency in palpitation which has been set off by some nervous excitement, when there is no organic disease of the heart ; and here also it seems homœopathic. Moschus is also occasionally useful in laryngismus stridulus affecting nervous children ; and should be remembered in hysterical asthma, and in hiccough. Dr. Guernsey considers it indicated in such conditions by the presence of great coldness. Its use in ataxic conditions occurring in acute disease seems beyond the range of our therapeutics.

Moschus is allied with *Ambra, Asafœtida, Castoreum,* and *Valerian ;* also with *Camphor* and *Nux moschata.*

I use the second and third decimal dilutions of the tincture. I believe that the odour of this medicine is of importance to its action, and that pilules and globules of it are useless.

I must now say a few words about the drug we call

Murex purpurea,

which is the colouring matter of the shell-fish so named. It is triturated for our use, being insoluble in water, alcohol, and ether. The British Homœopathic Pharmacopœia directs the whole mollusc to be used ; but this is surely needless.

Dr. Petroz proved Murex, in the fourth trituration, on three women. His results were published in the third volume of the *Révue de la Matière Médicale spécifique ;* and are translated by Dr. C. Dunham, with some additional matter, in the fourth volume of the *American Homœopathic Review.**

Murex evidently acts specifically upon the uterus, rendering the provers painfully conscious of possessing such an organ. It produces also in them the well-known sympathetic symptoms of sinking in the stomach and pains in the breasts, also great sadness and despondency : the sexual appetite moreover

* This article may also be found in his collected writings.

is greatly excited. It has proved curative in several cases of uterine congestion; and from one of these Dr. Petroz thinks it likely to be useful in "the inflammatory and fungous engorgements of the neck of the womb, whose degeneration, so rapid and so dangerous, often produces accidents and irreparable disorders." The co-existence of great depression of spirits may indicate it here.

One of the symptoms induced by Murex was "frequent need to urinate during the night; urine colourless." Acting on this hint Dr. Murray Moore gave it* in a case of polyuria, where the secretion was of this character, with rapidly curative results.

Murex evidently corresponds both as a medicine and as a natural product with *Sepia*. Dr. Dunham points, as a distinguishing feature, to the deficient catamenia of the latter, while the Murex patient is generally menorrhagic.

The dilutions from the fourth to the sixth were used in the cases cured.

I have now to speak of the salts of sodium we use in homœopathic practice—the carbonate, the chloride, and the sulphate. It is the old name for sodium—natron or natrum —which gives it this place in our alphabetical series.

The carbonate of soda,

Natrum carbonicum,

is triturated or dissolved in water for our use.

In the first edition of the *Chronic Diseases* Hahnemann published a pathogenesis of Natrum carbonicum, containing 308 symptoms, which from his preface we may infer to have been observed in patients taking the third trituration. The salt was then proved by Nenning and Schreter, and their results —making 625 in all—appeared in the third volume of the *Arzneimittellehre* of Hartlaub and Trinks. No information is given as to how they were obtained. In the second edition of the *Chronic Diseases* Hahnemann incorporated these with his own, and with some additional observations from three others, raising the total list to 1,082.

In spite of this extensive pathogenesis, Natrum carbonicum has found very little employment. Hahnemann says that it is useful in weakness of the stomach, leading to great discomfort from slight dietetic transgressions. Dr. Bayes has

* *Monthly Hom. Review,* xii., 305.

found it give relief in subacute inflammatory irritation of the whole alimentary mucous membrane, from the mouth to the anus; Dr. Madden thought well of it in deficient menstruation in adult females; Dr. Lippe commends it in headache from exposure to the sun or to gaslight, such as Glonoin benefits; and Dr. Guernsey in inflammation of the external nose, and the tendency to the formation of hydatidiform moles.* But it is hardly mentioned by the systematic writers on homœopathic therapeutics; and to this correspond the conclusions from recent experimentation that the soda salts, unlike those of potash, have little specific action upon the system.

I speak of the common preparations of soda, such as the carbonates and the acetates, which are used as antacids. But we are transferred into another region when we come to its combination with hydrochloric acid, the chloride of sodium, or

Natrum muriaticum.

We prepare this salt in the same way as the carbonate.

Natrum muriaticum has a pathogenesis in the first edition of the *Chronic Diseases*, consisting of 897 symptoms. A good many are supplied by three associates, and of these Hahnemann states that they were obtained on healthy persons by taking globules saturated with the thirtieth dilution. In the second edition the list has swollen to 1,349; and most of the additions are from Hahnemann himself, and pretty certainly (with his earlier contributions) observed on patients taking the same potency. Natrum muriaticum has also been thoroughly re-proved by the Austrian Society. Their experiments (in which many persons took part, using both the crude salt and the attenuations) were published in the fourth volume of the *Œsterreichische Zeitschrift*, and are amalgamated with Hahnemann's by Allen.

I wish I could tell you that the results of this exhaustive re-proving had rewarded the pains of the experimenters. They are to me rather disappointing. When I have said that the provers generally became constipated while taking the

* Dr. Jones, commenting on my light esteem of this drug, writes— " Dr. Hughes may some day get a patient having this symptom— ' Pressing in the abdomen, towards the genitals, as if everything would protrude, and as if menstruation would appear.' Belladonna will miss fire, Sepia do; and when some good repertory leads him to Natr. carb., we trust he will give that remedy in the 200th, and publish the result."

potencies; that the liver was usually somewhat affected, one prover having much biliary colouring matter in the urine; that the sexual desire was diminished and (in females) the menstruation delayed; that a weeping mood was induced in many; that pains in the thumb and forefinger were common, and the skin often showed signs of irritation, especially in the form of herpes labialis—I have summed up the main results of the proving. It gives us little more than what had been already elicited as the action of some form the symptoms experienced by those who had immoderately used it. These are a scorbutic degeneration of the blood and tissues; various eruptions and ulcers upon the skin; polyuria; delay of menstruation; and in one man genital irritability with its accompanying depression.

Nor has physiological experimentation added anything material to our knowledge. Münch and Plouriez have taken large quantities of salt for days together, with little effect on the blood, tissues, or secretions, save that the red corpuscles of the latter were somewhat increased in number.

Therapeutically, however, Natrum muriaticum holds a very respectable place in homœopathic practice; though hardly perhaps answering to Hahnemann's description of it as an heroic medicine, and one of the most energetic antipsorics. Like Graphites, the association of constipation and deficient menstruation are the features which chiefly suggest it; but, unlike that medicine, there should be much defective nutrition present, showing itself especially in emaciation with dry and ill-coloured skin. In a case of this kind which came lately under my care, and where suspicions of organic abdominal disease were entertained, a few occasional doses of Natrum muriaticum 30 changed the whole condition, and initiated a complete recovery. There was much depression of spirits here; and Dr. Bayes recommends the medicine strongly in a form of passive hypochondriasis. "There is," he writes, "a sort of despairing hopeless feeling about the future, accompanied by dryness of the mouth, irritable mucous membrane, often with sore tongue and slight ulcerations, and almost invariably chronic constipation, with hard stool."*

Save in these chronic morbid conditions, the only use of Natrum muriaticum which has established itself in homœopathic practice is in intermittent fever. Wurmb and Caspar

* See *Annals*, vol. viii., for some cases of constipation reported by this physician, with irritable mucous membrane, in which the medicine was strikingly beneficial.

spoke slightingly of it ; but Thorer, Neumann, and Hartlaub found it effective, and an experienced American physician— Dr. Pearson—writes : " If there be in our Materia Medica any such thing as a specific for intermittent fever, it is Natrum muriaticum."* It is of course in chronic agues especially that it is so useful, and in the malarial cachexia when assuming the features I have already described. But even when the disease is recent it is reported very effective if the characteristic symptoms are present. They are thus described by Dr. Guernsey : " exanthematous spots, looking like large peas, on the lips ; an excessive thirst before and during the chill, no thirst during the hot stage ; in the heat, or at its close, a headache as though a thousand little hammers were knocking upon the brain may begin, lasting a long time even after the perspiration has passed away ; the attack comes on in the fore part of the day ; after it passes off, the patient wishes to retain a recumbent position, does not feel able to get up, or go about anything." Dr. Mitchell, of the Chicago Homœopathic College, goes farther still. " The indications for Natrum," he writes, " are not always clear. Instead of being a remedy of feeble power over intermittents, as is asserted by some in our school, it is one of the most powerful. I formerly regarded it as most useful in chronic cases, and after Cinchona, but more extended experience with it convinces me that it is equally powerful in recent cases, and those that have not taken any quinine. Quotidians are most likely to be checked by it, but it affects tertians favourably in some cases. Profuse perspiration is a good indication. Thirst during chill is usually characteristic of Natrum. In this case "—that *apropos* of which his remarks were made— " it was not. Time of chill has not helped me in the selection of Natrum. I have not been able to verify Bönninghausen's 11 a.m. indication ; intermittents cured by Natrum have commenced both morning and evening." Bähr commends it in chronic cases where the patient has a greyish-yellow look, and the spleen and liver are very much enlarged.

This reputation of Natrum muriaticum in agues, gained—as it has been—with the higher dilutions of the drug, is not a little curious when we remember that salt is one of the febrifuges of repute in the old school, of course in substantial doses. Piorry was a constant advocate of its ·use ; and Dr. Willemin, in a report to the Board of Trade in Paris of his experience in the East, says that in Damascus common salt stopped the fever six times out of every seven ; two to four

* *United States Med. and Surg. Journal*, i., 211.

doses of half an ounce each being generally sufficient for the purpose. It was especially useful, he says, in anæmic individuals.*

Dr. Burnett has recently made a contribution of some value to our knowledge of Natrum muriaticum in the shape of a little monograph on the drug,† written to illustrate—by its efficacy—the development of power in substances ordinarily inert by the Hahnemannian process of trituration. The cases he relates, while confirming the usefulness of the medicine in chronic ague, and in conditions of defective nutrition manifesting themselves by ill-coloured skin, constipation, amenorrhœa, and depression of spirits, add thereto some new spheres of activity. Such are gouty and rheumatic affections, where elimination by stool and urine is imperfect; lithiasis and polyuria, when the other symptoms of the drug are present; but more especially morbid *coldness*, either of the whole body or of its lower half. It is a great thing to have a remedy which will promote the calorifacient function when depressed; and this cases 14, 19, 20, 24 and 25 of Dr. Burnett's series show Natrum muriaticum to be capable of doing.

In his first case he was led to the medicine by the fact that the neuralgia from which the patient was suffering was always worse at the seaside. A similar influence of marine air, but in the direction of amelioration rather than aggravation, enabled me, not long ago, to cure with Natrum a constipation of some years standing in a little girl. She had suffered from it since babyhood, her mother told me; and the only time that improvement had occurred was during a visit to the sea coast, and for two months afterwards.

The profound influence of Natrum muriaticum on nutrition and hæmatosis has led Dr. Lilienthal to suggest it as a promising remedy for such diseases as Addison's, for leucæmia, and for the cachexia which sometimes accompanies exophthalmic goitre. We have some actual experience with it in the last-named condition. Dr. Guernsey's symptomatic indications for it include, besides some of the foregoing phenomena, much headache on waking in the morning, disgust for bread and longing for salt, contraction of the anus, and sadness during the menses. Drs. Allen and Norton esteem it highly in many affections of the eye (Dr. Burnett gives a good case of strumous ophthalmia cured by it): they especially value it for the effects of the abuse of caustics. " Sharp pain over the

* See Pereira, fourth edition, *in loc.*
† *Natrum muriaticum; a test of the doctrine of drug dynamization.*

eye on looking down" is said to be characteristic for it ; and
in muscular asthenopia they reckon it "one of the most important remedies we possess, especially if there is a drawing,
stiff sensation in the eyes on moving them."

As analogues of Natrum muriaticum I may mention
Alumina, Graphites, Lycopodium, Plumbum, and *Zincum.*

As regards dose, I may cite the observation of Dr. Watzke,
under whose superintendence the re-proving was carried out :
—"I am, alas ! (I say alas ! for I would much rather have
upheld the larger doses which accord with current views)—I
am compelled to declare myself for the higher dilutions. The
physiological experiments made with Natrum muriaticum, as
well as the great majority of the clinical results obtained
therewith, speak decisively and distinctly for these preparations." All subsequent experience points in the same
direction.

Our third preparation of soda is the well-known "Glauber's
salt,"

Natrum sulphuricum.

It is prepared like the others.

Natrum sulphuricum has been proved by Schreter, and by
Nenning. Their results, with all else that is known of the
drug, have been collected by Dr. Hering into one of the
pathogeneses of his *Materia Medica.* Dr. Allen adds symptoms obtained by Lembke.

Dr. Hering's catalogue of symptoms is admirably arranged
for symptomatic prescribing, but is hardly helpful towards
enabling a definite conception to be formed of the special
action of the drug. It seems to cause disturbance of an ordinary kind in well-nigh every region of the body. Dr. von
Grauvogl, however, has made a beginning towards defining its
curative sphere. He thinks it one of the most important
remedies for what he calls the "hydrogenoid constitution,"
where the patients are hydræmic, and all their symptoms are
aggravated by damp weather or situations. In such cases a
gonorrhœal anamnesis is, according to him, nearly always to
be discovered ; and he connects the morbid state with the
sycosis of Hahnemann and his contemporaries, and with the
leucæmia of Virchow and Bennett. I shall have more to say
on this subject when I come to Thuja, which medicine is
generally used by him in the treatment of such patients. It

is only given occasionally, however ; while Natrum sulphuricum is continued persistently, four or five drops of the third
decimal dilution being taken several times a day. Dr. von
Grauvogl relates several cases illustrative of this treatment ;
and in the twenty-second volume of the *British Journal of
Homœopathy* you may read a cure of diabetes mellitus by it,
reported by Dr. Ægidi. Here the Natrum was evidently the
efficient agent, as only one dose of Thuja 30—chosen because
of the patient's gonorrhœal history—was taken.

Previous to von Grauvogl, it had been used in America in
high dilutions for phthisis, chronic diarrhœa, and flatulence
and sciatica, to the last of which its symptoms strikingly point.
It is also said to inflame the lower end of the ileum ; and to
have proved curative accordingly in a case of recurrent inflammatory colic, where the pain always commenced in the
right groin.

I have nothing further to say of analogous medicines or
dose.

And now a few words in conclusion about a medicine which,
though included by Dr. Hale among his new American remedies, we yet owe to one of our French colleagues. It is the
small-flowered yellow pond-lily—

Nuphar luteum.

The tincture is prepared from the whole plant.

The proving to which I have alluded, by the late Dr. Pitet,
of Paris, is given in Dr. Hale's second edition, with clinical
observations. It was conducted with the medium dilutions.

This proving confirms the ancient reputation of Nuphar as
an anaphrodisiac. It shows also its power to excite a diarrhœa,
which is most troublesome in the early morning. These are
the pathogenetic effects of Nuphar which have led to practical
results. Several cases of morning diarrhœa, and of atonic
spermatorrhœa, are reported in Dr. Hale's article in which the
medicine was used with very happy effects.

Agnus castus and *Rumex crispus* are the two medicines
which, between them, cover the double sphere of action of
Nuphar luteum.

The dilutions from the first to the sixth have been successfully used.

LECTURE XLV.

I devote this lecture to a drug whose name will ever be inseparably associated with homœopathy,

Nux vomica.

A tincture or triturations are prepared from the seeds of the fruit of the plant.

We owe the pathogenesis of Nux vomica almost entirely to Hahnemann himself. Of the 1,300 symptoms ascribed to it in the third edition of the first volume of the *Reine Arznei-mittellehre*, 1,200 are his own; the remainder are chiefly from authors. Dr. Allen, with numerous cases of poisoning and other sources of information before him, only gives some 300 more. We have but to add to Hahnemann's observations the account of the poisonous effects of the drug given by the ordinary treatises on Materia Medica, of which those of Pereira and of Trousseau and Pidoux are the best, and we shall have before us a complete picture of its action on the healthy. A hardly less complete *résumé* of its therapeutical virtues is given by Hartmann, in those *Practical Observations* of his to which I have several times referred.

The general physiological action of Nux vomica is on the spinal cord, or rather on the cranio-spinal axis; for, though it has no influence on the ideational centres proper, it obviously affects the motor and sensory tracts to their utmost prolongations. The condition set up by it is one of excitement and excitability. In its first degree it manifests itself by the patient becoming more susceptible to external impressions, as of light, sound, touch, and variations of temperature. With this there are tremors and twitchings of the limbs, with sense of weight and fulness, and some rigidity of the muscles if attempt is made to put them into action : at this time a sudden impression on the surface, as a tap on the ham, will induce a slight convulsive paroxysm. If the action go farther, a true tetanic condition is induced. The spasms come on from any exciting cause, however insignificant; or may even arise spontaneously. In the worst cases they go on to asphyxiate and kill.

This is in the main Pereira's description. Trousseau and Pidoux add some important features to the picture. The spasms, they say, are often preceded by rigors, and sense as of electric shocks in the sensory nerves. Formication also is frequently felt, which may go on to intolerable itching, beginning on the head and extending over the whole body. Vertigo, according to them, is the earliest symptom of the drug having taken effect.

I have said that these phenomena result from a direct action of the poison on the cranio-spinal axis. Claude Bernard led us to think that the morbid impression was first made upon the sensory nerves and carried by them to the cord, whence it was reflected upon the motor nerves and muscles. Later experimentation, however, has proved the primary action to be on the cord; and M. Bernard's facts are readily explained thereby, without the need of resorting to his hypothesis. Stimulation of a sentient nerve may give greater results than occur in health quite as well by increased excitability of the centre as by that of the conducting trunk. The former will also account for the preternatural acuteness of the senses noticed in poisoning by this agent, and the readiness with which the spasms can be excited by any impression on the surface — both which phenomena seemed strongly to countenance M. Bernard's theory.

The condition set up by Nux vomica in the nervous centres is described by Todd and Bowman as one of increased polarity. Drs. Ringer and Murrell,* however, while recognising its central action, will not allow that this is of an excitant character. They find similar tetaniform phenomena to occur in the course of poisoning by substances which are evidently paralysers of the spinal cord, as Gelsemium and the buxus sempervirens; and they maintain that they are due to a diminution or destruction of the *resistance* of the cord, " so that an impression conveyed through an afferent nerve can spread throughout the reflex portion of the central nervous system and produce tetanus." This is an important thought in relation to general considerations regarding pharmacodynamics; but it has no practical bearing on our study of the

* See *Medico-Chirurgical Transactions* for 1876, and *Journal of Anatomy and Physiology*, vol. xi.

action of the drug before us. Whatever may be the cause of such sensory and reflex excitability as culminates in tetanus, Nux vomica produces it in the healthy and will remedy it in the sick.

Further, as regards the circulatory disorder induced by Nux vomica in the nervous centres, it must be said that it is not in itself inflammatory, as is that of Belladonna ; although if the drug be given when there is a tendency to inflammation, as when blood has recently been effused, this process may be set up around the clot. There is, however, decided determination of blood towards the cord, so that the vessels become dilated, and even—as van der Kolk has observed—ruptured, causing effusion here and there. Moreover, probably from the intense molecular disturbance which is set up, softening of the nervous centres has been found after death.

I must say a few words about the preternatural acuteness of the senses caused by Nux vomica. Dr. Anstie, in his *Stimulants and Narcotics*, has given some striking instances of it. It displayed itself in hyperæsthesia of the surface ; photophobia, with flashes of fire before the eyes when looking towards a bright light, or even in comparative darkness after each dose of the medicine ; and painful sensibility to sound. Dr. Anstie well shows, however, that there is no increase, but rather a diminution, of the power of discriminative perception in these cases,—vision being impaired, and the effects of sounds being described as deafening.

These toxic phenomena are due to the two alkaloids which exist in Nux vomica—strychnia and brucia, the latter of which seems to be a feebler analogue of the former. But the vomic nut itself has a wider range of action than is manifested here; and this is exhibited by Hahnemann's provings, to which we will now betake ourselves.

I. Nux has, as I have said, no influence on the ideational and emotional centres. Illusion, mental aberration, rage, are unknown in its pathogenesis. The only phenomena of this kind are of sympathetic character, as anxiety, irascibility, sullenness, unfitness for mental exertion. But the cerebral circulation may show decided signs of being affected. In the first volume of the *Annals* Dr. Chapman relates the case of " a chemist who, by way of bravado, took one night three or four drops of the mother-tincture of Nux vomica. He awoke early next morning with a feeling as if his head would burst. He was so giddy that he could neither sit nor stand ; he had rushing sounds in his ears, intolerance of light and sound, and he could not see. His face was tumid, and he looked besotted, like a man reeling drunk." All these symptoms—the vertigo, the fulness and headache, and the intoxication—are reproduced by Hahnemann. The aching occurs most frequently in the occiput. The intoxication has also been observed by Dr. Anstie as a result of the medicinal use of strychnia. A man who was taking the sixteenth of a grain three times a day complained that the medicine " made him drunk;" and, half an hour after his dose, appeared with the uncertain gait, meaningless smile, and flushed perspiring cheeks characteristic of intoxication.*

II. Pereira shows that not the voluntary muscles only, but those also of the alimentary canal, the respiratory organs, and the urinary system, are affected by Nux vomica. This the provings entirely confirm. Spasmodic pains and irritable expulsive actions occur frequently in all these regions. But there also appear symptoms of irritation of the mucous membranes which are rarely or feebly seen in poisonings, or from strychnia. The combination of these two actions—in the moderate degree induced by the doses used for proving— gives several vivid pictures of dyspepsia and gastralgia. Constipation also is present to a marked degree ; and is generally accompanied with (ineffectual) urging to stool. With this there is much evidence, alike in liver, in abdomen, and in rectum, of portal congestion. In the respiratory sphere we have obstructive nasal catarrh, dry cough, and great constriction of the chest.

III. Trousseau and Pidoux affirm that Nux vomica produces troublesome erections, and more energetic venereal desires in both sexes. From Hahnemann it appears that the catamenia occur too early and too copiously under its use.

IV. His provings also reveal (what is indeed most probable) that the excitation caused by the drug affects the vascular nerves and the arteries, causing the febrile phenomena of chill, heat, and sweat. Modern experimentation has confirmed this observation, showing that strychnia contracts the arterioles and greatly increases the blood pressure ; and does this by direct stimulation of the vaso-motor centre at the base of the brain.

I have now to speak of the therapeutical uses of Nux vomica. Hahnemann found it in use mainly for dysentery and intermittent fever ; and since his time it has been given, on antipathic principles, for various forms of paralysis. But his proving showed that it was in head affections, in dyspepsia and other gastric derangements, and in constipation, that it was to find its chief sphere of usefulness ; and in these,

* *Stimulants and Narcotics*, p. 151.

and in spasmodic conditions generally, it has played its great part in homœopathic therapeutics. The knowledge of its usefulness in dyspepsia and constipation has leaked out into the other school ; and it now constantly finds a place in the complex prescriptions there dispensed. We shall endeavour to define its true place and action in these complaints. But first let us speak of the general characteristics of the curative operation of Nux.

These have been plainly put by Hahnemann, and have stood the test of large experience. It is specially suitable to vigorous persons, of dry habit, tense fibre, ardent and irascible temperament, and tenacious disposition ; to patients addicted to the use of much wine or coffee and highly seasoned (especially animal) food, and to those of sedentary habits combined with considerable mental exertion : lastly, where there is a tendency to sleep in the evening ; to wake from two to four a.m., and to be kept awake for hours by ideas crowding in upon the mind ; and then to sleep late in the morning. It is an indication for Nux, moreover, when the symptoms come on or grow worse at these early hours ; also when they are increased by taking food or by mental exertion. If you desire to follow up still farther these general characteristics of our drug, you will find them well put and illustrated in Hartmann's *Observations*. English experience has found the city man of business the typical patient for Nux. His troubles are all nervous and dyspeptic ; and their causes are worry, much mental with too little bodily exertion, and generally indulgence at his only real meal, which is a late dinner. Hence headache, sleeplessness, weight after food with flatulence and heartburn, constipation, and irritability. Of course Nux will not cure him unless he studies hygiene more ; but it helps him greatly.

M. Teste has called attention to the well-known toxicological fact, that Nux vomica affects carnivorous animals far more powerfully than it does the herbivora ; and connects this with the kind of human constitution on which it manifests its strongest influence.

We will now discuss the therapeutics of the drug in the same order in which its pathogenetics have come before us.

I. The striking similarity between the phenomena of strychnia poisoning and those of tetanus would of course suggest it on homœopathic principles as a remedy for the disease. Stillé cites eight instances of traumatic tetanus being cured by it, all of course of old school origin : the drug was given in the ordinary fractional doses. We have little recorded experience in the treatment of this disease from homœopathic sources; but Jahr states that in the insurrection of 1832 in Paris he treated a case of the traumatic form with Angustura 30, which soon controlled the convulsions. If he means the Angustura spuria, this is nothing but Nux vomica in disguise. However, the facts introduced above are sufficient to show that the homœopathic indications deducible from strychnia poisoning are well warranted. Dr. Bartholow writes :—" In certain forms of spasm strychnia sometimes achieves most important results. The evidence which has been accumulated as to its curative power in tetanus is certainly very conclusive."

While thus exquisitely homœopathic to tetanus, Nux would seem no less perfectly antipathic to paralysis, and upon such grounds has been largely used in its treatment. There seems no doubt but that in cases of functional deficiency, whether of motor or sensory nerves, the local employment of Nux vomica or strychnia has proved of decided service. Thus in simple amaurosis, in prolapsus ani, and in the enuresis of the weak or aged, the hypodermic injection of strychnia in the neighbourhood of the part affected has often been successful. Its action here may be considered as analogous to that of galvanism or of will-power, whose exercise has been shown by Dr. Roth to be so valuable in restoring the tone of paralysed parts.* But internal use of the drug as a remedy for paralysis of central origin has been fraught with disappointment; and has frequently wrought mischief when the condition of the nervous centres has been one of congestion or inflammation. Its employment under these circumstances is therefore now strongly deprecated in the old school : I need hardly point out that to us the warning becomes an indication, as far as it goes. Even in the old school they find it beneficial, if only they reduce the dose. Mr. Charles Hunter injects subcutaneously from one eightieth to one sixtieth of a grain of strychnia, and states that it removes the sensation of heaviness or weight and the muscular twitchings, spasms, or cramps of the paralysed parts. I need hardly remind you how readily full doses of strychnine *excite* these spasmodic actions in palsied limbs. Mr. Barwell objects to its use in cerebral or spinal paralysis, but we find that he injects from the twentieth to the twelfth of a grain. So Pereira says that when used locally for amaurosis it causes sparks to appear before the eyes, most in the affected one; while Hartmann recommends it when such sparks trouble the eyes, thinking it a symptom of cerebral congestion.

* See *Annals*, vol. viii.

II. From what has been said of the action of Nux vomica on the head, it may be readily conceived that it plays an important part in affections of this region. I will speak of three of these—delirium tremens, apoplexy, and headaches.

1. The strong resemblance of the cerebral symptoms of Nux to the effects of alcohol have led to its use in delirium tremens. It does not reach this disease when at its height, as Belladonna, Hyoscyamus, and Stramonium do; but in its forming stage and during convalescence it is very useful. It is also very good for the morning vomiting, the trembling hands, and other nervo-muscular affections of drunkards.

2. The character of the influence of Nux vomica on the nervous centres, while unfitting it for actual inflammation of the brain, makes it just the remedy for those congestive states of the organ which predispose to apoplexy. Even when sanguineous effusion has taken place, Nux is often the best medicine to give, unless the state of the local or general circulation is such as to call for Belladonna or Aconite. You will find these statements well illustrated in the cases of apoplexy recorded in Dr. Yeldham's *Homœopathy in Acute Diseases*.

3. Few medicines are more frequently used in headache than Nux vomica. You will see at once the chief form of the affection in which it is likely to be advantageous—the headache of strong, plethoric adults, with congestion, giddiness, flushed face, and constipation, the pain increased by taking food or by mental exertion. But it is also (in higher dilutions) curative of such cephalalgiæ as clavus and migraine, where the constitution suits Nux better than Ignatia. A number of cases illustrative of its value are collected together in Dr. Peters' *Treatise on Headaches*. To the headaches in which we esteem it Dr. Ringer has added those consisting in heat and weight at the vertex, whether occurring at the menopausia or otherwise. Dr. Schrön commends it when the headache begins with the vertigo spuria of Herz, which Nux causes as markedly as does Ignatia.

III. I come now to a still more important sphere of the action of Nux vomica—its influence over the disorders of the alimentary canal. We need here to be discriminating ; for the really great power of Nux in dyspepsia and constipation has led to its abuse and even discredit. It is no uncommon thing for homœopathic neophytes to take a pilule of Nux the first time their evacuations delay, and expect it to act like Aloes or Colocynth. They fancy, moreover, that it will clean their coated tongues, and disperse their bilious attacks, and indeed be a remedy for " indigestion " of all kinds. But the remem-

brance of the physiological action of the drug will save us
from this indiscriminate use. Nux acts here as elsewhere
mainly upon the nerves and muscles. Hence its true place in
gastric disorders. The acute dyspepsia in which it is curative
is that caused by taking indigestible food. There is no particular mucous disorder; but on the other hand pain, vomiting with much retching, and frequent scanty motions with
colic and urging are present. The chronic dyspepsia of Nux
is essentially the same, but of course presents more variety.
It is one in which the nervous and muscular energy of the
stomach is defective and perverted. The food either causes
pain and—less commonly—vomiting, or it lies like a load at
the stomach, oppressing the brain, and soon developing much
flatulence. The tongue is coated at the posterior part only:
Dr. Bayes thinks this a characteristic sign for Nux. It will
be seen that this is just the dyspepsia of men of business and
intellectual workers, when they perform their tasks with hurry
and worry, and give neither brain nor stomach fair-play. Dr.
Bähr, however, would extend the sphere of Nux to include
chronic gastric catarrh. The taste, both subjective and of
food, is either bitter or sour; and there are eructations of the
same kind. "The appetite is gone, yet there is a sensation
of hunger, which even increases to bulimia. . . . The region
of the stomach is sensitive, especially after a meal, and
generally distended. The pains in the stomach are more
especially a hard pressure, less frequently tearing or crampy
pains." He has here the concurrence of Dr. Ringer, who
esteems the drug highly in those catarrhal states of the
stomach which so often complicate organic disease elsewhere,
and also—from the homœopathic side—of Dr. Jousset. This
excellent writer, who touches no subject without illuminating
it, has published in his *Leçons Cliniques* (xvii.) two striking
cases of chronic gastritis cured by the drug in rare doses of a
high dilution. The sub-mucous tissue about the pylorus seems to
have been involved, so that thickening and obstruction occurred
here, leading to dilatation of the stomach and copious vomiting. I have myself great reliance on the drug under such
circumstances. In his comments Dr. Jousset characterises
the three leading affections of the stomach, gastritis, dyspepsia,
and gastralgia; and shows that Nux is the leading remedy
for them all. It is the principal stomach medicine. In
gastralgia I need hardly demonstrate its fitness, when the pain
is spasmodic rather than neuralgic. You will find records of
many cases treated by it in Hempel, and in the eleventh volume
of the *British Journal of Homœopathy*.

This is one of the affections in which our brethren of the old school are not unwilling to take a leaf out of our book. Dr. Anstie recommended the hypodermic injection of strychnia in doses of one hundred-and-twentieth of a grain to relieve the pain of cardialgia, saying that he knew no such remedy for it as this.

There are thus very few painful non-organic affections of the stomach which may not be helped by this precious medicine. The same virtues display themselves in the intestines. It is quite homœopathic to spasmodic colic from flatulence; but other medicines—as Colocynth and Cocculus—are more frequently used. *Constipation* is a well-known indication for Nux vomica in complex cases. As an idiopathic affection, moreover, it frequently requires this remedy. You may think that the use of Nux must be antipathic here, as constipation means atony of the intestines, and Nux is excitant and not depressant thereto. The therapeutists of the old school recommend it on these grounds. But I must point out that constipation by no means always depends upon atony of the intestines. Schroeder van der Kolk states that "long experience and a great number of post-mortem examinations have satisfactorily proved to him that chronic constipation is almost always dependent on constrictions in the descending colon." And of the Nux constipation Dr. Carroll Dunham well says,* "this medicine does not diminish the action of the intestine. It rather increases it, but at the same time renders it *inharmonious* and *spasmodic*—a hindrance, therefore, and not a help to evacuation. This is the reason why the constipation characteristic of Nux vomica is accompanied by frequent ineffectual desire for stool—the action of the intestine being irregular and spasmodic, and the constipation resulting from the irregularity of action, and not from inaction." It is probably in a similar way that Nux occasionally relieves ileus, and incarcerated, or even strangulated hernia. Dr. Imbert-Gourbeyre has studied the subject in *l'Art Médical* for 1860; and numerous illustrations of this property of the drug exist in homœopathic literature—Trousseau and Pidoux themselves admitting that the claim has been substantiated. Probably also the benefit occasionally obtained from this medicine in dysentery is due to its control over the tormina and tenesmus—which are nervo-muscular—rather than from any action on the mucous membrane. There is a form of diarrhœa, moreover, in which the undoubted usefulness of Nux seems explicable in this way. It is where artificial food disagrees with infants so far as to cause vomiting and purging, but without setting up actual gastro-enteritis. Here I suppose the same irritable state of fibre to be present which in the adult induces constrictions which impede free evacuation; but in this case it leads to impatience and frequent emptying of the intestinal canal. Dr. Guernsey regards the muscular irritability of the rectum of which I have been speaking as a " key-note " for the choice of Nux in affections of its neighbour, the uterus.

The action of Nux upon the portal circulation has been largely used in the school of Hahnemann. I cannot go so far as Bähr, who thinks that the drug has a more specific relation to the liver than to the stomach; but its hepatic influence is undoubted. In recent hyperæmia of this organ; in general abdominal plethora; and in hæmorrhoids, large and blind, hence resulting—Nux is an excellent remedy. In the two latter affections it is much aided by Sulphur.

In disorders of the respiratory organs Nux vomica plays a much less important part than in those of the alimentary canal. It is very good, however, for dry coryza—the so-called " stuffy cold ;" and for violent coughs, with little or no expectoration, jarring the head, and straining the abdominal muscles. Nux is obviously homœopathic to spasmodic asthma; and frequently plays an important part in its treatment. There is a brilliant case on record treated by Hahnemann in his early days, which teaches us that the medicine need not be used in infinitesimal doses for this malady at any rate. You may read it in his *Lesser Writings*. Dr. Kidd, also, states that he considers Nux our best anti-asthmatic. I think it best suited to purely spasmodic cases, where there is no bronchial lesion, but a standing reflex excitability of the pneumogastric to impressions made from without or through the stomach. I prefer here the lowest triturations.

Still less frequently is Nux vomica required when the urinary organs are affected. Its only uses here with which I am acquainted are for the irritable bladder of gout or alcoholism, and to relieve pain and spasm in the passage of urinary calculi.

The stimulant action of Nux upon the sexual organs has naturally led to its being employed in impotence; but the success seems rarely to have been more than temporary. With us it is much esteemed in irritable conditions of the male genital organs, whether primary or left behind by excess or masturbation, when the other symptoms correspond and the general characteristics are present. In the female sphere we find Hahnemann recommending it for the evils caused by too frequent and too copious periods. Its influence here reaches even as far as metritis. Hartmann writes : " Nux is a very admirable remedy in inflammation of the womb, and its virtues in this complaint are lauded by many experienced homœopathists, with whom I must join myself. Whether the metritis has occurred in the unimpregnated uterus, or during gestation, or after delivery, it matters not ; and just as little influence has the particular part of the womb which is affected." This would hardly be expected *à priori ;* but I must say that in two cases of metritis after parturition which I have had under my care, the effects of Nux were astounding. Dr. Lawrence Newton communicates a similar experience,* and Dr. Guernsey regards the remedy as "very frequently indicated."

The ancient repute of Nux vomica in ague has been fairly sustained in the school of Hahnemann. Its special indications are of course the accompanying gastro-intestinal symptoms ; though it is said that the paroxysm itself points to it when the heat precedes or mingles with the chill. Both Wurmb and Caspar and Dr. Lord place it high among the remedies required in actual practice ; and my own experience concurs with that of Fleischmann and Russell in thinking that Nux and Ipecacuanha in alternation most frequently control the impure intermittents which come under our treatment in non-aguish districts. In his *Lesser Writings*† Hahnemann describes such a fever as epidemic in Germany in 1809, and points to Nux and Arsenic as homœopathic to and curative of its only varieties.

There are, of course, numerous other applications of Nux vomica. You will always think of it when hyperæsthesia, irritability, or spasm is present ; when the patient presents the constitution characteristic of it ; and when his troubles own the causes and experience the aggravations I have mentioned. Thus you will often be led to it in hypochondriasis and spinal irritation ; and it will sometimes serve you well in photophobia, in alcoholic amblyopia, and in the vomiting of pregnancy. Stillé acknowledges its usefulness in this last affection "in very minute doses."

I will conclude by citing from Hartmann a typical case for the application of the medicine :—

"Mad. B—, some thirty years old, who had suffered for many years with a *troublesome and distressing cough*, lost her cough suddenly with-

* *Brit. Journ. of Hom.*, xxviii., 245.
† p. 628.

out any cause ; instead of the cough, she was afflicted with a constant pressure, which sometimes became a *griping*, in the gastric region, which was *aggravated after every meal*, and *after drinking coffee* became so much exacerbated, that she was obliged to sit completely bent over. She was at the same time afflicted with *constriction* and oppression of the chest, and could only make a short inspiration, with which a partial hiccough was always conjoined. *Water-brash* occurred frequently during the day : inappetence : *alvine evacuations hard, occurring every third or fourth day*. She had suffered from this complaint for full two years. I regulated her diet, and cured her entirely in four weeks by the administration of two doses of Nux vomica.* After this she could eat with impunity ; she could even occasionally indulge in coffee, without reproducing her complaint ; but she dared not make it her daily drink.''

Ignatia—through its common possession of strychnia—and *Opium* through its morphia and thebaia are the only true spinal analogues of Nux vomica ; unless we except *Atropia*. The tetanising action of Aconite, of Cicuta, and of Hydrocyanic acid is not so connected with increased reflex excitability. *Bryonia* acts most like Nux on the alimentary and respiratory organs, though stopping short of its spasmodic phenomena.

As regards dose, I must express my conviction that the full virtues of this medicine can only be obtained by a free use of all degrees of the scale of attenuation, from the mother-tincture or lowest triturations to the thirtieth dilution. The repute it has obtained in the old school, Hahnemann's case of asthma, and those of gastralgia cited by Hempel from Kopp's *Memorabilia*, show what it can do in substantial doses. On the other hand, all the earlier and many of the later homœo-pathic cures wrought by Nux, which have given it such a high place among our remedies, which make Hahnemann speak of it as "a polychrest most cherished and precious," were effected by the attenuations from 9 to 30, and mainly by the latter. My own experience makes me as fond of the thirtieth dilution as of the first decimal trituration, and I should not like to be without either in their proper places.

A word in conclusion about the chief alkaloid of Nux vomica,

Strychnia.—Mr. Henry Robinson has enriched the Materia Medica with two heroic provings of the liquor strychniæ, the one prover being a man, the other a woman. Besides the spasms, or attempts at spasm, which might have been ex-

---

* A similar case of chronic dyspepsia and constipation, with hæmorrhoids, cured with marvellous rapidity with Nux, is recorded by Dr Chepmell (*Op. cit.*, p. 97).

pected (these were especially sudden, severe, and painful in
the rectum), several other symptoms were produced. The
male prover became prostrated with a fever, which is compared
to the adynamic intermittents of India ; and, as this passed
over, great irritation of the urinary organs set in, culminating
in an attack of inflammation of the left testicle and cord, and
an abscess in the cellular tissue of the scrotum. We note
also continual full and bursting headache, with heat in the
eyes ; icy sensation all down the spine ; explosive cough ;
intense itching of the skin of the whole body, but especially of
the nose ; and sharp attacks of toothache, especially in the
upper teeth. You will find the record of these provings in
the twelfth and thirteenth volumes of the *Monthly Homœopathic Review.* Dr. Allen adds to their symptoms others obtained from cases of poisoning, giving a pathogenesis of 1,235
in all.

As Strychnia contains, in its most concentrated form, the
spasm-causing property of Nux vomica, it seems obvious to
use it as a homœopathic remedy for such conditions. I have
done so occasionally in the treatment of spasmodic asthma,
and should adopt the same course in tetanus. Dr. Ringer records a case of the " athetosis " of Hammond greatly benefited
by minim doses of liquor strychniæ, while aggravated by
hypodermic injections of gr. ᵢ₁₅ to ᵢ₁₀ of the drug. Liquor
strychniæ contains one part in 120. These are examples of
pure spasm. But in the more complex forms of disease in
which Nux is so beneficial, as in gastro-intestinal disorders,
I think we should suffer loss by substituting strychnia.

Dr. Walter Tyrrell, of Great Malvern, has published a series
of cases of epilepsy, in which the curative effects of strychnia
were not a little remarkable. He thinks that " its value lies
in the effect it has in deadening that condition of exalted sensibility and activity of the medulla oblongata, which most
recent authors consider to be the predisposing cause of the
disease." If it does this, it must be by homœopathic action ;
and so indeed Dr. Tyrrell admits. His success, as reported by
himself, is something marvellous : and the subject may repay
investigation. His doses are those usual in the old school.

NUX MOSCHATA, ŒNANTHE. OLEANDER, OPIUM.

I have yet another Nux to speak of—the nutmeg, called in the ordinary pharmacology Myristica, but by us

Nux moschata.

The homœopathic preparation is a tincture made from the nuts with rectified spirit.

Nux moschata was fully proved about 1833 upon twelve male and nine female subjects, by Dr. C. J. Helbig, who also experimented upon himself. The results obtained were published in a monograph, entitled " Heraklides," which contained also a compendium of all that had been said about the drug in previous literature. In the first volume of the *Révue de la Matière Médicale spécifique*, Dr. Roth has translated the proving, arranging the symptoms under the head of their subjects and also some of the cases of poisoning. Lastly, in his volume of *Materia Medica* (1873), Dr. Hering has made an exhaustive compilation of Helbig's and all later materials for the knowledge of the effects, pathogenetic and curative, of the drug. Allen's pathogenesis is based upon Hering's; it contains 571 symptoms.

Nutmegs are classed among the "narcotics;" but their narcosis is of a very distinctive character. Schmidius (1683) relates the case of a nobleman, aged 36, in whom four nutmegs seemed completely to overwhelm the nervous system. He remained in a state of *coma vigil* for three days, on emerging from which his memory was entirely lost. Continued fever supervened, with insomnia and palpitation ; and at length paralysis of all the limbs. Reason and recollection did not fully return till the expiration of eight days. This is an extreme case; but Cullen relates a similar one of shorter duration. In the latter, and in some other instances, delirium succeeded the sopor. Upon Purkinje the effects were very like those of Cannabis Indica,—the perception of time and distance being impaired in the direction of exaggeration.

Looking over Hering's collection of symptoms, one is struck by (besides the foregoing phenomena) loss of memory ; great tendency to laughter ; headache with drowsiness, or sense of looseness in the brain ; rush of blood to the head ; everything looking large and red ; chalky taste ; dryness of mouth and throat without thirst (Guernsey considers this a key-note of the drug) ; sensation as if something grasped the heart ; and pain in the shins as if the bone were smashed. To these I can add two curious sensations of a patient of my own after eating one nutmeg. These are—objects seem gradually to diminish in size while looking at them ; sense of coldness and emptiness under the heart, with distension.

The ordinary modern uses of Nux moschata are contained in Pereira's words : " Medicinally, nutmegs are used, like other spices, as stimulants and carminatives." The latter action seems to be of a specific nature, as the medicine is in increasing repute in the homœopathic school in the dilutions from the first centesimal upwards for *flatulent dyspepsia.* Where " everything turns to wind," as the patients express it ; where there is great bloating of the stomach, oppressing the heart and lungs, and causing pain behind the sternum ; where only high-seasoned food can be digested ; and in hiccough, Nux moschata is an excellent remedy. It is specially useful in nervous subjects, as hysterical and pregnant women ; and where unpleasant mental emotions will bring on the flatulence. The other uses of the medicine have hardly yet been defined ; but since it became a favourite one of Hahnemann's during his later practice at Paris, it must be borne in mind and consulted as having latent possibilities. Dr. Helbig considers women and children the most suitable subjects for it : and that it is indicated where drowsiness or disposition to fainting are present ; where the skin is cool and dry, and not inclined to sweat ; and where there is aggravation from cool moist air, and amelioration from external warmth. Teste recommends it in retrocession of gout to the stomach.

Allied medicines are *Moschus, Asafœtida,* and *Ambra.*

Helbig employed the second dilution mainly. Hahnemann would probably have given it in higher potency.

I have next to speak of the " hemlock water dropwort,"

Œnanthe crocata.

The root is the most active part, and our Pharmacopœia directs a tincture to be prepared from it with proof-spirit.

We know Œnanthe only by the poisonings of which it has been the agent (seventy-two of which are collated by Allen), and by a few experiments made with it upon animals. It is one of the group of umbelliferæ to which Æthusa and Cicuta belong, and is, as Christison justly says, the most energetic member of the series. Its special interest to us lies in the fact that the phenomena of its toxical effects resemble epilepsy more nearly than do those of its fellows. Dr. Bloc, a pupil of Dr. Imbert-Gourbeyre's, has lately made a study of the plant from this point of view, an account of which you will find in the thirty-second volume of the *British Journal of Homœopathy*. His experiments on animals entirely confirm the analogy suggested by the records of poisoning, and show material changes (inflammation and softening) at the central seat of the malady, the medulla oblongata and its neighbourhood.

We may, therefore, expect to find a place for Œnanthe among our remedies for convulsions of the epileptic type. Whether it will prove of service in genuine epilepsy, save when quite recent, is doubtful. Dr. Drysdale has wisely pointed out that agents curative of this malady are hardly to be looked for among those which provoke similar paroxysms in acute poisoning by them ; we have to combat the persistent proximate cause with medicines of firmer grip and longer action. Dr. Oehme has probably better applied Œnanthe for the purpose of checking the epileptiform convulsions of childhood and pregnancy, in which he has found it very effective.* He gives the third dilution.

I will now occupy you for a few minutes with the laurel rose, Nerium

Oleander.

The tincture is prepared from the fresh leaves.

There is a pathogenesis of Oleander in the first volume of the *Reine Arzneimittellehre*, containing 342 symptoms from Hahnemann and five others, and 10 from authors. Allen adds several fresh observations.

Oleander seems to be a narcotic of moderate intensity, and also a heart-poison like Digitalis. Hahnemann claims to be the first to introduce it into medicine, and, if he means in modern times, he is justified in so doing ; but Galen used it. Hahnemann thinks it likely to be useful "in certain kinds of

* *New England Med. Gazette*, June, 1877.

mental alienation, as distraction (*Zerstreutheit*) ; in some pain-less paralyses ; and in eruptions on the head and other affec-tions of the hairy scalp." The drug seems certainly to have an elective affinity for the skin. " The skin of the body is very sensitive all over : it becomes sore, raw, and painful, merely by the friction of the clothes : for example, the skin of the neck becomes so from the rubbing of the cravat, that of the thighs from the rubbing of wide trousers when walking." And again, " Forty hours after taking the dose, gnawing itching, as of an eruption over the whole body, while undressing." The scalp seemed to be a special seat of this sensation. Noack and Trinks say that Oleander has been found useful in "erup-tions on the hairy scalp ; at times scaly, at times humid, with burning itching." An excellent illustration of its power in such affections is related by Dr. A. R. Morgan, of Syracuse, in the fourth volume of the Transactions of the New York State Homœopathic Society (p. 332). Symptoms 122 and 123 are : " The power of speech is almost entirely lost, the breathing being natural. She attempted to answer when questioned, but she was only able to utter sounds, but no in-telligible words." They are taken from a narrative of poison-ing with the plant by Morgagni ; and have led to its recom-mendation for paralysis of the tongue. As I read the original, however, they merely express the extreme debility of the patient. From sympt. 189 Hartmann suggests it for lienteria. If China and Ferrum ever fail you in this disorder, Oleander might be worth a trial.

I can tell you nothing about allied medicines or doses, save that Hahnemann recommends the sixth dilution.

Our chief subject to-day is a drug which stands at the head of the list of the medicines of the old school, but occupies only a second-rate position in ours,

Opium.

A tincture prepared in the usual manner, or triturations, are recommended by Hahnemann, and used in our practice.

There is a pathogenesis of Opium in the first volume of the *Reine Arzneimittellehre*. Of its 662 symptoms, 144 only are from provings on the healthy ; the remaining four-fifths being taken from authors. The examination which Dr. Langheinz has instituted into a good many of these last shows them to be of very dubious purity, either as regards the mode in which the drug was given or the subjects of its influence; and the investigations by which I have completed his have led me to the same results. Hahnemann indeed depreciates them himself, saying that they are mostly secondary effects, and therefore (according to his view) not available for homœopathic application. But to add to his own and his (four) fellow-observers' symptoms we have two excellent provings of Opium in small but substantial doses. The one is by Professor Jörg and twenty of his pupils; the other by Dr. Eidherr, of Vienna, in which ten persons besides himself took part. The full record of the latter is given in the first volume of the Journal of the Austrian Homœopathic Society: its schema of results is translated in the twenty-second volume of the *British Journal of Homœopathy*. Dr. Allen, combining the symptoms from these sources, adds others from numerous fresh ones, so that his authorities are 350 in number, and his symptoms nearly 2,300.

Opium is, as you well know, a substance of very complex constitution. It contains a number of alkaloids—morphia, narceia, meconia, cryptopia, codeia, thebaia, and others—each of which has its own distinctive action. The effect of Opium is the result of the composition of the forces of these several ingredients. But, being so, it is for us the fact with which we have to deal. Opium is the form in which its constituents are given us in nature: as a single substance it has been proved on the healthy and tested on the sick. It thus becomes a medicine *per se*. So far as the pathogenetic effects of any of its ingredients are known, so far they too can be used therapeutically. But they cannot replace Opium, nor Opium them. Of one or two of their number I shall have to speak subsequently; but our concern just now is with Opium itself as a whole.

Hahnemann says of Opium that its effects are more difficult to appreciate than those of most other medicines; and so subsequent observers have found. Its action is as complex as its composition, and it has not been easy to unravel it. Various theories have been formed to account for the phenomena—as that the drug is stimulant to some parts of the nervous system, but depressant to others; that it stimulates at first, but narcotises afterwards; that it is a stimulant in a moderate dose, but a narcotic in a large one. None of these explanations has ever satisfied my own mind; and at various times during the last twenty years * my attention has been directed to the subject with the hope of penetrating its mystery. I think I am

* See *London Medical Review*, 1860; *Brit. Journ. of Hom.*, xxii.

clearer about it now than ever I was before : at any rate, you shall have my most mature thoughts on the matter. In giving you them, however, I must beg you to accept them *quantum valeant*, and simply as the expression of my own judgment. That they are not shared by all my colleagues sufficiently appears from the rather severe criticism they received, when first published *in extenso*, in the *Monthly Homœopathic Review*. The objections there raised I shall have before me while speaking to you to-day ; and you can hardly do better than refer to them subsequently in aid of your own conclusions. You will find the criticisms in question in the July and October numbers of the volume for 1876.

The facts are these. Taken in a moderate dose, Opium seems to act as a stimulant. This effect is especially felt in depressed and chilly conditions of the body, as in hunger and catarrh as described by Dr. Anstie,* or in the physical and mental wretchedness which often makes the poor resort to it, and which—occurring as a secondary result of its intoxication —drives the habitual opium-eater to " take a hair of the dog that bit him." There are some, however, who can induce the apparently stimulant effects of Opium in their ordinary condition of body. But larger doses are here required, and some approach to narcosis is often seen in the ending of the excitement in a comatose sleep.

Again, even when taken in quantities large enough to produce undoubtedly poisonous effects, Opium seems to excite some parts of the nervous centres. Hahnemann observes that it exalts the irritability of the voluntary muscles, and stirs imagination and courage ; and under these two heads the phenomena of what may be called its poisonous excitation may be classed. In the first division we have the observations, multiplying upon us of late, that in the lower animals and in the young human subject Opium is very apt to cause convulsions, sometimes of a clonic but quite as often of a true tetanic character. For the exaltation of the imaginative powers which it may cause we need not go beyond the " Confessions " of De Quincey ; and as to the emotions generally, it is well known that Orientals use Opium as the Western nations use alcohol, to spur flagging courage and excite desire.

On the other hand, it is confessed by all that the full effect of Opium is pure narcosis—that is, depression and paralysis of the whole functional activity of the nervous system. The sensory nerves may first lose their power, and dull aching

* *Stimulants and Narcotics.*

pains may accompany the process. But the brain itself soon shows it, first—it may be—in a low muttering delirium, but then in the supervention of that condition which at its height is called "coma." Coma is no intensification of natural sleep. It is not sleep at all, but a stupor; from which the patient may for a time be readily roused, going off again directly, but which ultimately deepens into entire unconsciousness. With these conditions of sensation and ideation, the motor powers are equally abolished : the respiration also becomes weaker, and the heart's action slow, until finally death ensues from the failure of the former function.

The difficulty is to account for the phenomena of stimulation which appear here and there in the action of a drug so unquestionably narcotic. Now of those which show themselves in the motor, imaginative, and emotional spheres, Dr. Anstie—who in his treatise on *Stimulants and Narcotics* has contributed so much thought and observation to this subject —gives, I think, a satisfactory explanation. He shows (what Hahnemann had noticed before him) that while the fancies and desires are aroused, the higher faculties of the mind are already dulled. He points out that in the normal state of being we keep down the animal within us ; but that in intoxication—whether with Opium or alcohol—our powers of control are relaxed, and the lower nature asserts itself loudly ere it too yields to the narcotic influence. This is confessedly true as regards alcohol, and it is an easy step to apply it to Opium. Again, Dr. Anstie argues that it is quite unjustifiable to assume that convulsion is an evidence of exalted motor energy. It may mean its irregular distribution and fitful discharge ; it may imply an unbalanced activity from withdrawal of the control of the higher centres or a diminished resistance to reflex excitation ; but in none of these cases is any exalted functional vigour present.

But I would now go a step farther than Dr. Anstie, though in the same direction. The apparent stimulation wrought by large doses, he maintains, is really paralysis of some parts of the nervous centres allowing undue manifestation of the rest. I think that the same explanation will account for the apparent stimulation (as of the mental and muscular powers) wrought by small doses, which in his eyes is a real one. It is to me inconceivable that a substance which in moderate quantity excites any function should in a somewhat larger one depress it.* I know well how this may be when the dose is an overwhelming one—as in the analogous case of an over-

* See the discussion on this subject in Lecture v.

strong galvanic current. But the question here is of the different effect of half a grain of morphia and of two grains.* No sudden shattering destruction of vital energy can be ascribed to the latter dose ; yet we are asked to believe that its influence is paralysing while that of the former is stimulating. I cannot think it ; and as there is no doubt about the paralysis, I question the stimulation. That is, I question whether the phenomena of stimulation (whose existence I have fully admitted, are due to a direct influence of this kind exerted by Opium on the organs w'.ich manifest them.

What part of the nervous system, then, is there whose depressed activity will account for excitement elsewhere ? I answer—the sympathetic. There is an apparent antagonism and contradiction between the nerves of this order and those of the cerebro-spinal class which accounts for many phenomena of drug-action and of disease. If we stimulate a sympathetic ganglion, the nerves animated by it cause the arteries they supply to contract. Less blood accordingly flows through the corresponding part of the body : it becomes cold, pale, and shrunken, and its nervous, muscular, and secretory activity is diminished. If, on the contrary, we divide the vascular nerves of any organ, precisely the opposite results occur. Its circulation is increased, and its functional energy for the time exalted, or, at any rate, more rapidly expended. If, therefore, a depressing agent makes its influence first felt in the sympathetic system, its earliest phenomena will be those of apparent stimulation, from the increased flow of blood thereby allowed.

That Opium does depress the sympathetic from the very beginning of its action I hold to be proved from a number of consentaneous phenomena, which we have not yet taken into account. Among these we have that diminished irritability of the involuntary (non-striated) muscles which Hahnemann noted as co-existing with excitement of the voluntary set. Constipation of the torpid kind is the well-known effect of opiates ; and Trousseau and Pidoux have called attention to the corresponding condition—sluggish and therefore difficult excretion—as induced in the bladder. Their careful observations, moreover, confirm the diaphoretic action of the drug, and show that the perspiring skin is also hot and flushed, which it would be from vaso-motor depression. The hot skin of Belladonna, which we have ascribed to tissue-irritation, is

---

* I mention these quanties because they were those taken by Dr. Anstie in his experiments on himself. A smaller maximum of dose would doubtless be safer for any one who sought to repeat them.

dry, as in scarlatina. In the face the same condition is shown by flushing, in the head by heaviness, giddiness, and somnolency, and in the eyes by injection of the conjunctiva and (as ophthalmoscopic investigation has shown) of the retina. But in this last region a phenomenon occurs which is yet more significant, and which alone seems to me a key to the whole condition.

I refer to the contraction of the pupil, so characteristic of Opium poisoning. It is, as Dr. Harley says, " in man the most constant of all the effects of Opium, and comes on in ten or fifteen minutes after the subcutaneous use of the drug. It occurs independently of hypnosis." What is its explanation ? Of late years the tendency of opinion has been to regard it as due to stimulation of the third nerve : this view is maintained by Harley, Ringer, and Wood. I am, however, quite unable to assent to it ; and must still maintain the position I took up in 1860, that it is the result of sympathetic depression. The difficulty which would arise from the continuance of the firm contraction even after the third nerve must itself have lost its energy is removed by the later researches into the structure of the iris, which have shown it to be more an erectile than a muscular organ. Thus the contraction induced by division or depression of the sympathetic is due to iridal congestion as much as to unbalanced activity of its circular fibres, and answers to the small pupil of plethora or apoplexy. With this accords the observation of Dr. Anstie, that shortly before death from Opium-poisoning the pupils dilate. The vessels are now emptied here as all over the surface, which is pale instead of flushed as heretofore.

Let us now, with this thought in our minds, read a few instances and descriptions of the early effects of Opium, and see if it will not explain them, and harmonise them with the well known phenomena which follow.

First, let Dr. Harley relate the results of injecting one sixth of a grain of morphia behind the trochanter of a patient suffering from sciatica. " After ten minutes," he writes, "there was giddiness and somnolency, and she fell asleep. On waking an hour after she complained of being very giddy, and said that everything was running round. The cheeks and forehead were hot and flushed, the hands hot ; she felt hot all over. The pulse was increased in volume and power. The pupils had contracted from $\frac{1}{5}$ to $\frac{1}{6}$ of an inch out of the light ; an hour later they were $\frac{1}{4}$. The tongue was clean and wet."

Next let us take Dr. Phillips' description of opiate poisoning. "When the quantity is very large, and the form such as to permit rapid absorption of the whole, the course of symptoms is as follows : the patient, if an adult, quickly becomes conscious of a sense of fulness in the head, which seems to commence in the nape of the neck, and to spread therefrom ; and in the course of a few minutes feels great and increasing drowsiness, and a sensation of general heat, which increases to an almost intolerable degree, and is then accompanied by sweating."

Passing now from health towards disease, we have Dr. Anstie's graphic description of the effect of a small dose of Opium upon himself when suffering from hunger or catarrh, to which I have already referred. In both these cases the surface is chilly, the arterioles are contracted ; and he notices especially the pleasant feeling of warmth which spread over his body as the drug began to take effect. Again, let us look at a patient in the first stage of the paroxysm of ague. The skin is pale, cold, and dry ; the circulation and respiration quick and feeble ; the pupils dilated : everythings shows vasomotor excitation. When in this condition, says Sir Thomas Watson, a full dose of laudanum was given (by Dr. Trotter), in most cases " after a few minutes an exhilaration of spirits was perceived : the pulse from being weak, quick, and sometimes irregular, became full, less frequent, and equal ; an agreeable warmth was diffused over the whole frame, and every unpleasant feeling vanished, sometimes in a quarter of an hour. The patients were themselves surprised at the sudden change in their sensations." Similar results have since been obtained (and even more rapidly) by inhalation of nitrite of amyl, which confessedly acts by relaxing the arterioles.

Lastly, I may mention one of the facts most frequently brought to light in the experiments conducted under the superintendence of Dr. Hughes Bennett to inquire into the antidotal action of meconate of morphia and sulphate of atropia.* It was that vessels turgid with blood under the influence of the former contracted considerably when the latter was administered ; and we have already seen that atropia, which characteristically dilates the pupil, is excitant to the sympathetic. Experimentation with morphia on animals has not always yielded consistent results ; but from its latest instance—that of Picard and Rebatel—I find that similar conclusions have been drawn, viz. : that morphia contracts the pupils and dilates the small vessels by sympathetic paresis.

* See *Researches into the Antagonism of Medicines* (Churchill), 1875.

I think, then, we may fairly conclude that Opium is throughout its action a direct paralyser of the nervous system, and that the apparent stimulation present during its earlier effects is due to the removal of the restraint exercised on the circulation by the vascular nerves. It is a phenomenon analogous to those observed in the face when the cervical sympathetic is divided, and to those which occur in the body generally when the ganglionic centres are depressed by ice-bags applied to the spine. We thus bring the whole action of the drug under one uniform and intelligible description, and this without any " obscuration," " ignoring," or " explaining away" of the facts. I use these terms because they have been freely applied to what I have written about Opium by my *Monthly Homœopathic* reviewer. You will bear me witness that I have not questioned the fact that the first effect of a moderate dose of Opium is often cerebral excitement. My difference with my critic begins when I come to the explanation of this excitement. He assumes that it can only be produced by a stimulant action of the drug upon the gray matter of the brain. I have pointed out another way of accounting for it, viz., by supposing a heightened cerebral circulation to be present through depression of the inhibitory influence of the vaso-motor nerves of the organ. I have argued that all the consentaneous phenomena show such a condition to exist, and to be so brought about, and that thus the cerebral excitement produced under some circumstances by Opium is of a piece with the rest of its operation, and needs no supposition of a reverse action of large and small doses to account for it.

Enough has been said on this score, and we have only now to consider the meaning of the changes in the respiratory and cardiac movements induced by the drug ; and to have brought before our minds the epiphenomena of its intoxication.

I. Opium kills, as we have seen, by suspending the respiration. The movements of the chest begin to slacken soon after its poisonous influence is established : breathing then becomes diaphragmatic only ; it is slow, sighing, and irregular, and at last stops. All this is easily accounted for by the gradual paralysis induced by the drug, first in the sensory excitants of respiration, and then in the motor agents of the process ; later, too, the breathing is affected by the congestive coma of the brain, as it is in apoplexy. The pulse is affected earlier still, viz., in the so-called stimulant stage of opiate action ; it is then full, somewhat quickened, and stronger. But it falls with the respiration ; and in the second stage of the poisoning is characteristically slow, while remaining full. Experiment appears to have demonstrated that this retardation of the heart's action is due to the inhibitory influence of the vagi; and the congested condition of the brain seems to explain how the cerebral centres of the nerves may well be excited, as they are, e. g., in acute hydrocephalus and (again) in apoplexy.

II. The after-effects of Opium, when the sopor has passed off, are very like those which follow an alcoholic debauch—nausea, anorexia, headache, chilliness, listlessness, sleeplessness, constipation. They are not contraries of the state previously induced, but merely alternating opposites, oscillations of the disturbed balance : the chilliness and insomnia imply the same depressed vitality of the nervous system as did once the heat and sopor. These epiphenomena are best seen in the unhappy subjects of opium-eating, whose whole life is spent in such morbid vicissitude.

We now come to the curative effects of our drug ; and must first inquire how far the induction of its physiological action is justifiable in disease. This would seem a strange question to the therapeutists of the old school, especially in these days of " hypodermic morphia." But, if you have followed me thus far, you will have seen that the great aim of homœopathic treatment is to avoid such physiological action, to induce it only up to the point at which it neutralises a similar condition already present, and then to stay the hand. To use Opium, therefore, to compel sleep, to allay pain or spasm, and to check excessive secretion, would with us be only tolerable when we had no similarly-acting medicines on which we could rely for the purpose ; and even then we should feel it a question for grave consideration whether remedy or disease constituted the greater evil.

Hahnemann has some excellent remarks on this subject. " A short cough," he says, " which has been occasioned by a cold, a recent trembling caused by fright, a diarrhœa which has been suddenly occasioned by fear, by a cold or other slight causes ; retching, which has come on in consequence of a moral emotion, as loathing, &c., may yield to Opium, and sometimes do yield suddenly, because all that Opium requires to do in these affections is to suppress them for a short while, in order to enable the organism to remove in the meanwhile all disposition to these affections, and to effect its restoration to health by means of its own inherent recuperative power." The same principles would apply to the treatment of recent and fugitive pains and spasms, and of the chilly and miserable state of commencing influenzal catarrh. But in morbid conditions of more permanent and recurring character it must always be a grave question whether we shall resort to the palliative medication of opiates. We are launching upon a boundless ocean when we once begin it; and the medical world teems with recorded cases (and still more unrecorded) of its pernicious influence.* Morphiomania, it is found, can be induced as readily as dipsomania; and what sort of nervous system will its subjects transmit to their offspring? God forbid that we should deny to the sufferers from *incurable* disease any relief from the pains which agonise them; but wherever cure is possible, I am sure that we are only diminishing our patients' chances and adding to their distresses by inducing the narcotism of Opium in their systems.

The abandonment of opiates must be to a new convert to homœopathy one of the hardest trials involved in his change of practice. He need not necessarily do it all at once. Let him feel his way. Let him see how far the more numerous and more potent specifics he now possesses will enable him to do without them. The cough, the diarrhœa, the neuralgia, which of old he hushed up by poisoning the nerves, now find in his new armoury their direct remedies. Let him keep his opiates for cases otherwise irremediable; and their use will become rarer and rarer. For myself, I can safely say that during twenty years of homœopathic practice I have not found one patient in five hundred who required them.

We turn, then, to the homœopathic applications of Opium, and find these more limited than might have been expected. Pereira indeed gives a long list of affections in which it is contra-indicated and objectionable; and these are of course the very conditions to which it is applicable according to the method of similarity. But his statements are too broad and general; and Hahnemann foresaw truly when he said :— "Opium is one of those drugs the primary effects of which seldom correspond homœopathically to the symptoms of disease." He moreover pointed out with great sagacity the two leading morbid conditions to which it really corresponds. "Opium is a specific," he wrote, "for certain kinds of the most obstinate constipation." It holds a high place among us in the treatment of this disorder, especially when the stools occur in round, black, hard balls, and the rectum is torpid : it reaches even to intestinal obstruction when of a paralytic

---

* "In 15 out of 55 cases of the hypodermic injection of morphia, the consequences were unpleasant, and in 7 death resulted, in none save one of which had the ordinary dose been exceeded." (*Brit. Med Journ.*, Nov. 16, 1878. See also *Lancet*, April 10, 1880).

nature, and to incarcerated hernia. We also esteem it the principal remedy for lead-colic, and suppose that it acts here by removing the constipation. In these latter uses we are at one with our brethren of the old school ; but this because they are herein unconsciously homœopathising. Opium is also a specific, Hahnemann continues, " for acute fevers characterised by a sopor bordering upon stupor, and by absence of any complaint, snoring with the mouth open, half-jerking of the limbs, and burning heat of the perspiring body." That it is actually homœopathic to the pyrexia may be inferred from the experiments with morphia on animals communicated by Dr. Oglesby to the fourth volume of the *Practitioner*, in which a rise of two or three degrees of temperature nearly always followed its adminstration. The cerebral symptoms also of fever quite as often remind one of the effects of Opium as of those of Hyoscyamus or Belladonna ; and in such cases it will be found very useful. The drowsiness of which this is the intensest form is always a special indication for Opium ; and may sometimes present itself as a morbid state *per se*, when there is little difficulty about the choice of the medicine. Thus Dr. Bayes recommends it in passive cerebral congestion, with somnolence after meals, in patients predisposed to apoplexy; and Dr. Drury finds it helpful in uræmic coma. Dr. Guernsey indicates it where the patient is very sleepy, but cannot go to sleep. Opium should also be occasionally serviceable in headaches like those it causes; and in the atonic dyspepsia of drunkards. It seems to paralyse the muscular fibres of the fundus of the bladder rather than those of its sphincter (herein just the reverse of Belladonna); and is accordingly remedial in paralytic *retention* of urine. It is especially serviceable in these (and perhaps in other) affections when they have occurred in consequence of a fright.

I have reserved the relation of Opium to two important cerebral affections, *delirium tremens* and *apoplexy*. Resembling as it does so very closely in its action that of alcohol, it ought to find a place in the homœopathic treatment of the drunkard's mania. I cannot, however, claim the ordinary use of it in this disease as an instance of the operation of the law of similars, as it is (or rather, was) given in full doses to compel sleep. There is very little recorded experience of delirium tremens in our literature. In the cases I have myself seen, Hyoscyamus or Belladonna was better indicated than Opium ; whose acute delirium, moreover, is without hallucinations. When, however, delirium tremens comes on as a consequence of the drunkard being deprived of his accustomed stimulus, the analogy of the sufferings of opium-eaters must be remembered. Stillé, describing from Libermann the chronic delirium into which they ultimately fall, says—" These images which, we are assured, are literal copies of the opium-eaters' phantasms, present a vivid resemblance to the more familiar spectral illusions of delirium tremens."—In apoplexy, Opium has been a good deal used in our school. It is, however, very questionable whether the symptomatic resemblance, undoubted as it is, warrants its adminstration here. What we have to treat in apoplexy is not the extravasation, which is irremediable, but that which has caused the rupture of the degenerated blood-vessel; and which, if allowed to continue, threatens to increase the mischief. This cause may be either an excitement of the general circulation or an active congestion of (*i. e.*, attraction of blood to) the brain. In either case, is Opium truly homœopathic to the morbid condition? Aconite is our substitute for the lancet in the former, and Nux vomica or Belladonna seems to me the true pathogenetic analogue to the latter. Where extravasation has not occurred, but active congestion is the beginning and the ending of the matter, these medicines seem to me to cover the whole malady. But I can conceive it possible that where extravasation has taken place, and the danger arises from oppression of the vital parts at the base of the brain, a few doses of Opium might be of service, as the drug would certainly be homœopathic to this portion of the disorder. In this connection the remark of Dr. Ringer must be borne in mind, that " effusion of blood into the pons Varolii will produce symptoms almost identical with those of opium poisoning."

Opium has a certain amount of reputation in the treatment of diabetes. If it does more than palliate symptoms, it must be, I think, in virtue of its homœopathicity to the disease. Dr. Coze, of Strasburg, wishing to determine its action on glycogenesis, injected fifteen grammes of a solution of muriate of morphia in distilled water into the jugular vein of a rabbit. The urine was not examined ; but the quantity of sugar in the liver was found more than doubled, and likewise that contained in the arterial blood.[*] Bernard, too, has lately informed us that morphia determines glycosuria after the same manner as woorara and puncture of the floor of the fourth ventricle, viz., by increasing the circulation through the liver.[†]

Another homœopathic use of Opium in the old school is the employment of it, in the shape of small doses of Dover's

[*] See *Brit. Journ. of Hom.*, xxiv., 255.
[†] *London Medical Record*, i., 725.

powder, to check the sweats of phthisis.* This preparation—compounded of opium, ipecacuanha, and sulphate of potash—is well known as a diaphoretic in ordinary practice.

Cannabis Indica is the only real analogue I know to Opium.

Save in intestinal affections, the higher attenuations seem most in favour.

* See *Brit. Journ. of Hom.*, xҳiii., 108; and *Practitioner*, Sept. 1879.

LECTURE XLVII.

OPIUM ALKALOIDS, ORIGANUM, OSMIUM, PÆONIA, PARIS, PETROLEUM, PETROSELINUM, PHELLANDRIUM, PHYSO-STIGMA, PHYTOLACCA.

Before leaving Opium, I must say something as to the distinctive action of some of its chief constituents.

Morphia, of all these, most nearly represents the full action of the parent drug, and I have freely used the observations of its effects when speaking of those of Opium. A full collection of them has been made by Dr. Allen, who cites from 73 sources. The only remaining ones I care to notice are the vomiting and the itching of the skin it causes. Of the former I shall speak under the head of Apomorphia. The latter is a frequent and marked effect of the alkaloid. It is rarely associated with any eruption; and should indicate morphia as a remedy in pruritus, in which I have several times given it with advantage.

Codeia very much resembles morphia, but the tendency to convulsive action is more pronounced under its influence than that which leads to coma. A pathogenesis of it, derived from several sources, is given by Dr. Allen in his *Encyclopædia ;* and in a note thereto two cases are mentioned in which involuntary twitchings of the eyelids were removed by it in the attenuations. I have myself had another.

Narceia, on the other hand, is a pure hypnotic; but its effects of any kind are feeble. Much the same may be said of *Meconia*, though it is a little more active ; and of *Cryptopia*, which Dr. Harley's experiments show to be more potent still. We could only use these substances in soporose conditions ; and nothing seems gained by substituting them for Opium itself.

Narcotia is moderately convulsive and hypnotic in its action; but the point of most interest about it is that it has anti-malarial properties like those of quinine. *Thebaia* seems to be the alkaloid in which the tetanising powers chiefly reside. The spasms resemble those of Aconite, of Cicuta, and of Hydrocyanic acid rather than those of Strychnia.

The last ingredient of Opium of which I shall speak is

Apomorphia, which indeed is no natural constituent of the
drug, but a derivative from morphia obtained by heating it
with excess of hydrochloric acid.   It has been found to contain in special intensity the emetic properties of morphia
itself.   Trousseau and Pidoux had long ago studied these,
and shown them to be most strongly manifested when the
drug was applied externally, and so to be of cerebral rather
than of gastric origin.   The same inference was drawn by Dr.
Wood from the fact that the sickness which follows intoxication by Opium is brought on whenever the patient raises his
head.   Apomorphia has been largely tested by Drs. Gee* and
G. Blackley† in this country, and by a number of foreign observers, and has been found to be a prompt and powerful
emetic, acting directly upon the nervous centre of the process.

When Dr. Blackley's paper was read before the British
Homœopathic Society, Dr. Cooper stated that he had succeeded in removing with Apomorphia the distressing vomiting
connected with a tumour in the brain.   Dr. Dyce Brown,
whose prescriptive right it seems to be to turn these new discoveries to homœopathic account, soon followed with a series
of cases of vomiting, in which Apomorphia, in the third dilution, proved promptly curative.‡   It was most beneficial, as
might be expected, when the vomiting was reflex ; but it
helped even the gastric form of the trouble.   It is now gaining quite a reputation as a remedy for sea-sickness.

Binz says that "the best preparation of it is the hydro-
chlorate, which forms beautiful crystals, and quickly and completely dissolves in water.   It turns dark green under the
action of light, but does not lose its efficacy in consequence."
Apomorphia itself is probably best prepared by trituration.

I now pass to some medicines of lesser interest.
Our information regarding the wild marjoram,

Origanum vulgare,

is derived from a paper by Dr. Gallavardin, of Lyons, published in *L'Art Médical* for 1865,§ and translated in the fifteenth
volume of the *North American Journal of Homœopathy*.

The oil of marjoram has long been in domestic repute as a
stimulating emmenagogue.   M. de Cessoles, who proved it on

* Transactions of the Clinical Society, vol. ii.
† *Brit. Journ. of Hom.*, xxxi., 497.
‡ *Ibid*, xxxii., 497.
§ See also his *Causeries Cliniques*, p. 15.

himself and two young women, found it produce in the latter considerable sexual excitement. Dr. Gallavardin has recorded eight cases of erotomania of various degrees in the female, in which the action of Origanum, generally in the third dilution, was most satisfactory. Dr. Bayes tells me that he has several times obtained excellent effects from Origanum in obscure nervous disorders in women, in which he suspected irritation of the sexual system as the exciting or maintaining cause. The tincture is prepared from the fresh plant.

I have next to mention the rare metal, called

Osmium.

Triturations are prepared for homœopathic use.

Dr. Hering has collected, in one of the pathogeneses of his volume of *Materia Medica,* all that was known of Osmium to that time (1873). In the sixteenth volume of its *Bulletin,* the Homœopathic Medical Society of France has, through Dr. Ozanam, put on record a recent case of poisoning in a worker with the metal ; and has also translated the experiments of Hoffbauer related in the third volume of the *Archiv.* This Hoffbauer, however, was the notorious Fickel, whose endeavour to palm spurious provings on Homœopathy makes anything from his pen suspicious. Dr. Hering does not include him in his list of authorities, among whom, nevertheless, are five provers of the metal, one of them Dr. Stokes, of Liverpool.

The workman I have mentioned died of the intense bronchopneumonia induced by the emanations from Osmium. But this action on the air-tubes—so far at least as the upper part is concerned—is not local only; for the provers had great hoarseness and cough. Gmelin's experiments on animals show the oxide to cause death in convulsions without signs of inflammation, evidencing an action on the nervous system. In the provers this is shown by headache, chiefly supra-orbital, and very marked dimness of vision. Osmium also acts on the kidneys, the urine being dark and scanty in the provers, and albuminous in the workman I have mentioned, in whom after death the so-called second stage of Bright's disease (that is, the large white kidney) was found established. This man had also a papular and desquamating eruption of the arms.

There is thus a good deal in the pathogenetic action of Osmium which, applied upon the homœopathic principle, promises good therapeutic result. It is comparable with *Manganum, Selenium,* and perhaps *Arsenicum.*

My next medicine is the peony,

Pæonia officinalis,

of which we prepare a tincture from the fresh root. This, it is said, must be gathered in spring; when August comes, its power has been lost.

There is a short pathogenesis of Pæonia in the twenty-first volume of the *Hygea*, mainly consisting of symptoms observed by Dr. Geyer on himself and three others, who all took substantial doses of the mother-tincture. There is little in it worthy of note, and the plant has scarcely received any medicinal employment. But one of its effects—" painful ulcer at the anus, with exudation of a fœtid moisture "—led Dr. Ozanam* to use it in a similar condition occurring idiopathically; and his success induced him to extend its application to other ulcers, with rarely failing benefit. Dr. Guérin-Méneville says that, " according to him, Pæonia would be efficacious in every ulceration seated below the umbilicus." But Dr. Ozanam only states that his experience had been limited to this part of the body; while he ends his paper with a fresh case in which an ulcer of the breast readily healed under its use. He used the first three dilutions, either externally alone, or also internally. Dioscorides and Pliny recommend it for nightmare, and it caused this affection in Dr. Geyer himself.

And now a few words about the " herb Paris," or true-love—

Paris quadrifolia.

The entire plant is used for the tincture.

Paris has a good pathogenesis—symptoms from provings of it by twelve persons (among whom was Hahnemann himself) being given in Hartlaub and Trinks' third volume, and in the eighth and thirteenth volumes of the *Archiv*. It has rarely received any therapeutic application; but I mention it that you may know its place in the Materia Medica, though I cannot tell you how the symptoms were obtained. Dr. Guernsey gives as characteristics of it—" great sensitiveness to offensive odours; imaginary foul smells. Cough with ex-

* See *Bull. de la Soc. Med. Hom. de France*, vol. viii. ; and *Brit. Journ. of Hom.*, xxvi., 53.

pectoration in the morning, without expectoration in the evening. Sensation of extension of size, *i.e.,* patient feels very
large. Collection of water in the mouth. Urine with greasy
cuticle on the surface." Hahnemann says that it removes
cramp in the stomach, and also (in large doses) causes it ; and
Allen emphasises (as verified) the symptoms—" it seemed as
though a thread were tightly drawn through the eye to the
middle of the head, which was very painful," and "a sensation
as if a great weight were lying on the nape." No other therapeutists mention the drug.

We have now a medicine of more importance—the rock oil,
oleum petræ, or

Petroleum.

We use the white variety, "mineral naphtha," which we dis-
solve in rectified spirit or triturate. Dr. Drysdale suggests
capsules where the pure substance should be given.

We owe the symptomatology of Petroleum almost entirely
to Hahnemann, who gives us 623 symptoms from it in the
first edition of the *Chronic Diseases* (where he recommends the
18th dilution for use), and 776 in the second. Allen adds
some effects of large quantities and of exposure to it in its
manufacture.

I have little to say of the pathogenesis, except that one of
its symptoms once guided me to the choice of the right medicine for an anomalous but annoying complaint, viz., a feeling
as if there were a cold stone in the heart. I would call attention, also, to the urinary symptoms, as presenting a pretty
close resemblance to some forms of vesical catarrh. The
workmen get the hair-follicles of their skins inflamed and indurated (comedones). The chief reputation of Petroleum in
our school has been as a remedy for *sea-sickness.* Hempel,
who in his first edition had recommended it, in his second
repudiates it as ineffective. But I must say that both myself
and friends whom I have supplied with it can testify to decided
benefit from its use ; and Dr. Bayes confirms this more favourable estimate of the remedy. In other forms also of nausea
and vomiting, as in that of pregnancy, it may prove useful :
Dr. Guernsey says that it has the aversion to fat food characteristic of Pulsatilla, and is "particularly applicable in all gastric
troubles of pregnant women." Diarrhœa occurring only in the
day-time is with him a special indication for the drug. Then

there are certain uses of Petroleum for which I was indebted to the experience of my friend Dr. Madden, but which I have frequently verified for myself. These are to check fœtid sweat in the axillæ; to relieve tenderness of the feet when these too are bathed in a more or less foul-smelling moisture (which it removes); and to modify that unhealthiness of skin which causes a general tendency to fester and ulcerate. Teste, moreover, recommends it in alternation with Ipecacuanha in dysentery affecting children. Dr. Drysdale* says that since he has used it in three-drop doses of the pure substance he has found it more efficacious than hitherto, getting excellent results in many chronic catarrhs (urethral, uterine, intestinal, bronchial), in chilblains and chaps, and in deafness with noises in the ear.

I commend Petroleum to your study as a medicine whose virtues have been as yet by no means exhausted.

I have, like Dr. Bayes, found a third decimal alcoholic attenuation answer every purpose in sea-sickness.

Petroselinum,

the common parsley, a tincture of which is made from the whole fresh plant, appears from its brief pathogenesis (which Allen gives from Bethmann) to have a decided action upon the urethral mucous membrane: and has been used accordingly in subacute gonorrhœa and gleet. You might be inclined to doubt the possession of active properties by this seemingly harmless esculent; but I may remind you that parsley seeds and their educt, apiol, have been found to affect the brain like quinine, and have been used with some success as a substitute for it in intermittent fevers and neuralgiæ.

The water-hemlock,

Phellandrium aquaticum,

of which we use the ripe fruit, has a pathogenesis of 373 symptoms in the second volume of Hartlaub and Trinks' *Arzneimittellehre*, mostly furnished by Nenning and obtained in his usual manner. Phellandrium appears to act as a poison similarly to its congeners Cicuta and Œnanthe. It was in considerable repute of old time for chronic suppurations occurring in the lungs and elsewhere, but it has fallen into

* See *Brit. Journ. of Hom.*, xxviii., 403.

disuse in the old school, and has found little place in the new.* Dr. Dudgeon, however, has published in the twenty-eighth volume of the *British Journal of Homœopathy* a case of severe and long-lasting headache cured by it, after the failure of more ordinary remedies. He states that he has given it with success in similar headaches since. The characteristics are " pain like a heavy weight, a stone, a lump of lead, on the top of the head, with aching and burning in the temples and above the eyes ; pain in the eyes, with congestion of the conjunctiva ; watering of the eyes ; intolerance of light and sound." It caused some stitching pains in the mammæ ; and Gross recommends it for nursing women when such pain is felt in the nipples on each application of the child.

And now, as we cannot go on to Phosphorus to-day, I will occupy the rest of this lecture with two other " ph"s—Physostigma and Phytolacca.

The first is a substance just emerging out of physiological into therapeutical interest, the ordeal bean of Old Calabar, the seed of the plant called

Physostigma venenosum.

It is not yet officinal ; but triturations of the whole bean seem the most suitable and active preparation.

A large collection of provings of Physostigma was presented to the American Institute of Homœopathy in 1874 by Dr. Allen, and published in its Transactions for that year. Besides all recorded experiments on the human subject made in the old school, it contains provings from homœopathic sources of a very extensive character. Forty-four persons took part in them, using the triturations from the first to the thirtieth. The full record of their trials is given here by Dr. Allen, and their symptoms in his *Encyclopædia ;* while he prefixes to his collection a very useful catalogue of the bibliography of the drug. The experiments which have been made with it on animals—chiefly by Dr. Fraser, of Edinburgh—are fully summed up by Wood and Ringer.

The Calabar bean has long been used—as its name imports —for purposes of justice in the African kingdom in which it is indigenous. Interest being excited in its properties by the reports of missionaries, they were investigated by Professor Christison, and subsequently, more fully, by Dr. Fraser.

* See, however, *L'Homœopathie Militante*, ii., 384.

Since their results were published (1855-1863) Physostigma and its active principle—physostigmia or eseria—have been tested on animals on a large scale, and on the eye in the human subject. Little clinical application has yet been made of the results ; but now that we have the more minute homœopathic provings to fill in the outline, we shall be inexcusable if we do not make that little expand into a great deal. There are certainly few drugs whose physiological action is so thoroughly known.

The normal poisonous action of the Calabar bean is to cause speedy general paralysis, and death from failure of respiration —consciousness being unaffected to the last. The seat of the paralysis is the spinal cord itself, the vital properties of the nerve-trunks and muscles being found intact. Reflex action is abolished, and also sensibility so far as pain is concerned ; but tactile impressions are perceived, and the muscular sense is perfect. The muscles themselves are the seat of tremors and fibrillary contractions of a very persistent character, which seem due to a direct action of the drug upon them. In those of the involuntary class this irritation goes on to active movements, so that the stomach, bowels, and bladder expel their contents with frequency,—the intestines being often twisted up in knots. All the secretions—sweat, tears, saliva, fæces, urine—are somewhat increased.

Two of the special actions of Physostigma are of peculiar interest,—those which it exerts upon the heart and the eye respectively.

1. In moderate doses the bean simply retards the heart's action, not regularly, but by prolonging the diastole, in which —when poisoning is induced—the organ stops. The retardation seems due to an exaltation of the inhibitory power of the terminal extremities (not of the central origin) of the vagi. It is accompanied by heightened arterial tension, and the power of the heart is not diminished. But a larger dose perceptibly weakens the cardiac impulse, and a very large one may paralyse it at once, leaving it after death flaccid, distended, and barely responsive to the strongest direct stimulation. General coldness and pallor are always noticed in poisoning by the bean.

2. Physostigma is almost the only drug besides Opium which contracts the pupil. It does this whether locally or internally exhibited. The careful investigations of von Graefe and Robertson have shown that the ciliary muscle is contracted as well as—and even before—the iris, so that accommodation is impaired, and myopia induced. There is

set up in the eye a condition precisely opposite to that caused by atropia, which produces dilatation of the pupil, paralysis of accommodation, and presbyopia. The rationale of the action is found by some in sympathetic paralysis; by others in excitation of the third nerve. I am unable to assent to either hypothesis; for I find none of the evidences of depressed sympathetic energy, as we have seen them from the influence of Opium, nor can I think that a drug which causes general paralysis can stimulate one of the nerves of the cranio-spinal axis. I should rather ascribe the condition to the direct action of the drug on the muscular substance of the iris, answering to that which we have seen it exerting upon other muscles. This is also Binz's view. Von Graefe says that on carefully watching the progress of the myosis, the iris is seen to contract convulsively with little jerks or twitches, which are so small and rapid that they easily escape observation. These seem analogous to the tremors of the voluntary muscles and the peristaltic agitation of the intestines. The action on accommodation (which consists in approximation of both the far and the near point of vision) progresses by the same spasms or jerks; and oscillation of the eyeballs has been observed.

A word as to the *sensations* which accompany these phenomena. In poisoning, they are those of extreme giddiness and faintness and utter powerlessness, with sluggish articulation. When more moderate doses are taken, severe pressure at the epigastrium, immediately below the sternum, is complained of; it is accompanied with eructations. It is compared to that which results from bolting large morsels, or swallowing indigestible food. The provers were mostly overpowered with drowsiness, and indisposed for mental work. Many had a severe frontal headache, with a feeling of tension in the muscles of the forehead. Though contraction of the pupils is caused by the internal use of the drug in sufficient quantity, no sensations of any moment are perceived in the eyes. But when it is locally applied, the myopia of which I have spoken occurs. Even near objects are not seen distinctly; and Mr. Bowman found when experimenting on himself that astigmatism was produced. Using the eyes for binocular vision (as in reading) causes pain, blurring, and sense of straining. Nervous achings may occur in the eyeball affected, extending along the supra-orbital nerves and over half the head; and towards the end of the myotic action there is experienced, even without provocation, a painful tension, partly in the equator of the ball, and partly in the ciliary region.

There are of course two possible applications of these facts—one on the principle *contraria contrariis*, the other on that of *similia similibus*. Upon the former Physostigma has been used in strychnia poisoning and in tetanus, and with occasional success. But such large doses are required to induce its physiological effects upon the cord that the heart often becomes dangerously affected, and even peril from paralytic asphyxia occurs. These inconveniences are well seen in a case reported in much detail in the thirteenth volume of the *Practitioner* (p. 338); and they were found by Dr. Hughes Bennett's Committee to render the bean useless as a standing antidote to strychnia. The excitant action of the drug on unstriped muscular fibre has led to its use in atony of the digestive and respiratory tubes (in one case causing "phantom tumour"); and its power over the eye has been utilised for the counteraction of the effects of atropia, and for the relief of mydriasis and weakened accommodation when otherwise arising. Its homœopathic application has been indicated by Dr. Ringer, who has given it with much benefit in general paralysis of the insane and progressive muscular atrophy. He administers the thirtieth of a grain of the extract, a whole grain being the ordinary dose. He has since (*Lancet*, Dec. 22 and 29, 1877) recorded several cases of paralytic disease in other forms in which it has proved useful, among them locomotor ataxy. That the benefit was generally temporary only seems inevitable, when we consider the "functional" nature of the paralysis induced by the drug. Dr. Woodyatt, of Chicago, has recently put the drug to a very important use, viz., for acquired myopia resulting from ciliary spasm, which he thinks a frequent and important factor in the affection. From Physostigma, given in the third decimal dilution four times a day, he has obtained "results favourable beyond expectation."* Dr. Woodyatt is a competent oculist, and his statements come to us with every recommendation. His pathology has been called in question by one of his own colleagues, but I think he has abundantly vindicated the soundness of his position. He might have quoted the corroborative testimony of Soelberg Wells, who writes :—" Dombrowsky and others find that rapid increase of myopia is often due to spasm of the ciliary muscle, which also causes asthenopia," and again—" Spasm of the ciliary muscle (apparent myopia) is not of such unfrequent occurrence as is often supposed. We have already seen that it may accompany myopia and astigmatism ; but it is most frequently observed in youthful hypermetropes who have strained their

* *United States Medical Investigator,* ii., 375 ; v., 390 ; vi., 44.

eyes much in reading, sewing, &c., without using convex glasses ; this continued tension of the accommodation producing a spasmodic contraction of the ciliary muscle, or apparent myopia. Such patients complain chiefly of two sets of symptoms, viz. : those of marked asthenopia during reading and fine work, and also that they are short-sighted."

Drs. Allen and Norton say—"Twitching of the lids should attract our attention to this drug, especially if combined with spasm of the ciliary muscle, as in one case in which there was twitching around the eyes, patient could not read at all without much pain, frontal headache aggravated by any light, Physostigma gave quick relief."

Eserine, the active principle of Physostigma, has of late found a good deal of tentative employment in ocular affections. Dr. Knapp, of New York, at one time proclaimed it as useful in acute glaucoma as atropine is in iritis ; and he still makes habitually a corresponding employment of it, though he admits that it only exceptionally cures. He also says that, as with atropine, its use in chronic glaucoma may set up an acute attack ; and that, in irritable eyes, its myotic effect is liable to induce iritis.* Mr. Walker, of Liverpool, has suggested the rationale of the action of eserine in glaucoma to be as follows. He considers that long-continued over-use of the ciliary muscle, causing spasm, may and often does cause the glaucomatous condition ; and hence that eserine, which can induce such spasm, does harm rather than good in most cases of the disease. After the cyclotomy which he practises, however, he finds it very useful ; and thinks that it acts by opening the discharge-pipes of the anterior chamber.†

I have little doubt but that the study of the provings of the Calabar bean will lead to further applications of it as time goes on. It compares well with *Gelsemium*, and perhaps with *Baryta acetica*. *Muscaria*, moreover, and the newly-discovered *Jaborandi* have many analogies with it in their action on the pupil and on secretion ; and, like Physostigma, are somewhat antidotal to Atropia.

We will speak next of the poke,

Phytolacca.

The P. decandra of America is the variety commonly used,

* *London Medical Record*, Feb. 15, 1879.
† *Essays in Ophthalmology*, 1879.

but the P. octandra of Australia seems to have the same
action.* The tincture is commonly prepared from the green
root ; but as there is some reason to believe that the berries
act medicinally, especially in rheumatism, it might be better to
employ the whole plant.

The original proving of Phytolacca appeared in the second
volume of the Transactions of the American Institute of
Homœopathy. It is collated with other provings—making
sixteen in all—and several poisonings and experiments on
animals, in an arrangement of the drug which appears in
Dr. Hering's *Materia Medica*. The article on the drug in
Dr. Hale's *New Remedies* is also full of information
regarding it, and Allen adds symptoms from some fresh
sources.

The interest of Phytolacca resides in three aspects of its
operation : its action on the throat, its power over certain
manifestations of syphilis and rheumatism, and its influence
upon the mammary glands.

I. Phytolacca is undoubtedly a specific irritant of the
throat. All the provers suffered more or less at this part.
The fauces appeared much, sometimes darkly, reddened, and
the tonsils swollen : one prover had thick white and yellow
mucus about the fauces. But it was a startling inference from
such premisses that Phytolacca would prove a valuable remedy
in *diphtheria*. Nevertheless, this inference Dr. Burt, one of
its provers, did make ; and his success and that of the many
American practitioners who have imitated his practice seems
to have justified him in so doing. Dr. Bayes has since introduced Phytolacca into English practice as the principal remedy
for diphtheria ; and again most gratifying results were
obtained both by himself and by many of his colleagues.†
The only dissonant note was struck by myself ;‡ and I fear I
must here prolong it.

That Phytolacca was curative in the cases recorded I do
not question for a moment. But on going carefully through
them I must say that I do not recognise in them the symptoms I have learned to dread in diphtheria. Some, indeed,
were instances of simple inflammatory ulceration of the
tonsils ; for when the so-called false membrane came away, it
left " large holes " behind it, which the diphtheritic pellicle
never does. The great majority, however, were undoubtedly
diphtheritic in nature. But they seem to bear to the really

* See Dr. Sherwin's remarks in *Monthly Hom. Review*, ix., 279.
† See *Monthly Hom. Review*, vols. ix. and x.
‡ *Ibid*, x., 169.

dangerous form of the disease much the same relation as scarlatina anginosa to scarlatina maligna. In no case among those recorded in America or in England is fœtor of the breath mentioned, save in two out of my own three ; and both these died. In nearly all there was high fever, with pains in the head, back, and limbs—symptoms which are never present, according to my experience, in bad cases of diphtheria. I apprehend, indeed, that it is the occurrence of these very symptoms which constitutes the special indication for Phytolacca. In a paper entitled "An Account of fifty cases of Diphtheria," which I read before the British Homœopathic Society in 1870,* I have related how this form of the malady first came before me in 1865, and how then and subsequently Phytolacca unmistakeably proved its specific remedy. Equally good results, I may mention, followed its use after Belladonna had failed in a case where, with these constitutional symptoms, the "large holes in the tonsils" followed the disappearance of the white patches. But then you will read how, becoming hopeful about the new remedy, I gave it assiduously in a case of what Dr. Hilbers graphically calls "stinking diphtheria." The throat certainly cleared under its use ; but the morbid process went on in the nose, invaded the larynx, and death from exhaustion closed the scene.

I have thus been led to conclude that Phytolacca is specific in diphtheria where high fever, with aching in head, back, and limbs, is present ; but is incompetent to cope with the malignant form of the disease. Nevertheless, the other variety is genuine diphtheria, for it is quite capable of leaving paralytic symptoms behind it ; so that Phytolacca is a real anti-diphtheritic. If Dr. Burt's urinary symptoms are confirmed, moreover, they go to show its essential homœopathicity to the disease ; for to the inflamed and patchy throat they add albuminuria. I am glad to find that Dr. Hale, in his fourth edition, while insisting strongly on this last point, agrees nevertheless with me as to the form of the malady to which the use of Phytolacca should be restricted. He states that in America it often occurs epidemically. Dr. Bayes now seems to think that the medicine acts as "a specific stimulant to those organs and tissues which are primarily depressed by the diphtheritic deposit—the throat, the heart, and the stomach." He lays much stress on its application by wash or gargle simultaneously with its internal administration.

II. Some of the facts mentioned in Dr. Hale's first account of Phytolacca indicated that it was a periosteal medicine, like

* *Brit. Journ. of Hom.*, xxviii., 731.

Mezereum. A recent case of overdosing with it, which is given at length in the "Symptomatology" of his fourth edition, shows its power of causing periostitis of the forehead and face, together with blotches, sore and painful, of the whole surface of the body, afterwards invading the mouth and the throat. The suggestion of secondary syphilis is here unmistakeable ; and we hear from time to time of its curing-rupia, ulcers of the feet, and other manifestations of this diathesis, but more especially that periosteal affection which is called syphilitic rheumatism. Extending its action in another direction, it has been found to act well in true rheumatism affecting the other fibrous tissues, as the sheaths of nerves and the fasciæ ; herein resembling Rhus. The tincture prepared from the berries seems especially serviceable here.

III. To the influence of Phytolacca on the *mammary glands* attention was first called by Dr. Hale himself in the twenty-first volume of the *British Journal of Homœopathy.* The article is reproduced in his *New Remedies.* It appears from this that the poke root is in constant use in the dairies to remove "caking," *i. e.,* inflammatory engorgement of the udders. Dr. Hale has used it successfully for this purpose in the human female, and finds it useful even after suppuration has commenced, and when sinuses have formed. I have myself never wanted any medicine but Bryonia in threatened milk abscess ; but when the mischief outruns the abortive power of that medicine I habitually rely upon Phytolacca. I have recently had a chronic case of mastitis in which it proved most beneficial. Dr. Hale commends this medicine also in irritable mammary tumours, and where the breasts are morbidly sensitive at the menstrual period or during suckling.

I once had a case where the adminstration of Phytolacca obviated any injury which might have resulted from a necessarily obscure diagnosis. In a baby of a few months old, a succession of restless nights occurred simultaneously with the development of a hard tender swelling about midway between the nipple and the sternum, but nearer the latter than the former. Whether the inflammation was affecting some of the elements of the undeveloped mammary gland, or whether it lay in the periosteum of a rib, appeared uncertain. In any case, however, Phytolacca was indicated. I gave it in the sixth dilution, and the malady rapidly disappeared.

These, I say, are the main spheres of the medicinal action of Phytolacca. But the breast is not the only gland it affects ; nor is diphtheria the only form of throat disease over which it exerts control. Several cases are on record proving its power to disperse enlarged lymphatic and salivary glands : and the following one reported by Dr. Allen will show what it can do in one form of chronic angina faucium.

"The patient, a man aged 45, had had chronic follicular pharyngitis for several years. No remedies had done him much good.

"Symptoms. — Physical : membrane lining fauces and pharynx, as well as the velum pendulum and the uvula, pale, puffy, and flabby. Uvula large, almost translucent. Rational: distressing sense of enlargement of the calibre of the pharynx and œsophagus from the choanæ to the epigastrium. This symptom much aggravated by exposure to damp winds. It then begins at the choanæ, and in twelve hours extends to the epigastrium. On reaching this point it provokes a cough, paroxysmal, extremely distressing, and accompanied with very profuse and exhausting expectoration of thick, starch-like mucus. The whole chest then feels like a big empty cask, as if its calibre were enlarged tenfold. Great constitutional debility along with these attacks, so that the patient, who is ordinarily intolerant of stimulants, can take whiskey to any extent, and with great temporary relief.

"Phytolacca decandra 6, a dose every other night for a month, cured this condition."

The analogues of Phytolacca are *Mezereum, Guaiacum, Kali iodatum* and *bichromicum, Mercurius* and *Rhus.* Its curative virtues have hitherto been obtained almost entirely from the mother tincture.

LECTURE XLVIII.

PHOSPHORUS.

I have to bring before you to-day one of our greatest poly-chrests—a medicine which will repay the utmost care we may bestow upon its study,

Phosphorus.

The pharmaceutical preparation of this peculiar substance is itself a large matter. In the old school, solutions in sulphuric ether and olive oil have generally been used. Mr. Ashburton Thompson has recently shown that the latter vehicle is very objectionable, as allowing of the free oxidation of the phosphorus, whereby hypophosphorous acid is produced, which is far more irritant than its base. He shows that all the unexpected poisonings which have deterred physicians from the medicinal use of Phosphorus have arisen from this preparation. The solution in ether, however, is all that can be desired. Hahnemann recommended it as an alternative to trituration; and the British Homœopathic Pharmacopœia, in its first edition, did the same, pointing out that the vehicle takes up almost exactly one per cent., thus making our first attenuation. In its second edition, it directs the primary solution to be of the 3x strength, making it either with absolute alcohol, or with equal parts of this and ether. Subsequent potencies may be prepared with rectified spirit. Mr. Thompson recommends the administration of Phosphorus in glycerine, instead of water to avoid decomposition. Another excellent preparation of it, according to this writer, is a solution in cod-liver oil, which takes it up freely, and does not—like the vegetable oils—allow of its oxidation.

A pathogenesis of Phosphorus was published by Hahnemann in the first edition of the *Chronic Diseases*. It contains 1,025 symptoms, of which 963 are his own—that is, as we have seen, observed upon patients taking the drug in infinitesimal doses. Soon after, additional provings from themselves and three others were published—without explanation of their origin—by Hartlaub and Trinks in their *Arzneimittellehre*. These, in the second edition of the *Chronic Diseases*, were incorporated by Hahnemann with his old and some new material, making a total of 1,915—the longest list in the collection, save that of Sulphur. 1,169 of these are his own, 662 from nine *collaborateurs*, and 84 from authors.

I must leave to your discretion what use you will make of this pathogenesis. I have already expressed my entire lack of confidence in the symptoms obtained on the principles avowed by Hahnemann, and mainly followed by his disciples, in the *Chronic Diseases* period. It is otherwise with many later provings of the school; and in the case of Phosphorus we have some excellent ones from Dr. Sorge and eleven associates. He has published these, with a copious collection of poisonings, of experiments on men and animals, and of cases cured by the drug, in his *Der Phosphor, ein grosses Heilmittel* (Leipsic, 1862), the prize-essay of the Central Homœopathic Society of Germany. For materials of later date I may refer you to a paper by Dr. Holcombe, "Phosphorus; a pathogenetic study," in the seventh volume of the *North American Journal of Homœopathy;* to another, "On the action of Phosphorus upon the Liver," by Dr. Madden and myself, in the twenty-first volume of the *British Journal of Homœopathy;* to Wegner's experiments on animals, translated from *Virchow's Archiv* in the thirty-first volume of the same journal; and to the treatise on *Free Phosphorus in Medicine*, by Mr. Ashburton Thompson (London, 1874), on whose pharmaceutical portion I have already drawn. Dr. Allen, including all pertinent matter from these sources, adds the symptoms of a number of fresh cases of poisoning.

The history of Phosphorus as a medicine has been curious and interesting. The primary stimulant influence which we shall see that it possesses, and which it exerts especially upon the nervous system, was for a long time all that was known of its action; and this property was made use of (often with success) in typhoid and other adynamic states. But so many accidents occurred from the large doses and (as we have seen) unsuitable preparations employed, that the drug became branded as dangerous, and, until lately, was seldom employed in the old school. Dierbach and Trousseau and Pidoux omit it from their works on Materia Medica; and it did not appear in Dr. Ringer's until its fourth edition. Its extinguished flame has recently been rekindled from the homœopathic territory, where its light had long been burning steadily and brightly ; and now it bids fair, in the sphere of the nervous system at any rate, to resume an important place among remedies.

Hahnemann, though speaking of Phosphorus as a very important medicine, was misled by the stimulant properties of the drug into denying its homœopathic applicability to states of depression, which he regarded as only secondary reactions. We shall see that they are its real and lasting pathogenetic effects. This mistake, and the unsatisfactory nature of his symptom-list, kept the medicine in the background for some time. But then Fleischmann, Arnold, and Liedbeck took it up, and showed its power and virtues ; and *pari passu* with the advance of knowledge as to its poisonous effects, its use in our hands as a remedial agent has widened and extended. For old-school therapeutics it is of no advantage to learn that Phosphorus congests the lungs, necroses the maxillæ, softens the nervous centres, liquefies the blood, and causes fatty degeneration throughout the body. But to us such knowledge is fruitful of practical results ; and has already raised the drug into the first rank of our medicines.

1. Before, however, we dwell upon these phenomena, let us speak of the stimulant properties of Phosphorus. This substance is one of those which enter into the normal composition of the body. It exists mainly in the nervous centres, in the form of a peculiar compound with fatty matter which has been named " protagon ;" just as iron is united with hæmatin in the blood. It actually forms more than one per cent. of the human brain, the amount gradually increasing from infancy to adult age, and then again decreasing in old age. Now the analogy of iron and lime suggests that, up to a certain point, Phosphorus may be a special stimulant to the tissue it goes to constitute ; and, the stimulation being in some sort that of a food, it need not be followed by reactive depression.

That Phosphorus has such an action on the nervous system— as iron has on the blood and (probably) lime on the bones—is beyond doubt. " About the second hour," writes Mr. Thompson, " after a dose of the twentieth or the twelfth of a grain, sensations of exhilaration begin to make themselves felt. The capacity for exertion, both mental and physical, is increased, and that condition which the French describe as one of *bien-être* is experienced. If the subject have taken the dose while in a state of fatigue, he finds his strength renewed ; if while in a state of despondency, he takes a more cheerful view of things. The pulse becomes firmer and a little more frequent. These effects pass off gradually in the course of a few hours, and a state of depression does not ensue." With this there is often increase of temperature, perspiration and diuresis, and sometimes venereal excitement.

It is this action of Phosphorus which made it available, given in full and frequent doses, in typhoid depression, and often rallied a patient from an apparently hopeless condition. It is a property of the drug which we may well employ, understanding clearly what it is—that we are giving it as we give alcoholic stimulants, and not as a medicine. After the same fashion it may be used, if it is needed, instead of a glass of wine for temporary nervous exhaustion ; remembering, however, that rest and food—if there is time for them—are far better remedies. But there is another application of the stimulant power of Phosphorus which has of late attracted much attention, viz., the relief and even cure of neuralgia obtained therefrom. Phosphorus causes and cures in minute doses its own form of neuralgia ; but this is rarely met with in comparison with that which requires Arsenicum, Belladonna, Aconite, Colocynth and Sulphur. The drug has hence occupied no prominent place in homœopathic therapeutics as an anti-neuralgic remedy ; but we have known how to use it when required. A cure of the intercostal form, wrought by one of us with it after long-continued unsuccessful treatment by an old-school practitioner, called the attention of the latter to the remedy ; and he and others tested it in various instances of the affection, and reported favourably of their results. It is here that Mr. Ashburton Thompson came upon the field. He treated some fifty cases with the medicine, with a 'success which leads him to regard it as an almost infallible remedy for pure neuralgia, wherever occurring, and as rapid in its action as it is lasting. But to obtain such result, he says, the medicine must be given in a full, *i.e.*, a stimulant dose, not less indeed than a twelfth of a grain every four hours. Thus its *modus operandi* seems to be that of food and wine, whose influence over neuralgic pain is so well known : only that its relation to nervous tissue gives it stimulant and perhaps nutrient qualities of a special kind. I think that medicine is much indebted to Mr. Thompson for working out this subject, as well as for his valuable contributions to the pharmacy and posology of the drug. We have, in most cases, remedies for neuralgia of more satisfactory kind ; but were we at a *non plus*, we might do worse than follow his practice.

But it is with Phosphorus as a neurotic as with iron as an

hæmatic : if too long continued, or taken in excess, it acts as a poison to the very tissues which it stimulates and feeds. Iron can in this way impoverish the blood, causing anæmia ; and Phosphorus still more surely impairs the vitality of the nervous centres, and gives rise to paralysis. In acute poisoning symptoms of this kind must be received with caution, as the effect on the nervous centres of an altered blood and a fattily degenerated heart must be taken into account ; and also the possibility of hæmorrhagic effusion into the membranes of the cord and the sheaths of the spinal nerves, which in a case of Bollinger's showing paralysis of the legs was actually found to be present. But, making all allowance for these facts, there are cases of acute poisoning by the drug which seem to exhibit pure paralytic phenomena. Among those given by Dr. Hempel, in one there was numbness of the extremities, with formication—the fingers having so little sensibility that they could not pick up a pin ; and in another there was amaurosis with widely-dilated pupils, and deafness. In an excellent study of " Phosphoric Paralysis," by Dr. Gallavardin of Lyons, translated from *L'Art Médical* in the twentieth volume of the *British Journal of Homœopathy*, two cases are given, in one of which the left arm, in the other the hands, became powerless. But the most striking instance of the kind presented by him is one in which, life being prolonged, there was progressive paralysis. It is cited from Huss's *Chronic Alcoholism*, as follows :—

"A man, æt. 39, who led an ordinary kind of life, occupied himself for three years in the preparation of phosphoric matches. He used to work in the room where he lived, and there he kept the materials and the product of his trade. He had suffered no inconvenience from it until a year ago, when a great quantity of Phosphorus and of phosphorated matches took fire, after a violent explosion. At the time, whilst trying to extinguish the conflagration, he so thoroughly respired the vapour of Phosphorus, that at last he fainted from suffocation. Immediately after this he experienced a sensation of weakness in the back, as if he were ready to sink ; then weakness in the extremities, and trembling at every effort ; creeping under the skin, and a sensation as if something were starting under the epidermis. At first, great sexual excitement, which afterwards diminished, and for the last six months gave place to impotence, with absolute impossibility of erection.

" Independent of that, he found himself well, with good appetite ; regular evacuations ; good health ; normal re-

spiration.   Nothing indicated any affection of the brain.
On his admission to the hospital, the following symptoms
were remarked : his two legs were so weak that he could
only walk a few steps, and even that he did with a tottering
gait, and as if he were not sure of himself; if he tried to
stand upright, his legs trembled and his knees bent; his
hands and arms trembled on making an effort.   In the state
of repose, the muscles started out all over the body, especially
in the extremities.   *They seemed to be twitching to and fro,
though painlessly; different muscles or bundles of muscles
twitched at different periods.   At times the twitching stopped,
but it was easily excited by contact.*   On the left arm, a
constant feeling of formication under the skin ; normal sensation over the general surface of the body.   The spine not
sensitive, nor painful, but so weak that the patient cannot
straighten himself, nor remain standing when once straight-
ened.   The faculties, both intellectual and moral, the functions of the heart, of the chest, and of the digestive organs,
normal ; but the pronunciation embarrassed (? paralysis of
the tongue).   The patient lived three or four years in the full
enjoyment of his senses, whilst the paralysis increased and extended ; but all the attempts at treatment were unavailing."

Dr. Gallavardin also mentions the experiments on animals
of Mayer.   The conclusions of this observer are—" Phosphorus
acts specifically on the nerves of voluntary motion, and on the
muscles themselves.   It impedes, diminishes, and at last
entirely destroys the power of movement, or rather it destroys
the irritability of the motor nerves, and the contractility of the
muscular fibres, and at last completely paralyses the powers."
He adds that it also " acts specifically on the nerves of sensation, destroying sensibility from the periphery to the brain,
the sensorium being in small degree disturbed."

To all this corresponds the condition of the nervous centres
commonly found in the animals poisoned by it, as you may
read in Sorge's treatise.   This is nearly always described as
" pale, soft, and bloodless," and Arnold found its prolonged
use to induce actual softening.

It follows that Phosphorus is truly homœopathic to paralytic conditions, when dependent on lowered vitality or even
softening of the centres ; and should be a valuable remedy
therein.   Dr. Gallavardin cites thirteen cases of the kind,
twelve from old-school and one from homœopathic sources.
Dr. Trinks has recorded another, described with his wonted
fulness and accuracy, which may be found in the nineteenth
volume of the *British Journal ;* and Sorge and Mr. Thompson

give some more.* They were nearly all of a "functional" nature—from amenorrhœa, seminal losses, exhaustion from acute disease, and such-like causes. In one case the loss of power involved only the third, in another only the sixth pair of cranial nerves. In softening of the brain from exhaustion Phosphorus seems acquiring quite a reputation in the old school; but it has long been in use for it among homœopathists. Jahr praises it also in corresponding cerebral conditions of less advanced degree, as "nervous vertigo" and hydrocephaloid. The muscular symptoms of the case I have narrated suggest the "fibrillary contractions" of "wasting palsy," the "progressive muscular atrophy" of Duchenne. With Phosphorus, indeed, we should not expect wasting of the muscles, but simply their fatty degeneration; and a form of the disease has been described by Duchenne which he calls "pseudo-hypertrophic paralysis," in which this very condition obtains. In a little treatise, *On the various forms of Paralysis*, which I published some years ago, I suggested Phosphorus for this malady; and Mr. Clifton has obtained striking benefit from its persevering administration in the third decimal dilution, in a well-marked instance of it. The girl, who could not walk six yards when she came to him, could, after a little over a twelvemonth's treatment, accomplish her four miles without difficulty.†

It is customary in the old school to speak of Phosphorus as a "tonic" in these cases. I have shown that, like other tonics, it weakens in health where it strengthens in disease. It is more plausible to argue that, like iron in anæmia, it acts as a food. It may do so under some circumstances. But I think that the evidence of dosage, which favours the hypothesis in the other case, is against it here. Jahr is as laudatory of his decillionths as Thompson of his hundredths of a grain in cerebral softening; and even the latter doses would not do much to feed an organ which naturally contains some three quarters of an ounce of the substance. So I think we must conclude that it acts dynamically and homœopathically here, and is entitled to our highest consideration.

II. I will take next the symptoms produced by Phosphorus in the male sexual organs, as these are probably a part of its influence on the nervous system generally. They are, however, of sufficient importance to merit special and distinct consideration.

* See another, post-diphtheritic, and with impairment of sensation, in Hoyne (i., 100).
† See the case in *Brit. Journ. of Hom.*, xxxvi, 127.

The sexual organs share in the general excitement caused by moderate doses of Phosphorus; but they manifest its influence in so marked a manner as to evidence a special action of the drug upon them, or upon that part of the nervous centre whence they derive their energy. That Phosphorus is an aphrodisiac has been known for a long time. It has displayed this property in a most unmistakeable manner among the lower animals. Leroy (quoted by Pereira) ascertained that it was aphrodisiac to drakes. In Dr. Sorge's experiments cocks, pigeons, dogs, and frogs were affected in the same way; the latter got those large growths on their fore feet that appear during their pairing season, and used them accordingly. But the same prover's experiments on the human subject show that this excitement is but temporary, and is followed by a much longer-continued depression, as we see in Dr. Gallavardin's case just cited, showing itself in absence of desire, imperfect erections, with too rapid ejaculatio seminis, and frequent involuntary emissions.

Phosphorus is thus a thoroughly homoeopathic remedy for that irritable weakness of the male sexual organs which is left behind by excesses in venery and by masturbation. Experience has over and over again confirmed the indications of theory in this matter. Phosphorus would also (in very small doses) be homoeopathic to satyriasis, which corresponds to its primary effects; for this Jahr recommends it from experience. Might it also be desirable to use it occasionally as a special stimulant, in full doses, as in impotentia senilis when offspring is much desired? The following observation from Dr. Sorge's collection shows that great caution must be exercised here :—" An old dog who had long lost his sexual power, after taking phosphorus rat-poison that was given to kill him, became sexually excited, *and died in the act of coitus.*"

III. I would now direct your attention to the well-known action of Phosphorus upon the jaws, as mainly seen in the workers in lucifer-match manufactories. The fullest researches instituted on this subject are those of von Bibra and Geist, of which, if you have not access to the original, you may read a full account in the eleventh volume of the *British Journal of Homœopathy.* The disease usually begins in a carious tooth, which gnaws and throbs, and sometimes shoots, with itching and bleeding of the neighbouring gum. Then gum-boils form, and discharge fœtid pus in which are found granules of bone. Then the teeth fall out, and the gums recede or melt away, and the bone appears in a state of caries or necrosis. Inflammation of the neighbouring parts and irritative fever are present : and the case often terminates in death. It is a moot point whether this effect of Phosphorus is produced by a local and chemical action on the parts, or whether it is a result of the dynamic influence of the poison. In favour of the latter being the true interpretation of at least some part of the morbid process is a case of poisoning by Phosphorus recorded by Dr. J. O. Müller, on the fourteenth day of which there came on painful boring burning pains in the bones, especially in the teeth, the jaws, and the nose.* They were removed by Mezereum, a drug which has cured the maxillary caries of the workers in Phosphorus.

This conclusion has been thought to be impugned by the recent experiments of Dr. Wegner ; but I am unable to draw such a conclusion from them. He finds that if rabbits are kept for some time in an atmosphere impregnated with the fumes of Phosphorus, in a small minority only does there appear periostitis and necrosis of the jaws, just as the same thing occurs in but a few of the workers in it. He fairly argues that there must be some personal causal condition in each individual case, in addition to the general influence to which all are exposed alike ; but I cannot follow him in his further assumption that this condition must be a local exposure of the periosteum from dental caries or injury to the gum. For he admits that in one only of his suffering rabbits could he find any such lesion ;† and that carious teeth are not always discoverable in the affected workers. Instead, therefore, of laying stress on the fewness of those exposed to the Phosphorus vapours whose jaws are affected without local access for the irritant, the fact that any are so affected should indicate that the influence is not local but constitutional.

Still more striking evidence to this effect is derived from the results obtained by Dr. Wegner from feeding the same class of animals with long-continued minute doses of Phosphorus—from one to three milligrammes according to one calculation, from the four-hundredth to the hundredth of a grain according to another, daily. Here an influence is produced upon the osteogenetic tissue (of which periosteum is the chief representative) all over the body, which leads to increased

---

* *North American Journ. of Hom.*, vii., 467.

† Dr. H. Wood's statement is thus quite incorrect that "Wegner found that when rabbits were kept in an atmosphere full of the fumes of the poison no necrosis ever occurred, unless, by means of an unsound tooth or an artificial wound, the atmosphere had access to the bone."

production of osseous matter, to thickening of the spongy and greater density of the compact substance of the long and short bones, and even in some instances to the obliteration of the medullary cavity by the continuous fresh formation. Dr Wegner himself cannot but see the analogy of all this with the effects on the jaws produced by the fumes. "Phosphorus," he sums up, "in minute doses in all probability is dissolved in the blood, and, circulating with it, operates on the osteogenetic tissue as a specific plastic irritant. Brought topically in the form of vapour into contact with denuded periosteum, in moderate concentration it provokes ossifying periostitis : while, if the fumes operate very energetically, the irritation becomes so intense that suppuration is added to the ossificatory process." I should have said that in the maxillary disease of the workmen and the rabbits there is always a combination of new osseous deposits with the necrosis of the old bone.

The results obtained by these small internal doses thus throw much light on the nature of the osseous affection induced by exposure to the phosphoric vapours ; but they are also of much importance in themselves. Dr. H. Wood represents them as if they evidenced merely a stimulant influence on the nutrition of the tissue. I cannot so read them ; nor does Dr. Wegner really regard them in this light. He connects them with alterations he finds the drug, when given in the same way, to produce in the stomach and liver—alterations which, as we shall see, are essentially of a morbid kind. "Older observations," he writes, "have taught that Phosphorus in large doses influences certain tissues, particularly the parenchymatous elements of the liver, of the kidneys, of the stomach, and of the muscles, as an extraordinary intense per-acute irritation, of such a violent nature that in a very short space of time a fatty degeneration, a necro-biosis of the same, follows. We have now seen that the same substance, given to the organism in a smaller quantity, while leaving the first-named parts perfectly immune, possesses an irritative influence on totally different kinds of tissue, on the osteogenetic substance, on the interstitial tissue of the liver and of the stomach ; an irritative influence which has not a degenerative, but essentially a formative tendency."

From the traditional point of view, the natural application of this power of Phosphorus would be to further bone-production in cases where it was defective, as in osteo-malacia and rachitis, or where it was needed in temporary excess, as in fractures, intra-periosteal resections, and transplantations of

this membrane. In the latter field Dr. Wegner has no doubt
of its beneficial operation ; and within certain limits the process is a physiological one. In osteo-malacia and rachitis he
can report no decided results ; and indeed in both the condition
is too complex for help to be expected from simple increase
in osteogenetic activity. He makes a remark, however, regarding the latter disease which is very suggestive to us.
" Under the simultaneous influence," he says, " of feeding with
phosphorus, and of the deprivation of the inorganic substances,
especially of lime, the mode of growth of bones is altered so
as exactly to correspond to what we are accustomed to call
rachitis." He then describes the result of such an experiment,
ending—" The conditions under which this artificial rachitis
arises are a not unwelcome confirmation of the theory which
an exact observation of the process has already set up, viz.,
that rachitis is conditioned by two factors ; first, an insufficient
quantity of inorganic salts in the blood, either from insufficient
ingestion of the same, or from their excessive elimination ;
secondly, a constitutional irritation influencing the osteogenetic
tissue." For us of course the inference is that we should use
Phosphorus as a medicinal agent here ; and indeed Phosphoric
acid already holds a high place in the homœopathic therapeutics of the disease. Other applications in this direction
of the osseous influence of Phosphorus are obvious. It should
be useful in some forms of periostitis and necrosis. Kafka
reports it to be a most efficacious medicine, in conjunction
with Natrum muriaticum, in interstitial disease of the
vertebræ and of the cancellous structure of bones in general
I have myself been led to its use in cases where the irritation
of a carious tooth is causing frequent gumboils and incipient
disease of the maxilla, and where for some reason or other
we are debarred from extraction of the offending member.
Here I have found it most efficacious. Dr. Bayes, also, praises
it highly in many affections of the teeth and gums. I may
mention that gingivitis, with looseness of the teeth, has been
observed, not only in acute poisoning by Phosphorus, where
it might be secondary to blood changes, but from its medicinal use.

IV. I have yet to speak of the action of Phosphorus in other
regions. Let us consider, first, what it does in the alimentary
canal and in the respiratory organs.

1. Phosphorus, in its unaltered state, is not a local irritant.
It does not set up gastro-enteritis as the corrosive poisons do,
unless (as I have said) it becomes oxidised in the stomach,
and hypophosphorous acid is formed. But however it is in-

troduced into the system, it is liable to set up what Virchow calls a gastro-adenitis, a swelling and shedding of the epithelial cells of the mucous membrane like that we have seen occasionally induced by Arsenic, and like that which obtains in cholera. The same process goes on in the intestines, and is accompanied there by diarrhœa, as in the stomach by vomiting. This is its acute action. But, when gradually ingested by rabbits, Wegner finds it to set up an irritation of the interstitial connective tissue of the stomach, causing a "chronic indurative gastritis, with thickening, analogous to cirrhosis of the liver." From one or other of these processes may occur the condition described by Taylor:—"chronic poisoning by the drug is accompanied by cardialgia, frequent vomiting, sense of heat in the stomach, diarrhœa, tenesmus, pains in the joints, marasmus, hectic fever, and disease of the stomach, under which the patient may slowly sink."

These facts should, I think, receive more homœopathic application than has yet been accorded to them. Chronic degeneration of the mucous membrane of the stomach may find in Phosphorus a potent remedy; the case recorded by Dr. Bolle,* and supposed to be of gastric cancer, may well have been of this kind. Phosphorus has a fair repute in Germany in chronic dyspepsia characterised by sour risings, heat at the epigastrium, flatulence, and canine hunger, of which several instances relieved by it are given by Sorge. Hahnemann himself mentions chronic diarrhœa, with soft and thin stools, as a special indication for it; it is of most service when this malady affects nervous subjects and delicate children. Mr. Proctor found it very useful in cholera, to check the drain of brownish fluid from the bowels which sometimes continued after the other symptoms had subsided.† But, next to the stomach, Phosphorus seems to act most powerfully upon the rectum. A prover, who took five drops of the tincture, experienced a severe attack of dysentery from his dose. "The passages were like the scrapings of the intestines, and almost constant, attended with tenesmus for upwards of two hours; involuntary passages occurred on the least motion; eight hours later, the passages changed to mucus, and mucus mixed with blood and slime, still involuntary. At the end of twelve hours, passages began to become periodical at every half-hour, and then every hour, still involuntary, with tenesmus at least an hour after each passage, when they became as far apart as two hours. During the second night," he says, "I was com-

* *Brit. Journ. of Hom.*, xii., 173.
† *Ibid.*, xxv., 95.

pelled to use the vessel a number of times, making my calculations to have a passage every two hours, as they were
involuntary the moment anything entered the rectum; this condition lasted for two days, and subsequently every time I went
from the warm room into the open air my bowels would
move." I quote from Dr. Allen, who emphasises the involun-
tariness of the discharges as having been clinically confirmed.
I have great confidence in it in chronic disease of the lower
part of the bowel. In one case I had under treatment a discharge of blood and pus, with tenesmus, had been going on
for eighteen months before I saw the patient. Phosphorus 30
effected speedy improvement, and in less than two months
entire disappearance of her symptoms; and she finished by
taking saccharum lactis for another month without any recurrence of her troubles. In another patient, the symptoms for
which he consulted me were those of incipient stricture of the
rectum, the fæces having already become flattened. There
was concomitant mucous discharge, and inquiry ascertained
that there had been an attack of acute proctitis about nine
months previously. Phosphorus 30 was curative here also, all
difficulty in defæcation and abnormal shape of fæces soon disappearing, and the discharge ceasing. An old-standing
urethral stricture was simultaneously much improved.

2. On the respiratory organs Phosphorus acts as a pure
irritant. I would not lay too much stress on the bronchitis,
emphysema, pneumonia, and pulmonary phthisis observed in
the workmen and rabbits exposed to its fumes, as these may
be but local effects. They are accompanied, however, with
the weakness, emaciation and hectic which characterise the
gastro-intestinal phenomena of the drug. But Magendie and
others have found hepatization of the lungs in animals poisoned by it; and the provers experienced decided symptoms
of laryngo-tracheal and bronchial irritation, and of pulmonary
congestion. For the last I may refer you to Dr. Holcombe's
thorough proving on himself. Its presence was evidenced by
great heat and oppression at the chest, obliging frequent
deep inspiration. Similar feelings were experienced by several
of the subjects of poisoning whose symptoms are given by
Allen, and in two of them the physical signs of pneumonia
were present. In the first—" percussion showed slight dulness on the right lower portion posteriorly, with diminished
respiratory murmur and fine vesicular râles; change of posture caused a change in the area of dulness; vocal fremitus
diminished beneath the line of dulness on the right posterior
portion of the ninth dorsal vertebra; on the fourteenth day,

after a second chill, the dulness extended upward half an inch, and bronchial breathing was distinct over the area of dulness." On the seventh day the dulness and râles had diminished, but the cough, which was at first dry, with scanty sputa, now became paroxysmal, accompanied by expectoration of tenacious, purulent mucus. In the other case " percussion over the lower portion of the thorax was dull on the right side, with indistinct bronchial respiration and numerous râles; on the left side vesicular murmurs and some moist bronchial râles."

Correspondingly, Phosphorus occupies a high place in the homœopathic therapeutics of respiratory affections. Pneumonia was the disease in which it won its spurs. First introduced by Fleischmann, of Vienna, his great success with it when made known led to its general use by homœopathists in this country. His own countrymen have hardly concurred so fully in his choice,—Wurmb and Caspar rejecting it altogether, Kafka thinking it suitable only to catarrhal (broncho-) pneumonia, and Bähr and Clotar Müller inclining to limit its appropriateness to cases in which the disease threatens to deviate from its normal course, and where " nervous " (*i. e.* typhoid) symptoms appear. I must admit that to the typical " croupous " pneumonia, excited in fairly healthy subjects by exposure to cold, and accompanied by much pain, Phosphorus is less homœopathic than Bryonia. But I submit that we comparatively rarely see the disease under such circumstances, and that it most commonly occurs in delicate persons, with lowered health, or secondarily to such blood-infections as typhoid and scarlet fever. The exudation here would be rather corpuscular than fibrinous. Under such circumstances Phosphorus is preferable to any other medicine, and the frequent English use of it in pneumonia is justified accordingly. It is no less suitable—after Aconite—to acute pulmonary congestion, even when effusion has taken place,—Bähr and Kafka both praising it in acute œdema pulmonum. I agree also with the latter author as to its perfect applicability to broncho-pneumonia—the catarrhal or lobular pneumonia of the nosologists. In this malady occurring in children it is the one medicine which has given me satisfaction ; and, in fact, so apt is bronchitis in these subjects to run on into pneumonia that I always employ Phosphorus, after Aconite, in its treatment. Otherwise, it does not play an important part in the therapeutics of bronchitis, either acute or chronic, nor in those of respiratory inflammations higher up, save when they occur in a subacute and lingering form in delicate, overgrown, or phthisical subjects. In these persons, hacking, dry coughs, with sensation of tickling and perhaps dryness and burning in the larynx, may often yield to the drug.

A word here about the use of Phosphorus in pulmonary phthisis. It is of great service in many ways in this disease. It keeps down the hyperæmia of the lungs, quiets the cough, and often moderates the diarrhœa. It may thus be actually curative in pneumonic phthisis; and I have often seen incipient symptoms of chronic pulmonary mischief clear away under its use, in the medium dilutions. I am unable, however, to credit it with any power of checking the deposit or development of true tubercle. Neither our small doses of the pure substance, nor Dr. Churchill's larger quantities of the hypophosphites, can be relied upon for this purpose.

I must reserve the consideration of the remaining actions of Phosphorus for our next lecture.

LECTURE XLIX.

PHOSPHORUS (*continued*)—PLUMBUM.

We resume our consideration of the several categories into which the effects of Phosphorus upon the organism naturally fall.

V. In nearly all cases of poisoning by this substance which have been recorded during the last thirty years (mainly from the ingestion of lucifer-matches), while symptoms of irritation have not been absent, another and a very different group of phenomena arrests our attention. The patient appears to be suffering from. what used to be called "malignant jaundice." The skin and conjunctiva assume a more or less yellow tint, and the stools are light; but with this there is a general typhoid prostration which is absent from ordinary icterus. Petechiæ and hæmorrhages occur in various parts of the body. The urine is scanty, high coloured, and loaded with albumen. Cerebral symptoms—delirium, convulsions, &c., somewhat like those of uræmia—supervene, and the patient dies in a few days in a state of coma. At the post-mortem investigation nothing is discovered in the brain save a little fulness. But the blood is found in a state of complete fluidity, non-coagulable, and with very few red corpuscles, while ecchymoses and sanguineous effusions appear everywhere. The liver, which during life had been (at any rate at first) enlarged and tender, presents profound alterations of substance. It varies in size; but fatty degeneration is found to have taken place in its secreting structure. The acini are sometimes found filled with fat, even to bursting ; but more commonly they are wholly destroyed, and oil and fat-globules fill their place. The secreting structure of the kidneys also is found to be undergoing fatty degeneration, and the ducts are sometimes filled with exudation matter. When the examination has been carried farther, this fatty degeneration is found to have involved other parts of the body, notably the heart and the muscles generally. Numerous experiments on animals have verified these observations, and have put it beyond doubt that these remarkable changes of tissue are really producible by Phosphorus in the space of a few days, or even sooner.

In the paper by Dr. Madden and myself in the *British Journal*, which I have already mentioned, you will find a detailed account of these remarkable phenomena.*

What is their rationale? I would answer, in the first place, that the fundamental lesion is an acute fatty degeneration, which Phosphorus has the power of causing in every part of the body susceptible thereof. In the second place, I would refer the neurotic and hæmatic phenomena to the suspension of the functions of the liver and kidneys, owing to the metamorphosis of their secreting cells. I attach most importance to the affection of the liver. Although the cerebral symptoms resemble those of uræmia so far that they suggest the retention of a similarly hurtful excretion in the blood, they could hardly be mistaken for them. Combined with the petechiæ and hæmorrhages they present a morbid condition only present elsewhere in what Frerichs calls " acholia," *i. e.*, a suspension of the functions of the liver, owing to a destruction of its secreting cells. The most prominent instance of this lesion is acute atrophy of the liver; but it also occurs occasionally in the course of cirrhosis, obstructive jaundice, and other chronic hepatic affections. The symptoms are those of blood-poisoning, to which the nervous phenomena are probably secondary. I do not want to wander too far into pathology; but I must call your attention to the very interesting speculations on the subject of Dr. Austin Flint, of New York. His theory is that cholesterine is the excrementitious material of the bile as urea is of the urine, and that the blood-poisoning of acholia is accordingly a cholesteræmia. But I must proceed to inquire into the therapeutic bearing of these curious facts.

1. Phosphorus unquestionably deserves the fullest trial in malignant jaundice, especially where, as in the great majority of cases, the pathological condition is acute atrophy of the liver. All observers, including Frerichs himself, are struck with the resemblance of phosphoric poisoning to the phenomena which accompany this lesion. I was myself at first inclined to question the identity of the two, seeing that in acute atrophy the fatty change of the secreting cells is by no means a prominent feature. But it is sufficiently marked to lead three pathologists (Engel, Wedl, and Bamberger) to explain the

---

* To the references there given the following are a few additions *Brit Journ. of Hom.*, xxi., 460; xxiii., 128, 280; xxv., 520; *United States Med. and Surg. Journal*, ii., 274.

destruction of the cells by a fatty degeneration arising from an acute exudation process. And while in acute phosphoric poisoning the liver is felt to be enlarged (probably from hyperæmia), Lebert and Wyss have ascertained that in slower poisoning animals have their livers very much diminished in size, and in a state which cannot be anatomically distinguished from that of acute yellow atrophy. A case, moreover, is recorded as occurring in a London hospital which was diagnosed during life as acute atrophy, but in which, after death, " the entire disappearance of the true hepatic secreting structure and its conversion into oil and fatty matter rendered it a remarkable case, justifying the term acute fatty degeneration.* I think, therefore, that we may with propriety, if not with confidence, combat this nearly always fatal disease with our Phosphorus.

2. Dr. Holcombe, who was the first to call our attention to these pathogenetic effects of Phosphorus, suggested its use where jaundice complicates toxæmic disorders, and notably in yellow fever. More recently Dr. Ozanam, of Paris, seeing a case of this form of phosphoric poisoning in which to the other symptoms black vomit was added, was forcibly struck by the resemblance of the phenomena to those of the typhus icterodes, and wrote accordingly. I feel a difficulty in acceding to these views, because, according to Frerichs, there is not in yellow fever (or in jaundice accompanying typhus and pyæmia) any destruction of the hepatic cells, but rather, if anything, polycholia. I should prefer Crotalus and the serpent poisons for such jaundice, which seems to me of different origin, *i. e.*, hæmatic rather than hepatic. In this Dr. Holcombe now agrees with me.†

3. In Phosphorus we evidently have a homœopathic remedy for that important pathological change known as *fatty degeneration*, wherever occurring. I need hardly enlarge upon the picture thus opened to us of the applicability of our medicine. It is most obvious when this morbid process attacks the liver or the heart. Dr. Bayes speaks from experience of its value in chronic cases of the former malady ; and I have seen undoubted evidence of its power of arresting the progress of the disease in the cardiac substance. Dr. Lade has recorded a striking case of the kind, in which, simultaneously with the cardiac symptoms, an *arcus senilis* disappeared.‡ Acute fatty

* See *Brit. Journ. of Hom.*, xxiv, 166 ; and also the case in vol xxviii, p. 409.
† See Transactions of Amer. Institute of Homœopathy for 1868.
‡ Hoyne, i., 107.

degeneration of the heart is apt to occur in typhus; and here Phosphorus must be remembered. I would also remind you that the same process is thought by many to constitute atheroma of the arteries and mollities ossium; to be an occasional cause of softening of the brain and cord; and, occurring in the bronchial tubes, to predispose to emphysema.

4. Before leaving the liver, we must take away the thought that Phosphorus has a very specific action upon it as an organ, and may often be found curative in its diseases. The disorder we have seen set up in it is a diffuse inflammation—as distinguished from the circumscribed hepatitis of tropical countries which is so liable to go on to abscess. But Dr. Wegner finds it capable of causing, when gradually administered, an interstitial hepatitis also, in which the organ is hard, enlarged at first but subsequently atrophied, and then often presenting the typical granular form, the classical cirrhosis of the liver. With all this there is chronic icterus; and in the latter event there occur the secondary disturbances so well known in human pathology—ascites and so forth.

For both these forms of hepatic disease Phosphorus may prove serviceable : in cirrhosis, Dr. Salzer, of Calcutta, speaks warmly of it. It should also be borne in mind for jaundice, not only when complicating such graver maladies, but when occurring to all appearance idiopathically. It has been found capable of setting up the catarrhal inflammation of the bile-ducts which is so frequently the cause of this disorder. In jaundice from nervous excitement, moreover, it may be the best medicine to give, as this is every now and then (especially in pregnant women) the beginning of an acute atrophy of the liver.

5. We have yet remaining the renal and hæmatic symptoms of this form of phosphoric poisoning. It may be thought that the affection of the kidneys is secondary to that of the liver, as in two of Frerichs' best-described cases of acute atrophy fatty degeneration was discovered in their glandular cells. I must mention, however, that there is one case on record in which there was no jaundice or cerebral disturbance during life, although the liver was found (*post mortem*) enlarged and fatty. In this case the urine during life was highly coloured and frothy, its specific gravity increased, and it contained albumen and exudation cells. After death, the cortical substance of the kidneys was granular; the Malpighian corpuscles resembled red points; and on a microscopical examination the uriniferous tubuli were found blocked up by exu-

dation matter. While I agree with Dr. Hempel that this is
not Bright's disease, it is nevertheless a very decided nephritis ;
and warrants the expectation that Phosphorus may find a
place in the treatment of the idiopathic affection. It would be
indicated in chronic tubular nephritis when occurring as a result
of long-continued suppurations, as Bähr suggests. It should
also obviously be given in primary fatty degeneration of the
kidneys. The indication for it here is strengthened by the fact
that in one of Dr. G. Johnson's cases this affection (which
came on in three weeks' time) appeared to be the immediate
result of sexual excess.

Yet more difficult is the question whether the dissolution
of the blood induced by Phosphorus is the result of a direct
hæmatic influence, or is secondary to the affection of the liver,
in whose idiopathic form it is a constant phenomenon. The
latter would seem, from physiological evidence, to be the true
alternative, as I can find no record of one set of symptoms
occurring without the other. It has been maintained, however, that both in acute atrophy and in phosphoric poisoning
the hepatic lesion is secondary to a blood-infection. There
are also therapeutic results which favour the hypothesis of a
primary hæmatic action on the part of the drug. I would not
lay too much stress on its value in purpura, as it is doubtful
whether the hæmorrhages here depend upon changes in the
vessels or in the blood itself. For what it is worth, however,
in relation to the present question, and for its own sake, let
me mention that Arnold, Clotar Müller, and other German
physicians esteem Phosphorus the great remedy for purpura,*
and that under it, in Dr. Jousset's hands, a case of hæmorrhagic small-pox made a good recovery.† But the symptom
in Hahnemann's pathogenesis, "small wounds bleed freely,"
which has led to the choice of Phosphorus in such cases, has
also conducted to very valuable and unexpected results in no
less a disease than *fungus hæmatodes.*

The first to report success with it was Dr. Constantine
Hering, his patient being a negro in Surinam.‡ Then the
editor of the *United States Medical and Surgical Journal*§ published a case under the title " What was it ? " in which a vascular bleeding fungus on the thigh, the seat of darting pain, got
rapidly well under Phosphorus 30. This narrative led me to
give the medicine in the following case.

* See *United States Med. Investigator*, vii., 396.
† See also a case in *Amer. Hom. Review*, v., 566.
‡ See *Archiv*, Bd. ix.. H. 3, S. 153.
§ See *Brit. Journ. of Hom.*, xxvi., 658.

Miss W., æt. 26, consulted me on May 23rd, 1870, telling the following story. Five years ago she noticed a small lump in the right breast. She showed it to a physician, but he told her not to be troubled about it. She thought no more of it till last winter, when it began to enlarge, and to be the seat of darting pains. Then a hole formed in the skin, through which matter discharged; and last a flat sore formed at the seat of the lump.

This was the condition of things when she came to me. I found a sore, not much depressed and not unhealthy-looking, near the nipple. The latter was not retracted, and there was no hardness at the base of the sore. The health was good; and the only trouble complained of was the soreness and occasional pain at the seat of ulceration. I prescribed (I hardly know why) Phosphorus 6, a drop night and morning; and Calendula lotion to the sore.

Miss W. came again on June 3rd, and, on displaying the breast, showed me, to my horror, a large bleeding fungus, which had sprouted from the sore during the ten days since I first saw her. It bled freely when dressed, and was the seat of frequent and severe darting pain. I now gave a drop of the 30th dilution every alternate night, and ordered the growth to be dressed with dry lint, and to be kept cool; pressure also was to be made upon it by means of a bandage.

June 10th.—The fungus has not increased since last week; and there is little pain now, and less bleeding than before. Continue.

June 18th.—No increase in size; the pain quite gone, and the bleeding only occasional. Continue.

June 25th.—Bleeding quite ceased; and the fungus, which was dark red at first, is now pale, and is suppurating. Continue.

So matters stood till August 4th; when, the size of the growth remaining unaltered, I thought I would try whether Thuja would help, and prescribed it in the 30th dilution. On August 9th Miss W. came again, saying that she feared the growth was increasing. It was certainly looking larger, and I found on one side of it a fresh red mass, which had evidently sprung from the root of the fungus, and was pushing the old and deadened portion up from beneath. There had also been an outburst of bleeding. As may be supposed, I returned to the Phosphorus 30, giving a dose every evening.

August 31st.—Miss W. has been taking the Phosphorus until now. The progress of the disease has again been checked; there is no pain or bleeding; her general health is excellent; and the axillary glands are unaffected.

September 24th.—There being still no diminution of size, I now once more resorted to Thuja 30, this time taking the precaution of giving the Phosphorus with it on alternate days.

On October 19th my patient exhibited the good effects of this proceeding. I found the fungus becoming detached at its root, and hanging only by the slenderest of pedicles. I directed her to continue the medicines, and to give the growth one daily twist upon itself until it should fall off, when she was to bring it to me. I designed to send it to some competent microscopist, that the question of its malignancy might be set at rest.

But I was disappointed; though my patient was not. On November 8th she returned to tell me that about a week after her last visit there had been a gush of blood from the breast, after which the fungus had rapidly withered away, and in a few days had disappeared. There was now nothing to be seen at its site but a small cicatrised sore.

I continued the medicines for a short time longer, and then left them off. I have seen or heard from her several times since ; and there has been no recurrence of the trouble.

That this growth was a " fungus hæmatodes " there can be no doubt, or there is nothing in the etymology of the phrase. But whether fungus hæmatodes is always soft cancer is another question ; though, if it be not, I know not what it is. I had hoped to have had an undoubted instance of that disease to report, as cured by Phosphorus. The growth sprang from the caruncula lachrymalis, and had completely covered and closed the eye. It was not very painful, but bled profusely. Under Phosphorus 30, a dose every other day, it diminished to less than half its size, and made vision again possible on that side. But the patient, a woman over sixty, showed coincident symptoms of break-up of constitution, and finally died hemiplegic and dropsical. I would not therefore lay too much stress upon the action of the medicine here ; but in the case cited it was unquestionable. The help rendered by the Thuja also seems palpable.

Dr. Broadbent published, some time since, a case of essential anæmia cured by our medicine, but its subsequent employment in this disease has not yielded satisfactory results.

There is one curious use of Phosphorus which does not fall within any of the above categories. It is its power of curing chronic mastitis, where sinuses have been left in the gland after extensive suppuration. There are several cases on record illustrating this power of the medicine. Bryonia has the same exceptional action on the mammæ. Has local affinity, I wonder, anything to do with it, both being such important chest medicines?

I must also say a few words upon the use of Phosphorus in diseases of the eyes. Its symptoms point to choroidal congestion and retinal depression ; and in affections of the fundus having these characters, especially when photopsies or chromopsies are present, Drs. Allen and Norton (and also Dr. Vilas) have found it very useful. Dr. Goullon has recorded a cure of amaurosis following cerebro-spinal meningitis wrought by it,[*] and it should be useful for this affection when brought on by excess in venery and perhaps in tobacco.[†] But its most important use in this sphere is its application to glaucoma. It is when this morbid change begins with recurrent neuralgic attacks, and seemingly depends upon the same nervous lesion as that which causes the pain, that it is suitable and effective.

[*] See *Brit. Journ. of Hom.*, xxxvi, 93.
[†] Dr. Usher has reported a case of this kind cured by it (Hoyne, i., 99).

Several cases of apparent cure with it have been recorded,* and in my own hands it has proved of no little efficacy in diminishing pain and checking the progress of degeneration in glaucomatous eyes.

I may mention, in conclusion, some of Dr. Guernsey's symptomatic indications for the drug. It is most suitable, he thinks, for tall, slender women (he is speaking only of that sex), who are liable to sensation of great weakness and emptiness in the abdomen, and of heat running up the back, with coldness of the feet and legs. They are generally costive, passing long, narrow, dry hard stools, difficult to evacuate. Upon the first of these characteristics Dr. Allen remarks that it by no means holds good universally, as in diseases of the nervous system requiring Phosphorus the patients are often fat ; as also in the fatty degenerations so obviously calling for it.† The "face like polished ivory," which Dr. Hoyne mentions as indicative of the drug, points to this morbid pro-cess in the system.

Phosphorus is so unique a drug that I cannot name a single genuine analogue to it.

As for dose : in the acute affections of the respiratory organs for which Phosphorus is so frequently required, I find the second and third dilutions answer every purpose. The first has been most used in paralysis and neuralgia, and I should not be disposed to go higher in malignant jaundice. The higher potencies have acted well in sexual irritability, and in chronic affections of the respiratory organs, alimentary canal, and mammæ.

I shall occupy the remainder of your time to-day with the important metal, lead, *Latiné*

Plumbum.

Either the precipitated metal itself, the carbonate or the acetate may be used to obtain the specific action of lead. They are all triturated for homœopathic use.

A pathogenesis of Plumbum was published by Hartlaub and Trinks in the first volume of their *Arzneimittellehre.* It con-tains 1,024 symptoms, of which 565 are cited from authors; being observations of the noxious effects of the medicinal or operative employment of lead. The remainder are the result,

* See *Brit. Journ. of Hom.* xxxii., 6-11.
† *Hahn. Monthly,* xiii., 486.

as is stated, of " a careful proving on the healthy by means of moderate doses of the acetate," in which five persons took part. The best pathogenesis of the drug, however, which we have hitherto had has been the well-known account given by Tanquerel des Planches of the phenomena occurring in workers with the metal.* A schema of the symptoms he enumerates was given by Dr. Black, in the appendix to the first volume of the *British Journal of Homœopathy*; and has been of great use. We have now, however, in Dr. Allen's *Encyclopædia* an amalgamation of the symptoms obtained from these two sources with those of upwards of four hundred additional observations of the same kind, making a total pathogenesis of 4,163 symptoms. An excellent account of the latest observations and studies of chronic lead-poisoning is given by Naunyn, in the seventeenth volume of Ziemssen's work.

I need hardly remind you that the earliest symptoms of saturnine intoxication are the well-known "lead colic," and the "wrist-drop" which results from paralysis of the extensor muscles of the fore-arm, accompanied by wasting of their substance. More profound poisoning of the system induces a kind of degeneration of all the tissues. The nervous centres are found indurated or softened; and headache, amaurosis, neuralgia, palsy, anæsthesia, epilepsy, occur during life. The muscular tissue throughout the body is wasted or contracted. The kidneys are small and granular. There is complete decay of the bodily and mental powers, with profound melancholia; and the impairment of nutrition shows itself in the anæmic and cachectic appearance of the subject, who presents commonly a yellowish hue of skin (icterus saturninus).

Let us consider separately each of these effects, or groups of effects, in connexion with the use of Plumbum as a medicine.

The division made by Tanquerel des Planches is that commonly adopted in describing lead poisoning, and we cannot do better than follow it. He classifies the phenomena as those of colic, of paralysis, of arthralgia, and of encephalopathy.

1. The colic of lead is a severe pain, consisting of occasional intense paroxysms, generally of shooting character, the intervals being filled up with a continued sense of griping and cramp. It is as a rule worse in the evening and night. It may occupy all parts or any part of the abdomen. It is always relieved by pressure, and the more the firmer this is made. It is accompanied by obstinate constipation, by retraction of the abdominal walls, frequently by vomiting and slight icterus, and by a slow, full, and hard pulse.

* *Traité des maladies de Plomb*, Paris, 1839.

Pathologically, this affection seems compounded of neuralgia and spasm. Naunyn and Eulenberg describe it as a neurosis of the intestinal plexus (iliac and cœliac), the peculiar pulse being due to reflex excitation of the cardiac nerves through the splanchnics. Stillé, describing the pain as " darting in every direction, to the back, loins, uterus, scrotum, and groins, or occupying the thighs and legs, or the muscles of the chest and of the upper limbs," says—" in a word, it has all the characters of a severe neuralgia whose greatest severity is expended upon the digestive organs." Spasm shows itself in retraction of the abdomen (and often of the testes); and Tanquerel " succeeded in feeling very energetic contraction of the rectum during an attack of colic, by digital examination." A similar condition is shown in the bladder by tenesmus or retention of urine, and by great hindrance to the passage of a catheter.

These abdominal phonomena of lead-poisoning at once suggest the metal as a remedy for colic and constipation, whether occurring separately or together. And indeed I know of no better instance of the truth of the law of similars than the beautiful action of Plumbum in such conditions. For obstinate habitual constipation, when the stools are dry and lumpy, and the intestines half-paralytic and half-crampy, I have the utmost confidence in it. It is no less valuable in what Dr. Copeman calls " obstipation "—that is, in impaction of fæces. Of this you may read a good instance by Dr. Lohrbacher in the twenty-ninth volume of the *British Journal of Homœopathy*. This use of lead, inexplicable save upon the homœopathic hypothesis, has been recently imported into ordinary practice by Dr. Thorowgood, as usual without acknowledgment of its source.* We carry it still farther, relying upon the medicine in any form of obstruction of the bowels that has not a mechanical cause, and in incarcerated and even strangulated hernia. You will do well to read the remarks of Drs. Baumann and Mayländer on this subject in the thirty-first volume of the *British Journal*. The latter generally succeeds in strangulated hernia with Belladonna and Nux vomica; but, if these fail, he resorts to the knife. Dr. Baumann considers that, before this extreme remedy is sought, we have a resource in Plumbum, and adduces good evidence for his belief, of which indeed there is no lack elsewhere.

Nor less when colic is the prominent point of similarity to the effects of lead is its medicinal power displayed. Of this Dr. Holland has put a striking case on record. The patient

* See *Brit. Journ. of Hom.*, xxxi., 376.

had been suffering from most agonising abdominal spasms for
two days, with vomiting, and suppression of stool and urine.
A grain of Plumbum aceticum, third decimal, was given ; and
in less than ten minutes the patient fell asleep, waking after
many hours free from pain, and able to relieve his bowels of a
mass of scybala.   The next day he was well. *   Most of us have
probably seen similar good effects from the medicine, though
under less striking circumstances.

The association of colic with constipation, and of constipation with colic, always forms the special indication for Plumbum as a remedy for either.   But such association is not
essential.   The habitual costiveness in which the medicine is
so efficacious may be quite painless ; and on the other hand
Bähr has related one case, and I myself another,† of what may
fairly be called neuralgic enterodynia cured by it, where the
bowels were regular enough.   In such cases the sense of retraction in the abdomen mentioned as characteristic by Dr.
Guernsey, or the actual hard and tense condition observed by
Bähr, may guide to its choice.   The latter author justly maintains that it is in neuralgic colic rather than that brought on
by cold (in which Colocynth is so valuable) that Plumbum finds
its place.   On the other hand, I think he errs in discouraging
the use of the drug in ileus, because the abdomen herein is
distended instead of—as in lead-poisoning—retracted. Naunyn
says of the latter condition :—" In not a few cases, however, it
is entirely wanting, and in its place there is swelling of the
abdomen."

2. Of the paralysis of saturnine intoxication I have already
spoken in its most familiar form of " wrist-drop," i.e, loss of
power of the extensors of the hands, which are affected more
than the flexors.   Manouvriez has shown that this may sometimes be a local effect of handling the metal (see S. 3089 of
Allen).   But, while much more frequently occurring in the
upper than in the lower extremities, yet lead paralysis every
now and then invades the latter.   It is rarely accompanied
with anæsthesia, though lead anæsthesia as an independent
affection is common enough.   The paralysis is preceded often
by a trembling (tremblottement saturnine) of the affected
muscles, sometimes by spasms and shooting or tearing pains.
It is partial rather than general ; and Tanquèrel des Planches
states that he was frequently astonished to find that muscles
were paralysed whose nerve supplied others also that were not
paralysed.   There is always marked atrophy of the affected
muscles ; and sometimes this condition becomes general, so

* Brit. Journ. of Hom.,xxxii., 79.   † Ibid, xxii., 239.

that the patient resembles a walking skeleton. The muscles, when examined post mortem, are found wasted and very pale, and have sometimes the appearance of white fibrous tissue.

It is impossible not to be reminded here, even more than with Phosphorus, of the disease known as progressive muscular atrophy or wasting palsy. The local selection, the predominant atrophy, the presence of trembling (fibrillary contractions) and absence of anæsthesia correspond in the two. Trousseau admits that the differential diagnosis is attended with difficulty ; and can only adduce by way of distinction the different behaviour of the muscles when submitted to the electric stimulus, and the history of the evolution of the symptoms. The former is a mere matter of degree, and as to the latter, M. Trousseau is inconsistent with himself. " In the lead-disease," he says, " palsy precedes atrophy," leaving it to be understood that in wasting palsy atrophy precedes loss of power. But he himself had already made the following remark on the case of the latter malady which gave rise to his clinical lecture. " You may remember that Dr. Duchenne himself, who honoured us with his presence during our round, had shown that most of the muscles of the arm and fore-arm still contracted under the influence of electricity, whilst the patient could not voluntarily move his hands or his fore-arms. One could not but suppose, therefore, that previous to any anatomical change, which seemed not to exist then, the peripheral extremities of the nerves had undergone a modification, in consequence of which they had lost the power of rousing muscular contraction. *A loss of excitability of the peripheral extremities of the nerves would therefore precede the degeneration of the muscular fibres*, a fact perfectly in accordance with pathological physiology."

Consider, then, the experiments on rabbits which are related in the seventeenth volume of the *North American Journal of Homœopathy*, and which point strongly to the same analogy. Read, moreover, the series of cases of muscular atrophy given in the first volume of the *Practitioner* to illustrate the effects of electricity in its treatment. In several of these it remained doubtful to the last whether the poison of lead was not the exciting cause of the disease. I think that, in the face of this evidence, you will warrant me in recommending from the homœopathic point of view the persistent trial of Plumbum in the first instance of wasting palsy which comes under notice. I may mention, for your encouragement, two cases in which this recommendation of mine (first made in 1869*) has been

* *On the various forms of Paralysis*, p. 43.

acted upon with advantage. One was treated by myself. The muscular wasting, which had been going on for two years, was completely checked by the use of Plumbum, in varying dilutions, during a space of three or four months ; though I have been disappointed in my expectations of a restoration of power. The second is reported to me by Dr. Reginald Jones, of Birkenhead. The patient "presented the appearance of a living skeleton." The presence of fibrillary contractions in the paralysed muscles led him to the use of Plumbum, which he gave in the sixth attenuation. "The results," he writes, "have been most gratifying."

But I have already reminded you, when speaking of Belladonna, that wasting palsy is a member of a group of paralytic diseases dependent upon the same pathological alteration in the nervous centres, and differing only in the seat of its occurrence. Accordingly, a further study of plumbic paralysis brings features to light which correspond with the symptoms of other spinal paralyses. I will content myself for the present with referring you to the remarks of Erb, in commenting on the wrist-drop of lead under the title of "musculo-spiral paralysis" in Ziemssen's *Cyclopædia* (vol. xiii.). It cannot be doubted, he says, that the seat of paralysis should not be looked for in the muscles : and we have here a primary lesion of the nervous system. He then discusses the question whether the lead-paralysis is peripheral or central; and concludes—"The spinal origin of the paralysis thus appears to be a *possibility* ; and I am at present inclined, on various grounds, to regard it as more probable than the peripheral origin, partly on account of its obvious analogy with the spinal paralysis of children, with regard to distributive atrophy of muscles and electrical relations, partly on account of the regular symmetrical affection of the same nerve-regions, partly on account of the merely partial paralysis of definite fibres of the same nerve-trunk (the supinator longus remaining free), and, lastly, on account of the sensibility remaining unaffected." Naunyn concurs in the same conclusion.

The paralytic conditions in which Plumbum has hitherto been used in the school of Hahnemann are principally those resembling its wrist-drop. Drs. Dudgeon,[*] Sharp,[†] and Chalmers[‡] have each recorded a cure of a case of this kind ; and Dr. Bayes speaks of having seen others. But Dr. Jousset has made the commencement of an application of Plumbum to the

* *Brit. Journ. of Hom.*, xxix., 612.
† *Essays on Medicine*, pp. 388, 456.
‡ *Monthly Hom. Review*, xiii., 145.

inflammations of the cord by curing **a** case of acute spinal
paralysis with it. You will find the narrative at p. 465 of his
Leçons de Clinique Medicale. He gave the 30th dilution.
That paralysis may occur as early as the third day after the
first exposure to lead (Tanquerel) shows it to be perfectly
suitable to such cases. But I should expect to find it still
more useful in chronic inflammations of the brain and cord,
whether seated in the nervous substance itself or in the neur-
oglia. Some of the symptoms of multiple cerebral sclerosis
are very obvious in its pathogenesis, and in one case observed
by Renaut (occurring in a worker) the ataxy characteristic of
posterior spinal sclerosis was present. Mr. Thorold Wood
lately communicated to the British Homœopathic Society* a
case regarded by him as of this kind, occurring in a child, in
which Plumbum 6 was curative. I cannot quite agree with
his diagnosis, but unquestionably spinal paresis was present.

3. The neuralgic and spasmodic pains of lead-poisoning,
which we have already seen in its colic, are also manifested in
the limbs. They occur even in acute poisoning by the acetate ;
and among the workers are the symptoms most frequently
seen after those of the abdomen. They are the *arthralgies* of
Tanquerel, who explains that he uses ἄρθρον in the sense of
limb, not of joint. He describes the pains as sharp in
character (Naunyn says burning and tearing) ; not precisely
following the track of the nervous cords (Dr. Bartholow thinks
that the intra-muscular sensory nerves are their seat) ; constant, but becoming acute by paroxysms ; diminished by
pressure and increased by motion ; and accompanied by
cramps, which are always a very marked feature of the pains
of lead. They are sometimes felt in the thorax also, but
very rarely in the face—in one only of all the observations
collated by Allen. They have once at least been described as
"lightning-like" (S. 3,300 of Allen), suggesting the *douleurs
fulgurantes* of locomotor ataxy.

The neuralgic pains of Plumbum have hardly found their
application to practice ; but it plays an active part in our
hands in the treatment of local spasms. Dr. Stokes has put
on record a case of cramps of the calves of long standing
rapidly cured by it.† Drs. Chapman‡ and Cooper have
illustrated its value in spasmodic conditions of the rectum and
anus, and Teste has removed with it painful retraction of the
testicles. Dr. Dyce Brown has called our attention to the im-

---

* See its *Annals,* viii., 375.
† *Brit. Journ. of Hom.,* xxvi., 128.
‡ *Ibid,* iii., 170.

portant observation that vaginismus has been observed as an effect of lead-poisoning,*—a fact which may yet be turned to practical service, though I found the medicine inoperative in a case in which I gave it. In an incurable paralysis which I once treated with it, it almost entirely removed the cramps which constituted the most distressing element of the case.

4. The "encephalopathy" of lead-poisoning embraces its cerebral symptoms, which, though of diverse kinds, always appear as a connected group. They are doubtless sometimes uræmic, from the renal mischief of which I shall presently speak; but more commonly they are primary. Violent headache and amaurosis are the usual prodromata; then maniacal or melancholic conditions may supervene, but most frequently eclampsia. The convulsions are quite epileptiform in character, and coma or delirium may fill up their intervals.

This epilepsy of lead-poisoning has hardly received sufficient attention hitherto. Occurring, as it generally does, in the "secondary saturnine intoxication," it implies the existence of some amount of degeneration of the nervous centres, thus rendering Plumbum as truly homœopathic to chronic as Hydrocyanic acid to recent epilepsy. I agree with Bähr in ranking it with Cuprum as the remedy from which most is to be expected in confirmed cases of the disease. Dr. Burnett has recorded† a striking cure of epilepsy of 13 years' standing by it: the patient's general condition was one to which the medicine was exquisitely homœopathic. He gave the 30th dilution.

Besides these recognised forms of lead-poisoning, I must speak of certain other manifestations of its influence.

5. The first of these is its action upon the urinary organs. In the first place, we have Dr. Ringer's statement that after the administration of its salts there is an increased amount of mucus in the urine, with signs of irritation of the lining membrane of the bladder, even to the extent of inducing a catarrhal condition. Correspondingly, Teste claims to have cured with Plumbum several chronic affections of the urinary organs. But of still greater interest is the action of the poison on the kidneys. These are found, as I have said, small and granular: there is present the contracted kidney which constitutes the most serious form of Bright's disease. So frequently does this lesion occur in the subjects of plumbism, that Dr. Dickinson states that it was found in twenty-six out of forty-two workers in lead who died from various causes in St.

* *Monthly Hom. Review*, xiii., 574.
† *Ibid*. Jan., 1878.

George's Hospital. During life, albuminuria is an evidence of the mischief being set up; and it has been thought that the saturnine epilepsy and amaurosis may sometimes be due to it.

Another effect of the renal degeneration induced by lead is that the separation of urates from the blood is checked, so that the uric acid of the urine is diminished while that of the blood is increased. This is the pathological condition which, according to Dr. Garrod, excites gouty inflammation; and he and Dr. Ringer agree in stating, from experience, that if to a gouty person, free at the time from the special manifestation of the disease, a salt of lead is administered, it developes an acute attack of gout, with its usual symptoms of severe pain and high fever. Dr. Garrod accounts in this way for the frequency with which gout appears among workers in lead as compared with those following other occupations. Of all this there need be no question. But it is another thing to suppose that lead causes its renal degeneration through the intermediary development of gout. That its kidney is the "gouty kidney" is unquestionable; but only, I think, because both it and the gouty poison have the same renal action. It is admitted that in many instances the granular kidney is the only gouty manifestation present in the subjects of lead-poisoning; and Dr. George Moore has entered into a thorough examination of the evidence in a paper contributed to the twenty-fourth volume of the *British Journal of Homœopathy*, the result of which is entirely adverse to the causation of true gout—or rheumatism—by lead.

We conclude, then, that lead causes granular degeneration of the kidneys by a direct and specific action; and should be a hopeful remedy for the disease, whether of gouty or other origin. No medicine, moreover, so closely corresponds to the general phenomena of the malady—as the atheroma, the cachexia, and the depression of spirits: the amaurosis also of the two is precisely similar. The only recorded (old-school) experience of the use of lead in renal disease is that of Lewald, as given by Dr. Ringer. He found it constantly diminish the albumen in the urine, though only by nine or ten grains in the twenty-four hours. The diminution appeared to hold no constant relation to the quantity of lead administered. At the same time, and with the same absence of quantitative relation to the drug, the amount of urine was increased in the same period by 200 cubic centimétres. The form of the renal mischief here is not stated, but Dr. Ringer thinks with reason that the large white kidney existed. I have myself tried the treat-

ment in two well-characterised cases of granular degeneration. In one the effect was *nil*, save to relieve an accompanying constipation. In the other great improvement in general
health ensued for a time ; but a chill caused pericarditis and
death. Dr. Samuel Jones has recorded an apparent cure in
the twelfth volume of the *American Observer*.

6. The other affection I have now in my mind is the
amaurosis of lead-poisoning. It is sometimes (as I have said)
secondary to renal mischief, when it is either a temporary anæmia
of the retina, or a more lasting retinitis albuminurica. It may,
however, occur as a substantive change, and then appears to
consist in an optic neuritis, with its central scotoma. This
action of the metal has not yet been, but ought to be, applied
in practice.

In these six categories I have included the main effects and
uses of Plumbum. But other conditions of body every now
and then come across us in practice which remind us of lead-
poisoning, and in which we may expect benefit from its use.
Such is the melancholia religiosa of which two cures by it are
recorded by Dr. Chapman,* and with which great constipation
is generally, as there, associated. Dr. Sharp also speaks of
using it beneficially here. Dr. Winter points out its homœopathicity to chlorosis, and gives instances of its successful
use.† Bähr suggests its employment in chronic encephalitis,
and I have seen good results from it in chronic dull headaches,
with depressed spirits and constipation. Again, the effects of
drinking water contaminated with the metal must be taken
into account as homœopathic indications for the use of the
drug. An interesting series of such cases has lately been
communicated to the *British Journal* by Dr. von Tunzelmann.‡
In one amblyopia with double vision occurred ; in another
icterus and (nocturnal) vomiting ; a third had renal congestion,
a fourth anasarca and paralysis ; in another pulmonary con-
solidation with wasting occurred ; and in yet another hæmoptysis and epistaxis—all these troubles passing off as the
noxious influence was removed. It is also worth noting that
in a case related in *Frank's Magazin* a quarter of a grain of
the acetate three times a day caused swelling, pain, and great
weight in the testicles ; and Dr. Rutherford has lately ascertained that it is a direct depressant (*i.e.*, not through the
medium of purgation) to the secretion of bile.§ Plumbum is

---

* *Brit. Journ. of Hom.*, iii., 170.
† *Ibid*, p. 218.
‡ Vol. xxxii., p. 17.
§ *Brit. Med. Journ.*, Dec. 28, 1878.

another medicine whose remedial effects seem to me far from
having been exhausted.

Alumina, Opium, Platina and *Zinc* are more or less closely
allied medicines.

LECTURE L.

I have to speak to-day of three medicines,—two of the second or even a lower rank, but the third of primary importance. They are Platina, Podophyllum, and Pulsatilla.

First, of

Platina.

Our preparation is made by triturating the precipitated metal. It would more correctly be called Platinum.

There is a pathogenesis of Platina in the second edition of the *Chronic Diseases.* It contains 527 symptoms, most of which are credited to Gross. They are taken from a proving instituted by this physician, chiefly on "a damsel, both bodily and mentally healthy and blooming, though somewhat excitable," who took doses of the first trituration equivalent in all to between two and three grains of the metal. This proving (or rather the symptoms thereof) is recorded in the first volume of the *Archiv.* An admirable study of Hahnemann's pathogenesis, and of the clinical uses of the metal, by Dr. Veith Meyer, was translated in the second volume of the *Philadelphia Journal of Homœopathy* by Dr. Dunham, and will be found in the first volume of his collected writings. Upon this study mainly my remarks will be based.

The chief action of Platina appears to be upon the nervous centres—the symptoms, when allowance is made for the temperament of their chief source, being generally characterised by depression. There is a strong tendency to paralysis and anæsthesia, localised numbness being a frequent sensation ; and in the emotional sphere there is anxiety and apprehension, even to the fear of death. With this—perhaps through an action upon the abdominal and pelvic plexuses—there is torpor of the intestinal canal, shown in flatulence and constipation ; and also premature menstruation. As is usually the

case, many spasmodic and neuralgic phenomena are mixed up
with those of paralysis and anæsthesia ; the pains are
mostly crampy, and associated with numbness and coldness.

In accordance with these pathogenetic indications, Platina
has hitherto been used mainly for hysteria and melancholia
in females, connected with deranged uterine health. It has
cured even religious melancholy in these subjects; and altogether may be said to be to women what Aurum is to men.
In corroboration of this remark, it may be observed that
Platina holds the same place in the treatment of chronic
ovarian disease as Aurum in the corresponding affections of
the testicle. Hering recommends it for induration of the
ovaries (Hahnemann had already mentioned a similar condition in the uterus as indicating it); and Mr. Harmar Smith
has published a case of chronic ovarian irritation with sterility
in which it was curative.* The distinguishing feature between
Platina and Pulsatilla in these cases is that with the former
there is menorrhagia, with the latter the reverse. Menorrhagia itself is often helped by Platina, especially, Dr. Guernsey
says, when a black and thick condition of the menstrual flow
is present. Sexual excitement, both psychical and physical,
is apt to accompany such phenomena ; and Platina is much
esteemed for this, even when it reaches to nymphomania. It
is also useful in such a condition in the opposite sex, while
below puberty; I mean to subdue the morbid excitement
which keeps up the habit of masturbation in young boys who
have been inducted into it. For this purpose Dr. von Grauvogl commends it highly. Dr. Meyer thought much of it in
the treatment of hysteria, when the patients are depressed ;
herein contrasting with Ignatia, whose subjects are keenly
impressionable and capricious. He notes the "hysterical
asthma" and the clavus as frequent among its symptoms.

Dr. Guernsey lays more stress, among the mental symptoms of Platina, on the sense of exaltation of self and contempt for others as characteristic of it. He also frequently
reports "horrifying thoughts" among its key-notes.

Platina has also some points of usefulness which remind us
of those of Plumbum, to whose effects it has been suggested
as an antidote. It is useful in some superficial neuralgiæ,
accompanied with torpor and numbness. Hahnemann mentions "constipation while travelling" as indicating it ; and in
this trouble when occurring in women whose uterine health is
imperfect, it is often helpful. Dr. Guernsey describes its stools
as putty-like, so hindering their own expulsion.

* Brit. Journ. of Hom , xxv., 157.

The chloride of platinum has been used successfully in the old school in the treatment of chronic syphilis and of condylomata, acting very much like the chloride of gold.* Höfer, who has introduced it here, found six grains to produce in himself a violent but short-lasting headache, chiefly occipital. A very severe and obstinate syphilitic headache in a woman, which iodide of potassium alone seemed unable to cure, went on rapidly to recovery when I gave the chloride of platinum (five drops of the third decimal dilution twice daily) as an alternating remedy. I was led to its selection by the profound depression which was present. As to condylomata, Teste long ago classed Platina with Thuja as an anti-sycotic.

The analogues of Platina are the *Aurum, Pulsatilla, Ignatia,* and *Plumbum* I have already named. You will find their points of resemblance and difference well pointed out (together with those also of Asafœtida and Crocus) in Dr. Meyer's article.

Platina has generally been used in the higher potencies, from the sixth to the thirtieth; but Dr. Meyer professes himself quite satisfied with the second and third triturations, in which I agree with him.

My second medicine is one which we homœopathists took many years ago from the so-called " eclectic " practitioners of America, and of which ordinary medicine has since made the acquisition from the same source—the mandrake, or Mayapple,

Podophyllum.

We use a tincture prepared from the root of the P. peltatum. Podophyllin, which is now so much used as a cholagogue, is a resinoid derived from the plant, and seems to contain its active virtues. It is triturated, or dissolved in rectified spirit, for our purposes.

Podophyllum was proved, in the 1st, 3rd, and 15th dilutions, by Dr. Williamson in 1844; and his results published, with a few symptoms from five others, in the *Materia Medica of American Provings.* But the knowledge of the action of the drug is best learned from its toxical and curative powers, as Dr. Hale records them in his *New Remedies;* and from the numerous experiments on animals which have been made with it during the last twenty years. Allen's *Encyclopædia*

* Like this metal, it appears able to excite some salivation.

gives symptoms from twenty human subjects, obtained in various ways.

Podophyllum came to us with the reputation of a chola-gogue purgative, resembling calomel. The three sets of experiments which have been made with it on the lower animals —those of Dr. Anstie,* Dr. Hughes Bennett,† and Dr. Rutherford‡—bear especially on this question. Dr. Anstie found an increased quantity of bile in the evacuations a comparatively rare phenomenon; but the liver in most of his autopsies is stated to have been somewhat congested. Dr. Hughes Bennett found purgation by the drug, as by other agents, diminish the flow of bile through a biliary fistula; but even when the dose fell short of producing this effect, the solid elements of the secretion were reduced in quantity, though its fluid portion was somewhat increased. Both observers seem to infer that Podophyllum has no action on the liver; but I cannot think that such a conclusion is fairly deducible from their facts. On the contrary, they seem to be such as to invite further experimentation, especially upon human subjects, with the view of following up their hints. My own expectation is that Podophyllum will be found to act here as we have seen Mercury doing in the mouth, i.e., that its irritant influence on the duodenum (which will presently come before us) leads to a copious flow of bile from the gall-bladder and liver; but that it may also act on the liver itself, congesting it, and so impairing its function. The former part of this hypothesis seems confirmed by the recent experiments of Dr. Rutherford, who, on introducing Podophyllin into the duodenum of fasting dogs found it increase the amount both of the solid and fluid elements of the bile.

However this may be, there is—as with Mercury—a consensus of opinion as to its therapeutical virtues which no physiological evidence can set aside. Doses much too small to induce purgation—from the fourth to the hundredth of a grain or even less—have been shown by practitioners of both schools to act with the best effect in relieving hepatic torpor and partial stagnation, to the great benefit of the patient. I would refer you especially to the observations of Dr. John Moore in the thirty-first volume of the *British Journal of Homœopathy*, and to those of . Dr. W. A. Allen in the fourth volume of the (American) *Homœopathic Times*. The latter believes it the great remedy for rectifying the hepatic disorders occurring under malarious influences; and it cannot

* *Med. Times and Gazette*, 1863, i., 326.
† *Brit. Med. Journ.*, 1869, i.,418. ‡ *Ibid*, 1875, ii.

act as a "cholagogue" in his hands, as he gives it in doses which could only avail for a truly homœopathic operation, viz: the second and third attenuation where constipation is present, the thirtieth and higher where there is diarrhœa. Whatever may be its *modus operandi* here, it seems evident that, so long as we stop short of its purgative effects, no harm is done.

We get on clearer ground when we come to the intestinal influence of the drug. That it readily caused vomiting and purging was well known ; but the experiments of Dr. Anstie have enabled us to define this action with great precision. He found, in numerous experiments on dogs and cats, that an alcoholic solution of Podophyllin, when introduced into the peritoneal cavity, caused no inflammation there, but set up in the small intestines an intense hyperæmia. The duodenum was chiefly affected, and actual ulceration was more than once developed there. The lining membrane of the whole small gut was generally found covered with bloody mucus. The inflammation usually ceased at the ileo-cæcal valve, but occasionally invaded the large intestine. The frequent stools consisted of glairy mucus, sometimes stained with bile, but more commonly with blood.

These are very important results. They give us in Podophyllum another medicine to add to Arsenic, Kali bichromicum and Uranium nitricum as acting specifically on the duodenum, and capable of controlling ulceration therein. And more, they give us a remedy truly homœopathic to enteritis affecting the jejunum and ileum, which neither these nor Mercurius corrosivus are. The first enabled me once to cure a duodenitis, which was resisting Arsenic. The latter shows a local affinity for the diarrhœa of typhoid, in which, and in simple enteritis affecting the same parts, the drug may do good service.

No action on the rectum was manifested in the animals poisoned by Dr. Anstie ; but in the human subject—especially in children—this part is readily affected by the drug, as shown by tenesmus and prolapsus recti complicating the diarrhœa. The feeble affinity of Podophyllum for the colon makes it unsuitable for ordinary dysentery, which has its seat there. But when dysenteric diarrhœa appears to depend on inflammatory irritation of the rectum, it will give rapid relief. Such a malady is not uncommon in children, and is generally accompanied by painful prolapse of the rectum at each stool. Dr. Hale speaks of having seen two such cases caused by the over-use of the drug ; and I have recorded one, and Mr. Harmar Smith another,* of speedy cure by it. In simple pro-

* *Brit. Journ. of Hom.*, xxiv., 673 ; xxix., 399.

lapsus ani from debility, moreover, when occurring in childhood, beautiful results are almost always attainable from
minute doses of the drug.

Besides enteritis of the small intestine, and dysentery of the
rectum, Podophyllum is useful in several forms of diarrhœa,
both acute and chronic.* Drs. Ringer and Phillips concur
with us in praising it here, adding the necessary caution that
it must be administered in very small doses. The former,
moreover, confirms what homœopathists have always regarded
as a main indication for the medicine in chronic diarrhœa,
viz., its recurrence especially in the early morning. It is often
serviceable in cholera nostras and cholera infantum; but its
place in their therapeutics is hardly yet defined. It is very
useful when the stools are too frequent, and yet natural—a
not uncommon complaint in children, and generally associated
with some amount of wasting.

A good deal of evidence has accumulated of late, showing
a power on the part of Podophyllum of benefiting prolapse
of the uterus as well as of the rectum. I know not whether
it is by a direct action that it accomplishes this. Dr. Guernsey
speaks of a·sense of falling in the abdomen as especially
indicating it.

In the fourth edition of his *New Remedies*, Dr. Hale gives
two interesting communications on Podophyllum, one from
Dr. Scudder, an "eclectic" practitioner, evidently "almost
persuaded to be a" homœopathist; the other from a prominent
writer of our own school, Dr. Searle, of Brooklyn. The former
gives, from his experience, certain peculiar symptoms as indicating the choice of the drug. They are, fulness of the
superficial veins; dull, unpleasant pain, or weight, in the hypogastric region; a sharply defined ache in the sacro-ischiatic
foramina, with tenderness on pressure; and pain in the course
of the ulnar nerve. He also mentions a peculiar stool as
characteristic of it,—the first part being large and hard, but
then fluid and wind following. Dr. Searle compares the
morning diarrhœa of Podophyllum with that of some other
medicines. " In the morning aggravations of the bowel symptoms," he writes, " Podophyllum resembles Aloes and Sulphur,
but may easily be differentiated from these. The stool of
Aloes is a windy spurt of watery or slimy yellow fæcal matter,
the desire for which can hardly for an instant be controlled
from a seeming if not real weakness of the internal sphincter.
Sulphur demands equal haste from tenesmus. It has a brown
stool, not especially flatulent, and neither so scanty as that

* See *Brit. Journ. of Hom.*, xxvi., 654.

of Aloes, nor so profuse as that of Podophyllum. Podophyllum gets its victim up early, but not in so great haste as the others; and has a very profuse, yellowish or greenish, stool—so profuse, indeed, that one wonders whence so much can come. It often contains undigested food, and is very offensive to the smell, having sometimes the odour of carrion."

Dr. Searle might have mentioned *Apis, Nuphar* and *Rumex* as additional analogues to Podophyllum in respect of morning diarrhœa. In its general action it resembles *Colchicum, Iris, Leptandra,* and *Mercurius*.

The third attenuation of Podophyllin seems to give us all its strictly homœopathic applications.

My last medicine is the meadow anemone, pasque flower, or wind flower—

Pulsatilla.

It was the P. nigricans which was introduced into medicine by Stoerck, and proved by Hahnemann; and which accordingly is used in homœopathic practice. The American species has been found, as we shall see, to possess similar properties; but though chemical research has discovered that the P. pratensis also contains the alkaloid anemonin, it is not proved that this is its active principle, and as a fact the English indigenous species has little medicinal power. The Pharmacopœial tincture is made from the entire plant.

The pathogenesis of Pulsatilla is in the second volume of the *Reine Arzneimittellehre*. It contains 1,153 symptoms, all except about a hundred of which are Hahnemann's own, the remainder being supplied by five provers and a few authors. Hahnemann states that his own symptoms were obtained from very moderate doses, and are therefore primary effects of the drug. He has bestowed great attention upon the pathogenesis, annotating it freely, and pointing out the connection of the various symptoms. For an excellent commentary on these I may refer you to Dr. Carroll Dunham's remarks on Pulsatilla in the second volume of his lectures. Dr. Allen adds provings, with the mother tincture, by Lembke and Wenzel, and, with the dilutions, by Robinson. The American species—Pulsatilla Nuttalliana—has been proved by Drs. Burt and C. Wesselhœft. You may read the experiments of the former in the second edition of the *New Remedies*, of the latter in the Transactions of the American Institute for 1868. They include observations on several women Dr. Allen, of course, presents them all.

Pulsatilla was one of the plants introduced into medicine by the celebrated Baron Störck. He found it very useful in chronic affections of the eyes, as cataract, spots on the cornea, and amaurosis; in secondary syphilis; and in cutaneous diseases. It has fallen into entire disuse in the old school; and though homœopathy has preserved it in full employment, its provings and small doses have not led to these applications of the drug. But an American (old-school) physician, Dr. W. H. Miller, of S. Paul's, Minnesota, using the native variety in full doses, has obtained the same results. It will be for us to consider how far we can follow his practice with advantage.

Little was known of the physiological action of Pulsatilla until Hahnemann proved it. Some German therapeutists (quoted by Dr. Hale) speak of its causing, in over-doses, nausea and vomiting, slimy diarrhœa, profuse and offensive sweats, vesicular and pustular eruptions, coryza and cough, increased urinary flow, and peculiar pains and dimness of the eyes. But the homœopathic provings show that, besides these affections of the mucous membranes and the eyes, Pulsatilla exerts much influence on the synovial membranes, the veins, the ears, and the generative organs of both sexes.

1. In the mucous membranes Pulsatilla sets up the catarrhal process. The dry stage is short and little marked (except sometimes in the respiratory tract); and much mucous secretion is the rule. As symptoms of this condition the pathogenesis gives us—in the *alimentary canal*, raw throat, coated tongue, furred mouth, fœtid smell of the breath, taste deadened or variously altered (bitter, sour, salt, even putrid), foul or acid eructations, nausea and inclination to vomit, sensation as if the stomach were spoiled, weight and pressure in the stomach, and mucous diarrhœa; in the *respiratory tract* green or yellow discharge from the nose, and cough with much expectoration* (often tasting salt or bitter); in the *urinary mucous membrane* frequent micturition with tenesmus, and jelly-like sediment in the urine.

2. Pulsatilla seems to fall just short of the true serous membranes, but compensates itself by acting powerfully upon their near relatives, the *synovial membranes*. The joints chiefly affected are the knees, the ankles, and the small joints of the hands and (most especially) the feet. The rheumatico-gouty action thus displayed is also manifested in pains of divers kinds in the nape of the neck and the extremities.

3. The *veins* seem to lose their vital resistance under the

---

* The dry cough of Pulsatilla I am disposed, from clinical experience, to set down as sympathetic, *i.e* as a " stomach cough."

action of Pulsatilla ; so that varicosis readily occurs, especially in the rectum.

4. Pulsatilla manifests its affinity for the *eyes* mainly by affecting the lids, which it inflames greatly, causing them to be agglutinated in the morning, and to pour out quantities of mucus. It causes also, however, considerable aching pain in the eyeballs, and many disturbances of vision. Temporary obscurations of sight often occur ; fiery circles or haloes are seen ; and after sleep there is a feeling as if something were hanging over the cornea which could be wiped away. The sensation is only subjective, and disappears spontaneously.

5. The *ears* suffer from the action of Pulsatilla even more than do the eyes. In some provers the concha and external meatus were inflamed, with purulent discharge. In others deafness, generally with noises of various kinds, was present. The seat of the latter symptoms is indicated by Dr. Burt, who suffered from " snapping noises in the ear," and " drawing pains along the right *Eustachian tube.*" Others yet suffered from mere pain in the ear, generally of a jerking character.

6. The action of Pulsatilla upon the *generative organs* of both sexes is very marked, but is not easy to define. The pathogenetic symptoms of its action in this sphere are, in the female, contractive pains of the uterus, leucorrhœa of various kinds, and scanty, delayed, and often painful menses. The abdominal pains are too vaguely described to enable us to discern any irritation of the ovaries ; but their analogues in the male, the testes, swell up and become painful,—the spermatic cord also being involved.

The febrile condition which accompanies most of these ailments is marked by predominant chilliness.

This is the best outline I can give you of the physiological action of Pulsatilla. It has little interest in itself, being hardly capable of a rational exposition ; but it is amply available for therapeutic applications. Before, however, I turn to these, let me cite some of Hahnemann's remarks upon the symptoms of the drug. Of certain of the pains caused by Pulsatilla, he says that they are "a short-lasting drawing tension, which always terminates in a darting analogous to tearing, somewhat as if a nerve were put upon the stretch, and then let loose again suddenly, causing a painful jerk." Of others he says that they feel as if there were an internal ulcer present. Of all save these he notes that they are relieved by pressure. He points out, moreover, that its symptoms are generally worst when at rest and in a warm room, while they are relieved by motion in the open air; and that they tend to appear on one side only of the body.

Hahnemann has also done much to fix for us the character and temperament to which Pulsatilla best corresponds. " The medicinal employment of the drug," he says, " will be the more salutary when, in the maladies to which this plant corresponds as regards bodily evils, there is at the same time a timorous tearful state of mind, and tendency to inward depression and quiet grief, or at least to passiveness and resignation, especially if in health the patient was kindly and pleasant (or even of light and changeable disposition). It therefore especially suits the lymphatic constitution, and is consequently but little appropriate to men quick at their course of action and energetic in their movements, even though they appear kindly disposed." He gives, moreover, as indications for it—frequent chilliness, absence of thirst, retarded menstruation, long delay in getting to sleep, and the aggravation of the symptoms towards even- ing. Teste adds, as regards constitution, that it is "particu- larly suitable to persons who, by the relative predominance of the adipose tissue in their composition, by the whiteness of their flesh, the roundness of their forms, the mildness of their disposition, and their fitful moods, exhibit all the marked features of the female sex."

I see no reason for supposing that Pulsatilla has any gene- ral influence upon the nervous system or upon the blood. I shall arrange its therapeutic virtues under the headings already adopted for the physiological outline.

1. Pulsatilla plays an important part in gastric disorders. In dyspepsia, whether acute or chronic, the prominence of *mucous* derangement—*i.e.*, white tongue, nausea with little vomiting, and absence of much pain—indicates this medicine in preference to others, such as Nux vomica.* The tongue calling for Pulsatilla is thickly coated with a white roughish fur, very different from the milky white of Antimonium cru- dum, or the yellowish brown of Kali bichromicum. The acute dyspepsia in which Pulsatilla is curative generally arises from the ingestion of fat or other rich food, as the pork specified by Hahnemann. In chronic gastric disorder it does better when heart-burn than when water-brash is present, in which it again contrasts with Nux. Dr. Marston, however, says

* There is a good case illustrating its action here by Dr. Marston in the twelfth volume of the *Monthly Homœopathic Review*, following upon a differential diagnosis between this medicine and Nux. You may also refer to that one which Hahnemann himself has recorded in the preface to the second volume of the *Materia Medica Pura*.

that when the fluid of water-brash is sour or foul tasted Pulsatilla is quite equal to its removal. Indeed, bad taste, whether subjective, of the ingesta, or of eructations, is a special indication for our remedy. Dr. Bayes considers it indicated in dyspepsia by a great feeling of tightness after a meal, so that the clothes must be removed or loosened. The diarrhœa for which Pulsatilla is suitable is a passive mucous flux, with little pain, occurring chiefly at night. The stools, Dr. Guernsey says, often vary in character from one to the other. These gastro-intestinal symptoms are frequently present in the febrile affections of childhood, as in mumps and varicella ; and a few doses of Pulsatilla are useful accordingly. In two of these diseases our medicine is indispensable, viz., measles and re-mittent fever. Having no control over the fever itself—which requires in the former case Aconite, in the latter Gelsemium—it aids powerfully to recovery by cleaning the tongue and (in measles) checking the diarrhœa and moderating the catarrh. Pulsatilla has less influence when the respiratory mucous membrane is affected. Nevertheless, it is of considerable utility in chronic nasal catarrh, with thick aud bland dis-charge.* It is often a valuable palliative in nocturnal loose coughs, as of phthisis ; and is sometimes the best medicine in subacute and chronic bronchitis occurring in delicate persons, and accompanied with much mucous expectoration. Dr. Hirschel says that it is also specific for a cough which is loose by day, but becomes dry and tickling on lying down at night. So in disorders of the urinary tract Pulsatilla is far less fre-quently indicated than Cantharis, Cannabis, and Belladonna ; yet is sometimes useful for the dysuria of pregnancy, and for chronic catarrh of the bladder.

Dr. John Brunton, an old school practitioner, recently (1876) made a communication to the Medical Society of London,† recalling their attention to this neglected remedy. He related a series of acute nasal, bronchial, vaginal, vesical, and conjunc-tival catarrhs "so rapidly and successfully cured by it as to be, so to say, cut short," and mentioned that he had also used it with benefit in some chronic affections of the mucous mem-branes (as dyspepsia) and in amenorrhœa. Dr. Routh con-curred with him in esteeming it in the last-named malady.

2. The action of Pulsatilla upon the joints has led to its use in suitable forms of gout and rheumatism. The disorder of digestion, which lies at the foundation of gout, is just that to which Pulsatilla corresponds. Hence it is well calculated to

---

* See cases in *Brit. Journ. of Hom.*, xxxi., 370 ; and Hoyne, i., 295.
† *Proceedings of the Med. Soc. of London,* iii., 67.

effect radical benefit in recent cases of this malady. In the
paroxysm itself it is generally superseded by Colchicum;
though I know of one case in which the timely administration
of Pulsatilla has several times seemed to blight an incipient
attack. It is said to be indicated especially when the pains
fly from place to place. In subacute rheumatism with little or
no fever occurring in delicate persons it is extremely useful,
especially when the knees, ankles, or small joints of the hands
and feet are affected. In idiopathic inflammations of these
joints, moreover, Pulsatilla is the best remedy while the mischief is yet recent. But perhaps the form of arthritis to which
Pulsatilla most closely corresponds is *rheumatic gout*, using
this term to signify the independent malady so named. Dr.
Fuller has pointed out the much preponderating frequency
with which the female sex is invaded by this disorder, and its
intimate relations with menstrual derangements. Pulsatilla is
almost specific in its acute form; and even in chronic cases
may sometimes be given with advantage. Jahr recommends
it in the analogous gonorrhœal rheumatism.

3. In affections of the veins Pulsatilla occupies much the
same ground as Hamamelis. It is superior to that medicine
in crural phlebitis following parturition, but yields to it in
venous hæmorrhages. In piles and other varicoses—as of the
spermatic cord or the lower extremity—Pulsatilla will act
well when the general condition of the patient seems to call
for its use.

4. It was for diseases of the eyes, as I have said, that Pulsatilla was first brought prominently forward by Störck. The
more modest claims to service here warranted by our experiments can be amply sustained. Pulsatilla is most useful in
affections of the lids. In recent blepharophthalmia, with
profuse lachrymation and meibomian secretion, it is the best
medicine. It will blight a stye almost as effectually as Belladonna will a boil: but I have not found it prevent their tendency to recur. For the twitching of the eyelids, with dazzling
of sight, with which some persons are annoyed, I know no
remedy so useful as Pulsatilla. The aching of the eyeballs
produced by it is rather such as occurs in some forms of headache than an idiopathic affection. For a further presentation
of what Pulsatilla can do in diseases of the eye I may refer
you to the article on the drug of Drs. Allen and Norton. They
commend it in ophthalmia neonatorum, and even in strumous
ophthalmia where the discharge is profuse and bland, and
there is not much photophobia; also in superficial ulcers of
the conjunctiva corneæ.

5. Few medicines are used in our practice in affections of the ears more frequently than Pulsatilla. Its curative virtues are most evident in the ear-ache which so often troubles children, and which is generally a subacute inflammation of the middle ear; and in recent catarrhal deafness, with noises in the ears. But it has also been used with good results in acute inflammation of the auricle and meatus, in neuralgia of the nerves of the ear, and in non-scrofulous otorrhœa with deafness when the discharge is thick. Drs. Houghton and Cooper, moreover, concur in giving it the highest place among the remedies for acute inflammation of the middle ear.

6. I now come to what is perhaps the most important sphere of the operation of Pulsatilla,—the generative organs of both sexes. In the male subject you will find it invaluable in acute orchitis, however caused (this property of the drug has lately been vouched for by two practitioners of the old school,* who admit that they got the remedy from us); and in prostatitis (with Thuja). It is one of the medicines (with Graphites and Rhododendron) which have cured hydrocele. But its fullest powers are displayed in the female organism. When in girls of mild disposition puberty is unduly delayed, or the menstrual function is defectively and irregularly performed; when they grow pale and languid, and complain of headache, chilliness, and lassitude, Pulsatilla (with or without Ferrum) is a most excellent remedy. Dr. Guernsey recommends it for the painful lumps which sometimes form in the breasts of these subjects,—the pain extending to the corresponding arm. When the menses have been suppressed by a chill, if the time for Aconite has gone by, Pulsatilla will generally restore the discharge. This property of the drug Störck had indicated. I believe it to be as good a remedy for ovaritis as it is for orchitis; and far superior to most of those ordinarily recommended. In simple mucous leucorrhœa it is often curative; and in dysmenorrhœa when the little blood which flows is black and coagulated, and when diarrhœa is wont to occur at the periods. It presides in a most beneficial manner over the function of parturition. Given daily for a month or so previously, it greatly facilitates the process in women whose labours are tedious and difficult. In labour itself, when the pains are irregular, tardy, and defective, yet ergot is hardly called for, Pulsatilla will often do good service; as also when from the same cause the placenta is unduly retained. There are several cases recorded which leave little doubt but that in false presentations Pulsatilla favours spontaneous version

* See *Hom. Times*, May, 1878.

After labour, it is very useful in promoting the secretion of milk, when this is deficient, or in improving the quality. Altogether, the weaker sex has much for which to thank homœopathy in its gift of Pulsatilla.

You may smile at one of these properties I have ascribed to our remedy, namely, that of rectifying false presentations. But you must remember that in these cases spontaneous version is not so very uncommon an occurrence, which shows that nature has means of effecting the change, and may well be helped thereto by an appropriate drug-stimulus. The evidence that Pulsatilla does render such aid comes from several practitioners, both in France and in America.* And if you suggest that the cures they report may have been instances of the spontaneous version of which I have spoken, I will adduce the testimony of Dr. Mercy Jackson, (late) of Boston. In a communication made by this experienced lady to the American Institute of Homœopathy in 1875, she relates fifteen successive cases of false presentation, being all that had occurred in her practice from a certain time onwards. In every one she administered Pulsatilla, and in every one the body underwent rotation and the head came to the fore. It is beyond all probability that these fifteen cases should have been a series of coincidences; so that they seem to establish the power of the drug in question.

Dr. Bayes, whose article on Pulsatilla is one of the best in his book, speaks of its predominating action on the left side of the body, and recommends it accordingly in clavus, hemicrania, and infra-mammary pain having this seat. He also advises it in constitutional disturbance in children associated with copious excretion of urate of ammonia in the urine, an experience which I have often confirmed.

Pulsatilla is also one of the leading remedies for chronic intermittents. It is indicated where its temperament, gastro-intestinal symptoms, and circumstances of aggravation and amelioration obtain; and also where a condition of hydræmia and chlorosis has been set up.

Pulsatilla, like the polychrests generally, has no true analogue. The medicines which most frequently come up for comparison with it in practice are *Actæa, Antimonium crudum, Caulophyllum, Conium, Cyclamen, Hamamelis* and *Sepia.*

Again like the polychrests generally, Pulsatilla requires to be given in various potencies to obtain all its virtues. I have little experience with the mother-tincture or first dilutions,

* See *Bull. de la Soc. Med. Hom. de France*, xviii., 544.

though with the former Dr. Phillips seems to get all the good effects of the medicine, and our old-school colleagues of whom I have spoken cured their cases of orchitis. In dysmenorrhœa only, I have myself gone as low as the 1st decimal. But I can recommend to you the 3rd decimal in gastric disorders and inflammations of the testicle or ovary, the 3rd centesimal in affections of the eyes and ears, and in rheumatism ; while the 6th and 12th I believe to be best suited for gout, for affections of the veins, and for ovario-uterine disturbances.

RANUNCULUS, RATANHIA, RHEUM, RHODODENDRON, RHUS,
RUMEX, RUTA.

We shall be able to dispose of all the drugs beginning
with the letter R to-day. They are a succession of vegetable
medicines of various degrees of importance.

The first will be the several varieties of Ranunculus. Two
of these, Ranunculus bulbosus and sceleratus, have received
a very fair proving. As I see no essential difference between
their properties, I shall treat of them indiscriminately here
under the title of

Ranunculus.

The tincture of either variety is prepared from the whole
plant.

The provings appear in Stapf's *Additions*. That of
Ranunculus bulbosus was undertaken by Dr. Franz and two
others (one being a woman), all using full doses of the pure
tincture. Ranunculus sceleratus was proved on himself, in
the same form, by an anonymous physician. Dr. Allen adds
a proving of the former (on a woman) by Stapf, and of the
latter by Schreter.

The Ranunculi are intensely irritant when applied locally,
causing inflammation and vesication, with burning itching.
It is not evident from the provings whether this effect—so
much resembling that of Rhus—is, as with that medicine,
dynamic and specific in nature. But this may be inferred from
Franz's experiment, in which contact with the juice produced
not only an immediate eruption of bullæ, but a subsequent
development (a fortnight after these had healed) of a series of
herpetic patches, the vesicles being dark blue, and itching and
burning intolerably. No eruptions were developed by the
internal use of the plant, though there was a good deal of
subjective cutaneous irritation. The most characteristic and

lasting effects of both were exerted upon the walls of the chest. The symptoms from the 175th to the 212th of Ranunculus bulbosus, and from the 117th to the 138th of Ranunculus sceleratus, are composed almost entirely of the various kinds of pain and soreness experienced by the provers in the sternum, ribs, intercostal spaces, and hypochondria.

Correspondingly, the Ranunculi have been used with the utmost success in *pleurodynia*, whether rheumatic,* neuralgic,† or myalgic.‡ I cannot *à priori* diagnose for you their place in these maladies as compared with that of Actæa racemosa and of Arnica : you must be guided by the accompanying symptoms, *i.e.*, by the absence of the nervous or uterine disorder of the former, and by the greater acuteness of the pain than in the cases suitable to the latter. I know of no other standing uses of Ranunculus. I once treated a case of chronic dysentery in a domestic servant accompanied by infra-mammary pain on both sides. After a fruitless trial of Mercurius corrosivus and Kali bichromicum, I was led by the pains to give Ranunculus bulbosus in the third dilution. Under its use the intestinal symptoms rapidly subsided, and the pain disappeared from the left side, but persisted in the right, from which it was at length dislodged by Nux vomica. Two or three returns of the malady have been rapidly checked by the same drug.

In conclusion, Ranunculus should be borne in mind in some cases of sciatica, and other rheumatic neuralgiæ : also in herpes and eczema. It ought to be a very efficient medicine for shingles, covering as it does the intercostal neuralgia as well as the eruption. Dr. Markwick says he finds it very useful here ;§ and Drs. Allen and Norton mention a case involving the supra-orbital region, in which the success consequent on the use of this drug was " exceedingly brilliant." Dr. Bayes praises it in pleurisy and hydrothorax of the right side, and Dr. Guernsey in leucorrhœa at first mild, but afterwards acrid and corrosive.

Rhus, Clematis, Euphorbium, Croton, Mezereum, Sabadilla and *Staphisagria* are the analogues of Ranunculus.

The dilutions from 1 to 3 seem to have been generally used.

And now a few words about a medicine which is ordinarily

---

* *Brit. Journn. of Hom.;* xxiv., 160 ; ii., 274.
† *Ibid,* ii., 274.
‡ *Monthly Hom. Review,* x., 752 ; Bayes, *sub voce.*
§ *Ibid,* xv., 64.

known only as an astringent, and not often used even in that capacity at the present day, the Krameria root,

Ratanhia.*

The tincture is prepared from the dried root.

There is a pathogenesis of Ratanhia in the third volume of Hartlaub and Trinks' *Arzneimittellehre*. Some additional symptoms are furnished by Teste, in his article on the drug, and by Allen.

I can give no general account of the symptoms ascribed to Ratanhia. One of them only, so far as I know, had (until lately) led to practical results,—" sensation as of a skin before the eyes." Acting on this very slight hint, Dr Madden tried it in a case of *pterygium*, and with success. I have myself used it with curative results in three cases of this disease— one in the human subject, and two in the lower animals (a dog and a cat respectively). Several other cases of success with it have appeared in the *Monthly Homœopathic Review* during the last few years.

Another symptom of Ratanhia, " dry heat at the anus, with sudden stitches which the patient compares to stabs with a penknife,"† makes it possible that it is somewhat homœopathic to the fissure of the anus which the French physicians profess to cure with it. Dr. Allen has confirmed this supposition by the cure of a bad case with the third dilution.‡ He thinks it indicated in preference to Graphites when the pain is cutting and lancinating rather than a sensation of smarting and soreness, and to Nitric acid when such pain is felt more after than during the passage of the motion. Teste recommends it in uterine pains following retrocession of an eruption situated on the lumbar region.

I can say nothing about medicines allied to Ratanhia.

For dose I have always used the second dilution ; but the first decimal has been employed with benefit.

And now we come to an old enemy of the childhood of

---

* In his paper subsequently referred to, Dr. Allen says that this name should be spelt " Ratania," but in his *Encyclopædia* he prints it as above.

† This is given by Teste, as observed by himself; but omitted by Allen.

‡ *North American Journ. of Hom.*, May, 1878.

most of us—happily unknown, as a drug, to our own children
—Rhubarb, *Latiné* Rhabarbarum, or

Rheum.

Our tincture is made, like the common one, from the dry
root.

The pathogenesis of Rheum is in the second volume of the
Reine Arzneimittellehre. It contains 194 symptoms from
Hahnemann and five others, and 14 from authors. It was
also one of the medicines tested by the Vienna Provers'
Society; whose results you may read in the sixth volume of
the *British Journal of Homœopathy*, or in Hempel.

None of these provings add anything of import to the
knowledge previously existing of the action of Rhubarb on
the alimentary canal. Of this Hahnemann writes :—" It is
not an easy, liquid, and copious stool, or a painless diarrhœa,
which is the primary action of Rhubarb on the bowels, but
rather a colicky and sometimes ineffectual urging to altered
evacuations, which are nevertheless always fæcal." To the
same effect is the testimony of all therapeutists. Rhubarb
is considered to stimulate the muscular fibre of the whole
length of the intestine, purging without causing serous
effusion, and never—however far its action may go—inflaming
the mucous membrane. Dr. Rutherford has ascertained that,
like Podophyllum, it increases both the liquid and the solid
elements of the bile. The constipation which often follows
the purgation of Rhubarb seems due to an after action of the
tannin it contains.

A corresponding form of diarrhœa is occasionally met with,
especially in children : a sour smell has been found characteristic of it, and was noticed by Gross in the course of his proving. When this morbid condition occurs, Rheum—from the
second to the sixth dilution—will give you every satisfaction ;
and you will feel glad that you can use it to remove children's
troubles instead of to cause them.

Dr. Allen emphasises repulsiveness of food as characteristic
of this remedy.

My next medicine is the beautiful Siberian rose,

Rhododendron chrysanthum.

The dried leaves and flower-buds are the officinal portion of
the plant.

A proving of Rhododendron, conducted by Dr. Seidel on himself and several others with moderate doses of the mother-tincture, is given in Stapf's *Additions*. Dr. Allen adds some symptoms by Lembke.

The most characteristic effects of Rhododendron are the pains which it excites in the muscular and fibrous tissues, and the swelling and tenderness of the testes and epididymis. In practice it has been found useful accordingly. It has a high native reputation for gout and rheumatism; and homœopathic experience shows it to be specifically curative in many forms of these maladies. It seems especially serviceable in rheumatism of the cervical and thoracic muscles, and in rheumatic neuralgia of the extremities. The pains are worse at rest, and at the approach of stormy weather. I have myself used Rhododendron with much benefit, acting on a hint from German experience, in rheumatic face-ache.* Relief of pain during and after eating seems characteristic of it here. Drs. Allen and Norton mention a case, apparently of incipient glaucoma, in which the aggravation of the (recurring) pains before a storm led to the choice of Rhododendron, which not only relieved these, but checked the disease, and materially improved the vision. Chronic affections of the testes—as orchitis and hydrocele—have also been frequently cured by Rhododendron.

The stools characteristic of this drug are loose, but require much pressure for their expulsion.

Rhus and *Clematis*, and perhaps *Ranunculus*, are analogues of Rhododendron. The diagnostic marks between it and Rhus are fully given in the second volume of the *American Journal of Homœopathic Materia Medica* (p. 247). Briefly, they are that, with Rhododendron, the pains do not admit of the limbs being at rest, and moving relieves at once; while, with Rhus, the first movement aggravates the pains, and continued motion only relieves. Again, the pains of Rhododendron are aggravated in the night indeed, but more towards morning; those of Rhus more towards evening and night. Once more—Rhus corresponds to rheumatism in the cold season, Rhododendron in the hot; and the symptoms of the former are worse after, the latter before rain.

The dilutions from 12 to 30 were given in the cases which Dr. Seidel prefixes to his pathogenesis; but in rheumatic prosopalgia my experience is that of the German physicians, who prefer the 1st and 2nd decimal.

---

* See *Brit. Journ. of Hom.*, xxvii., 149.

I have now to introduce you to the medicine, which, whatever the species of the plant we use, is known as

Rhus.

Under this name we include the Rhus toxicodendron, the sumach, or poison oak ; Rhus radicans, the poison ivy or vine ; and Rhus venenata, the poison wood or ash. The last, by the way, must not be confounded (as it sometimes is) with the Rhus vernix of Linnæus, which grows in Japan. The leaves of the two former species, and the juice which exudes from incisions in the bark of the Rhus venenata, are used to make their tinctures.

Rhus toxicodendron was proved by Hahnemann. The second volume of the *Reine Arzneimittellehre* contains a pathogenesis of 976 symptoms, of which more than half are his own, the remainder being supplied by nine fellow-provers and some authors. Rhus radicans was proved by Dr. Joslin and ten others : the record of his experiments is contained in the first volume of the *American Homœopathic Review*. Dr. Allen unites the symptoms of R. radicans with those of R. toxicodendron, and adds numerous observations of the effects of handling the plant. The effects of Rhus venenata have been very fully ascertained by Drs. Burt, Hoyt, and Oehme, both by taking the drug internally and by exposing themselves to contact with its juice or emanations ; as you may read in Dr. Hale's pages. Here too Dr. Allen adds much fresh matter in his *Encyclopædia*.

The poisonous influence of the juice of all the sumachs has been found to reside in a volatile acid which it contains. Hence exposure to the emanations has almost as potent an effect as actual contact with the juice. I will describe the results of either in the words of a late Lecturer on Materia Medica at the Medical School of the Westminster Hospital :—

"The effects produced by Rhus are redness and swelling of the affected parts, which, if the exhalations be the exciting cause, are more particularly the face and eyes. Subsequently there is pain, and often a considerable increase of temperature, and the inflamed surface is generally studded with vesicles. Combined with these symptoms, there is an almost unbearable amount of itching, which is not confined to the patches of inflammation, but diffuses itself, more or less, over the entire surface of the body, the hairy portions appearing to be very specially affected. The condition induced thus

appears to be of an erythematous or erysipelatous type. It
is superficial, but spreads rapidly over the surface, and speedily
involves large areas of the body; eventually extending to the
mucous membranes, as indicated by redness and swelling of
the throat and mouth, with, ordinarily, great thirst, irritable
cough, nausea, vomiting, vertigo, dulness and stupefaction of
head, and colicky pains throughout the abdomen. These last
are chiefly experienced during the night, and are aggravated
by eating or drinking. Diarrhœa frequently ensues, accompanied by tenesmus, and the stools are often bloody. There
is often retention of the urine, or else diuresis, and the water is
frequently accompanied by blood.

"Rhus also induces pains, apparently of a rheumatic kind,
and which are felt not only in the limbs but in the body,
though most especially about the joints. Pain and stiffness
in the lumbar region are often induced, and to these affections
is often added a sense of numbness in the lower extremities.
The structures most powerfully affected appear to be the
fibrous ones. The pains in question are accompanied by a
very slight amount of swelling; and, singular to say, they
become intensified by rest and warmth. Sleep is greatly
disturbed, the patient becoming restless, constantly turning
about, and often suffering from great nervous depression.

" The fever which sometimes accompanies the effects of
Rhus, though by no means an universal symptom, usually
occurs, when present, in the later stages, and generally partakes
of a typhoid character. It is often attended by delirium ;
the lips are apt to become dry and parched, and to be covered
with a brownish crust. Sometimes it assumes an intermittent
character, and is then usually marked by profuse perspiration.

" The above-described effects of Rhus, though so distressing to whoever may have to endure them, appear, however, to
be very seldom fatal ; and it is remarkable that a certain
constitutional predisposition appears requisite to their occurrence, so that it is only individuals who are in danger.
Were it otherwise, a plant so common in its native country
as the present would be a perpetual source of trouble to the
persons dwelling near. I have myself witnessed several
instances of the poisonous influence, and can personally vouch
for the manifestation of nearly all the phenomena that have
been indicated."*

I have thought it well to cite this account from an author
not partial to the homœopathic doctrine, as I shall have to

* *Materia Medica and Therapeutics. Vegetable Kingdom.* By
Charles Phillips, M.D., &c.

show that the efficacy of Rhus as a medicine is displayed in the very regions in which it is so active as a poison. We shall see it as a remedy for many cutaneous affections, for rheumatism, and for typhoid conditions of several kinds.

I. The action of Rhus on the skin is obviously of a very acute and specific kind. Teste well describes it as that of "a corrosive caustic, which, from its extreme subtilty, has a tendency to invade large surfaces, rather than to penetrate deeply into tissues." He compares it with Arnica, which dips deeper down ; and with Ledum, whose influence is more localised. Severe boils followed the primary symptoms in two of the provers of Rhus venenata. An additional value for homœopathic purposes is given to these effects by the fact mentioned by Dr. Phillips, that they only occur in a certain number of those who are exposed to the influence of the plant, *i.e.*, they are contingent upon special susceptibility. Dufresnoy, moreover, states that persons, not constitutionally susceptible to the disorders induced by Rhus as a poisonous agent, are not so likely to receive benefit from it if used as a medicine. It points in the same direction when we hear from Trousseau and Pidoux of the symptoms first appearing twenty-five days after inoculation with the juice, and from Fontana of their recurrence at intervals subsequently.

Correspondingly, in cutaneous affections, especially when acute, Rhus naturally takes high rank as a remedy. The members of the order vesiculæ—herpes (especially h. zoster), eczema, and pemphigus—are the forms of eruption to which it is most suitable. I have frequently cured these affections with Rhus, and indeed rarely require any other remedy for them. Dr. Hedges, physician to the Half-Orphan Asylum of Chicago, says that 75 per cent of all the cases of eczema occurring therein have been cured by this remedy. Itching with burning is a characteristic indication for it here, and also (according to Dr. Guernsey) the presence of an inflamed margin around the spots of eruption. Dr. Dunham recommends it in eczema impetiginodes, and Dr. Wesselhœft has communicated cases of prurigo senilis and vulvæ cured by it.* Still more closely do the effects of Rhus correspond with erythema and erysipelas. When this latter malady goes on to the formation of vesicles and bullæ (vesicular erysipelas), Rhus is the standard remedy among homœopathists ; and I have often seen it act here in the most beautiful manner. Teste seems justified in recommending it as the best medicine to be given in extensive but superficial burns.

* See *Brit. Journ. of Hom.*, xxiii., 563.

It was the accidental cure of an old herpetic eruption by the development of the cutaneous symptoms of Rhus poisoning that led to its first introduction into medicine, by Dufresnoy of Valenciennes. His memoir on the subject (of which you may read a full account in the twenty-eighth volume of the *British Journal of Homœopathy*) relates several cases of a similar kind in which he gave the drug internally with distinguished success. Like so many other valuable pieces of practice, however, this use of Rhus had perished in the old school, but has been maintained in homœopathy, to which it legitimately belongs.

II. The rheumatoid pains described by Dr. Phillips as occurring in Rhus poisoning are seen in an especial degree in the provers of the drug. From Rhus venenata the joints, as well as the fibrous tissues, were affected—especially the knees, ankles, feet, and hands ; but there was no genuine synovial swelling, as with Bryonia and Pulsatilla. It is chiefly to these rheumatoid pains that Hahnemann's well-known observation belongs, that, unlike those of Bryony, they are most violent when the part affected is in a state of perfect rest. He extends the statement, indeed, to the symptoms produced by the drug generally ; and the recent provings of Rhus venenata support his 'statement.

Rhus has thus come to occupy a high place in homœopathic therapeutics amongst the remedies for rheumatism. It is not often indicated in rheumatic fever. It would be so where, as in a case mentioned by Dr. Bayes, restlessness and constant desire to change the position were present. Dr. Phillips also says that " in the after stage of acute rheumatic fever, when aconite may have been employed, and when the temperature has fallen to 100°, or below it, and where the patient still suffers from wearing stiffness, and aching in the neighbourhood of the joints, rhus is positively invaluable." But in various subacute and chronic rheumatic affections it is a most precious remedy, especially when they can be traced to a *wetting*. Herein it resembles Dulcamara, and differs from Aconite and Bryonia, whose local rheumatic symptoms are rather such as dry cold produces.* Its action is mainly, if not entirely, upon the fibrous tissues—tendons, fasciæ, sheaths of nerves, &c.—and perhaps the muscles. I do not think that it controls the rheumatic affections of the synovial membranes, but only those of the ligaments external to the capsules of the joints. Nor do I think that it acts upon the nerves them-

* See a case of rheumatic pleurodynia in Hoyne (i., 128) illustrating this point.

selves. Its undoubted value in rheumatic sciatica* depends, I take it, upon its influence on the fibrous sheath of the nerve, which is so often the seat of the pain. It is powerless in pure neuralgia here or elsewhere. It is certainly the best remedy in most cases of lumbago, at any rate after Aconite :—I suspect that here the lumbar fascia is the part affected rather than the actual muscles. It is thus especially indicated when lumbago and sciatica are present together. In rheumatic lameness of the lower extremities, depending largely upon the state of the fascia lata, Rhus has made brilliant cures.†—In all these maladies the characteristic features, "worse at rest, relieved by motion," are of immense weight in determining our choice of Rhus. Dr. Neidhard has added the important observation that on first moving after rest the pains are increased. It is not until the parts have been moved for some little time that relief ensues. With Bryony, on the other hand, the longer the movement continues, the worse the pains become ; and with Rhododendron, as we have seen, movement relieves from the first. Dr. Carroll Dunham has drawn out these characteristics of the pains of Rhus in a very interesting manner, in some observations on the drug which you will find in the first volume of his *Lectures*. "The rheumatic symptoms of the drug," he says, "come on with severity during repose, and they increase as long as the patient remains quiet, until, at length, their severity compels him to move. Now, on first attempting to move, he finds himself very stiff, and the very first movement is exceedingly painful. But as he continues to move, however, the stiffness is relieved and the pains decidedly decrease, the patient feeling much better." He goes on to point out that this improvement does not continue indefinitely ; for weariness readily comes on in such patients, and then rest is at first grateful, only after a while to be disturbed by a recurrence of the aching pain. As chronic rheumatisms of muscles, ligaments, and fascia are generally of this character, Rhus is by far the most frequently indicated remedy for them, and in my own hands has made many a cure.

The action of Rhus on the white fibrous tissues has led to its being used in the treatment of sprains. Hahnemann says, —"I have recognised in these latter years that Rhus is the best specific against the consequences of muscular strains and contusions." He does not say what relation it bears to Arnica

---

* See case in *Brit. Journ. of Hom.*, xi., 146 ; and another in Hoyne, i., 136.

† *Ibid*, xxv., 661.

here ; nor do I know that general experience has found it
superior or even equal to that medicine, save when its own peculiar symptoms of aggravation and amelioration are present.   In
so-called " rheumatisms," however, having these features, and
where severe or continued strain seems to have been the
originating cause, Rhus is of undoubted value.

III. The fever of Rhus poisoning is at first sympathetic
with the dermatitis that is set up.   But later here, as pointed
out by Dr. Phillips, and perhaps primarily (as suggested by
the provings) from the internal use of the drug, a febrile condition of low and nervous type is set up, with diarrhœa and
prostration.   Hahnemann was led hereby to use Rhus as a
principal remedy for the epidemic fever which ravaged Germany in 1813.   Whether it was true typhus, or (as Dr. Russell
thinks) relapsing fever, is doubtful ; but this at least is certain,
that while the mortality under the ordinary treatment was
considerable, Hahnemann treated 183 patients without a single
death.*   He also recommended it, in alternation with Bryonia,
in the consecutive fever of cholera.†

Rhus has accordingly taken rank as an important anti-
typhoid remedy in homœopathic practice.   Drs. Wurmb and
Caspar, from their experience in the Leopoldstadt Hospital at
Vienna, define its place in typhus and enteric fever.   It corresponds, they say, to an erethistic type of the malady, such
as, when more severe, requires Arsenic.   Dr. Dunham points
out that a corresponding condition is apt to supervene in the
course of measles‡ and scarlatina ; and that here Rhus is no
less indicated and beneficial.   In the latter disease, he says,
it is still more strongly called for " if there be an œdematous
condition of the fauces, soft palate, and uvula, with vesicles
upon these parts, and a singularly annoying itching, smarting,
and burning."   Epidemics of influenza sometimes present this
condition of the throat, with great debility ; and here also
Rhus is remedial.   A red triangle at the tip of the tongue is
said to indicate it in typhoid states.

Another variety of scarlatina in which I have much confidence in Rhus is that in which rheumatic symptoms appear.
I speak of the " scarlatina rheumatica " of this country ; but
I should think the remedy equally applicable to the epidemic
disease which sometimes bears this name—the " dengue " of
America and the Indies.   I would suggest the Rhus venenata
here, on account of the implication of the mucous membrane

* *Lesser Writings*, p. 712 ; see also p. 328 of this *Manual*.
† *Ibid*, p. 847.
‡ See case in *Brit. Journ. of Hom.*, xxx., 587.

of the mouth and throat, which is seen most prominently in the pathogenesis of this variety. On this account I gave it once, and with much success, in a relapse of Ceylon fever in a patient lately returned from that island.

These cutaneous, rheumatic, and febrile disorders form the main sphere of action of Rhus in homœopathic practice. Of its anti-paralytic virtues we have not, perhaps, sufficiently availed ourselves. Dufresnoy first brought these to light by accident. Giving the medicine for a hemiplegia, under the supposition that it was caused by a repelled eruption, he cured his patient, though mistaken as to the origin of the malady. He therefore gave it in other paralytic affections, often with benefit; and his practice was followed with the same results by Alderson in England. Improvement, as with Collin's use of Arnica, was generally preceded by pains and other sensations in the affected parts. It is doubtful whether Rhus acts homœopathically here. The paralytic symptoms of its pathogenesis are rather those of general prostration than of special depression of the motor centres; and the only recorded experience of its value in the school of Hahnemann is that of Trinks, who gave it in increasing doses of the mother-tincture. The paralysis in all these cases is described as painless. But there is a paralytic condition which is far from being painless, viz., the rheumatic form; and in the minute doses commonly used by homœopathists it is here that Rhus has been chiefly used. It will often result from exposure of the back or seat to damp cold. Dr. Dunham suggests that paraplegia occurring in young children is generally thus caused; and states that it readily yields to Rhus, and an occasional dose of Sulphur.[*] Of the same kind is the paresis of one or more of the muscles of the eyeball which sometimes results from damp cold; and here Rhus vies with Causticum.

Rhus is, moreover, thoroughly homœopathic to affections of the mucous membrane resembling those which it causes on the cutaneous surface. The late Sir James Simpson has well shown that conditions answering to erythema and eczema of the skin are not uncommon on the lining membrane of the bowels and other parts, especially in women. Rhus is also beneficial in diarrhœa and dysentery associated with low general conditions, as typhus[†] and scorbutus. Dr. Guernsey says that it is "almost, if not quite, a specific in dysentery when the pain runs in streaks down the limbs with every evacuation." This is in children. The mucous membrane it in-

[*] See case in *Brit. Journ. of Hom.*, xxviii., 793.
[†] *Monthly Hom. Review*, xvi., 733.

fluences most powerfully is the conjunctiva. In the sixth volume of the *British Journal of Homœopathy* Dr. Dudgeon has collected numerous testimonies, from both old and new schools, to its value in strumous ophthalmia. Perhaps the phlyctenular character of the affection has something to do with its usefulness here ; and it is noteworthy that there is often an association of general eczema of the face. When this occurs, Rhus is doubly indicated.

Drs. Allen and Norton have considerably extended the sphere of action of this medicine in ocular disorders. They account it " a remedy of the first importance," " *the* remedy," in orbital cellulitis, saying that some alarming cases of this disease occurring in their own experience have been promptly arrested by it. They praise it in ophthalmia neonatorum and suppuration of the cornea, and say that " the grandest sphere of its action is to be found in suppurative iritis, or in the still more severe cases in which the inflammatory process has involved the remainder of the uveal tract, especially if of traumatic origin, as after cataract extraction." It is thus in suppurative inflammation of the eye, especially of its deeper parts, that it plays such an important part in their hands. Great œdema of the eyelids is said to be symptomatic of such morbid processes, and to be a special indication for the remedy. They recommend the employment of the higher dilutions at first, as " we cannot afford to produce an aggravation in a sensitive subject ; " but that " if most prompt results are not obtained in a few hours," we should resort to the lowest.

In favour of this power of Rhus over acute suppurative processes is a case of poisoning with the " radicans " variety observed by Dr. Helmuth,* in which " the symptoms were all those belonging to septicæmia. Suppuration had taken place in the ankle, which was affected with severe synovitis. Besides the symptoms above-mentioned, the patient had vesicles in the mouth and throat, . . large and purple bullæ over the leg, which was immensely tumefied and red, together with a toxæmic expression, which was remarkable in every respect."

Several other facts about Rhus, and applications of it as a medicine, may be gleaned from Dr. Dunham's study of the drug, which I cannot too warmly commend to your notice. His observation as to the acridity communicated by it to all the fluids and secretions of the body is especially worthy of notice. I was led by this symptom to give it in a case of gouty ophthalmia, to the very great relief and improvement of the

* *System of Surgery* (4th ed.), p. 67.

patient. Dr. Guernsey's chief indication for it, in addition to the characteristic rheumatic pain I have already described, is bodily restlessness, so that the patient cannot remain long in any one position, and finds momentary relief from any change. It has been recommended in intermittents when a tearing cough occurs during the chill.

The medicines most allied to Rhus are *Croton, Ranunculus, Ledum, Rhododendron* and *Bryonia*.

In recent cutaneous affections I recommend the 6th dilution : in chronic, from the 1st to the 3rd decimal, as also in shingles and erysipelas. In chronic rheumatism the higher dilutions seem to have made the best cures; while in paralysis and strumous ophthalmia the material doses of Old Medicine have given the drug its reputation. Hahnemann says that the action of Rhus is slow; and that improvement is rarely perceived (I hope he means in chronic cases) until thirty-six hours after the administration of the dose.

Once again we turn to America, as she sends us the yellow dock,

Rumex crispus.

The fresh root is used in the preparation of the tincture.

The original proving of Rumex, by Dr. Joslin, is in the second volume of the *American Homœopathic Review*. Several persons took part in it, using both the tincture and the dilutions. The pathogenesis is given, with numerous clinical cases, in the second edition of Dr. Hale's *New Remedies ;* and by Allen, who adds symptoms from three other provers.

Rumex has some influence on the skin and alimentary mucous membrane, causing in the former an itching which is increased by exposure to cool air, and relieved by warmth (herein contrasting with that of Sulphur and Mercury), and in the latter a sense of weight at the stomach, and a morning diarrhœa. Its main action, however, is exerted upon the respiratory mucous membrane, and especially that of the larynx ; where it diminishes secretion while exalting sensibility. Hence changes in voice, and dry titillating cough. The action hardly goes on to inflammation.

Rumex has cured some cases of gastric and intestinal derangement characterised as above, especially morning diarrhœa. It should be thought of in prurigo, where the itching has the unusual characteristic of that excited by the drug.

Dr. Searle communicated to the third volume of the *United States Medical and Surgical Journal* an account of the contagious prurigo, or " army itch," so frequently observed during the American civil war. After trying several ordinary remedies in vain, he found Rumex crispus its specific. He gave several drops of the first decimal dilution for a dose.

But the chief use of Rumex is in laryngo-tracheal cough, of which quite an array of cases may be read in Dr. Hale's article. The symptoms are those of catarrh, with excessive irritability of the laryngo-tracheal mucous membrane, causing a violent, incessant, and fatiguing cough, with little expectoration. Pressure, talking, and especially inspiration of cool air, cause aggravation. There is often a sense of excoriation behind the sternum. I have several times prescribed Rumex with success in this kind of cough, but quite as often with entire failure, though it seemed thoroughly indicated. When it cures, it does so with almost magical rapidity.

The analogues of Rumex in the respiratory sphere are stated by Dr. Carroll Dunham to be *Lachesis, Belladonna, Causticum* and *Phosphorus.* His sketch of the laryngeal symptoms of the five medicines respectively (given by Dr. Hale)* is a model of delicate application and discriminative comparison. I would add to his four analogues a fifth, *Spongia.* In its relation to morning diarrhœa, Rumex corresponds to *Apis, Nuphar, Podophyllum* and *Sulphur.*

Nearly all the recorded cures have been made with the dilutions from the 6th to the 30th.

My last medicine to-day is the common rue,

Ruta graveolens.

The tincture is prepared from the whole plant, which should be quite fresh.

The proving of Ruta is in the fourth volume of the *Reine Arzneimittellehre.* It contains 26 symptoms from Hahnemann, 259 from eight others, and 3 from authors. Dr. Allen adds some further provings, and some poisonings.

" Hardly any medicine," writes Stillé, " was more frequently employed of old, or with greater confidence in its virtues, than this now neglected plant." Its poisonous action shows it to be an acro-narcotic, with a special action upon the uterus. This last has lately been studied by Dr. Hélie, of Nantes, who finds it cause both active determination of blood to the

---

* See also *Homœopathy the Science of Therapeutics,* p. 417.

organ, and contraction of its muscular walls. Rue is thus emmenagogue and abortifacient, which properties of the plant have long been known and utilised in domestic, and to some extent in professional, practice. We of course turn them to account by giving Ruta, not in amenorrhœa, but in meno- and metrorrhagia ; and not to cause miscarriage, but to avert it. In the former use of it we have the countenance of an old-school celebrity, M. Beau of La Charité, who appears quite unconscious of the homœopathicity of his practice.*

In Hahnemann's proving the chief symptoms elicited were pains in the bones, joints, and cartilages, especially of a " bruised " character. " Ruta seems," he remarks, " to excite many pains in the bones or the periosteum." It has accordingly been used in the treatment of rheumatism, especially of the wrist and ankle ; and in bruises of the periosteum. Dr. Henriques has published an interesting case in which an un-united fracture in a cachectic patient rapidly took on healing action under its influence.† The tenesmus which the provings show it to cause in the rectum and bladder—even to prolapse of the former—well corresponds to its action on the uterus, and should receive homœopathic application. Dr. Guernsey recommends it in constipation with prolapse of the rectum before or during the stool.

Yet another virtue of rue is its undoubted power in dimness of vision caused by over-exertion of the eyes. Hahnemann mentions it as commended by Rosenstein, Swedjaur, and Chomel in this trouble, and points to S. 38 and 39 in his " Observations of Others," as showing that the drug causes what it cures. A Hungarian physician, Dr. Elgâjaki, has lately drawn attention to the same double series of facts. Ophthalmology has not yet ascertained for us what is the precise pathological condition induced by Ruta or removed by it (Drs. Allen and Norton consider it to be asthenopia); and meanwhile we must content ourselves with phenomenal indications. You will remember that it was " with euphrasy and rue" that Milton's angel purged Adam's visual nerve, that he might see.

" All parts of the body upon which he lies, even in bed, are painful, as if bruised (after 17 hours) " is a symptom of Hartmann's emphasised by Allen's type, and worth bearing in mind.

Crocus and Sabina in the uterine sphere, Mezereum and Phytolacca in the locomotive organs, and perhaps Euphrasia

---

* See Brit. Journ. of Hom., xxi., 343.
† Ibid., x., 445.

in the eyes, correspond to Ruta. M. Beau says that rue is to savin what Ipecacuanha is to Tartar emetic.

The second dilution is recommended by Hahnemann. In Dr. Henriques' case the twelfth was given.

LECTURE LII.

SABADILLA, SABINA, SAMBUCUS, SANGUINARIA, SARRACENIA, SARSAPARILLA, SCILLA, SECALE, SELENIUM, SENECIO, SENEGA.

The medicines beginning with the letter S, on which we now enter, will occupy us a much longer time than those which have R for their initial.

We will commence with the Indian barley,

Sabadilla.

A tincture and triturations are prepared from the dried cap-suled seeds as imported.

The proving of Sabadilla is in Stapf's *Additions*. It appears to have been a thorough one, having been conducted with the mother-tincture on upwards of eleven healthy persons.

Sabadilla contains veratria, of which we shall speak when we come to Veratrum album ; and besides the virtues of that alkaloid, it has acrid properties of its own. Its proving exhibits many well-characterised symptoms, but it has been very little employed in disease. Stapf writes :—"among the many important and characteristic symptoms of Sabadilla which every observing physician will easily recognise, the Sabadilla fever is especially remarkable. Sabadilla is not only a specific for a certain kind of very bad angina, and to a rare kind of pleurisy (where no inflammatory fever or thirst is present, and the patient complains of coldness mingled with isolated flushes of heat), but also for some forms of ague where the chilliness sets in with nausea and inclination to vomit, recurs frequently, and sometimes alternates with flushes of heat ; and where the heat is more perceptible in the face and on the hands than on the rest of the body. There is absence of thirst both in the cold and in the hot stage." Dr. Bayes communicates some unique experience with it in hay-fever, in which he regards it as of the greatest possible use. " The method," he writes, " I have found most serviceable for its administration has been to order the olfaction of the third decimal tincture several times a day, and the taking of one drop two or three times a day in water. By this means I have cured a number of severe cases, and have made many firm converts to our system of medicine." He has also used it in other cases of coryza, with severe frontal pains and redness of the eyelids, with great benefit ; and I have had good results from it in two cases of chronic nasal catarrh.

Sabadilla is a medicine to which you will more frequently be led by a repertory than by *à priori* knowledge of its action. When, however, you are directed to it by its homœopathicity to the morbid condition before you, you may employ it with confidence.

Staphisagria and *Veratrum album* seem somewhat analogous medicines.

We come next to a better known medicine in the shape of savin, the Juniperus

Sabina.

The tincture is prepared from the fresh leaves and green tops ; or from the oil distilled from the same, dissolved in ether,—it is not satisfactorily soluble in alcohol. Sometimes the oil is triturated with sugar of milk.

The proving of this drug also is in Stapf's *Additions*. Ten experimenters are mentioned ; but nothing is said about the doses they took. Dr. Allen adds some symptoms from poisonings and over-dosings.

Savin is a general irritant, stimulating the circulation and congesting the brain and lungs, and also inflaming the kidneys by which it is eliminated, so that the urine becomes bloody and albuminous. It further manifests a specific influence over the pelvic organs, causing strangury in front, bloody stools behind, and between the two metritis with hæmorrhage, and (in pregnant women) abortion. This uterine action of the drug has given it its chief therapeutic application. It is, of course, used in the old school as an emmenagogue, and enjoys some little repute in that capacity. Dr. Madden has shown that it may occasionally be used without harm in this way.*

* See case in *Brit. Journ. of Hom.*, xxiv, 301.

But it must be remembered that it acts here as a purgative opens the bowels ; and its use in our hands must be correspondingly exceptional. On the other hand, it is a most valuable homœopathically acting remedy for ovario-uterine excitement ; as in menorrhagia where the blood is bright red, in metrorrhagia, in threatened miscarriage from irritation, and in metritis—in a case of which disease in an acute form I have seen it effect a most satisfactory cure. The presence of consentaneous rectal and vesical irritation adds weight to the indications for the choice of Sabina in these disorders. M. Beau, whom I have already quoted as a witness to the value of Ruta in uterine hæmorrhage, extols savin as its chief remedy. He will have it exactly homœopathic, moreover ; for it is in "hæmorrhagic metritis," "metritis accompanied by flooding," that he gives it. One grain of the powder is given for a dose, and very often needs no repetition.[*] Pain going through from the sacrum to the pubes, and discharge of blood half fluid and half clotted, are Dr. Guernsey's chief indications for it. He also praises it in thick, corrosive leucorrhœa, which probably connotes a similar state of the uterus (see Allen, S. 267).

Sabina caused in the provers an unusual number of symptoms relating to the joints, even so far as to set up heat, redness, and swelling. It has been used in both schools for what are vaguely called "arthritic affections." The connection which has been traced between rheumatic gout and the uterine functions makes it probable that this is the malady in which, especially when recent, Sabina would be curative. I have used it once or twice upon these indications with very satisfactory results. It has occasionally relieved the paroxysm of true gout.

As allied medicines to Sabina I may name *Belladonna, Crocus, Pulsatilla, Ruta* and *Trillium*.

All dilutions, from the 1st to the 24th, and even the crude oil or powder, have in various hands proved efficacious. I myself am very well satisfied with the 2nd and 3rd decimal.

The next name on my list is the common elder,

Sambucus nigra.

The fresh inner bark of the young branches is used for the tincture.

[*] See *Brit. Journ. of Hom.*, xxi., 342. Aran had recommended it before him (vol. iii., p. 416). Recent therapeutists attempt to make out that it is in atonic menorrhagia that Sabina is curative ; but M. Beau is against them.

There is a pathogenesis of Sambucus in the fifth volume of the *Materia Medica Pura*, containing 20 symptoms from Hahnemann, and 99 from five others.* The articles in Hempel and Teste also should be consulted, and the additions made by Allen to the symptomatology.

The only facts about the physiological action of Sambucus to which I can assign importance are that it is a powerful sudorific ; and that it has caused asthmatic phenomena.† Its therapeutic use accordingly has been to moderate excessive sweating, and to relieve asthma, laryngismus stridulus, and the obstructive coryza of infants. I have myself found it of great use in checking those debilitating perspirations which often retard convalescence after delivery. I think, too, that I have seen some benefit from it in asthma : Dr. Jousset praises it in the paroxysm. Dr. Bayes writes :—"in the suffocating cough of children, waking them up in the middle of the night, and accompanied by rough sibilant wheezing, and great dyspnœa, but without croup, I have found small doses of Sambucus φ of the most rapid service." It has some repute among us in laryngismus stridulus, similarly occurring. Dr. Searle, who contributes an excellent paper on this disease to the ninth volume of the Transactions of the New York State Homœopathic Society, gives the determining symptoms for this remedy as—" burning, red, hot face, hot body, with cold hands and feet, *during sleep. On waking*, the face breaks out into a profuse perspiration, which extends over the body, and continues, more or less, during the waking hours ; then, on going to sleep again, the dry heat returns." When these peculiarities are encountered, he says, Sambucus is pretty sure to cure, and almost as certain to fail if they are absent. I may remark that such symptoms, as well as those described by Dr. Bayes, often depend (in children) upon nasal obstruction ; and that for this trouble, when the nostrils are dry, Sambucus is (as I have said) much esteemed among us.

Teste describes some neuralgic pains in the forearms which it cures.

Aconite and *Ipecacuanha* are allied remedies.

The 1st decimal is the dilution I have used in diaphoresis and asthma, and Hahnemann himself recommends the pure juice to be given.

---

* As Dr. Allen did not receive my notes on Hahnemann's cited symptoms in time for this medicine, I would mention here that the "dropsical swellings " of his S. 94 should be " œdematous state of the parts to which it is applied."

† See Hahnemann's sixth symptom.

America again comes forward to furnish us with our next medicine, the blood-root,

Sanguinaria Canadensis.

The tincture is prepared from the rhizoma.

Sanguinaria has been proved principally in the old school, as you will see from Allen's pathogenesis of it.   Some homœo-pathic experiments, however, are given in the *Materia Medica of American Provings*.   Dr. Hale's article in his *New Remedies* should be consulted.

The physiological effects of Sanguinaria are not very distinctly known.   It seems to be an emetic, a general irritant of mucous membrane, and a depressant of the circulation.   It comes to us from the eclectic practitioners of America with a high reputation in the treatment of affections of the respiratory organs ; in which it excited in the provers many symptoms of irritation.   It is said to have proved curative in homœopathic practice in membranous croup and œdematous laryngitis, in chronic cough with hectic, and even incipient phthisis. Dr. Hale recommends it in the third stage of pneumonia (grey hepatisation) ; and Dr. Drysdale also in pulmonary abscess.*

But a more frequent application of the drug which has been made in the school of Hahnemann is to *migraine*.   Dr. C. Hering was the first to indicate its suitableness thereto, but many others have followed in his wake.   Among them is Dr. Jousset, who in the new edition of his *Elements de Médécine Pratique* styles Sanguinaria the principal remedy for this malady.   It corresponds, he says, to violent hemicrania, relieved by lying down and by sleep, accompanied by bilious vomitings, toothache, earache, pains in the limbs, electric shootings in the head, and shiverings.   Migraines connected with the catamenial period, especially in women whose menses are profuse, are peculiarly appropriate for Sanguinaria.   He gives the dilutions from the 12th to the 30th.   One of our latest homœopathic journals, the *American Homœopathist*, has in its third number two good cases of sick headache reported by Dr. Mills, of Chicago, in which Sanguinaria was very effective.   He describes the form of migraine indicating it (as Hering does) as a " sun-headache," *i.e.*, increasing in violence with the ascent of that luminary, and decreasing as it declines.   It is generally, he adds, preceded by scanty urine

* *Monthly Hom. Review*, x., 349.

and passes off with profuse aqueous diuresis,—which last he regards as a "key note" for the drug. He thinks it specially suitable to women at the climacteric age, for whose flushings indeed Dr. Gray, of New York, had already recommended it.

Dr. Lucius Morse, of Memphis, in his excellent treatise on *Nasal Catarrh*, speaks well of Sanguinaria in chronic affections of the mucous membranes of the nose and throat, when there is present " a sensation of stinging and tickling, accompanied by irritative swelling of the parts, with or without free discharge." He gives the third trituration. A patient of my own, in whom these symptoms have co-existed with frequent attacks of migraine, has been much benefited in respect of both her troubles by the remedy.

Dr. Guernsey commends Sanguinaria in catamenial or other headaches when the pain ascends from the nucha into the head.

Dr. Hale compares Sanguinaria with *Phosphorus* and *Lycopodium :* to me *Scilla* seems its closest analogue.

Both high and very low dilutions seem to have been used with advantage.

I would now say a few words upon the pitcher-plant,

Sarracenia purpurea.

A tincture of the root, or triturations of the whole dry plant, seem the best preparations.

Provings of Sarracenia, instituted by three persons, with substantial doses, are contained in the second edition of Dr. Hale's *New Remedies*, and in the therapeutic portion of the fourth edition you may read its clinical history.

Sarracenia came into medical practice some fifteen years ago with a high repute among the American Indians as a remedy for smallpox. Several English and American practitioners reported most favourably of its virtues : it seemed to promote eruption at first, but to check maturation afterwards, so that unvaccinated subjects recovered as if they had only had varioloid. Mr. Marston's trial of it at the London Smallpox Hospital, however, proved unsuccessful ; and it has fallen out of use in the old school. Its homœopathic provings showed a power of developing feverishness, with pains in the bones and soreness of the limbs, not unlike that with which variola sets in ; and Dr. Miracas in Spain, Dr. Cigliano in Italy,* and Dr. Mouremans in Belgium have

* This physician has also proved it, as may be seen in Allen's *Encyclopædia*.

published reports of its use which seem to show it possessed
of no little efficacy. We need further experimentation to
fix its place in the treatment of this disease.

The dilutions from the 1st decimal to the 3rd centesimal
have been those in which Sarracenia has been used.

Next, of

Sarsaparilla,

of which also triturations, or a tincture of the root, are prepared in homœopathic pharmacy.

There is a pathogenesis of Sarsaparilla in the fourth volume
of the *Reine Arzneimittellehre*, containing 34 symptoms from
Hahnemann, and 111 from four others. Nenning then proved
it for Hartlaub and Trinks' *Arzneimittellehre*, the second
volume of which contains 347 symptoms from him. In the
Chronic Diseases all these are incorporated, together with
some new symptoms from Schreter, making 561 in all. An
arrangement of these materials, with clinical observations
interspersed, appears in Dr. Hering's *Materia Medica*.

It has long been said in the old school that while surgeons
swear by this medicine, physicians despise it. Dr. Clifford
Allbutt has lately proved an exception to his class in this
respect; for he has come forward to show the benefits of the
practice followed in the Leeds Infirmary of giving Sarsaparilla
in large doses—from twelve ounces to a pint of the compound
decoction daily.* In this way he is able to benefit old
syphilitic patients whose condition would otherwise seem
hopeless—" patients," he says, " whose constitutions have been
undermined by want of nourishment or by excesses, who have
gone through many courses of mercury, whose irritable mucous
membranes will not bear any more iodide of potassium, and
who are so sallow, so worn, so broken down, so eaten up by
disease as to seem fit only for the grave." The large quantities
required, and the fact that the compound decoction (which
seems always the preparation employed) contains also mezereum, guaiacum, and sassafras, show that, whatever use we
may make of such practice, we are not thereby turning to
account any specific properties of the drug.

The proving shows considerable irritation of the urinary
organs, and Dr. Hering gives many testimonies to the power
of Sarsaparilla to relieve the sufferings attendant on gravel.

* *Practitioner*, iv., 257.

It seems also to have some relation to asthma—the association of this trouble with gravel, and their mutual dependence on gout, must be remembered. In another direction, we find it acting well in gonorrhœal rheumatism. Dr. Guernsey gives as its "key-note"—"much pain at the conclusion of passing water, especially in women." Schreter found a gravedo of six months' standing lessen, so that his head became free, from the first day of his proving.

Dr. H. C. Allen has related a case in which, a mother having given her four children teaspoonful doses of a preparation of Sarsaparilla, daily, for some time, they all became affected with herpes.

Teste makes a curious statement about this drug, which I give you for what it is worth. "When a child with red hair takes Sarsaparilla for three months (three teaspoonsful a day of a solution in four ounces of distilled water of three drops of tincture at the eighteenth), his hair absolutely changes colour. From red it becomes a light flaxen. It is to be remarked that Sarsaparilla in such a case causes no appreciable organic trouble: the health of the child is in no way affected."

The higher potencies only have been used.

We will now speak of squills, under the name of

Scilla maritima.

A tincture is prepared for our use from the recent bulb.

There is a pathogenesis of Scilla in the third volume of the *Reine Arzneimittellehre*, containing 86 symptoms from Hahnemann, 172 from seven associates, and 30 from authors.

The acrid properties of squill, which are manifest enough on the skin or in the stomach from its local application, remain in it when absorbed, and manifest themselves more or less everywhere: it sets up irritation in the nervous system, in the respiratory and urinary organs, and on the cutaneous surface. It is in the second and third of these regions that its influence is most felt; so that it is ranked in old-school therapeutics as expectorant and diuretic, in either action being qualified as "stimulating." Studied physiologically, we find that in its mildest operation it excites (as Hahnemann says) the muciparous glands of the trachea and bronchi, and the urinary secretion so far as its aqueous portion is concerned. When it acts more powerfully, inflammatory symptoms are manifesteu in both regions, going on to bronchitis and pleuro-pneumonia in one, and to nephritis, strangury, and suppressed —or scanty, bloody, and albuminous—urine in the other.

Squill being thus expectorant and diuretic in ordinary practice, it has been used by homœopathists mainly for coughs with excessive secretion, and for diabetes insipidus. In both these conditions I can commend it highly. But there is no reason why it should not be used, on the principle of similarity, in those higher degrees of irritation which it causes. The presence of inflammatory action is always held to contra-indicate it in ordinary practice; and, as I have often said, their *contra* corresponds to our *pro*. Hahnemann justly characterises as merely palliative its action in chronic dropsies with scanty urine. But in an earlier treatise* he had pointed out that it was quite homœopathic to rapid acute dropsical swellings with suppression of urine. He also says that in and before his time it was much used in pneumonia and pleurisy, and that its good effects are only explicable upon the same principle. It has received some employment in his school as a remedy for the latter malady; and Professors Wood and Chapman from the other camp recommend it very strongly in cases of serous effusion into the pleura dependent upon chronic inflammation of the membrane.

The narcotic, emetic, and cutaneous action of Scilla, and the power of retarding the heart's action which it shares with Digitalis, must be taken into account in our selection of the drug; but have not themselves been utilised in our practice.

I know of no other medicine which has the same characteristic range of action as that of Scilla.

I have myself used the first dilution for coughs, the second and third for diuresis.

Our next medicine is the ergot of rye, which we (incorrectly) call

Secale cornutum.

Incorrectly, I say; for it is not the rye which we use in medicine, but the fungus which has developed at its expense. Of this "ergot," freshly gathered, we prepare a tincture. We also use ergotin, which is not an alkaloid, but a "concentrated preparation" analogous to macrotin and leptandrin. It is usually triturated.

* See *Lesser Writings*, p. 348.

No proving has been made of Secale in the homœopathic school ; but the numerous observations extant as to the effects of eating the spurred rye—"ergotism"—have been collected by Trinks (in his and Hartlaub's *Annalen*) and by Buchner : the latter's collection of symptoms was translated in the appendix to the fourth volume of the *British Journal of Homœopathy*. Dr. Allen has enriched the pathogenesis of Secale from numerous other sources, giving it over 1,000 symptoms. A full account of later experimentation, physiological and clinical, is given by Dr. Horatio Wood.

It has long been known that when rye in which ergot has been developed is taken for some time as food, a train of poisonous symptoms is developed. These appear in two forms —the "gangrenous" and the "convulsive." In the former the first symptoms are " deep, heavy, aching pains in the limbs, an intense feeling of cold with real coldness of the surface, deep apathy, and a sense of utter weariness. Then a dark-red spot appears on the nose or on one of the extremities ; all sensation is lost in the affected part; the skin, perhaps over a large surface, assumes a livid red hue, and in the foci of local changes bullæ filled with serum appear. . . . . The gangrene is generally dry, the parts withering and mummi-fying; but sometimes it is moist. . . . The toes are most generally the portions destroyed, but it may be any one or all of the extremities ; and the nose, lips, ears, and even the buttocks sometimes bear the brunt of the disorder."

The rationale of these remarkable effects was very obscure until it was discovered that Ergot exerts a specific influence upon unstriped muscular fibre throughout the body, exciting a persistent and long-lasting contraction. Hence its well-known effect upon the uterus, of which I shall speak presently. But, finding as it does this kind of muscular fibre in great abundance in the coats of the arteries, it has the same influence upon them, diminishing their calibre and so reducing their current of blood. It is in this way it seems to cause gangrene : the mortification induced by it is like that which appears in senile gangrene, or which results from embolism or from frost-bite. The general coldness which is noted points in this direction ; and also the fact that when suckling women are ergotised the milk is dried up, and young women get amenorrhœa.

It seems to be an open question whether this action of ergot on unstriped muscular fibre is exercised directly, or through the ganglionic nerves ; but I myself incline strongly to the former hypothesis. Division of the sympathetic does not materially affect the vascular contraction, according to Brown-Sequard. The drug would be thus the precise opposite of Amyl nitrite. The arterial spasm caused is more persistent than that which results from cold, and there is less tendency to reactive dilatation. In acute poisoning, however, the latter may be seen, as in a case cited by Dr. Wood, where the face became intensely congested and purplish red, and pain in the head was felt.

The other form of ergotism is the convulsive or spasmodic. The symptoms here are those of the nervous system. Formication and numbness, going on to complete anæsthesia, commence the morbid history. Then follow violent and painful tonic contractions all over the body, but especially in the flexors of the extremities. More or less paralysis mingles with the spasms, and the same condition is manifest in the cerebral and optic centres, where disturbance of vision often goes as far as amaurosis, and giddiness, epileptic paroxysms, delirium and idiocy reveal the low estate of the brain.

These phenomena, I say, belong to the nervous centres. The voluntary muscles and the nerve-trunks are found after death in their wonted integrity. But it is another question whether they arise from any direct action of the poison upon the nervous substance. It seems to me more probable that they are the result of the profound anæmia induced in the brain and cord by the arterial contraction caused by the drug. Gaspard's experiments on frogs, indeed, cited by Buchner, showed much congestion and softening of both centres ; but this condition is so unlike that induced in warm-blooded animals, and which Dr. Brown-Sequard has experimentally demonstrated in the spinal cord under the influence of ergot, that I cannot lay any stress upon them.

These gangrenous and spasmodic phenomena constitute the chief effects of ergot on the healthy body. They are somewhat intermingled in chronic poisoning by it, and still more in acute. In the former, moreover, they are both accompanied by gastro-intestinal symptoms, of which the most characteristic is a ravenous hunger, which may persist even till death. The frequency of abortion in pregnant women suffering from ergotism directed attention to the action of the drug upon the uterus. It was found to be powerfully stimulant to its muscular fibres, having therefore little effect upon it in the unimpregnated state or in early pregnancy, where these are but little developed, but acting as an abortifacient in the later months, and as an ecbolic during parturition. There is some reason, moreover, to believe that it is capable of causing

3 F

an inflammatory state of the organ, when given for such conditions as leucorrhœa; it certainly does so in experiments on animals, and has several times produced such effects when given to menstruating or pregnant women, as Allen shows.

This power of ergot to contract unstriped muscular fibre as it is found in the arteries and in the uterus has led to its extensive therapeutic use in ordinary practice. It is employed to arrest hæmorrhage, to occlude aneurisms and varices, to starve fibrous tumours, and to diminish congestion of the brain and cord. You know, also, its value to the accoucheur, who with it aids the expulsion of the fœtus or the placenta, and prevents *post-partum* hæmorrhage by inducing immediate contraction of the uterine walls and vessels. There is nothing to prevent your use of it for these purposes, under the usual rules and with the obvious precautions. It is a potent agent you are handling; and you must take care not to asphyxiate the child you would deliver by making the pains too continuous, or (as an American colleague of ours has lately done*) irremediably destroy the whole nutrition of your patient while you are aiming at her morbid growth. You will also do well, here as elsewhere, to consider whether you cannot cure by the more excellent way of homœopathy ere you avail yourself of a purely antipathic agent.

Not much, however, has been done with Secale as a homœopathically-acting remedy. Persistent arterial contraction is not a common idiopathic morbid state. It is certainly present in Asiatic cholera, and here Secale has some reputation,—Dr. Russell expressing great faith in it in some of the worst varieties of the disease, especially when occurring in women. It is not unlikely, moreover, that the anæmic condition which is now regarded as the basis of "spinal irritation" is thus caused. The cramps and dysæsthesiæ which accompany this affection are very like those of Secale, and are often amenable to its use.† Senile gangrene, frost-bite, and other forms of sphacelus are phenomenally at least like the effects of ergot; and it should be borne in mind in their treatment. Dr. Jousset speaks of having cured a case of senile gangrene with it.

But the chief use of Secale in the school of Hahnemann has been derived from its action on the uterus. To check the tendency to miscarriage it is generally the best remedy in the later months of pregnancy, when the muscular tissue of the womb is largely developed. Frequent labour-like pains, without discharge, indicate it here. It will also relieve after-

* See *Brit. Journ. of Hom.*, xxxiv., 391.
† See *Ibid*, xxvi, 218.

pains, when these are continuous and unintermitting. Its tendency to inflame the uterus shows that it *may* be homœopathic to hyperæmic and even hæmorrhagic conditions of the organ. There is a general agreement among those who use the medium and higher dilutions that it will, thus given, check many a menorrhagia when the other symptoms of the patient suggest it. Bähr and Kafka, moreover (and also Guernsey), recommend it in inflammations of the uterus when symptoms of putrescence appear. It has also proved useful in prolapsus uteri.* In a woman three months pregnant, who took a large quantity, " the uterus, that had previously been in a normal condition, descended so that it almost protruded from the labia " (Allen, S. 538). It is said to be used in the Leopoldstadt Hospital with much benefit to relieve the pain of uterine cancer.

More difficult of belief are the statements of the practitioners I have mentioned as to the efficacy of high potencies of the drug to restore labour-pains, when these are flagging from general or uterine exhaustion. Experienced accoucheurs like Leadam, Croserio, and Guernsey, however, seem to have no doubt on the subject ; and experience must always outweigh theory. I can only leave you to test the question for yourselves. Dr. Guernsey thinks the remedy best suited to thin " scrawny " women, in a weak, cachectic state. In such subjects he commends it in several forms of disease, especially excessive discharges of dark colour and bad character. In acute affections he considers it much indicated when the patient, through cold, cannot bear to be covered. One of the observations collated by Allen exhibited this symptom in its subject,—one affected by ergotism.

Secale has also some repute in paralysis of the bladder (which it has caused), when there exists a continuous sensation as if the organ were imperfectly relieved of its contents.

Caulophyllum probably acts on the uterus in a manner similar to that of Secale. Its myotic influence is unique.

I have mentioned the affections in which the higher dilutions have been found useful. Otherwise, Secale has usually been given in the lower potencies.

I have but little to say about my next medicine, which is another of the rare metals,

Selenium.

It is of course prepared by trituration.

* *Brit. Journ. of Hom.*, i., 407.

There is a short pathogenesis of Selenium in the twelfth volume of the *Archiv*, purporting to have been obtained by Dr. Hering on himself, but without explanation as to the manner of his experimenting. He has revised and augmented it for Allen's *Encyclopædia ;* and some experiments by Schreter and others are added there.

Selenium appears from this pathogenesis to have some influence upon the larynx and the male genital organs. A similar concatenation appears in the pathogenesis of Spongia : it is interesting, from the physiological connection between the two parts, as seen in the changes which occur at puberty. Dr. Meyhoffer writes of it :—"few as are the laryngeal symptoms of the proving of this mineral, the raising of small lumps of blood and mucus, and the tendency to hoarseness, are sufficiently characteristic to show its specific affinity for the vocal organ. Moreover, Selenium, when combined with alkalies, appears to possess a powerful energy, according to the experiments of Rabuteau, and an almost exclusive affinity for the breathing apparatus. Rabuteau operated on seven middle-sized dogs : he introduced from 10 to 50 centigrammes of selenite or seleniate of potash or soda diluted in water or milk, either directly by injection into a vein, or by causing it to be absorbed from the stomach. The animals died ; but whether death occurred within half an hour of the introduction of the poison into the system, or some days later, they all expired with the symptoms of asphyxia. The lungs were found extensively and intensely congested, the air-tubes injected, the trachea choked with froth, and the blood in the arteries dark-coloured." He esteems the medicine highly in the milder forms of follicular and the incipient stage of tubercular laryngitis, preferring the seleniate of soda, from the third to the sixth decimal, to any potencies of the pure metal.

Selenium has also been found useful, in higher attenuations, in impotence.

I must now say a few words upon the

Senecio aureus,

of which we make a tincture from the entire plant.

There are provings of this plant by three persons, in substantial doses of the mother-tincture, in the second edition of Dr. Hale's *New Remedies ;* and the therapeutic part of his fourth edition tells us all that is known of its curative virtues.

These provings evidence a good deal of action upon the kidneys, as shown by pain in the loins and bloody urine. Senecio has occasionally proved curative in renal dropsy, and in congestion and even inflammation of the kidneys; also in one case of chronic inflammation of the neck of the bladder. It is popularly known as "female regulator" and "false valerian," names which indicate its kind of action. It has not been proved upon a woman, but appears likely to be beneficial in some forms of amenorrhœa. It also seems to act upon the respiratory organs somewhat like Sanguinaria. Its exact place in practice has yet to be defined.

Helonias, *Pulsatilla* and *Sanguinaria* seem its closest analogues.

The clinical results mentioned above have been mainly obtained from the mother-tincture.

My last medicine to-day is the snake-root, Polygala

Senega

We make a tincture from the dried root.

Stapf's *Additions to the Materia Medica* contain an exhaustive monograph on Senega by Dr. Seidel, which includes provings by eight persons, carried out with the powdered root and the mother-tincture. Dr. Allen adds symptoms from Lembke and from eight experimenters of the old school.

Senega is commonly known and used as a "stimulating expectorant." The drugs so-called are generally, if not always, specific irritants of the respiratory mucous membrane. Such is Senega. The proving reveals that it has a special affinity for this tissue, causing a great deal of cough, mostly dry, and pains of all kinds about the chest; while Schroff found senegin to produce irritative cough and secretion of mucus, lasting several hours. You will find prefixed to the pathogenesis some good cases of chronic bronchitis, thus characterised, in which Senega proved curative. I myself have often prescribed it with the utmost benefit in the bronchitis of old people, when the cough is irritating and shaking. One patient to whom I gave it compared its effects to that of an opiate. That in such cases it acts homœopathically we have the testimony of one of the old school, Dr. H. Dobell.* "Senega,"

* *On Winter-cough.*

he says, " irritates the cough. If it already is frequent, it does harm." I have seen it cause this aggravation even in the first dilution. Dr. Meyhoffer commends it when the phlegm is very adhesive.

This is the main sphere of the action of Senega. But it undoubtedly has something to say also to the *eyes*. In the provers, the lids were much inflamed, and there were aching pains and sense of tension in the balls. From Dr. Seidel's citations, it seems that Senega was in high repute of old among the German oculists for various affections of the eyes, on which they regarded it as exerting a specific action. Dr. Emery has mentioned its value in hypopyon ;* and Dr. Seidel gives some cases of iritis and specks upon the cornea treated by it. Dr. Allen cured with it a paralysis of the third nerve, affecting especially the superior rectus muscle, so that the patient could only see clearly by bending the head backwards.†

In one of his interesting *Causeries clinicales* Dr. Gallavardin has illustrated the value of Senega in pleuritic effusion and hydrothorax ;‡ and in the twenty seventh volume of the *British Journal of Homœopathy* you will find some cases of pneumonia and of vesical catarrh in which it proved efficacious. To the last-named affection symptoms 274-278 of the proving plainly point.

Bryonia and *Hepar sulphuris* are the medicines which most resemble Senega in their influence upon the respiratory organs.

I have always used the second dilution where the drug was perfectly homœopathic ; but higher potencies seem to have acted well.

* See *Brit. Journ. of Hom.*, xxiii., 341.
† See New York State Society's Transactions, x., 194.
‡ See *l'Art Médical*, xxvi., 127, 290; and *Brit. Journ. of Hom.*, vi., 338.

LECTURE LIII.

SEPIA—SILICA.

The subjects of my lecture to-day are two of those medicines whose extensive use is so marked a *differentia* of homœopathic practice.

The first is

Sepia,

or, more fully, Sepiæ succus. It is the blackish-brown fluid contained in the pouch of the mollusc so named, which in its dried state is so largely used by artists. In this condition we triturate it with milk-sugar for medicinal use.

Hahnemann published a pathogenesis of Sepia in the first edition of the *Chronic Diseases*. It contained 1,242 symptoms, obtained (of course) from patients taking it in the attenuations from the third upwards. In the second edition 413 additional symptoms are given, of which about 160 were from five fellow-provers: the remainder were his own. Sepia was the medicine selected for re-proving by the American Institute of Homœopathy in 1874; and the report of the experiments made with it is contained in the Transactions of that body for 1875. Thirty persons took part in them, all of whom tested the drug on their own (healthy) bodies. Ten of these were women. The experiments were superintended, and their faithfulness and accuracy are vouched for, by the lecturers on Materia Medica in the homœopathic colleges of New York, Cincinnati, Philadelphia, and Boston. The attenuations from the third to the two-hundredth were employed. Uterine examinations and urinary analyses were made when required. Out of the thirty persons twenty-six experienced effects, more or less decided, from the drug; and the total register shows 517 symptoms to have been elicited. These have, of course, been incorporated with Hahnemann's by Dr. Allen.*

* See also a single but interesting experiment with the drug in *Brit. Journ. of Hom.*, xxxvi., 397.

The objections which have hindered me from drawing any conclusions from the pathogeneses of the *Chronic Diseases* exist in fullest force in the case of Sepia. When, therefore, I refer you to the study of its symptoms by Dr. Veith Meyer, which is translated from the *Vierteljahrschrift* in the thirteenth and fourteenth volumes of the *British Journal of Homœopathy*, it is with this reservation. Nevertheless, it is an instructive paper. He attempts to give unity to his subject by assuming that the primary and essential action of Sepia is to cause *venous congestion,* first in the portal system, and then throughout the body ; and that its local effects are to be ascribed to this general condition. The hypothesis corresponds well with the curative action of the drug, and may be used with advantage as a tentative clue to its pathogenetic phenomena.

It does not appear what led Hahnemann to introduce the juice of the cuttle-fish into medicine. He rightly says that he was the first so to employ it. But it is a curious fact that broths and other preparations made from the mollusc itself were (as Teste points out) used by the ancients in many of the affections of the generative organs, of the urine, and of the skin, in which Homœopathy now finds the juice so beneficial. I need hardly say that for many centuries its use has been quite unknown. Here, as in so many other instances, that holds good which our laureate says—

> " Is it so true that second thoughts are best ?
> Not first, and third, *which are a riper first ?*"

I. Ever since its introduction into the list of medicaments Sepia has been reputed a valuable remedy in disorders of the female sexual system. Since now we have for the first time an undoubted proving upon healthy women, we look with great interest to see what symptoms are manifested in this sphere. They are of much importance.

1. The catamenia were always diminished in quantity, and either dark or pale in colour. The one exception to this rule was a woman whose menses for some time past had been scanty and dark ; in her case, under the influence of the drug they flowed freely, and were brighter in colour. The period was often, but not always, delayed; sometimes, indeed, it anticipated.

2. Considerable pain was experienced by several of the female provers in both ovaries and uterus. In the former the pain was sometimes a dull and heavy ache, sometimes a series of sharp shootings. The uterine pains are commonly described as a general sense of distress within the pelvis, with bearing

downwards; they were relieved by pressure from without or by crossing the thighs. One prover had severe uterine cramps before each of the two periods which occurred while taking the drug.

3. With three of the female provers the effect on the uterus seems to have been very intense. The first was a widow, æt. 41, who took doses of the 200th dilution, at intervals, between January 5th and 24th. She was examined by Dr. Emma Scott, an intelligent young " lady-doctor " of New York, whose acquaintance I had the pleasure of making during my stay there, and whose competence I can attest. She was perfectly healthy at the commencement of the proving ; but at its close, after experiencing a great deal of dull pelvic pain, with pressure to pass water, a yellowish leucorrhœa appeared. Dr. Scott examined her, and reports, "uterus congested, and a yellowish leucorrhœa pouring from it ; beginning to prolapse ; slightly displaced." The second case was that of a married woman, who took six doses of the third trituration on three successive days. The only effects at that time seemed to be a sense of prostration and " goneness," especially referred to the stomach. After an interval of nearly four weeks, of which no account is given, she again took a powder, with the same results, and also much aching in the pelvis. The uterus was then (it would seem) examined, and found prolapsed, with inclination of the fundus to the left side : there was also tenderness of the os. This report is too scanty ; but as it is presented by Dr. Conrad Wesselhœft, there can be no doubt of its validity. The third case, though given on the same authority, is less satisfactory. Dr. Wesselhœft notes,—" This patient (Miss H—) has suffered from enlargement of the womb, ' a tumour cured by galvanism,' at our hospital." He does not say when, or in what state the uterus was left after the disappearance of the tumour. We must therefore take the proving provisionally for the present. Its subject took four doses of the third trituration on as many successive mornings. Flushing of the head and face, with frontal headache, followed each dose ; and there gradually supervened weight and bearing down in the pelvis, which lasted some days after the proving ended. It was resumed a fortnight later, and a dose of the same potency taken every morning for thirteen days. The pelvic symptoms reappeared, but more severely, and on the eighth day leucorrhœa set in, at first yellowish, then creamy, then glairy and offensive—with the last two kinds blood also being intermingled.

These effects of Sepia show its power of congesting the

uterus even to inflammation, and hence of favouring its prolapse or displacement. The provers in whom they appeared
report many of such sympathetic sufferings as would be expected to occur in these conditions. But they are best marked
in the case of the first in order of the female provers, who took
Sepia 200 for three days together. Pelvic distress, of an out-
pressing character, speedily set in, and with it came vesical
irritability, feverishness (temp. 99⅔ at noon), thirst, tenderness
of the mammæ, and sensitiveness at the epigastrium. The
urine was strongly acid, and of sp. gr. 1,030 nearly throughout
the proving.

Such facts confirm the appropriateness of Sepia to affections of the female sexual system which is so generally recognised in the school of Hahnemann. It has indeed found its
chief employment in homœopathic practice in chronic diseases
affecting the female sex during the period of ovario-uterine
activity. It is considered especially suitable to women of
dark complexion, of fine delicate skin with red or yellow tint-
ing here and there, and of great sensitiveness to all impressions. In such subjects it renders eminent service in many
derangements of the sexual apparatus. Pelvic congestion, of
passive venous type, is the pathological condition specially
calling for it; and from this source spring most of the symptoms which indicate its employment. No medicine is more
frequently beneficial in leucorrhœa owning such origin : the
discharge is either greenish and thick, or profuse, watery, and
offensive. It will often remedy uterine displacements connected with congestion of the organ. Dr. Bayes strongly
recommends it in dysmenorrhœa with insufficient loss. I
myself find it the best medicine for gonorrhœa in the female,
after the acute symptoms have subsided ; and it is praised for
follicular vulvitis. In pregnancy it is often useful to relieve
constipation, and to remove such sympathetic troubles as
vomiting and toothache. At the climacteric age it is very
helpful in reducing the congestions which are incident to the
failure of the monthly relief of the system. Altogether, no
medicine save Pulsatilla is so useful to the weaker sex as
Sepia.

The venous congestion which characterises all these Sepia-
affections of the uterus may be primary. But it is very often,
I think, secondary to abdominal plethora. The uterine veins,
indeed, open into the vena cava, and are consequently not
directly affected by portal obstruction. But the womb may
be indirectly influenced by such cause through the rectum.
When in this way constipation, prolapsus ani and hæmorrhoi-

dal fulness are induced in women, and then the uterine health becomes impaired, Sepia is indicated for the whole group of symptoms; and will do much towards removing them.

Some observations on the drug appended to the American proving would seem to extend its virtues beyond those commonly ascribed to it, at any rate in this country. They are from the pen of the late Dr. Mercy B. Jackson, of Boston. I had the opportunity of a good deal of conversation with this lady during my visit to America, and can quite corroborate the high estimation in which she was held by her colleagues of the other sex. She was advanced in life, and had had large experience in the maladies of women and children. Her remarks are so brief and to the point that I will read them to you in full.

"For more than twenty years," she writes, "I have found Sepia indispensable in the treatment of uterine diseases. There has been no other medicine used by me that has been beneficial in so many cases.

"The symptoms and conditions which most surely call for Sepia, in my opinion, are *misplacements*, whether by prolapse, or ante-version, or flexion on itself forward and backward; Sepia will in most cases restore the uterus to its normal position, if given in the 30th or higher potencies, daily or every second day, and persisted in for sufficient time, without manual interposition, and the cure is generally permanent.

"But in order for it to be useful in any case the subjective symptoms must correspond to its pathogenetic symptoms.

"Those most characteristic are turns of prostration and sinking weakness running suddenly over the patient, resembling fainting, but not going so far as to destroy consciousness. I have rarely, if ever, found a case of uterine disease in which these turns were frequent, in which the other symptoms of Sepia were not found, and when it did not do a great deal for the sufferer.

"Another characteristic symptom is a burning pain in the small of the back, accompanied by a dragging sensation there, continuous or often recurring.

"Bearing down in the pelvis is another symptom that calls for Sepia, and when this and the first-mentioned symptom are wanting, it will rarely or never be useful.

"Yellowness of the skin and brown spots on it corroborate the other symptoms and make the choice more easy.

"Profuse leucorrhœa, rather watery and offensive, is almost always improved by Sepia, and if to these indications are added a brownish colour, and acrid character of the discharge, it is still more sure to be successful.

"I have felt it in procidentia restore the uterus so rapidly that its movement was plainly felt returning to its place, as if raised by a power within the pelvis, and have often seen cases restored by it in a few minutes, in my practice, and so great is my confidence in its power to do this, that in recent cases of prolapsus I never resort to manipulation, but prepare some in water and give one teaspoonful every few minutes till the sufferer is relieved, and then continue it at longer intervals, until it is given only once a day to complete the cure.

"Of course the patient is placed in a favourable position, on the back with the knees elevated and the feet resting on the soles.* In many cases of recent origin, Sepia will entirely cure, but in cases brought on by lifting, Calc. carb. is often needed to aid the Sepia.

"I have found in many cases of chronic disease in women, where the symptom first mentioned of sudden prostration with sinking faintness was often experienced, that Sepia was a very important remedy, and I think that symptom is the most characteristic of any in its pathogenesis."

Professor Henderson mentions such an attack as occurring in a gentleman to whom the medicine was given (in the 30th dilution) for a cutaneous eruption.† Dr. Guernsey adds several other symptoms as indicating Sepia. As belonging to the pelvis he mentions—a sensation of bearing down so considerable that the patient feels she must cross her legs and "sit close" to keep something from coming out of the vagina ; pains shooting upwards in the os uteri ; a feeling as of a weight or heavy lump in the anus (this, he says, is very characteristic) ; and fœtid urine, so offensive sometimes that it cannot be suffered to remain in the room, "depositing a reddish, clay-coloured sediment, which adheres to the bottom and sides of the vessel as if it had been burnt on, like burnt clay." Elsewhere he notes that the Sepia patient has very cold hands and feet, and complains of a great sense of emptiness at the pit of the stomach. You may remember this symptom in connexion also with Ignatia and Phosphorus ; but with those medicines it is of nervous origin, here it is uterine.

II. The influence of Sepia upon the portal system has always been recognised, as Meyer's generalisation of its action shows. It has not hitherto been much employed in substantive hepatic affections, save when connected with uterine derangement. But Bähr recommends it in lithic acid dyspepsia and hepatic engorgement occurring in females, even without such complication ; and the American proving makes it promise much usefulness in this sphere. You are aware of the close connexion between hepatic disorder and lithiasis, as so well described in the late Dr. Murchison's Croonian Lectures on *Functional Derangements of the Liver.* Now among the re-provers, besides many symptoms referable to the liver and digestive organs, marked alterations in the urine were observed. This point was specially studied by Dr. Allen, who made the six provers of his class examine their urine daily.

* It is no less "of course" open to question whether the posture adopted had not as much to do as the Sepia with the restoration effected in these *recent* cases.—R. H.

† *Homœopathy fairly represented,* 2nd ed., p. 240.

All noticed a great increase of the urates in the secretion, which was very acid, deeply-coloured, and of high specific gravity. An amorphous sediment, either of brick-dust or whitish colour, was deposited ; and examination proved it to consist of urates. The significance of this symptom (already noticed in the instance of Lycopodium) was at once appreciated. The last practical contribution to our literature of the lamented Carroll Dunham was on the subject ;* and he relates two excellent cases of sub-acute hepatic congestion, with lithiasis, in which the action of Sepia (30th trituration) was very rapid.

III. Sepia has always had some repute in cutaneous affections. The re-proving displayed a considerable action of the drug on the skin. Perspiration was increased in one person, having an unpleasant odour ; abrasions were slow in healing in two ; and in five a rash appeared. It was generally vesicular, but a tendency to pustulation showed itself : itching accompanied the vesicles, and the pustules in one case were painful.† It has been mainly when the skin has been discoloured in connexion with derangement of the general health that Sepia has been employed, as when " liver-spots " and other maculæ have appeared, or a yellow saddle has formed across the bridge of the nose ; and the presence of such phenomena is always considered an indication for it. In Professor Henderson's case, however, a " scaly eruption on the legs, on a dark dusky redness of the skin," of fifteen years' standing, disappeared in a few weeks after the single dose whose effects I have mentioned ; and Dr. Drury, who has had much experience in diseases of children, expresses great confidence in it in recent ringworm.

IV. The most important action of Sepia, however, beyond that which it exerts on the abdominal and pelvic organs, is its power over migraine. There is a general agreement among the German writers as to its great value here ; among others Trinks states that he has made several radical cures by it. It is in patients of the sex and characteristics already mentioned, and of venous and bilious constitution, that it proves most useful. The pain is generally very severe, of rending character, and increased by any excitement. You will find several statements and illustrations relative to this matter in Peters' *Treatise on Headaches.* Tietze points out the " sudor hystericus," a peculiar odorous perspiration in the axillæ and

* See Transactions of N. York State Hom. Society for 1876-7, p. 87.
† Cutaneous symptoms were also experienced by the prover referred to in the note to p. 807.

soles of the feet, as an unerring guide to its selection here; and Dr. Clotar Müller says* that he has given Sepia with happy results in other maladies when this symptom was present.

The following are Dr. Meyer's conclusions :—

" 1. Sepia has its sphere of action in the portal system, in which it causes obstructions.

" 2. Most of its symptoms indicate a high degree of venous congestion.

" 3. It is characterised by torpidity and depression, often ending in perfect exhaustion of the vital powers.

" 4. Hence it is suitable in mild and easy dispositions, and therefore especially for women.

" 5. The affections arise and increase in severity, mostly in the evening and at night, during and immediately after a meal.

" 6. The affections either disappear during, or are alleviated by, active exercise, and by pressure of the painful part.

" 7. The affections are often accompanied with chilliness.

".8. There is great sensitiveness of the skin to cold air."

I may add that the re-provers experienced much dulness of the intellectual powers and diminution of energy ; and that amelioration of most of their subjective symptoms was usually observed (contrary to Dr. Meyer's canons) from eating and after repose.

Dr. Hoyne says that he has cured more cases of chronic nasal catarrh with Sepia than with any other remedy ; and Drs. Guernsey and C. Wesselhœft warrant it in enuresis nocturna, when the wetting of the bed always occurs during the first sleep.

The only real analogue of Sepia with which I am acquainted is *Pulsatilla*. *Lycopodium*, *Lilium* and *Murex* have points of contact with it.

Sepia is a medicine which has been almost exclusively used in the higher dilutions. I know of no records showing it to possess much activity from the third downwards. I myself nearly always employ the twelfth.

My second medicine is one of equally strange origin, and of no less therapeutic virtue. It is common flint,

Silica.

Thus, and not Silicea, it should be styled : " silicea " is an

* See *Brit. Journ. of Hom.*, xxi., 16.

adjective, whose substantive is " terra," the two being conjoined in the *Chronic Diseases*. Chemically, it is of course
silicic acid, an oxide of silicon. In the Pharmacopœia you
will find Hahnemann's directions for obtaining the pure
Silica in powder, but I suppose that any other approved
process, or even that of Berzelius which makes the flint
soluble, would give us what we want. The ordinary form is
triturated for our use.

The original pathogenesis of Silica appeared in the first
edition of the *Chronic Diseases*. 567 symptoms are ascribed
to it there, which seem to have been observed on patients
taking the attenuations from 6 to 12. In the second edition
the list has swelled to 1,193, about 150 of the additions being
contributed by seven others. A short proving of the soluble
Silica, in a preparation of strength about equivalent to our
second dilution, is translated in the twenty-eighth volume of
the *British Journal of Homœopathy*. Dr. Allen adds symptoms from provings made with the dilutions, instituted by
Ruoff and Robinson, raising the total of his pathogenesis to
1,903.

It seems that flint was first used as a medicine by Paracelsus, and praised by him and his followers in renal and
vesical calculus, in suppression of milk and of urine, and in
some nervous disorders. But its employment had become
quite unknown when Hahnemann, encouraged by the
success of triturating the otherwise inert metals, applied the
process to it also; and thereby gave us a most valuable
remedy.

The genuine physiological action of Silica is quite unknown.
No Meyer has sought to define its central point, and no association has selected the drug for re-proving. Dr. Becker's
experiments with silicated water were slight, and, owing to
his imperfect health, gave curative rather than pathogenetic
results. We will turn at once, therefore, to therapeutics,
where Silica plays a well-understood and very important
part.

Silica influences the nutrition rather than the functional
activity of the tissues which come within its range of action :
it is hence suited to organic changes rather than to functional
disorders. Its deep and slow action, moreover, makes it
appropriate to chronic rather than acute diseases ; though
we shall see some of the latter in which it acts rapidly enough.
Teste says it is especially suited to fat people, of a lymphatico-
sanguine temperament. Such is its general character ; and
now to descend to particulars.

I. The first great property of Silica is its power over *suppuration*. It does not act like Mercury in averting this process when threatening ; and it is inferior to Hepar sulphuris for promoting it when inevitable. But when it is once established, and by its excess or long duration is causing mischief, the effect of small internal doses of Silica in checking it is something magical. You cannot do better than read in illustration the two cases related by Dr. Noack, jun., as translated from *L'Art Médical* for 1865 in the twenty-third volume of the *British Journal of Homœopathy*. Both were severe and extensive (one caused by dissecting wound), and purulent infection was threatening ; but Silica 30, internally and externally, changed the whole aspect of affairs, and effected a speedy cure. I have seen it no less efficacious in purulent infiltration of the tissues of the neck, following carbuncle : here the sixth dilution internally was all that was given. In carbuncle itself, when the inflammatory stage is past, and matter has already begun to form, Silica will often stay all further progress : and many an abscess will become absorbed under its use. So also with whitlows, which it will often blight if given early enough, and whose tendency to recurrence it will check.* The same property makes it curative (according to Teste) in impetigo capitis and (according to Bähr also) in chronic purulent bronchorrhœa, such as the " stone-cutters' phthisis."† Dr. Vilas recommends it in purulent otorrhœa.

It is probably in virtue of a property of the same kind that Silica promotes the healing of some ulcers, as in the leg and on the cervix uteri. It is the " simple ulcer " alone which it benefits ; and its local use is generally necessary, though this need not be in greater strength than that in which it is prescribed constitutionally.‡

II. From these forms of perverted nutrition we rise to those of more general character ; and find Silica one of the chief medicines in the two great dyscrasiæ of childhood—rachitis and scrofula. In Sir William Jenner's graphic account of the phenomena of rickets, you will find two symptoms which are very characteristic of Silica, viz., the perspirations about the head only, and the tenderness of the general surface. The tendency which obtains, moreover, to defective formation of bone and increased growth of cartilage in this disease calls loudly for Silica. Dr. von Grauvogl pointed out

* A case of this disease cured with it (by Dr. Stens) is given by Hoyne (i., 493).
† See Hoyne, i., 507.
‡ See Goullon on Scrofula, *sub voce*.

that the only chemical difference between cartilage and bone is that flint is present in the latter but not in the former ; and he has given a good case of enchondroma of the fingers in which, acting upon this suggestion, he administered Silica 3 with most satisfactory results. I have already expounded to you his theory about " tissue remedies," of which this bit of treatment is an instance. I can speak no less confidently of the power of the drug when, as in rachitis, the enchondromatous tendency is general. I am accustomed to prescribe it in the earliest manifestations of the diathesis, which are generally unhealthy evacuations, sweats of the head, and tenderness of the surface ; and with the best results. In scrofula we have so eminent a therapeutist as Dr. Jousset proclaiming it the chief of remedies. I should myself have placed it below Sulphur and Calcarea ; but in Dr. Goullon's treatise on the disease you will find quite an array of instances of it in which Silica has proved curative.

It is chiefly when scrofula manifests itself in the bones and joints that Silica proves its remedy. There is abundant testimony to its value in periostitis, when non-syphilitic in origin ; and it is no less valuable when the bone itself is affected, as shown by caries or necrosis. In the scrofulous joints—the " white swelling " of the old authors, where all commend it, it is probably most useful when the mischief has begun in the bones or cartilages, rather than in the synovial membrane. If in any of these cases matter is already discharging, do not neglect the local use of the remedy.

III. Another very important influence of Silica is that which it exerts upon the nervous system. It is probably the nutrition of the centres which it affects ; but, whatever be its *modus operandi*, its remedial powers are unmistakeable. The first (so far as I know) to direct attention to this property was Dr. Black, in the second and fifth volumes of the *British Journal of Homœopathy*. He there states that Silica exercises a powerful action on the brain and spinal cord, especially the latter ; indicates nervous exhaustion, as from over-study, as the condition specifically calling for it ; describes two forms of headache characteristic of it ; and relates three cases of spinal paresis in which it proved curative. The first was an instance of Pott's disease of the vertebræ ; the other two of long-delayed ability to stand or walk in strumous children. We have next a valuable contribution on the subject from Dr. Dunham, which you will find in the Transactions of the New York State Homœopathic Society for 1871. His chief point here is that " with evidence of exhaustion furnished by the

3 G

sensation of weakness, paralysis, &c., there is," with Silica, " an exalted condition of susceptibility to nervous stimuli. The special senses are morbidly keen, the brain cannot bear even moderate concussion, nor the spine either concussion or pressure, and the whole surface is unnaturally tender and sensitive. Cold aggravates and warmth relieves." This " erethism conjoined with exhaustion" may, as he further shows, go on to spasm ; and he relates a case of epileptiform spasms, with great nervous irritability, cured by it. It had been caused by a fall on the supra-orbital region, whose feel suggested that some fracture had occurred there ; pain was felt at the spot on stooping, or when the upper spine (which was tender) was pressed upon. All these symptoms, after lasting some months, and resisting other medicines, yielded rapidly to Silica.

Dr. Dunham subsequently recorded two cases of chronic headache cured by the drug, in both of which great sensitiveness to pressure, noise, motion, and light were present, and relief was obtained from warmth, as from wrapping the head in a shawl.* He has further described the Silica patient as one who " feels as if he could not possibly do this or that, but, when urged to the doing, goes off in a paroxysm of over-doing." Dr. Samuel Jones, who reports this last observation, has put on record a striking cure of chronic headache, with nervousness and loss of memory, resulting from overwork, in which the patient (himself a medical man) was led to the remedy by it.† The description of his headache given by this sufferer is typical of that to which Silica corresponds. It " commenced low in the back of the neck, with a feeling as though the muscles could not support the head, gradually increasing until there was a sensation as if the neck had been severely bruised (as struck with a club), but it was not sore to the touch. Gradually the pain would work up over the head, leaving in the vertex a sensation of heat, as though one had caught cold in the scalp ; finally settling in the forepart of the head, and at times involving the eyeballs and making them sore."

I think you will now see that there are (as Dr. Jones says) many neurolytic conditions which Silica promises to benefit. The headaches of spinal patients, of students and governesses, of the subjects of masturbation and indeed of any whose nervous centres are debilitated and at the same time hyper-æsthetic, find in it one of their best remedies ; and it will

* See Hoyne, i., 487.
† See Brit. Journ. of Hom., xxxvi., 196.

prove "tonic" as well as "sedative" to them. To its virtues of this kind I can testify from my own experience. Whether it will reach to the profounder effects of such causes, as paralysis and epilepsy, one cannot yet say. It will have been observed that in the two chief cases of this nature which I have mentioned, the lesion lay in the osseous surroundings of the brain and cord rather than in their substance itself.

I should add Teste's observation, that in the nervous disorders calling for Silica there is often present a sense of great prostration, causing a craving for food to remove it, and that the symptoms are always the worse for abstinence.

IV. In suppuration, in scrofula and rickets, and in neurolytic conditions, we have the more general sphere of action of Silica; but it has several miscellaneous properties, which I must now detail to you.

1. Dr. Dudgeon has put on record a striking case in which Silica arrested the progress of inflammation of the lachrymal sac*, and I have myself had another precisely similar. It is said, also, to have caused the healing of lachrymal fistula.† Drs. Allen and Norton confirm these virtues of the drug, but add that to check dacryo-cystitis it must be given before suppuration has occurred, and that a lachrymal fistula to be healed by it must be a recent one.

2. In the lower extremities Silica finds frequent employment in "housemaid's knee," where the testimony to its usefulness is very general. Another use of it in this region has regard to perspiration of the feet, which is an affection of no uncommon occurrence, and, from the tenderness it causes, and the offensive odour it often exhales, is a cause of considerable distress. If, moreover, it be violently suppressed, not only are the feet left cold, but various constitutional affections are apt to supervene. Of these one of the most frequent is weakness of sight, and the cause of such weakness has more than once been found to be opacity of the lens. Now Silica controls this entire series of occurrences. We have already seen its influence over the constitutional condition which manifests itself in perspiration about the head; and Dr. Guernsey notes, as one mark of difference between it and Calcarea here, that the sweat is apt to be offensive. No less power does it display in checking similar perspirations of the feet. But—and this is the important point—when the exhalation has been suppressed from without, and systemic troubles have hence arisen, Silica will make the feet warm and moist again, and wil'

* *Brit. Journ. of Hom*, xiii., 135.
† Hoyne, i., 488.

cause the morbid symptoms to disappear. Some of Dr.
Becker's cases treated by silicated water illustrate these statements. But their best evidence is a series of instances
recorded by Dr. Gallavardin in *L'Art Médical* for 1866.[*] The
local use of atropia, as introduced by Dr. Ringer, to check
these perspirations is becoming so general, that we shall
probably have frequent occasion to resort to our Silica as a
remedy for the consequences.

3. Dr. Hering has found Silica of frequent value against
bad effects resulting from vaccination. It is of course
especially suitable when these are of a suppurative character,
as porrigo capitis ; and in such conditions I have found it
most serviceable. But Dr. Hering extends its use, as in some
cases he has mentioned, to convulsions thus arising. [†]

4. Dr. Cooper recommends it in cutaneous eruptions
itching only in the daytime and evening, not at night. It
has been little used, however, in affections of the skin, save
when suppuration has been their leading feature.

5. Dr. Guernsey lays much stress on a form of constipation,
as not only itself curable by Silica, but as indicating the
remedy when present among other symptoms. It is where
the fæces form in hard lumps, which remain long in the
rectum, and are difficult of expulsion ; while sometimes, after
long straining, the protruding part suddenly recedes again.
He sets this down to deficient power on the part of the rectum,
but Dr. Dunham seems to ascribe it to spasm of the sphincter
ani. Besides this " key-note " for the drug, Dr. Guernsey
mentions—in women—paroxysms of icy coldness during the
menses, and—in children—frequent grasping at the gums
during dentition.

6. The great sensitiveness of the surface characteristic of
Silica led Dr. Ludlam to give it, with success, in a distressing
cough occurring during convalescence from spinal meningitis,
where the slightest current of air set going in the room provoked the paroxysms.[‡] In the same category is probably to
be placed a cure of vaginismus wrought with it, as reported
by Dr. Skinner.[§]

So far speaks Homœopathy ; and I think you will admit
that, if these statements can be substantiated, it possesses in
Silica a most precious remedy. But there is something more
to be said about the drug.

Silica is a constituent of several mineral waters, among

* See also his *Causeries clinicales homœopathiques,* nos. iv. and xix.
† See Hoyne, i., 502.   ‡ *Ibid,* p. 492.
§ See *The Organon,* i., 76.

others those of Teplitz and Gastein, where it exists in the proportion of from three-fifths to three-tenths of a grain in the pound. But it forms a much larger percentage of the Missisquoi and Bethesda springs of America, the former of which contains ˙016000 parts in a thousand. Now these waters have a great reputation in their own country for cancer, tumours, diabetes, and albuminuria. Dr. Tuthill Massy called our attention to them in the *Monthly Homœopathic Review* for 1870 ; and, as they are largely impregnated with lime, their action was supposed to be due to this ingredient, and to be of a piece with the experience of Drs. Hood and Spencer Wells with pulverised oyster-shells, of which I have spoken under Calcarea. But Dr. Fowler Battye has recently communicated to the *Edinburgh Medical Journal** a series of cases of chronic disease which he has treated with finely powdered Silica. He does not explain how he was led to employ it ; but the fact that his cases consist entirely of those in which the Missisquoi waters have gained their repute speaks for itself. A side-wind of the high estimation of the medicine in homœopathic practice may also have influenced him ; but this would not account for his choice of cases, as they are quite outside the range of our employment of the drug. Dr. Battye's results are very important. The pains of cancer abate greatly or cease within ten days of commencing the drug, and sometimes a withering of the growth occurs. Fibroid tumours of the pelvis greatly diminish ; and both sugar and albumen disappear from the urine, with corresponding improvement in the general health. These last effects seem certainly due to the dynamic action of the drug ; and Dr. Battye's grain doses night and morning point in no other direction.

As allied medicines to Silica we have *Fluoric, Phosphoric* and *Picric acid, Calcarea, Hepar sulphuris, Mercurius* and *Phosphorus.*

The dilutions from the sixth to the thirtieth have been those most commonly employed by homœopathists. It may be that to get Dr. Battye's results we most employ his more material doses. I have verified his experience with Silica as an anodyne to the pains of cancer, giving the 1x and 2x triturations.

* Vol. xx., p. 420

LECTURE LIV.

SPIGELIA, SPONGIA, STANNUM, STAPHISAGRIA, STRAMONIUM.

My first subject to-day is a very interesting, and—beyond the homœopathic range—little-known medicine, the pink-root,

Spigelia.

The tincture is prepared by maceration from the dried root of the Spigelia anthelmia, the Demerara pink-root, which was that proved by Hahnemann. The Carolina pink-root—S. Marylandica—seems to have the same properties, and Hahnemann has admitted symptoms produced by it into his list, though Allen isolates them.

The proving of Spigelia is in the fifth volume of the *Materia Medica Pura*. Thirteen persons co-operated with Hahnemann therein, and added 525 symptoms to his own 130, and to 17 which he cites from authors. Large doses seem to have been used, as in his preface he speaks of having observed the effects of 60, 80, and 100 drops of the tincture; and the symptoms are very full and pronounced.

Spigelia was introduced from America as a medicine for destroying lumbrici, and is in use there for such purposes to the present day, though it is little known elsewhere. Struck, probably, by the narcotic effects observed from over-doses, Hahnemann thought well to prove it; and in view of the "varied and great powers" it presented predicted that it was destined to accomplish results much more important than the destruction of worms. His prophecy has been fulfilled, but only among his own disciples: the common practice is content to know this valuable remedy only as a vermicide.

The effects of over-dosing with Spigelia are somewhat like those of the mydriatics. There are dilated pupils; flushed and swollen face; quickened pulse; heat and dryness of skin: spasms of the facial muscles, especially of the eyelids; and subsultus tendinum, which may even go on to convulsions and death. The irritation of the nervous centres here displayed is in the provings shown especially in their sensory portion. Pain, usually of a shooting character, is stirred up in many parts of the body, but especially in the head, face, and chest; and in all very predominantly on the left side.

Spigelia has hence taken a high place in homœopathic practice in the treatment of neuralgia, especially of the trigeminus. When headaches take the form of supra-orbital neuralgia, especially on the left side; when the pain recurs at regular intervals, tends to spread to the face or neck and to involve the eyes, is aggravated by the least concussion or motion, but especially by stooping, and is associated with pale face, restlessness, and palpitation—in such circumstances Spigelia, in almost any dilution, will prove strikingly curative. Thirteen cases of the kind are cited in Peters' *Treatise on Headaches;* and others are scattered throughout our journals. It is no less effectual when the pain is seated in the infraorbital and maxillary branches of the nerve; so that Bähr gives it the first place among the remedies for prosopalgia, and Hoyne has collected several cases of cure by it. The pain is relieved, according to Dr. Guernsey, by firm pressure. It must be observed that the supra-orbital neuralgia I have described here is not true migraine: in this disease Spigelia has accomplished little.

The most marked actions of the drug, however, which Hahnemann's provings display are those which it exerts upon the *eyes* and the *heart.* The first of the two had been observed by several of the authors whom he cites. Pain in and over the eyes, redness and injection of the whites, sparks before the sight and distortion and irregular movements of the balls are symptoms taken from Linning, Chalmers, Wright and Browne. His own provers confirm them; and add still more decided evidences of inflammation, the severe pain accompanying which indicates the sclerotica and iris as the tissues chiefly affected. The symptoms of the heart are those of great pressure on the chest, shooting pains through it and down the left arm, and violent palpitations.

All this reminds us of Aconite; and has led to the use of Spigelia as an auxiliary to that great medicine in several affections of the eyes and heart. It is especially when these organs are attacked by acute rheumatism that its powers are called into play. When "rheumatic ophthalmia" is very painful, Spigelia will act most satisfactorily in the process of its cure. Still more important is its control over the cardiac

inflammation of rheumatic fever. Decisive testimony is given
on this score by Fleischmann. He treated, he says, in the
Gumpendorf Hospital at Vienna fifty-seven cases of rheumatic
" carditis " (evidently including under that name all forms of
inflammation of the heart) with but one death, and Spigelia
was the only medicine employed.* Dr. Russell writes—" In
the few cases of pericarditis I have treated it has done all
that medicine could do, and I have the utmost confidence in
it."† Dr. Bayes expresses (and substantiates)‡ equal satisfaction in its power over endocarditis. Thus Spigelia becomes a
most useful addition to our *armamentarium* in combating
acute rheumatism. Dr. Phillips even commends it for the
joint affection itself, when it shifts rapidly : the drug seems,
he says, to centre and steady it.

But you must not suppose that it is only in true rheumatic
affections of the eyes and heart that Spigelia is beneficial. It
is much praised in the primary, neuralgic stage of the "arthritic
ophthalmia " of the old ophthalmologists, which is probably
acute glaucoma. Dr. Angell commends it in several inflammatory conditions of the eyes in scrofulous children, where,
with photophobia, there is severe ciliary neuralgia. It is the
presence of this last trouble, whether alone or in association
with inflammatory affections of the eye, which chiefly indicates
Spigelia, and which leads to its best results. The pains
radiate from a point, and are increased by movement of the
eyes and at night. As regards the heart, Dr. Bayes relates
one case and Dr. Kendall§ another of angina pectoris, in
which it proved curative,—Dr. Jousset also speaking of frequent success with it ; and Dr. Yeldham has shown what great
benefit a heart chronically damaged by rheumatism can receive
from the free and persistent administration of the drug.‖ In
all these affections it is the darting, shooting, stabbing, or
lacerating pain which indicates Spigelia, and which is relieved
by it.

I think that Teste is well borne out in saying that Spigelia
—at any rate in infinitesimal doses—acts best in anæmic and
debilitated subjects.

Aconite is the medicine most nearly allied to Spigelia. Like
Cina it has numerous symptoms in its pathogenesis which
resemble those of helminthiasis ; and it may possibly act in

* *Brit. Journ. of Hom.*, xiv., 23
† *Ibid*, xii. 569.
‡ *Monthly Hom. Review*, June, 1867.
§ *Brit. Journ. of Hom.*, xxvi., 157.
‖ *Annals*, iii., 539.

this condition with the same inexplicably beneficial results which we have already recognised in Cina itself. Like that medicine, moreover, it will prove as beneficial in disordered states simulating helminthiasis as if worms were actually present. Stillé writes:—"there is a state of intestinal derangement presenting all the symptoms of lumbricoid ascarides, and which is most frequently observed among strumous, feeble, and precocious children. They have fever, a dry hot skin, furred tongue, tumid and confined bowels, capricious appetite, and nervous irritability. These symptoms are often dissipated by the influence of spigelia, and without causing the discharge of any worms, to the presence of which they are most commonly attributed." You will remember Dr. Chepmell's similar testimony to the usefulness of Cina. Dr. Guernsey commends it here when the child refers to the navel as the most painful part, and where palpitation is a coincident symptom.

The higher dilutions in neuralgia, the lowest in cardiac affections, have been those generally given. Hahnemann, who recommends the thirtieth, says that even a small dose acts for four weeks, and that its effects go on progressively increasing for the first week or ten days. This observation, which of course belongs only to chronic disease, needs confirmation

Our next medicine is the Spongia marina tosta, or, more briefly,

Spongia.

You will observe that it is Spongia *tosta*, not usta. Hahnemann justly directs that it shall only be roasted brown, and not burnt black, so that its natural constituents shall not be too greatly altered. In this condition it is treated with alcohol to make a tincture. Triturations would seem a better preparation, considering the many mineral ingredients of sponge ; but they have not been used, and all I shall have to say of the homœopathic employment of the medicine belongs to it as made into tincture.

The proving of Spongia is in the sixth volume of the *Reine Arzneimittellehre.* It contains 156 symptoms from Hahnemann, and 235 from ten others. Dr. Hering's volume of *Materia Medica* contains an arrangement of the drug embodying much of the clinical experience gained with it.

1. Burnt sponge has been used, ever since Arnold of Villanova introduced it in the fourteenth century, as a remedy for goitre. Hufeland and all the authorities of his time express the utmost confidence in it; and Joseph Frank says that it is as sure as Cinchona in intermittent fever. Since the discovery that it contained Iodine, and that this agent by itself displayed marvellous anti-goitrous properties, sponge has fallen into disuse in ordinary practice,—Vogt alone among modern therapeutists protesting that it will often cure when Iodine fails. In homœopathic practice it has not undergone this neglect. Hahnemann says that the endemic bronchocele of the inhabitants of valleys, being always essentially the same affection, ought to be curable by the same specific; and this he considers Spongia to be. He states that one or two doses of the attenuated tincture (he does not specify how far attenuated) suffice for the purpose. If this is spoken from experience, it ought to be tested more widely than it has been. Dr. Hering can only find three cases of cure by it in infinitesimal doses, and Dr. Hoyne reports but one more ; and of these one alone answers to Hahnemann's description. I know, however, of another ; and probably many testimonies could be borne to it.

As to the rationale of this action, all that I have said while upon Iodine holds good. Spongia itself has caused swelling, pain and tenderness in existing goitres ; and one of Hahnemann's provers reports—" The region of the thyroid gland is as if hardened." These symptoms, and the cures of the disease—however occasional—wrought by infinitesimal doses, show that Spongia is sometimes at least homœopathic to it. When it is preferable to Iodine in its treatment we have not yet learnt to predict beforehand.

2. Hahnemann proved Spongia in order to learn its relation to goitre ; but he thereby brought to light a much more important action of the drug, viz., that which it exerts upon the larynx. Hoarseness, tenderness, dry and painful cough, and obstruction of respiration as if a plug were there—these were the symptoms produced ; and Hahnemann at once inferred the applicability of the medicine to *croup*. By the time the second edition of his *Materia Medica Pura* was published, he could speak of this as the most remarkable curative application of Spongia which homœopathy had made. You may first lessen the local inflammation, he says, by a dose of Aconite ; and you will sometimes, but rarely, need the aid of Hepar to complete the cure. Such has been the experience of homœopathists generally, as you may see from the series of cases

given by Dr. Hering, or those collected in the fifth volume of the *British Journal of Homœopathy*. Bönninghausen's celebrated "powders for croup" consisted of two of Aconite, one of Spongia, and two of Hepar,—a powder to be taken every two hours. Dr. Hale in his excellent *Lectures on Diseases of the Chest* has recently taught the same practice; and I can myself recommend you nothing better. The same process has indeed been gone through with croup as with goitre. Koch, in 1841, suggested that Iodine was the active ingredient of sponge in the former as in the latter case; and I have already told you, on the authority of Elb and Meyhoffer, how actively Iodine can influence this disease. But so also, as we have seen, can Bromine; and Spongia contains them both in a state of natural combination which may be superior to our artificial preparations of either. It may be that, as with goitre, Iodine will cure some cases of croup, Bromine others, and Spongia óthers again; and that we may yet learn how to distinguish them *à priori*. At present we must be content to hold the remaining members of the group in reserve in case of the failure of the first chosen; and that, from its traditional claims, may well be Spongia. Dr. Guernsey says as to its indications,—" the cough is dry and sibilant, or it sounds like a saw driven through a pine board, each cough corresponding to a thrust of a saw. Spongia is particularly indicated when there is no mucous rattle. The cough is dry and hoarse, and causes pain in the throat, but no mucous rattle."

But whatever may be thought about membranous croup, there can be no question as to the eminent value of Spongia in simple inflammations of the larynx, from the lightest catarrh to the severest laryngitis, with all their manifestations of hoarseness, aphonia, and barking cough. It is in the dry form or stage of these affections that Spongia finds its place; and it rapidly promotes resolution. I have seen it so prompt in removing laryngeal symptoms in a phthisical patient that I can well believe the reports of its value in laryngeal phthisis. Indeed, Spongia bears to phthisis pulmonalis itself the same relation as Iodine—both Neumann and Hufeland warning that its incautious use is liable to set up this affection, in which Dr. Hering esteems it highly as a remedy. The cough of Spongia is said to have the characteristic of being relieved by eating and drinking.

3. Hahnemann observed from Spongia aching swelling of the testes and a similar condition of the spermatic cord. Dr. Hering gives several cases of chronic orchitis and epididymitis in which the drug proved highly efficacious.

4. But perhaps the most important action of Spongia after that which it exerts on the larynx is displayed in the cardiac sphere. This was first brought to light by Dr. P. P. Wells, of Brooklyn. A sufferer from organic affection of the heart ate and swallowed a piece of newly roasted sponge. It produced a frightful attack of pain, palpitation, and dyspnœa, with livid lips and fear of approaching death. On recovering from this a remarkable relief of her wonted cardiac distress ensued, and lasted for several weeks. Dr. Wells was thus led to give it, in minuter doses, in several cases of heart-disease. He is led to think it the most valuable medicine we have where there is fibrinous deposit upon the valves. He states that he has repeatedly found the bellows-murmur disappear, as well as the subjective symptoms become relieved, under its use. Sudden waking in the night, with a sense of suffocation, is the symptom which especially leads him to its choice; and others have noted orthopnœa as indicating it. In another case it greatly relieved the cough and other concomitants of an aneurism of the descending aorta. I must say that, for removing the valvular lesions of endocarditis, I have found Spongia very inferior to Naja.

5. Teste's recommendation of Spongia in all serous inflammations—pleurisy, pericarditis, peritonitis, &c.—with or without effusion has not been confirmed.

Allied medicines are *Iodine* and *Bromine* (of course), *Hepar sulphuris, Kali bichromicum* and *Selenium.*

In croup and laryngeal affections Spongia seems to act well in all dilutions : I myself find the first and second decimal to answer every purpose. In cardiac disease the higher attenuations alone have yet been used.

We will speak now of metallic tin,

Stannum.

We use the purest tin-foil ; and, having reduced it to powder, triturate it with milk-sugar for medicinal use.

The proving of Stannum appears in the sixth volume of the *Materia Medica Pura.* It contains 204 symptoms from Hahnemann, 5 from authors, and 451 from seven fellow-observers. The pathogenesis in the *Chronic Diseases* is but a reproduction of this, with the preface abridged and the notes omitted ; so that it would be better if translators would give us the original draught. Dr. Allen adds some effects of the bichloride, and an observation of poisoning from food cooked in a new tin pan.

Stannum is one of the few Hahnemannian medicines regarding which we have any information as to the doses used in the proving. In a note to Gross's first communication, we are told that his symptoms were obtained from a male and a female prover, taking increasing doses of a trituration of five grains of tin to a hundred grains of milk-sugar till the man had consumed three and the woman two grains of the metal. The inference that the rest of the proving was conducted with similar quantities is supported from another source. In the case of Stannum alone among medicines does Hahnemann recommend a lower potency than before to be used. Writing so late as 1827, he says that he has hitherto used the sixth attenuation; but now finds it unnecessary to go above the third.

Tin is known to modern medicine only as a vermifuge. It is generally supposed to act mechanically; but Hahnemann showed that such an hypothesis was untenable upon the facts known in his day, and it has since been affirmed that water in which tin has been boiled (or cooled after heating) is anthelmintic, and that several compounds of the metal have the same property. Hahnemann thinks that tin acts in tapeworm by stupefying the parasite, and so enabling purgatives to dislodge it : he asserts that even in the third trituration it produces this effect. Teste says that both lumbrici and ascarides come away often in large quantities after the use of the dynamized metal.

The frequent causation of nervous disorders—as epilepsy and chorea—by worms led to the use of tin in instances of the kind where such origin was suspected. But it not unfrequently happened that no worms were brought away, and yet epileptic fits were much alleviated. Thus the medicine grew in favour for a time as directly influencing the disease ; and Hahnemann can justly cite Fothergill (though not Monro) as commending it, and Quincy as saying that we possess no more potent antiepileptic than this metal. Hahnemann's 409th symptom among the "Observations of Others," if taken (as it is in some translations and compilations) without its bracket and note, would seem to show that tin was capable of producing actual epilepsy in the healthy. The observation he cites is one of a boy, who suffered frequently from convulsive attacks, especially in the morning fasting. Tin was given to destroy the worms which were supposed to be present ; and thereupon the fits increased and multiplied to perfect epilepsy. More satisfactory is the evidence of the neurotic influence of tin derived from the observed effects of the chloride. Pereira's account of this salt is naively homœopathic. "When taken as a poison," he writes, "it causes convulsive movements of the muscles of the extremities and of the face, and sometimes paralysis. It has been used . . . . as an anti-spasmodic in epilepsy, chorea, and other convulsive diseases, and as a stimulant to paralysed muscles in paraplegia." Orfila, who is Pereira's authority for the physiological part of this statement, relates one instance in which a cataleptic state was induced in a dog by the introduction of this salt.

In homœopathic practice, the neurotic properties of Stannum have been turned to effect mainly in certain neuralgiæ. It produced a good deal of nerve-pain among its provers. Hahnemann says that this is usually of a "drawing pressing or pressive drawing" character; and Gross notes as a general condition of such pains that "they commence lightly, increase gradually and to a very high degree, and decrease again as slowly." From these indications Stannum has often been given with success in neuralgia (chiefly supra-orbital) and headache. You will find some interesting cases of the kind by one of our Russian colleagues, Dr. Villers, in the seventeenth volume of the *British Journal of Homœopathy*, and another by Dr. Dudgeon in the twenty-ninth volume. I have myself found it very beneficial in migraine having this *crescendo decrescendo* character, the vomiting supervening at the acme. Another nervous disorder in whose treatment Stannum has found a place is hypochondriasis. Albrecht and Geischläger found it useful here, says Hahnemann ; and he points to some of his provers' symptoms as very like the abdominal spasms and diaphragmatic pains of these subjects. He also says that it is indicated by intolerable uneasiness, so that the patient knows not what to do with himself. Hartmann, in harmony with this, urgently recommends Stannum in hypochondriasis where the abdominal pains are relieved by walking about, while on the other hand the sufferer is so weak that he is fain to rest, whereupon his distress returns. *Apropos* of abdominal pains, I should mention that Dr. Guernsey strongly commends Stannum in the colic of young children (whether from worms or not) when firm pressure affords relief.

Before the anthelmintic and neurotic properties of tin were known, it was in some repute as an anti-hectic, and as a remedy for what Hahnemann calls "ulcerous phthisis." (A preparation of it constituted the "anti-hecticum Poterii," and is much commended by Muraltus, Hoffmann, Vogel, and others.) He means chronic bronchial and pulmonary conditions characterised by profuse muco-purulent discharges and general colliquative symptoms. He quotes Stahl's statement that tin "causes marasmus and phthisis," and points to several of the symptoms observed by himself as suggesting the same action. Thus the use of the metal in such conditions has survived in the homœopathic school, while it has become unknown elsewhere. We regard it as indicated by great abundance of the sputa, especially if they have also a greenish colour and sweetish taste; and also by a sense of great weakness and emptiness of the chest, so that a slight exertion of voice causes much fatigue. This last Dr. Guernsey considers a general "key-note" of the drug. Dr. Meyhoffer has found much benefit from it in dilatation of the bronchi. Even in phthisical cases where it cannot cure, Stannum will often do a good deal to moderate the exhausting sweats and expectoration.

While homœopathy has preserved this use of the drug, it has initiated another. The sensations experienced by a female prover have suggested its use in relieving the sensation of "bearing down" so often complained of by women, and even in benefiting prolapsus uteri. I have hardly ever known it fail to effect the former purpose; and I have been quite astonished at its power over prolapsus. It seems to strengthen the uterine ligaments.*

Sepia in the two latter spheres of action, and *Argentum*, *Cuprum* and *Zincum* as neurotics, are analogues of Stannum.

While Hahnemann's experience seems to show that there is no advantage in going beyond the third, I must say that, like Drs. Bayes and Drury, I have seen higher dilutions act well.

We have as our next medicine one which we have turned to more noble purposes than that of destroying lice, the "staves-acre," Delphinium

Staphisagria.

The tincture is prepared by maceration from the seeds.

The proving is in the fifth volume of the *Materia Medica Pura*. It contains 283 symptoms from Hahnemann, and 438 from twelve others.

Up to Hahnemann's time Staphisagria was little known save

* This observation, however, I find not to be new. Hoffmann quotes Muraltus as saying that tin "uterum corroborat."

as an external application for phthiriasis—a use of it which, in the form of the oil of the seeds (ascertained by Mr. Squire to be the active element), still survives. Dioscorides, however, had praised it as a masticatory for toothache ; and Schulze had experienced a frightful aggravation of the pain when so employing it. Hahnemann was thus, perhaps, led to prove it ; and he found it so powerfully to affect the healthy body that he thought it likely to prove a great medicine. His pathogenetic results have been substantiated by the active properties found to belong to the two alkaloids of stavesacre—delphinine and staphisagrine ; but his therapeutic expectations have hardly been realised as yet. Staphisagria, in fact, is one of those drugs which one hardly ever thinks of in connection with the treatment of the ordinary forms of disease. Every now and then, however, the consultation of a repertory leads us to choose it as the *similimum* to the group of symptoms, and in time, perhaps, it will attain a forward place in therapeutics ; for its provings evidence its possession of a very extensive range of influence. In the meantime I would call attention to its effects upon the genito-urinary organs. Putting them all together, they present a perfect picture of that form of *spermatorrhœa* so well described by Lallemand, in which the prostatic portion of the urethral mucous membrane is the seat of chronic inflammatory irritation, which sometimes extends into the ejaculatory canals and seminal ducts. I have used it several times in this malady with great benefit, and Bonjean commends it highly. The provings, moreover, confirm the suggestion of the experience of Dioscorides and Schulze as to the specific influence of the drug on the teeth and gums. The teeth ache and decay, get loose, and even show black streaks in their substance under its use : the gums become retracted and white. Odontalgia in persons so affected readily yields to Staphisagria ; and the tendency to such decay of the teeth may in other maladies be an indication for its use. It here resembles Kreosote

The writer who seems to know most of the curative virtues of Staphisagria is M. Teste. He gives a long list—like those of Hahnemann for his antipsorics—of morbid conditions in which it has proved beneficial. Of these I may especially mention nausea from vertigo, as in sea-sickness. From experiencing this combination of symptoms in himself he was led to try the medicine in the *mal de mer*. Of twenty persons whom he supplied with a single dose of three drops of the sixth dilution when starting on a voyage, and from whom he received a report of the result, five only derived no benefit. In seven the trouble was absolutely avoided, and the remaining eight expressed themselves as greatly relieved. The medicine must be taken, he says, before vomiting ⌐as set in, at the moment when the dizziness and nausea commence. He also speaks of it as the best remedy for another form of sympathetic nausea and vomiting, viz., that of pregnancy. Dr. Phillips, who gives the drug in doses of from five to twenty drops of the tincture, confirms these recommendations of Teste's, and also those which he makes of it in regard to ophthalmia tarsi, chronic amenorrhœa, periostitis, and shifting pains in the long bones. Bähr has much confidence in it in chronic blepharitis, and to prevent the recurrence of styes, in which last recommendation he is joined by several other writers.

Mr. Clifton has lately given us one of his practical communications as to Staphisagria, in which—among other things —he speaks of its usefulness in chronic gout in atonic subjects, in caries, neuralgia, and chronic tonsillitis and prostatitis.[*] Dr. Guernsey considers the subjects best suited for it to be those who are extremely sensitive alike to mental and physical impressions. It was ranked by the older homœopathists as one of the antidotes to the after effects of Mercury, and also to those of indignation and chagrin.

Dr. Turnbull found delphinia, when taken internally, to cause heat and tingling in various parts of the body ; and used it with benefit in some forms of neuralgia. Dr. Bayes praises Staphisagria itself in this malady, having once obtained striking relief from it in tic-douloureux itself. All this reminds us of Aconite ; and it is like Aconite that (according to Böhm) delphinia affects the heart. It has been given as a " sedative " to the circulation in acute rheumatism.

Teste classes Staphisagria with *Causticum, Coffea*, and *Cocculus ;* to which I would add *Kreosote*, and Dr. Hering *Colocynth.*

The dilutions from the sixth to the thirtieth have given most satisfaction.

We will conclude to-day's lecture with a few words upon the thorn-apple, Datura

Stramonium.

The tincture is prepared from the entire herb in the usual manner.

There is a pathogenesis of Stramonium in the third volume

[*] *Monthly Hom. Review*, xxi., 469.

3 H

of the *Reine Arzneimittellehre*.   It contains 96 symptoms from
Hahnemann, 90 from two others, and 383 from authors.
Among these last I must caution against any dependence on
citations from Stoerck and Greding, as they were taken, in
the same wholesale way which we have heretofore seen, from
patients treated by them.   Dr. Hering has given us a very
full arrangement of the symptomatology of Stramonium in
his *Materia Medica*, incorporating many fresh cases of poisoning.   The English materials of this nature which he has used
may be read at length in Dr. Berridge's " Pathogenetic Record,"
now publishing as a supplement to the *British Journal of
Homœopathy*.   Dr. Allen adds symptoms from some 150
more observations of the kind.

To the therapeutists of the old school Stramonium must
be a greater puzzle than even Hyoscyamus.   Pereira's article
on the drug might have been written by an avowed homœopathist.   It is "used to produce intoxication for licentious
purposes," *i.e.*, as an aphrodisiac ; and—" Wendt used it to
lessen venereal excitement, as in nymphomania."   In fatal
doses " the leading symptoms are   .   .   .   delirium (usually
maniacal) ;" and—" the diseases in which Stramonium has
been principally used are *mania* and epilepsy."   " In some
cases of spasmodic asthma smoking the herb has given at
least temporary relief ;" but—" the practice requires great
caution, as it has proved highly injurious.   .   .   .   Aggravation of the dyspnœa   .   .   .   is one of the evils said to
have been induced."   We may fairly look under these circumstances to the systematic account of the drug which
Homœopathy enables us to give.

Stramonium acts chiefly on the brain, and in a manner
closely resembling that of Belladonna and Hyoscyamus.   The
delirium it causes is more furious than that of either ; but
the determination of blood to the head, while greater than
that of Hyoscyamus, is less than and not so inflammatory as
that of Belladonna.   With the delirium are hallucinations ;
dilated pupil ; amaurosis ; diminished general sensibility ;
extreme mobility of the muscular system, with loss of
voluntary control ; sexual excitement ; spasmodic dysphonia
and dysphagia ; great dryness of throat ; and frequently a
bright red eruption over the body.   If the poisoning goes on,
congestive sopor and general palsy set in.   I have already
discussed the rationale of these phenomena, when speaking
of Belladonna.   Stramonium is evidently an almost pure
neurotic.   The only parts besides the brain which show any
signs of tissue-irritation are the throat and the skin.

Correspondingly, the use of Stramonium as a therapeutic agent has been nearly exclusively confined to affections of the brain and nervous system. The only exception is *scarlatina ;* in some forms of which Stramonium may be preferable to Belladonna. The distinguishing characteristics of the two drugs in relation to this malady are well given by Dr. P. P. Wells, in the fifth volume of the *American Homœopathic Review.* He lays most stress on the presence of an extreme degree of nervous erethism—convulsions, trembling, restlessness, &c.—as indicating Stramonium.

There are few neuroses in which Stramonium is not more or less useful. It is our chief remedy in acute mania, to which it is more homœopathic than the inflammatory Belladonna ; and is hardly less valuable in delirium tremens, when assuming the active form described as " mania-à-potu " by the older writers. Numerous cases of these maladies in which it proved curative are recorded by Dr. Hoyne. The constant association of hallucinations with its delirium makes it very appropriate here, and wherever else they occur. You will not be surprised that a homœopathist should speak thus ; but it is curious to hear the same practice advocated, and on the same grounds, by an eminent alienist of the old school—I refer to Dr. Moreau.* Stramonium is sometimes indicated for the cerebral manifestations of typhus and typhoid, but less often than the other mydriatics and Opium. But in nymphomania and in puerperal mania it stands highest among remedies, owing to its special action on the sexual functions. In epilepsy brought on by a fright, and yet recent, it may prove very useful. It is, as Hahnemann points out, exquisitely homœopathic to hydrophobia, even more so than Belladonna. In a child of Dr. Duffin's poisoned by the seeds,† not only were the symptoms during life strikingly analogous to those of this disease, but after death " a slight unusual blush pervaded the pharynx and œsophagus to about one third of their extent ; the larynx was similarly injected, and the rima glottidis thickened and very turgid." It appears that in China the different species of Datura, and among them the D. Stramonium, are in popular use as prophylactics against hydrophobia. Extracts from reports of missionaries on this subject are given by Dr. Ozanam in the eighteenth volume of the *Bulletin de la Societé Medicale Homœopathique de France.* It is stated to be necessary that enough of the plant should be taken to provoke an attack of " rage ;" the patient is then

---

* See Trousseau and Pidoux, *sub voce.*
† See Berridge, Case 2.

safe. We have no certain experience with Stramonium when
hydrophobia has actually set in, for in the case recorded by
Dr. Ozanam the symptoms (which came on the day after the
bite) might have been the effect of fright. But I should be disposed to trust to it rather than any other medicine when, as it
generally is, the tendency to death arises mainly from the exhaustion produced by the incessant delirium and restlessness.

Nor is Stramonium less beneficial when the nervous
erethism, just stopping short of inflammation, which these
maladies imply within the cranium, manifests itself in the
spinal cord. In chorea it is one of the best vegetable medicines; though it rarely cures cases of any standing without the
aid of the minerals Arsenic, Cuprum, Zinc, &c. Stammering
is a kind of local chorea; and in this affection great good may
often be obtained by the persevering use of Stramonium.
The recommendation is Teste's; and it is sustained by many
published cases.* Dr. Cooper has found the drug curative of
a similar morbid state in the bladder; though the vesical condition which best indicates it is, according to Dr. Guernsey,
one in which the urine dribbles away slowly and feebly,
though without pain. It is, like Ignatia, frequently indicated
in spinal convulsions : you may read a good case of the kind
by Trinks, where they originated from concussion of the spine,
in the nineteenth volume of the *British Journal of Homœopathy*. But it goes beyond Ignatia in reaching also to true
eclampsia, as infantile and puerperal convulsions. In the
latter Dr. Guernsey gives the following indication :—
"parturient women show such signs of fear as to cause them
to look frightened and to shrink back from the first objects
they see after opening their eyes. If they have had no
spasms, they soon will have after betraying such symptoms,
unless Stramonium be immediately administered." This
symptom is, according to him, very characteristic of Stramonium in many disorders. The other mental symptoms
which he assigns to it are great loquacity, expressing (it may
be) wild and absurd fancies; desire for light and society;
and an imploring and beseeching mood.

You will find abundant evidence of these and other curative powers of Stramonium in Dr. Hering's arrangement.

As allied medicines, besides its blood-sisters *Hyoscyamus*
and *Belladonna*, Stramonium has *Agaricus*, *Chamomilla*,
Cannabis Indica and *Ignatia*.

For dose, I am very well satisfied with the dilutions from
3 to 6.

* *Brit. Journ. of Hom.*, xv., 399.

LECTURE LV.

SULPHUR.

I shall occupy your time to-day with a medicine which, if not the most important, is perhaps the most frequently used of all we have—

Sulphur.

The washed "flowers of sulphur" of commerce, again washed in distilled water, are used in our pharmacy; and are of course prepared by trituration. A "tincture of Sulphur" is also in use; it is made with absolute alcohol, which (at a temperature of 60°) retains nearly one per cent. in solution. If this form is desired, it must be prescribed as such. Its strength is uncertain when exposed to lower temperatures. It is now only used in its primary preparation, which is designated as the "tinctura fortissima;" but at one time Hahnemann employed it for making the subsequent attenuations.

The pathogenesis of Sulphur appeared first in the fourth volume of the *Materia Medica Pura*. In the second edition of that work (1825) it contains 755 symptoms from Hahnemann himself, and 60 from his son Friedrich and some authors. As the medicine is recommended to be given in the second trituration, it is probable that the symptoms were obtained from this or lower potencies; though their subjects are doubtful. In the first edition of the *Chronic Diseases* (1830) another pathogenesis is presented, to which Hahnemann adds upwards of 300 symptoms; and in the second edition (1839) the list has swollen to 1,969, a few only of the additions being taken from a proving by Nenning which had appeared in the third volume of the *Arzneimittellehre* of Hartlaub and Trinks. The source of these later materials is obvious, as Sulphur was in constant use at the time in the treatment of chronic affections. Much more satisfactory information is supplied by the splendid re-proving undertaken by the Austrian Society, and reported by Dr. Wurmb in the first volume of the *Zeitschrift des Ver*

Hom. Aerzte Oest. It is translated in the fifteenth and six-teenth volumes of the *British Journal of Homœopathy.* Twenty-four persons took part in the experiments, which were conducted with full doses of the crude substance and of the tincture, as well as with the attenuations. Dr. Allen in-corporates their symptoms with Hahnemann's, adding a few from later observations. Dr. Casanova has also enriched the pathogenesis of the drug by some observations of the effects of the sulphureous waters of Harrogate.*

Sulphur has long been reputed as a stimulant to the capil-lary circulation of the skin and mucous membranes, and to the venous system of the pelvis. Dr. Wurmb's proving con-firms and illustrates the ancient opinion. The drug excited a peculiar itching of the whole surface, giving an agreeable sen-sation on rubbing or scratching, and increased notably by the warmth of bed. With this were various eruptions, mostly papular, but sometimes vesicular, and occasionally closely re-sembling that of scabies. Boils, too, frequently result from the use of Sulphur. I know of a lady who accompanied her husband to Harrogate ; and, although herself in good health, joined him in drinking the waters. When she returned home, she came under treatment covered with boils. After the skin, the mucous membranes feel most severely the influence of Sulphur, especially those of the eyes (conjunctiva oculi et palpebrarum), bronchi, urethra, and rectum. Burning with itching, and mucous discharge, are the characteristic symptoms here.

Besides these more general effects, the use of Sulphur pro-duces other pretty constant phenomena, as follows :—

1. There is a decided determination of blood to the head. Fulness with aching was experienced by nearly all the provers : vertigo by some. The Harrogate waters, if drunk largely and incautiously, appear to be capable of bringing on apoplexy. Part and parcel of the above is the erysipelatoid inflammation of the nose so frequent among the provers, and mentioned also by Dr. Casanova.

2. The sexual organs are always excited by Sulphur, even to swelling of the external parts. The catamenia in one prover came on profusely ; and were black, clotted, and gluey, as with Crocus.

3. Although Sulphur in massive doses is a mild aperient, its dynamic action is manifested by constipation, from which nearly all the provers suffered. The alternative, diarrhœa, is very rare.

* *Brit. Journ. of Hom.,* xxi., 353.

4. Rheumatoid pains were very common among the provers; most of whom were troubled also by awaking early in the morning, and finding it impossible to go to sleep again.

5. In two provers there was painful swelling of the tongue

Unless we add to these the countless symptoms of the pathogenesis in the *Chronic Diseases*, we seem to have but a narrow basis on which to rest the vast fabric of the therapeutic applications of Sulphur. But this drug has attained a unique place among homœopathic medicines, of which the relation of Mercury to syphilis affords the only—and that a faint—resemblance. This is owing to the famous " psora theory " of Hahnemann, of which I must here take notice.

The first volume of Hahnemann's *Chronic Diseases* is devoted to an exposition of this theory of his. He begins by assigning one eighth of these maladies to syphilis and its ally sycosis. He points out that each of these diseases depends upon a specific and contagious " miasm." This, being received into the organism, after a period of incubation developes an external sign—the chancre and the condyloma respectively. If these are left alone, or cured from within by small quantities of their appropriate specific (Mercury in the one case, Thuja or Nitric acid in the other), no general evils result. On the other hand, the suppression of the external sign is followed by the well-known constitutional symptoms. The maladies thus set up are far more difficult to cure, and are only curable at all by the same or similar specifics—selected not merely on the ground of their homœopathicity to the existing symptoms, but also because of their relation to the primary taint, in like manner ascertained. Thus (the illustration is my own) it would be useless to attempt to cure a syphilitic angina with Belladonna, or a syphilitic psoriasis with Arsenic.

In the remaining seven-eighths of chronic diseases, Hahnemann says that he found the same impossibility of effecting a permanent cure with the common homœopathic specifics. He sought therefore for some constitutional miasm or miasms which should explain the protean changes and inveterate duration of these maladies, as the syphilitic poison explained the character of the disorders resulting therefrom. In the common itch (psora or scabies) he thought he had found what he sought. Numerous authors testified to the evils resulting from repercussion of the itch eruption—these evils including nearly every ill to which flesh is heir. Again, many of his chronic patients confessed to having had the itch, and in many

others he ascertained the same fact by inquiry of parents and
nurses. The itch was a specific disease, very contagious, having a period of incubation after infection, and then manifesting itself by one or more vesicles at the point of contact,—in
all these features resembling syphilis and sycosis. Unable to
discover any other chronic miasm but this to account for
the host of chronic diseases which were neither syphilitic nor
sycosic, Hahnemann propounded the theory that they were all
psoric. Hence followed the treatment. Recent itch could
nearly always be cured in a reasonably short time, by one or
more infinitesimal doses of Sulphur; and the same medicine
was curative of many of the consequences of the suppression
of the eruption. But these were too multifarious to be homœopathically covered by any one remedy. Hence a number of
other medicines were, on various grounds,* classed with it as
antipsorics;" and with these, selected according to the law
of similars, all chronic non-venereal diseases were to be combated.

I think that the above is a fair presentation of Hahnemann's
theory. For a fuller account of it, and of the criticisms it has
provoked, I may refer you to Dr. Dudgeon's *Lectures on
Homœopathy.* But I would strongly recommend you to read
Hahnemann's own exposition of his doctrine. It is a marvel
of erudition, of thought and of reasoning.—if only the premisses were sound.

But here is the fatal flaw. Hahnemann lived at a time
when the parasitic nature of scabies had been forgotten. His
contemporaries Rayer and Biett regarded it as questionable;
and Hoffmann, Juncker, Wenzel and Autenrieth had gone
before him in tracing numerous diseases to the repercussion of
the eruption. Now, however, no reasonable doubt can exist
but that the reception of the acarus is the proximate cause of
the whole phenomena of scabies. The disease is invariably
treated by external applications. chiefly Sulphur ointment;
and the extensive experience of such men as Hebra and
Erasmus Wilson may be taken as conclusive when they say
that they have never seen any ill effects from the practice,
which, I may add, is as freely used by homœopathists as by
others.

Is there then no truth in Hahnemann's theory? Just the
reverse; as I have already pointed out in one of my introductory lectures to this course, and as I shall now further attempt
to show.

Although Hahnemann undoubtedly based the logical super-

* See *Chronic Diseases* (Hempel's transl.), I., 185.

structure of his theory upon the distinct entity, scabies,* yet
ever and anon he includes other cutaneous affections under its
name. Thus he considers the ancient leprosy to hold the
same relation as scabies to chronic diseases; and in another
place he speaks of "tinea capitis, crusta lactea, herpes, &c.,"
as "varieties" of itch. He is thus standing upon the truth
which is every day becoming more generally recognised, that
many cutaneous diseases are external manifestations of a constitutional taint. To say nothing of the syphilitic exanthemata, who does not know how frequently the gouty, rheumatic,
or scrofulous diathesis comes before us represented solely by
an eruption on the skin? Nor would it be denied that the
suppression of such eruptions from without would greatly
favour the development of internal disease. The same thing
would happen, though more slowly and mildly, as that which
follows the retrocession or even the non-development of the
rash in the acute exanthemata. Again, there is no doubt but
that the repulsion by external applications of any cutaneous
eruption is liable to cause disorder of the internal organs in
its immediate neighbourhood. Lallemand reports cases of
spermatorrhœa thus induced,† Beer of amaurosis,‡ and
Weitenweber of aphonia§—in the two latter the itch itself
being the exanthem in question.

A still more important point is made if we accept the
doctrine of many French pathologists—among whom, besides our own Tessier, I may name Bazin, Chomel, and
Gueneau de Mussy—as to the existence of a "dartrous," or
"herpetic," diathesis, distinct from the ordinarily recognised
constitutional vices which manifest themselves on the skin.
To this "herpetism" Bazin would refer all cutaneous disorders not purely local (as those of parasitic origin), and
which cannot be traced to scrofula, syphilis, or gout. An
interesting account of these views is given by Dr. Jousset, in
the first volume of his *Elements de Médécine Pratique*.
"Dartre," he says, is characterised by cutaneous and visceral
affections which alternate or coincide. The cutaneous affections, under the title of "dartre séche" and "dartre humide,"
embrace all the ordinary diseases of the skin; they are superficial, mobile, and of variable type; they are accompanied

* This has been denied; but I think it cannot be doubted by any one
who studies his argument as a whole. It was this that led him to reject
an hereditary origin for his psora, which would banish scrofula from the
category of its representatives.
† *On Spermatorrhœa* (Engl. tr.), p. 83.
‡ *Brit. Journ. of Hom.*, iii., 255.
§ *Ibid*, vi., 314.

with intense itching. The visceral affections of herpetism are chronic catarrhs of the mucous membrane, whose discharges —whether serous or purulent—are also provocative of great itching; ophthalmiæ, neuralgiæ, migraines, and asthmas. In severe cases of long standing, the visceral mischief may become cancerous. There are "anomalous" and "larvaceous" forms, in which the cutaneous affections are slight or absent; and in which the character of the visceral disorders, the absence of other causes for their development, and the family history of the patient (for "dartre" is hereditary) are our only guides to its recognition. This is evidently "psora" under another name, and with a more limited range; and one must regret to see that the French pathologists give no credit to Hahnemann for his exposition of the subject.

Now the point of main interest to us here is, that for all these disorders alternating with skin eruptions or resulting from their suppression, Sulphur is confessedly the principal remedy. Dr. Jousset of course esteems it (with Arsenic) the great remedy for the dartrous diathesis. But the same practice prevails in the old school. Beer's amaurosis was removed by it—the eruption returning. Dr. de Mussy recommends the Eaux-Bonnes (which are sulphur springs) as the best treatment for the chronic throat affections which (especially when assuming the form of follicular pharyngitis) he traces to herpetism. Lallemand cures his cases by sulphuretted baths. Dr. Casanova maintains that the reason why Harrogate waters cure some cases, and utterly fail in others apparently similar, is that in the former the symptoms may be traced back to the suppression of some eruption, while in the latter they have originated from other causes. He gives two pairs of cases strikingly illustrative and confirmatory of his doctrine. And in chronic gout and scrofula—diatheses in which the skin is so frequently involved—Sulphur stands at the head of our remedies; while in other constitutional maladies, such as rachitis, which have no cutaneous determination, it plays no useful part.

This is the "antipsoric" action of Sulphur. You will see that it is not peculiar to the homœopathic school, though it is there that it has received its fullest development, both theoretical and practical. Of the theory of it I have spoken at sufficient length : let me now turn to the practice.

There are very few chronic diseases in which the treatment may not be advantageously commenced by a few doses or a short course of Sulphur. This is well illustrated by the facts mentioned in Jahr's *Therapeutic Guide*, the result of his forty years' practice. You will continually find in that work the first and earliest place given to Sulphur in the treatment of chronic disease, and will hear of some even of the most unlikely character yielding to it. Of these I may specify the nocturnal enuresis of childhood, in which I have several times verified Jahr's praise of it. Still more obviously appropriate is the practice when diathetic disorders are present. I shall speak of rheumatism presently; but as regards gout, Dr. Acworth, who made this malady a special study, said that he knew of no better medicines for the diathesis than Sulphur and Calcarea. In scrofula in all its manifestations (except in the bones) the occasional exhibition of Sulphur is most useful. And besides such definite maladies, we frequently meet with cases presenting numerous symptoms of ill-health, which rapidly clear up under the influence of the drug. I suppose that in these patients there is or has been some tendency to cutaneous eruption; in a word, that they are "dartrous." Many observers, moreover, testify to the striking results of giving a dose or two of a high dilution of Sulphur in the course of such diseases as inflammation of the brain and lungs, and in almost any disorder where improvement flags or relapses occur. In all these instances the drug seems itself to effect a certain amount of improvement, while it renders subsequent medicines more efficacious. Curiously enough, however, it rarely cures alone. If it be continued, in chronic disease, above a week or two, the progress made towards cure is generally arrested, and even becomes retrograde. Hahnemann says— "Sulphur, when administered in a small dose, seldom fails in effecting an incipient cure of the chronic non-venereal diseases. I know a physician in Saxony who obtained a great reputation for curing such maladies by adding, without knowing why, flowers of Sulphur to every one of his prescriptions. In the beginning they produced a good effect, but only in the beginning, for, in a little while, the good effects ceased.

There is one of the diseases now under consideration, however, in which Sulphur plays a more permanently curative part. This is rheumatism. Here the medicine has the highest reputation—alike in the domestic practice which carries it in the pocket, or takes it as "brimstone and whisky" or the " Chelsea Pensioner"; in its local application in the old school to muscular and tendinous rheumatism and sciatica; and in the internal use of homœopathic therapeutics. "I almost always," writes Dr. Russell, "commence the treatment of chronic rheumatism by the administration of Sulphur in some form; and sometimes I find it useful to persevere with this one remedy for months. I believe that in this I merely act in accordance with the general practice of all experienced homœopathists." Dr. Bayes says that he has found it very beneficial in chronic lumbago and sciatica in patients of venous constitution. Sulphur seems to act here rather in virtue of its immediate homœopathicity than by any relation it bears to the rheumatic diathesis at large. It caused much rheumatoid pain in its provers; one of whom, being sceptical as to its influence, tested it by alternately omitting and resuming the drug, when he found his pains invariably showing a corresponding decline or increase. The cutaneous manifestations of rheumatism—of which erythema nodosum may be taken as a type—are hardly those for which Sulphur is suitable. It lends force to this view that it is in the lower potencies that Sulphur has done most for rheumatism, while the higher best bring out its virtues as an antipsoric.

In passing now to the local actions of Sulphur, I would note that the "venosity" of which Dr. Bayes speaks is a recognised character of the subjects and maladies in which it displays most decided influence. Hempel says that it is to the venous radicles what Aconite is to the arterioles, with èqual force dissipating their engorgements. We may with advantage take this thought with us as we proceed.

1. For many *cutaneous diseases* Sulphur is the best medicine we have. It readily cures recent prurigo, when the itching has the characteristic of that induced by the drug. It clears the skin of the anomalous eruptions which infest it in unhealthy children. It is good for acne, where also its local application in some form is useful; and in the closely allied "molluscum" Dr. C. Wesselhœft has found it curative.* Teste commends it for favus, Chepmell for eczema, and Hempel for crusta serpiginosa. It is almost an unfailing preventive of the recurrence of boils; and only less so of that of styes and whitlows. In scabies we of course use Sulphur in the usual manner to destroy the acarus. But since the eruption often spreads far beyond the burrows of the parasite, and endures after its destruction, we need an internal remedy homœopathic to it; and this our provings show that we possess in Sulphur. I would add that dry porrigo capitis and psoriasis discolor disappeared during the Austrian provings; and that Dr. Clotar Müller (as also Jahr) esteems Sulphur the principal remedy for old ulceration of the legs.

2. Sulphur is very useful in many affections of the *eyes*. It acts most upon the conjunctiva, and is of course best indi-

* See Hoyne, i., 169.

cated when inflammations of this membrane take place in unhealthy subjects. Its chief place is accordingly in strumous ophthalmia, for which at some time in the treatment it is indispensable, which it will indeed at times cure single-handed.* But it also, says Dr. Dudgeon, possesses in acute catarrhal ophthalmia an efficacy almost magical; and has been used with more or less success in inflammation of nearly every texture of the visual organs. I refer you to his able series of papers in the sixth and seventh volumes of the *British Journal of Homœopathy*, for cases illustrative of its value. Drs. Allen and Norton rather minimise its efficacy in affections of the deeper parts of the eye; but their experience has been mainly gained with the higher dilutions, while the older observers who have reported its power in "arthritic ophthalmia" have given it in the lower triturations. Our authors bear high testimony, however, to its value in every form of strumous ophthalmia, whether affecting the lids, the conjunctiva, or the cornea; and also in acute and chronic ophthalmia catarrhalis. Sharp pain, as if pins were sticking into the eye, and dislike to the use of water, which aggravates all the symptoms, are their chief subjective indications for it. It has removed, to their knowledge, pterygium, pannus, hypopion, "ground-glass" cornea, the adhesions of iritis, and opacities of the vitreous.

3. Another chief seat of the influence of Sulphur is the *rectum*. It is very good for itching and burning of the anus; and for piles, especially when dependent upon abdominal plethora (with Nux vomica). I can recommend you nearly always to *begin* the treatment of chronic constipation with Sulphur, especially when piles are present. But here, also, you will generally have to go to some other medicine to complete the cure. Often, delighted by the wonderful improvement effected in these cases by a week's course of Sulphur, I have continued its administration; and as often have seen the benefit gained steadily disappearing until I changed the medicine. Dr. Brown, as you have probably learnt, finds it very effective to give a pilule of the tinctura fortissima every night to patients who, while being treated for other affections, think they "need an aperient." There are also cases of chronic diarrhœa, the evacuations occurring chiefly if not entirely in the early morning, and being very urgent, in which Sulphur is curative. It must be remembered that, as Dr. R. Bell has lately pointed out,† this morning diarrhœa is frequently a

---

* See a lecture on Sulphur, by Dr. Dyce Brown, in the *Monthly Hom. Review*, vol. xx., p. 552.

† *Lancet*, Feb. 14, 1880.

symptom of chronic retention of fæces ; and hence, possibly, the efficacy of Sulphur in its treatment. The laxative effect of this drug does not present urgency of evacuation among its features. Hahnemann, in the *Materia Medica Pura* (and therefore when he was using the second trituration), recommends it in autumnal dysentery with fatiguing tenesmus, worse at night. Here its action on the rectum comes in.

4. Not less specific is the influence of Sulphur on affections of the *respiratory organs*. I cannot better exhibit its homœopathicity here than by bringing before you the experience obtained with the sulphurous springs of Eaux-Bonnes. Pidoux, who had great opportunities of observing their effects, writes :—" It is rare that after three or four weeks' use at the most of these waters, patients do not experience sharp heat in the larynx and isthmus faucium, a peculiar dry, stifling, or choking (*etranglée*) cough, with a constrictive irritation at the entrance of the respiratory passages, some dyspnœa, mingled with a feeling of weight and contraction of the thorax, vague pains in the walls of that cavity, principally under the clavicles, and so forth."   A further account of these effects of the Eaux-Bonnes is given in a communication made by Dr. Leudet to the eleventh volume of the *Practitioner*. He describes the effect of the medication in a case of chronic bronchitis, characterising it as " a kind of congestive *poussée* towards the respiratory organs, with nervous and circulatory stimulation throughout the whole of the system. It seems as if the bronchial disease resumes an acute character under the exciting impression of the sulphurous water, and that in order to heal and disappear it requires this ephemeral revivification."   In another place he says—" There is no doubt that the Eaux-Bonnes may bring on spitting of blood in phthisical subjects, since they are capable of producing the same result in individuals whose air-passages are quite unimpaired."*   And again—" The Eaux-Bonnes stimulate the muscular coating of the bronchi, excite its contractions, and may go so far as to create artificial asthma."

To these actions of the drug (which are fully substantiated by our pathogeneses) its use in homœopathic practice precisely corresponds. At the Leopoldstadt Hospital in Vienna Sulphur has for many years held a very high place among the remedies for pleurisy and pneumonia. In pleurisy it is given (after Aconite) in the acute plastic form, where it is said rapidly to disperse the effusion. Nor has it less power, according to the able physicians who first conducted the Hospital—Drs. Wurmb

* Dr. Bayes has seen Sulphur produce this effect more than once in the 30th dilution ; and Dr. Madden related to me a similar experience.

and Caspar—, in promoting the resolution of pneumonic hepatisations. It is at the end of the second stage of pneumonia that it is indicated;—that " period," as Bähr well says, " of anxious expectation to the physician, because he cannot decide whether re-absorption or a purulent dissolution of the exudation will take place. . . . . Now is the period for the exhibition of Sulphur, and it is astonishing with what magical rapidity the organic reaction is sometimes kindled by this agent." Dr. Russell considers Sulphur a most important remedy for asthma; and points out the frequent alternation of paroxysms of this disease with fits of gout and attacks of lepra and psoriasis. I know indeed of no remedy so frequently beneficial in chronic asthma. Dr. Meyhoffer, in his classical treatise on *Diseases of the Respiratory Organs,* gives several illustrations of the value of Sulphur in chronic bronchitis, especially in gouty, rheumatic, or otherwise unhealthy subjects. Dr. Bayes praises it in phthisis when the skin is eruptive. As regards this disease I would again refer you to Dr. Leudet's interesting paper. While showing that the good effects of the sulphurous waters are primarily due to their local affinity and substitutive action, he goes on to say that the forms and varieties of phthisis in which they are most beneficial are those in which " the patient is not only phthisical, but something else besides—rheumatic, gouty, or herpetic." These old " organic habitudes," he says, " are stirred up and brought to life by the sulphurous medication. They had been vanquished by the more destructive and fatal tubercular diathesis; but now, revived, they in turn prove antagonistic to it, and suspend its course." This is just the " antipsoric " use of Sulphur in other words.

. It is worth remembering that of the diseases most frequently ascribed to the repercussion of itch by Autenrieth and his fellows asthma and phthisis occupy the highest place.

5. A neurotic action has only lately come to be ascribed to Sulphur. Dr. Robert Cooper, one of our most industrious therapeutic workers, has been labouring at this subject for some years past. In a pamphlet published in 1869,* he endeavoured to establish the specific power of the drug over " an intermittent periodical neuralgia, in which an aggravation takes place every twenty-four hours, generally at 12 or 1 o'clock, either in the middle of the day or at midnight, gradually increasing up to this point, and then as gradually diminishing." In subsequent communications, mainly to the

* *Sulphur as a remedy for Neuralgia and Intermittent Fever.*

British Journal of Homœopathy,[*] he shows that he has been led to extend the use of Sulphur to almost every form of neuralgia, and with rarely failing benefit. It is in his hands what we have seen Phosphorus to be in those of Mr. Ashburton Thompson ; and, like that, has hardly proved so successful elsewhere. Several cures by it, however, have already been published by other practitioners ;[†] and further experience will doubtless enable us to fix its place in the therapeutics of the disease, and so to have another useful agent at our command in its treatment. It is possibly when neuralgia is of " dartrous " origin that Sulphur is its remedy.

Dr. Cooper would extend the neurotic action of Sulphur to intermittent fever, and considers that we have in it an "anti-periodic" of the first order. I can hardly think that the evidence yet adduced is sufficient to warrant this conclusion. But some of the cases he has related [‡] do show that we have in it a valuable remedy for the malarial cachexia, as we often meet with it in those who have returned from tropical climates ; and as this, too, is a new use of the drug, Dr. Cooper merits our best thanks for having added to our knowledge of its virtues and put new means at our disposal for the aid of our patients. He considers the subjects best suited for it as those whose complexion is dark, muscular system flabby, hair long and lank, and skin moist.

6. Lastly, I would speak of the use of Sulphur in the form of sulphurous acid, as obtained by burning it in the atmosphere the patient breathes, or spraying a solution into the air-passages. This medication has been brought before the profession by Dr. Dewar, of Kirkcaldy,[§] and Mr. Pairman, of Biggar.[‖] In affections of the respiratory organs they obtain the same benefits which we have seen as resulting from the internal use of the drug ; and find that Sulphur can thus cause asthma as well as cure it, just as the Eaux-Bonnes do. But their most important result is to show—what was indeed partially known previously—that the fumes of Sulphur constitute one of the most potent disinfectants known ; and in this capacity operate most beneficially in the management of all infectious diseases. In those of animals such a mode of treatment seems to promise great things ; and there is no reason why, especially in the form of spray, sulphurous acid

* See vol. xxix., 664 ; xxx., 274.
† As in *Monthly Hom. Review*, xvi., 93.
‡ *Brit. Journ. of Hom.*, xxviii., 192 ; xxxiii., 698.
§ *On the Application of Sulphurous Acid.* 1868.
‖ *The Great Sulphur Cure brought to the test.* 1868.

should not be helpful in destroying the germs of contagious maladies in the human subject.

It is curious to find Dr. Dewar and his friend as enthusiastic about Sulphur, as being almost a panacea for all diseases, as if they were complete adherents of the psora-doctrine.

There may yet be forms of disease—especially old congestions, as of the brain and liver—in whose treatment Sulphur finds a place ; but I think that from what I have said you will have gained a fair idea of most of its properties. I would only add Dr. Guernsey's suggestions for the use of the drug. " The indications for this remedy," he writes, " are to be found rather in general characteristics than in local symptoms." These " general characteristics " he specifies thus :—" heat on the top of the head, general flushes of heat, weak, fainting feeling; very hungry and faint about 11 o'clock a.m. ; awakens frequently at night, and feels very weak and faint in the morning; very cold feet, sometimes burning in the soles of the feet at night in bed." In another place he says that the sleep of the Sulphur patient may, instead of being broken, be heavy and exhausting. The itching and eruptive state of the skin and the muco-cutaneous outlets are also given due weight by him as indications for the medicine. The flushings of which he speaks suggest those of the menopause, and I am informed that for these the drug is in constant use in America.

As an " anti-psoric," Sulphur is a unique drug. Otherwise, it best compares with *Arsenic* and with *Sepia*.

All dilutions seem to act well; but in rheumatism and asthma the lowest triturations seem most in favour. Dr Cooper's cases were all treated with the tinctura fortissima.

LECTURE LVI.

TABACUM, TARAXACUM, TELLURIUM, TEREBINTHINA, TEUCRIUM, THUJA, URANIUM.

WE are now beginning to see the end of our journey. Sulphur is the last medicine which will require any lengthened treatment; and in two or three more lectures I hope to complete all I have to say about the Materia Medica Homœopathica.

My first topic to-day will be the "weed" dear to smokers, Nicotiana

Tabacum.

We make a tincture from the leaves of the Virginian plant.

There is a proving of tobacco in the third volume of the *Arzneimittellehre* of Hartlaub and Trinks, contributed by Schreter and Nenning, and seemingly obtained from substantial quantities on the healthy subject. To this Dr. Allen adds numerous effects of poisoning with or excessive use of the plant.

Most of those who listen to me are, probably, smokers. I need not therefore remind you of the ordinary effects of tobacco on unsophisticated frames. They form the group of symptoms—pale face, cold and perspiring skin, salivation, faintness, sinking at the stomach, small, frequent, and irregular pulse—which, with the distressing sensation of sickness itself, constitute the condition called "nausea," as we have seen it induced by Tartar emetic and Lobelia. With it—and more from tobacco than from the others—is general muscular relaxation throughout the body. I have already said that physiology has not yet explained the rationale of this condition, save by referring it to the emetic centres at the base of the brain; and that pharmacology accordingly can only deal with it phenomenally. It is important, however, to know that the ordinary depressant and relaxant effects of tobacco—whether as smoked by a novice or as injected in infusion into the rectum—belong to the state of nausea. For its actual direct effect upon the heart, muscles, and nervous centres is of a somewhat different character, as experiment has ascertained and poisoning by it occasionally shown. It is—in the form of its alkaloid nicotine —a tetaniser to both voluntary and involuntary muscles, including the heart, intestines, and uterus ; and it contracts the pupil. In large poisonous doses it affects the cerebral functions, causing a semi-apoplectic condition and *(post mortem)* much congestion of the brain, especially about the pons Varolii and medulla oblongata.

Beside these effects of tobacco, we have those of its long-continued use *in excess*. Palpitation and intermittent action of the heart are among the most common of these ; and in extreme instances even angina pectoris may be induced, as observed by M. Beau.* Amaurosis, from white atrophy of the retina (without preceding neuritis), was for some time among its more dubious effects : but the observations of Mr. Hutchinson seem to have established the reality of the connexion between the two.† In *Le Progrés Medical* for June 2nd, 1877, M. Guelliot has defined the characters of the tobacco amaurosis, as observed by him. It always commences in one eye, generally the right; at first the patients see as through a mist, with a central scotoma, then from time to time they see objects yellow : there is no confusion of colours : the patients see worse in the evening : the pupils are contracted and immoveable. Alcoholic amaurosis, on the other hand, commences in both eyes at once : there is confusion of colours, sometimes pain, and the patients see better in the evening. In a case recorded by Lallemand, spermatorrhœa with all its attendant evils seems to have been induced by continued exposure to the emanations of tobacco.‡ Then we have observations upon the state of health of workmen in cigar manufactories, some of which you will find in a paper by M. Teste translated in the seventeenth volume of the *British Journal of Homœopathy*. It produces in these subjects a peculiar dull grey complexion (evidently of hæmatic origin, as it is removable by the preparations of iron), loss of flesh, and dyspnœa probably asthmatic. Last, we get such effects as those described in the *Edinburgh Medical Journal* of August, 1864, where long-continued tobacco-eating (!) caused complete marasmus, paralysis, and death.

* See Phillips, *sub voce.*
† See *Medical Times and Gazette*, Sept. 28, 1867.
‡ *On Spermatorrhœa*, p. 233.

Shall I add to these unquestionable symptoms any derivable from what is called the "moderate" use of tobacco? As I am no smoker myself, I must be careful to preserve impartiality here. I believe that the use of tobacco stands on the same footing as that of tea and coffee.* They are all medicinal agents; all produce violent symptoms of poisoning when taken in large quantities; and all, when habitually used in excess, disorder the functions, especially those of the heart and nervous system. But the experience of all of us goes to prove that tea and coffee may be taken daily without any appreciably disturbing effect on the health. This is the "moderate" use. Its figure can only be ascertained by experience, and probably differs with different persons. So also with tobacco. Only I suspect that the *quantum* allowed themselves by most smokers is beyond the safety-point of moderation. Teste says :—" all smokers of long-standing, or almost all—for I admit exceptions—have their slight or severe ailments which would immediately cease were they to leave off smoking." It is easy for any one who suffers, but does not as yet mistrust his pipe, to try the experiment for himself. I think that any one who will read M. Teste's cases (including his own experience) as related in the paper I have mentioned will feel inclined to do so. Dr. Dyce Brown's recent advocacy of moderate smoking† in no way conflicts with these views. I cannot, however, agree with him in supposing that to the healthy body tobacco is ever a "stimulant," however small the dose. His own experiences of its action of this kind are entirely taken from morbid conditions; and he himself admits that if he smokes when not fatigued or depressed his usual allowance will make him "seedy."

I can say little at present about therapeutical uses of Tabacum. To poison people with it for the sake of obtaining muscular relaxation is of course no part of our practice; and even in the old school has been rendered unnecessary since chloroform has become known. Its employment in tetanus *may* rest upon another foundation. If the drug is given to cause relaxation through nausea, it is of course used antipathically, and is sufficiently perilous. But, as we have seen, it is in another mode of its action perfectly homœopathic to the tetanic condition; and some of the success claimed for it

* I do not mean, as my *Monthly Homœopathic* reviewer supposes, that their action is similar. Tea and coffee are stimulants, and the effect of large doses of either is morbid excitement; while tobacco I apprehend to be a sedative throughout.

† See *Brit. Journ. of Hom.*, xxxiii., 496.

here (in the form of nicotine) may be due to this *modus operandi*. It ought to be an occasional remedy for sea-sickness; my trials of it, however, have hitherto yielded only negative results. Teste's observations would show its homœopathicity to some forms of gastralgia and enteralgia. Dr. Edward Blake commends it in the insomnia of dilated heart,* and Dr. Jousset in what he calls "essential vertigo" —the "vertigo a stomacho læso" of the old authors. In the very interesting little *brochure* he has lately published, entitled "On Deafness, Giddiness, and Noises in the Head," Dr. Woakes has shown cause for believing that it is through the labyrinthine circulation that any gastric disturbance causes vertigo in patients thus affected ; and he cites the effects of smoking tobacco as another instance of the same morbid state. He adds, from his own observation, to the features of mild tobacco-poisoning "feeling of tightness in the head, as though a band were stretched around it," and "aching and feebleness of the arms."

As allied medicines we have *Antimonium tartaricum, Digitalis* and *Lobelia*.

We next come to the dandelion, Leontodon

Taraxacum.

Our tincture is prepared from the expressed juice of the recent plant.

Hahnemann obtained five provers for Taraxacum, though he did not experiment with it himself. Their results, making 264 symptoms, appear in the fifth volume of the *Reine Arznei-mittellehre*.

This pathogenesis presents little that is characteristic. The coating of the tongue with a white skin, which peels off in patches, leaving a raw surface ; diuresis ; and profuse perspiration throughout the night, are the only symptoms which strike me. A case of over-dosing with the drug, cited by Hempel from the *Lancet*, shows its power of causing an exanthem like a mixture of lichen and urticaria, with fierce itching and constitutional irritation.

We have no experience of Taraxacum confirmatory of the hepatic action ordinarily ascribed to it, but which the experiments of Dr. Hughes Bennett, and also those of Dr. Rutherford, render very questionable. Dr. Phillips thinks its medi-

* *Monthly Hom. Review*, xix., 94.

cinal efficacy is due, not to any action on the liver, but to a "tonic" influence which it exerts on the stomach and duodenum.   This may well be, as Pereira says that "where the digestive organs are weak, and readily disordered, Taraxacum is very apt to occasion dyspepsia, flatulency, pain, and diarrhœa." It ought to be serviceable in such dyspepsia, when accompanied with patchy tongue. It might be useful, moreover, in some cases of diuresis, of night-sweats, and of recent cutaneous disorder.   Dr. Frédault finds it useful in the affection he calls "tympanite hysteralgique."*

For dose Hahnemann advises a drop of the pure juice, *i.e.*, two drops of his mother-tincture.

Another of the rarer metals now comes before us in the shape of

Tellurium.

The precipitated metal is triturated for our use.

A monograph on Tellurium, containing provings on twelve persons mainly instituted with the lower triturations, is contributed by Dr. Hering to the fifth volume of the *American Homœopathic Review*.   Dr. Allen incorporates with these a few later observations.

Dr. Hering tells us that he proved Tellurium on the same day in the morning of which, for the first time in his life, he saw the metal and took it into his hands.   "Everything of the kind," he says, "must, with me, pass as soon as possible over the mucous membrane of the tongue, mouth, and pharynx; and I then listen with a more attentive spiritual ear than if a symphony of Beethoven were being performed. I listen eagerly to hear what kind of an answer may be forthcoming from the unknown depths of the human body and life."   He did not hear much that was significant in his experiments on his own person; but two of his fellow-provers —Drs. Metcalf and Carroll Dunham—got very striking results. Several provers had prickling itching of the skin, with papular eruption; but Dr. Metcalf had besides two or three well-marked patches of herpes circinatus.   Dr. Carroll Dunham found, after some days, his left ear beginning to itch, burn, and swell.   "There were aching and throbbing pains in the external meatus, and, in the course of three or four days, a copious watery discharge from the ear, smelling like fish pickle.
* *L'Art Médical*, vol. xlvii.

The discharge was acrid, and caused a vesicular eruption on the lower lappet of the ear and on the neck, wherever it touched the skin. The inflammation of the ear generally was not vesicular. The colour was a bluish red, and the ear had the appearance of being infiltrated with water." This affection lasted nearly three months; and left the prover with his hearing permanently (though but slightly) affected.

Both Dr. Metcalf and Dr. Dunham report much success from using the drug in accordance with these indications. I can myself confirm the experience of the former as to its value in herpes circinatus; and Dr. Houghton, of New York, who is giving much attention to aural disease, tells us that Tellurium is as specific for otitis media with thin acrid discharge as Pulsatilla when it is thick and bland.*

Another effect of the drug on Dr. Dunham was great superficial tenderness of the spine, from the last cervical to about the fifth dorsal vertebra, with an irritation radiating therefrom upwards, outwards, and forwards. This lasted for some two months; and should cause the metal to be remembered in spinal irritation.

As Tellurium was proved mainly in the third and fourth triturations, it would seem that it should not be given lower in disease. Dr. Metcalf used the third potency in his cases, Dr. Dunham the thirtieth.

I must next direct your attention to the place occupied in homœopathic practice by the oil of turpentine,

Terebinthina.

We make a solution of the oil in rectified spirit.

Terebinthina has received hardly any proving; but observations of over-dosing with it are so numerous that Dr. Allen can give it, from these, a pathogenesis of 326 symptoms.

The rubefacient effects of turpentine when applied to the skin suggest its local action on the stomach and bowels when swallowed, though it is commonly hurried too quickly through the alimentary canal to set up inflammation. Given in conditions of passive inflammation and ulceration of the digestive mucous membrane, the same local influence, acting substitutively, becomes curative. Hence its repute in typhoid fever, when the ulceration of the bowels becomes active (as shown mainly by the dry and glazed tongue), or lingers too long into the stage of convalescence, provoking recurring diarrhœa.

* See *Brit. Journ. of Hom.*, xxxiv., 356.

When absorbed into the blood, turpentine acts as a general stimulant, causing intoxication and a febrile condition, and setting up inflammatory irritation at the seats of its elimination, which are the urinary and respiratory organs and the skin. I will speak of these *seriatim*.

1. By far the most important sphere of the action of Terebinthina lies in the region of the kidneys and urinary mucous membrane generally. It is an irritant throughout the tract. Acting on the kidneys, in very small doses it is diuretic : in larger quantities, it sets up congestion going on to inflammation of these organs, with hæmaturia, albuminuria, and sometimes complete suppression of urine. Dr. Goodfellow* records a case in which its inhalation seems to have induced renal dropsy. It inflames also the bladder and urethra, and often causes strangury. All this is so well known, that any application of turpentine to urinary inflammations must be admitted to be homœopathic. So Pereira says, " In blennorrhœa of the urinary apparatus, it seems to set up a new kind of irritation in the affected membrane, which supersedes the previously existing disease." It is indeed our chief remedy in hyperæmiæ of the urinary organs. In simple renal congestion, which is almost as common as the corresponding affection of the liver, it is well nigh infallible. When this condition goes on to complete suppression of urine, turpentine will often restore the secretion ; as in a case of Dr. Yeldham's in the first volume of the *Annals* (p. 386). When it manifests itself by hæmaturia, you will generally find turpentine the best styptic. But the relation of the drug to true inflammation of the kidneys requires more detailed consideration.

There is a typical case of its pathogenetic effects in the eleventh chapter of Dr. George Johnson's book on Kidney Diseases. Besides the evidences of inflammation of the urinary passages, there was considerable hæmorrhage, which the presence of blood-casts of the renal tubes proved to have come from the kidneys themselves. But it should be observed that albumen was found only when blood was present, and that no desquamation of renal epithelium could be discovered. These are, as I have satisfied myself, the usual effects of turpentine upon the kidney. They signify, I take it, that its main influence is expended upon the Malpighian bodies, causing their congestion, and hence (as we have seen) hæmaturia or ischuria. In nephritis, accordingly, it would be preferable where the congestion predominated over the desquamation. This obtains, according to Dr. Dickinson, in the nephritis

* *Diseases of the Kidneys*, p. 44. See also Allen's S. 172.

from cold as distinguished from that of scarlatina. Our experience with the drug fairly corresponds with these pathogenetic indications. A paper of Dr. Kidd's on Bright's disease, published in 1855,* first brought it prominently forward as a remedy. The first case in which he gave it was one of albuminuria of some months' standing, with great anasarca, from cold. The urine was scanty and smoky, sp. gr. 1018 ; under the microscope blood-globules only were observed. Complete recovery took place under four-drop doses of the pure spirit three times a day. The other case was apparently one of granular degeneration. But it had begun with hæmaturia from mechanical violence ; there was much anasarca, with hydrothorax ; and the urine contained fibrinous casts and blood-discs. Terebinthina ϕ, gtt. j ter die, removed the anasarca and hydrothorax, and the general health improved ; but the urine remained slightly albuminous and of sp. gr. 1012 only.† Nor do the cases of post-scarlatinal nephritis adduced by Drs. Henderson and Yeldham‡ lead to any different conclusion. In all the immediate effect of the turpentine is to make the urine freer and clearer ;—i.e., it liberates the Malpighian capillaries from their congestive torpor, so that the aqueous portion of the urine is freely secreted, and the loaded tubes flushed of débris and cleared for action. I myself, however, prefer Arsenicum and Cantharis in this form of the disease.

Two excellent cases illustrating the sphere of Terebinthina and Cantharis respectively in the post-scarlatinal renal affection were contributed to the Transactions of the British Homœopathic Society in 1878 by Dr. Wolston, of Edinburgh, and appear in the eighth volume of the *Annals*. They entirely conform to the canons I have just laid down. The action of Terebinthina in acute nephritis, from cold, has also found another recorded example in the *Comptes rendus* of the Paris Congress of 1878 (p. 91). Dr. Cartier, of Lyons, was its employer ; and he gave it in doses similar to those of Dr. Kidd.

In other affections of the urinary mucous surface Terebinthina is homœopathic enough, but is hardly used so frequently as its analogues in our practice.

2. That turpentine is exhaled by the breath is evident to

---

* See *Brit. Journ. of Hom.*, xiii., 560.

† In his recently published *Laws of Therapeutics*, Dr. Kidd writes— "The cure in this case was not permanent. Some months afterwards he took cold, with symptoms of pleurisy. The country doctor bled him, and in a few days he died" (p. 144).

‡ *Brit. Journ. of Hom.*, xiv., 1 ; *Annals*, i., 386.

the senses; and it is allowed by all that where the bronchial mucous membrane is the seat of chronic catarrh, the medicine in passing through it exercises a modifying influence for the better. But it is not clearly recognised that this influence is of the same character as that which we have seen in the urinary sphere—that it is a true instance of "substitution," *i.e.*, of homœopathy. Trousseau and Pidoux, however, make this plain. "The mucous membranes," they say of those under its influence, "are dry, as if in the first stage of catarrh : they are injected, turgid, and hot. There is frequently herpes labialis, heavy sub-sternal pain and tickling in the trachea, as at the commencement of bronchitis : the subjects have been seen to bring up phlegm streaked with blood."

3. Turpentine, as it is eliminated by the skin, causes redness and even scarlatiniform eruption there. No use, however, has yet been made of its cutaneous action.

There are three other properties of turpentine which require consideration, and which do not obviously spring from its physiological action.

The first is its anti-hæmorrhagic virtue, which is unquestionable. Whether it is homœopathic or no, I cannot say. We have certainly seen it causing hæmaturia and hæmoptysis, and Stillé says that females inhaling the oil suffer from menorrhagia and dysmenorrhœa. To such bleedings, then, it is a *simile ;* but I cannot yet affirm that this is its *modus operandi* when curative of the hæmorrhage of gastric and intestinal ulceration, or of purpura, as it is said to be.

Secondly, turpentine is well-nigh specific for tympanites, as it occurs in typhoid fever and in puerperal disorders. Here the evidence of homœopathicity is stronger ; for Trousseau and Pidoux specify meteorism among the effects of swallowing a drachm of the oil, as observed by them.

These writers also show that the same account is to be given of another singular property of turpentine, viz., its power over sciatica. "In certain cases," they say, "it causes an exquisite sensibility, especially in the lower extremities— a general painfulness of the parts, but existing especially along the track of the great nerves." I suspect that its value in rheumatic ophthalmia, as established by Carmichael and others, rests on the same foundation ; though this has not yet been demonstrated. Dr. Henderson has suggested that, to ascertain this point, the drug ought to be proved on a rheumatic subject. He mentions a case of a gentleman who had taken a quantity of turpentine for rheumatic sciatica, and who thereupon became affected with iritis ; but whether *post* or *propter hoc* cannot be asserted. Dr. Liebold esteems it highly in this complaint ; and Dr. Norton has communicated several cases to the *American Observer*, in which, given because of the urinary symptoms present, it removed ophthalmic troubles.

Cantharis and *Copaiba* are the chief analogues of Terebinthina, though many others might be named.

The lower dilutions only have (to my knowledge) been employed. I use from the third to the first of the decimal scale according as the case is acute or chronic.

I have now a few words to say about the cat-thyme—

Teucrium Marum verum.

The tincture is prepared from the whole plant.

The pathogenesis of Teucrium is in Stapf's *Additions.* The proving was conducted by four persons, but their manner of proceeding is not stated. In Allen's *Encyclopædia* this medicine appears under the name of Marum verum.

There is little that is distinctive in the list of symptoms produced by Teucrium. It was reputed of old in polypus narium, used locally in the form of snuff ; and homœopathy, discerning some specific action on the Schneiderian membrane, has preserved the tradition, giving the drug as an internal remedy. But its chief value is as a remedy for ascarides, against which it operates in the same curious manner as we have seen Cina do. I prefer it to the latter when these parasites cause much irritation of the rectum. It rarely fails, when given in small doses of the mother-tincture or one of the lower dilutions, to neutralise their effects and promote their expulsion.

I have next to bring before you a medicine of some importance, which is quite strange to ordinary practice. It is the product of the evergreen known as " arbor vitæ," the

Thuja occidentalis

of Linnæus. Our tincture is prepared from the young shoots.

The pathogenesis of Thuja was published by Hahnemann in the fifth volume of the *Reine Arzneimittellehre*. It contains 334 symptoms of his own, and 300 from ten fellow-observers. For this drug also we have the advantage of one of the admirable re-provings of the Austrian Society. It was carried out upon twenty-six persons, of whom eighteen were men, five women, and three children. The doses were pushed even to as much as 1000 drops of the tincture. The full record of the proving was published by Dr. Mayerhofer in the second volume of the *Austrian Journal*, accompanied with a complete account of its clinical history. This valuable monograph may be read in English in Metcalf's *Homœopathic Provings*. Dr. Allen adds some few other observations ; but I regret that he includes among these the report of the enthusiastic Wolf, who took a single globule of Jenichen's 1000th potency, and then recorded every deviation which occurred in his health for the next two years as the result of this violent dose. All symptoms in Allen's pathogenesis marked [12] only must be regarded as dubious until otherwise confirmed. A number of them (as S. 2819-2825) are quite beyond the range of the drug's action, and S. 2990 is obviously an attack of variola.

The Austrian provings, which are entirely confirmatory of Hahnemann's, show that the main action of Thuja is on the genito-urinary organs, with the anus, and on the skin. It causes copious and frequent urination ; burning in several parts of the mucous tract; pains of various kinds in the penis ; inflammation of the prepuce and glans ; ulcers, tubercles, and other excrescences on the sexual organs, with itching and profuse sweating ; and—in the female—leucorrhœa. The sexual appetite was depressed, and the catamenia retarded. Burning, itching, swelling, and mucous discharge occurred at the anus ; and on the skin generally, but especially in the ano-genital region, tubercles and warts were developed. In the neighbouring mucous membranes similar phenomena appeared, but naturally of moister character.

Hahnemann found Thuja almost unused in practice ; and the few recommendations of it contained in the older writers were of the vaguest character.* The symptoms he observed it to produce in the generative organs led him to recommend it as the most appropriate—because most homœopathic—remedy for the non-syphilitic form of venereal disease, which he called " sycosis." I do not think that his doctrine on this subject is generally understood : I can certainly say for myself that only lately I have come rightly to apprehend it. In those days gonorrhœa and chancre were generally regarded as products of the same poison ; and in his treatise *On Venereal Diseases*, published in 1788, Hahnemann adopted the same opinion. But in later times he saw reason to modify his views in favour

* See ch. ii. of Mayerhofer's monograph.

of the now received doctrine of their essential distinctness, which had already been maintained by Bell, Autenrieth, and others. His attention was also drawn to the condylomatous excrescences or fig-warts which—perhaps more frequently then than now—were apt to accompany the contagious blennorrhœa of the urethra. He formed the opinion that these were the chancre of the non-syphilitic venereal miasm ; and, like that, constituted the vicarious local manifestation of the internal evil. If cauterised or otherwise destroyed, they either returned in the same spot ; or " similar excrescences broke out in other parts of the body—whitish, fungous, sensitive, flat elevations in the cavity of the mouth, on the tongue, palate, and lips, or large, elevated, brown, dry tubercles in the axillæ, external neck, scalp, &c. ;" or other bodily sufferings came on, which, with the exception of contraction of the flexor tendons, especially of the fingers, he does not specify.

The pathology of this subject, so far as condylomata are concerned, still remains obscure. Jahr, who was a devoted follower of Hahnemann, differs from him about it, holding the common view that condylomata, with the mucous patches in the mouth described as connected with it, are products of syphilis ; while Drs. Skae, Wallace and Rose Cormack agree with Hahnemann. The first,* who from his experience at the Edinburgh Lock Hospital spoke with some authority, states that the condylomatous form of venereal disease is known in some parts of Scotland under the distinctive name of "sibbens." There seems no doubt that a true chancre not uncommonly sprouts into condylomatous vegetations before disappearing, or becomes transformed *in situ* into a mucous patch ; and that both fig-warts themselves and mucous tubercles like them may occur as manifestations of syphilis. But it is also certain that condylomata are frequently met with in connection with gonorrhœa, and even without any other venereal sign whatever. Dr. Skae relates that, when so occurring, they may be communicated by contagion ; and that secondary symptoms accompany them in the shape of whitish elevations on the mucous membrane of the mouth and fauces, a husky tone of voice, and perhaps some cutaneous eruptions. He evidently, with Hahnemann, considers that condylomata, with or without gonorrhœa, are themselves the primary phenomenon of a specific venereal taint. His successor, Dr. Gillespie, has observed the same secondary phenomena, though he thinks the condyloma the result of local irritation and non-contagious. I have taken the above facts from his interesting communica-

* *Northern Journal of Medicine*, vol. i., 1844.

tion on the subject in the second volume of the *Edinburgh Medical Journal.*

However this may be, the point of interest to us here is that Thuja is the great remedy for all sycosic manifestations. When indeed these occur in connexion with syphilis, the mercurial preparations,* or Nitric acid, which seems to occupy a sort of middle ground between the two diseases, will generally answer every purpose. But even here, when the condylomata are acuminated and dry; and invariably when they come alone, or in connexion with gonorrhœa, Thuja has proved of striking efficacy. Dr. Mayerhofer has shown by numerous citations how large has been its success both in allopathic and in homœopathic hands, and in all dilutions. The local use of the drug seems generally helpful—Hahnemann himself recommending that in old cases the larger excrescences be touched once a day with the mother-tincture. This treatment has been forgotten of late years, and was perhaps never known in this country. But since Dr. Phillips has recommended it in his treatise—of course as an original product of his own experience—it is likely to gain ground in British practice, to the saving of much cauterisation and snipping.

These fig-warts being hypertrophies of the cutaneous papillæ, Dr. Petroz has argued that other growths of like nature—as warts and polypi—are also products of the sycosic virus.† While this is doubtful enough, I think he is justified, both from theory and from practice, in claiming for Thuja a like efficacy in their treatment. He gives cases of polypus of the uterus and larynx which came away spontaneously under its action; and both he and Mayerhofer relate numerous instances of its cure of warts. One of these is especially interesting, as showing how the drug acts in the same direction as the disease. A woman had four horny and painful warts on her hands, of three years' standing. After taking from six to ten drops of the mother-tincture of Thuja daily for a month, first one and then another crop of new but painless warts appeared on the hands. After leaving off the drug, these soon disappeared, and the old ones vanished simultaneously, leaving her hands quite free. I have myself had most successful results from Thuja in warts. If one or two only are present, they should be painted with the mother-tincture daily. But when they come in crops, the internal administration of the

---

* Dr. Gillespie says that he has " seen the effects of Mercury on the lips and tongue very closely resemble the milky patches of condyloma."

† *Mémoire sur la Sycose,* in his collected works (ed. Cretin).

the drug is the proper treatment. I have more than once seen large collections of these excrescences, of long standing, disappear in a few weeks under infinitesimal doses of the medicine.* I have also obtained the detachment of an aural polypus from its use,† and the rapid withering of an elevated and enlarging nævus on the thigh in a child of five months old. Dr. Drysdale removed with it a vascular tumour of the cornea.‡ Nor does it fail us when the morbid growth is of the serious character known as "epithelioma." This is—histologically at least—identical with warts and polypi, and feels similarly the action of Thuja. Dr. Quin has recorded a case of cauliflower excrescence of the os uteri, in which the medicine was strikingly beneficial ;§ and it served me equally well to complete the cure of a bleeding fungus of the breast, after Phosphorus had brought its activity to a standstill.‖ You will also consider the celebrated case of Radetsky, in which a fungous tumour in the orbit seemed to disappear under its use.¶ But I must not further multiply instances. Suffice it to say that, whatever you may be led to think of the sycosic theory (which, I should mention, Dr. Jousset also holds, calling the condition a "diathése epithéliale") the presence of excrescences on skin or mucous membrane may always suggest to you the use of Thuja.

Dr. von Grauvogl would extend the range of sycosis farther still. He thinks that the leucæmia of Virchow, with its enlarged spleen and lymphatic glands, is an effect of the poison ; and that many complex cases of chronic disease can be traced back to an initial gonorrhœa. Acting upon this view, he treats them with Thuja and—as its ally—Natrum sulphuricum ; and reports excellent results, even such forms of disease as locomotor ataxy and diabetes recovering hereby. You may read a further exposition of his views in the prize essay on Thuja, lately written by Dr. H. Goullon, which has been translated in the twenty-fifth volume of the *North American Journal of Homœopathy*. You will see that an additional connection is established here with the so-called "hydrogenoid" constitution described by von Grauvogl, in which the patient is morbidly hygroscopic, so that damp air and the neighbour-

* See also a case in *Brit. Journ. of Hom.*, xxvi., 491. In this a concomitant enuresis of long standing disappeared while the medicine was being taken.
† *Monthly Hom. Review*, xiii., 536.
‡ *Brit. Journ. of Hom.*, vii. 244.
§ *Annals*, vol. i.
‖ See p. 746.
¶ See *Brit. Journ. of Hom.*, vol. i.

hood or use of water are highly inimical to him. The Natrum sulphuricum is the agent to which he mainly trusts in combating this diathesis ; while the Thuja antidotes the specific infection of sycosis.

But I have been carried away from my primary subject, which was to establish the specific relation of Thuja to gonorrhœa and its condyloma. I have shown this as regards condyloma ; but it is no less true in respect of gonorrhœa itself. Dr. Dudgeon shall tell us what the drug can do in causing the phenomena of the disease.

" On the 10th of July last, when taking a walk, I happened to pass a Thuja tree laden with green cones. I plucked one, chewed it a little, and thought no more about it. That same evening I observed a very disagreeable scalding on making water, which continued all next day, and I was horrified to observe on undressing that my shirt was spotted all over in a manner extremely repugnant to one's notions of respectability. I found a considerable gleety discharge from the urethra, which was evidently swollen and inflamed, as the stream of urine was small and split, and the burning had increased. I had quite forgotten the circumstance of having chewed the Thuja cone the previous day, and I could not imagine what could have produced in me, a decent paterfamilias, such a very incongruous complaint. The following day the discharge had become yellow, while the other symptoms remained as before. I now remembered the cone-chewing on the 10th, and regarded the malady with more composure. I resolved to take no medicine to interfere with its course. The discharge still continued, though in a diminished degree, until the 15th, but the scalding and interrupted stream of urine were by that time gone, and on the 16th I was again quite well."

This is a more decisive picture of acute gonorrhœa than the provings present, and warrants the use of the medicine even in this condition. Hitherto it has rather been reserved for lingering and chronic cases, especially when the prostate is involved. Dr. Böhm writes that an extensive experience has taught him that the prostate is more or less affected in all gonorrhœas which have lasted longer than six or eight weeks, and that this condition of the gland is itself the cause of a good half of all chronic cases of the disease. In such conditions he has the utmost confidence in Thuja. He says that he could produce more than twenty cases from his own practice, which, though of long standing, and treated with the most varied remedies, have yet yielded rapidly and perfectly to Thuja alone. My own experience is quite in favour of the specific influence of Thuja on the prostate. I have derived unequivocal benefit from it in several cases of acute and chronic inflammation of the gland. It should be useful, also, for balanitis, and for some affections of the pudenda feminæ, for which indeed Dr. Guernsey commends it. I have recently obtained a pretty cure with Thuja, to which—had it not been for its relation to gonorrhœa—I should not have been led. The patient consulted me about his voice, which, being an amateur of no mean pretensions, he desired to have in good order. For a twelvemonth it had become thick, and reedy in its high tones. Every morning he had to clear away (by coughing) a large quantity of dense blackish mucus. Further enquiry ascertained that he had frequently incurred gonorrhœa, and was liable, on the slightest chill, to a return of urethral discharge. His health was otherwise good. Under Thuja 30 and 12 improvement soon set in, and in a few weeks the mucus had almost entirely disappeared, and the voice had become satisfactorily clear. He has continued well since : a cold brings back some slight laryngeal catarrh for a time, but the urethra is no longer liable to irritation.

Drs. Allen and Norton consider that Thuja has a special action on the sclerotic coat of the eye, and is of great use in its diseases. They also call it " a grand remedy " in syphilitic iritis.

Bönninghausen and others have thought that Thuja has some specific action in small-pox, even so as to prove prophylactic against it, as Belladonna against scarlatina. More evidence seems required here ; though I should mention that Dr. Drury in this country esteems it highly. But there is no doubt that the medicine has proved curative of "grease" in horses, which many think of the same nature as vaccinia and variola. I take this opportunity of saying that Thuja has often been of eminent service in veterinary practice, as in the treatment of farcy and of the warty vegetations of the surface so common in the lower animals.

In the thirteenth volume of the *Monthly Homœopathic Review* Dr. Gibbs Blake narrates one case, and refers to four others, of ranula, in which Thuja was curative. Dr. Guernsey considers that the drug has a special influence on the left ovary, and is indicated when this is chronically inflamed, or is the seat of dysmenorrhœic pain. The suffering in it is aggravated by walking or riding, and often becomes so severe as to compel the patient to lie down.

Cannabis, Cantharis, Copaiba, Mercurius, Petroselinum and *Pulsatilla* resemble Thuja in its influence on the genito-urinary organs. *Nitric acid* is its only ally as an " anti-sycosic."

All dilutions seem to have acted well : perhaps on the whole the balance is in favour of the higher.

My next medicine is as novel as the last.   It is yet another of the rare metals,

Uranium.

The nitrate is the salt generally used, and is best prepared for use by aqueous solution, or (less suitably) by trituration.

Dr. Edward Blake has carried out an excellent proving of Uranium nitricum, three human subjects and nineteen animals having been the subjects of experiment, and full doses being taken.   His results, first published in the twenty-sixth volume of the *British Journal of Homœopathy*, have been wrought by him into a monograph upon the drug which constitutes the second part of the *Hahnemann Materia Medica.*

Our attention was first called to Uranium as a medicine by a statement in the *British and Foreign Medico-Chirurgical Review* for 1851 that " Leconte always found sugar in the urine of dogs slowly poisoned by small doses of nitrate of uranium " (vol. xix, p. 44).   This fact, curious only in the eyes of an ordinary reader, was to a homœopathist pregnant with suggestiveness.   Its import was first pointed out by Dr. F. S. Bradford, in the eighth volume of the *North American Journal of Homœopathy.*   He gave no cases ; but stated generally that, in diabetes, "two or three grains of the third trituration, administered morning and night, will, in a short time, reduce the quantity of urine passed to nearly a normal standard, and, after a continued use, the proportion of sugar is materially lessened."   He also commended it in simple diuresis, especially when the urine was apt at times to become acrid.   In the tenth volume of the same journal, Dr. E. M. Hale—ever to the fore when " new remedies " are concerned —published three cases of supposed diabetes in which he gave Uranium nitricum, in one with great amelioration, in the other two with cure.   Unfortunately, the urine was not tested for sugar, nor was even its specific gravity taken ; so that the cases are open to question, and Dr. Blake maintains that the two which were cured resemble Bright's disease rather than glycosuria.   Of this you will form your own opinion.   But in the twenty-fourth volume of the *British Journal of Homœo- pathy* you will find three cases of my own of undoubted dia- betes mellitus, in which the beneficial effects of the drug were unquestionable,—all dietetic influences being eliminated. From this time onward numerous communications appeared testify-ing to the value of the remedy. Dr. Blake's monograph con-tains those from Drs. Lowder, Curie, Jousset, Bähr, Drysdale, and John Blake, which had appeared up to the time of its publication. I have myself published two additional cases ;* and Dr. Cornell, of America, another.† Drs. Zwingenberg and Fischer have spoken of successful results with it ;‡ and Dr. Magdeburg has related two severe cases in which the muriate proved most beneficial.§ Another cure has since been reported by Dr. Koeck, of Munich.‖ The practice has even been adopted in the old school; and in the *Lancet* of June 13th, 1874, Mr. Carey narrates an instance of its success. He ended his paper with a frank acknowledgement of the source of his prescription ; but this the *Lancet*, with characteristic dishonesty, omitted.

Such evidence appears highly satisfactory, both as to the positive value of the remedy and as to the homœopathicity of its action. Dr. Blake's experiments, indeed, seemed to cast a doubt on the latter point ; as in none of his subjects, human or brute, was sugar eliminated in the urine. But he was rather hasty in assuming therefrom that " glycosuria was quite put out of court, as a condition theoretically calling for the use of nitrate of uranium." He might have remembered that it was in *dogs* that Leconte obtained his results ; while he himself employed in seventeen out of nineteen experiments cats and rabbits. The non-appearance of sugar in two pup-pies and three human subjects is no warrant that it might not be found in the next instance of either kind. In the latter, this warning against rash conclusions from negative results has already received an illustration. Dr. Magdeburg says— " I have satisfied myself by my own experiments that after several weeks' ingestion of small doses of Uranium muriati-cum or nitricum by healthy persons sugar can be found in their urine."¶ On the other hand, I think that Dr. Blake may be right in suggesting that the marked action on the stomach which (as we shall see) he found Uranium to possess may account for its usefulness in the treatment of diabetes. My own experience leads me to believe that it is best suited to cases originating in dyspepsia or assimilative derangement ;

* *Brit. Journ. of Hom.*, xxxi., 369. Blake, Case 21.
† *Ibid.*, xxvi., 661.
‡ *Ibid.*, xxxiii., 544.
§ *Ibid.*, xxxiv., 67.
‖ *Ibid.*, xxxvi., 86.—See also vol. xxxvii., pp. 356, 360.
¶ Dr. Curie, also, states that he has verified Leconte's experimen⸴

while Phosphoric acid excels it where the starting-point of the disease was in the nervous system.

The whole question, both as to the physiological and the therapeutic action of the metal, seems likely soon to be tested on a wider field. Among the subjects of experimentation for which grants have been made by the British Medical Association is "The action of Uranium salts in glycosuria ;" and the results obtained are announced to be published in the *British Medical Journal* as soon as complete. They have not yet appeared ; but I look forward to them with much interest and equal confidence. In the meantime I may refer you to the article on diabetes in the second edition of my *Manual of Therapeutics*, where you will find further testimony to the value of the drug, and a substantiation, from Senator, of the existence of the distinct type of the malady to which I have indicated it as suitable. You should also read Dr. Black's observations upon Uranium in the essay on diabetes to which I have already referred.*

The action of Uranium in Dr. Blake's proving was rather to increase the total quantity and specific gravity of the urine —the excess being either in urates or chlorides ; and also to render it more irritating, causing burning and mucous discharge. It is thus homœopathic to the diuresis described by Dr. Bradford ; another instance of which, with incontinence, is related as cured by it in the twenty-fourth volume of the *British Journal of Homœopathy*. But the most important result obtained was the production of ulceration of the pyloric end of the stomach and of the duodenum. This was well-marked in three of the rabbits and one of the cats experimented upon ; and in ten more of the remaining fifteen animals the pylorus was found more or less affected, while in none was the drug introduced directly into the stomach. These results show an unquestionably specific action of the drug ; and indicate it in gastric ulcers and in those which occur in the duodenum after burns. Dr. Drysdale has already turned the facts to good account by curing a case of ulcer of the stomach with Uranium.†

Phosphoric acid is the only medicine which has (presumably) the same relation as Uranium to saccharine urine. *Kali bichromicum* and perhaps *Arsenicum* correspond to its gastro-duodenal action.

The lowest dilutions only have hitherto been used, save in one case of cure of diabetes reported by Jousset, in which the 6th attenuation was employed.

* *Brit. Journ. of Hom.*, xxxvii., 122, 354.   † *Ibid.*, xxvii., 307.

LECTURE LVII.

URTICA, UVA URSI, VALERIAN, VERATRUM ALBUM AND VIRIDE, VERBASCUM, VIOLA ODORATA AND TRICOLOR, XANTHOXYLUM, ZINCUM.

MY first medicine to-day is the common stinging-nettle,

Urtica urens.

The tincture is prepared from the entire fresh herb.

There is a proving of Urtica, conducted by two persons with increasing doses of the first decimal dilution, in the second edition of Dr. Hale's *New Remedies*.

The most interesting result of this proving was to show that Urtica, taken internally, can produce on the skin an affection very similar to that occasioned by its external application, and which, when occurring idiopathically, is called nettle-rash (urticaria, hives). Both provers also had dysenteric stools, and continuous pain in the right deltoid muscle. A case of poisoning from an infusion of the plant was reported by Dr. Fiard to the French Academy of Medicine, in which the upper half of the body was affected with extremely distressing burning heat, with formication, numbness, and violent itching. Great œdema of the sub-cutaneous cellular tissue ensued, and bullæ developed, which on rupture exuded much serum. The urine was suppressed for days; but the breasts swelled and formed a quantity of milk. The woman had had no children for upwards of three years, and had not nursed those she had previously borne.

Urtica is the favourite homœopathic remedy for burns of the first degree, *i.e.*, where the injury does not involve the cutis. It should be used both internally and externally. Its employment in nettle-rash is obvious : it is reputed by many the best remedy for this affection, though I myself have always been satisfied with Apis. It is also useful to relieve the rectal irritation caused by ascarides ; and might act well in acute dropsy, as from a chill. Dr. Terry speaks highly of it in deficiency of milk in nursing women.*

* *Hom. Times*, April, 1877.

Apis, Rhus and *Cantharis* are analogous medicines. I can say nothing about dose.

And now a few words about the bear-berry, Arbutus

Uva ursi,

of which we prepare a tincture from the leaves.

There is no homœopathic proving of Uva ursi ; but as there is no doubt that it specifically affects the urinary mucous membrane, it has found a place in our Materia Medica. It is spoken of in old-school therapeutics as a " stimulant astringent ;" and Dr. Phillips states that in large doses " it produces inflammatory irritation of the lining membrane of the bladder and of the urethra, accompanied by tenesmus, and often by a bloody discharge, and later on, by a purulent and bloody one." I do not know upon what authority he speaks ; but I need hardly say that this is the very condition in which it is reputed curative : as the same writer says—" The principal value of uva ursi is shown in chronic affections of the bladder, attended by mucous, bloody, or purulent discharges, with burning in the urethra during urination ; and especially when these symptoms are produced by calculus."   Pereira says of its use in this affection :—" in some cases, the benefit obtained by the use of it is marked ; whereas, in other instances, it is of no avail."   It is my own impression that it acts more on the kidneys than on the bladder, and is most useful in vesical complaints when these are symptomatic of renal disease. It has cured renal hæmaturia and pyelitis ; and has much repute in the West Indian chyluria.

We come now to a well-known medicine,

Valeriana.

The tincture is prepared with dilute alcohol from the root.

A short pathogenesis of Valerian appeared in the *Fragmenta de viribus.*   Hahnemann did not take it up again ; but Stapf, Gross, Franz and Wislicenus proved it, and their symptoms, with his, appear in the *Additions to the Materia Medica* of the first-named. Valerian was also proved by Jörg and his pupils, twelve in all.   Dr. Allen adds yet further experiments.

Valerian appears to exert a direct influence on the nervous

centres, of the same kind as, but more enduring than, that of Ambra, Asafœtida, Moschus, and the other nervines. It especially affects the brain and the organs of sense. It causes headache, giddiness, and mental excitement, with (as Heberden observed) "agitation and hurry of spirit"; and, in the visual sphere, sparks and flashes of light, even to the extent of objects seeming to be on fire. The motor centres are also agitated, as shown by restlessness and even spasmodic movements; and in the sensory sphere there is formication of the hands and feet, and a sensation about head and spine which has been compared to the *aura epileptica*. Franz suffered a good deal in the eyes; and Jörg and all his pupils had turbid urine, the sediment being now bran-like, now of brick-red sand, now of slime.

It is thus evident that Valerian is perfectly homœopathic to those conditions of nervous erethism for which it has so long been in repute. As Hahnemann says—"It is not to be wondered at that Valerian in moderate doses cures chronic diseases with excess of irritability, since in large doses, as I have ascertained, it can exalt so remarkably the irritability of the whole system."* It has not been much used for them in the homœopathic school; but in the other camp it seems to retain its credit. Dr. Ringer commends it especially in that modification of hysteria which appears at the menopausia— "flushings of the face, hot and cold perspirations, restlessness, nervousness, depression of spirits, sensation of suffocation at the throat, throbbing at the temples, fluttering at the heart." Dr. Phillips, who states that "perseverance in its use for too long a period induces a decided tendency to low melancholy and hysterical depression," says that "in hypochondriasis, it calms the nervousness, abates the excitement of the circulation, removes wakefulness, promotes sleep, and induces sensations of quietude and comfort; sadness is removed, and the hypochondriac state of the mind in general abates." He commends it also in the globus, headaches, flatulence, and coughs of hysteria. In the only homœopathic record of its use with which I am acquainted,† it removed in one case hysterical dyspnœa, coming on paroxysmally, and in another a choreic condition accompanied with typhoid symptoms. In both its effects were very marked. Dr. Guernsey mentions a curious symptom as indicating it—"sensation as if a thread were hanging down the œsophagus from the pharynx," causing frequent urgings to vomit.

* *Lesser Writings*, p. 316.
† See *Philadelphia Journ. of Hom.*, ii., 715.

The properties of Valerian seem due to two constituents, valerianic acid and an etherial oil. The latter, in experiments on animals, is found to be sedative to reflex excitability, which is hardly the physiological action of the whole plant. Valerianic acid, on the other hand, in combination with zinc or ammonia, seems to produce all the nervine effects of the drug : it is in this form that Dr. Ringer commends it, though Dr. Phillips pronounces it untrustworthy. Dr. Bartholow says that the valerianic acid of pharmacy is derived from the oxidation of amylic alcohol, and is not identical with that existing in Valerian. I shall have more to say about the combination of valerianic acid with zinc when I come to the latter medicine.

Besides the nervines I have mentioned, *Ignatia* and *Stramonium* compare well with Valerian.

The first decimal dilution answered well in the cases I have cited.

I have now to speak of the white and green hellebores, Veratrum album and viride. These, though called vernacularly by the same name, are both botanically and medically very different from the black hellebore, which has already come before us. They were at first supposed to owe their activity to veratria. But further investigation has shown that the substance so described as existing in them is not identical with the veratria of Sabadilla, though so like it in physiological action as to be called "veratroidia ;" and that other alkaloids are conjoined with it—"viridia" in the green variety and "jervine" in the white—which have properties of their own. I shall therefore speak of either Veratrum as a separate entity in itself, using the results obtained with the alkaloids as illustrative only.

We will take first the white hellebore,

Veratrum album.

The tincture is prepared from the root-stock.

The proving of Veratrum (so called ordinarily among us) is in the third volume of the *Reine Arzneimittellehre,* and is an enlargement of one which had already appeared in the *Fragmenta de viribus.* It contains 315 symptoms from Hahnemann, 154 from five fellow-observers, and 247 from authors. The majority of these last are from Greding ; and, being observed upon melancholico-maniac patients, must not be received without qualification. Lembke and Schelling also have proved it, as you may see from Allen.

Some instructive cases of poisoning by Veratrum are contained in Dr. Hempel's article on the drug. The picture they present is decidedly choleraic. There is general coldness, with prostration going on to collapse, embarrassed circulation, copious watery vomiting and purging, cramps in the extremities, and severe spasmodic colic. The experiments cited by Christison had already shown that the vomiting and purging of Veratrum are specific, appearing however the poison may have been introduced into the system. The more recent investigations of Schroff have further proved that these evacuations do not depend upon gastro-enteritis, as Veratrum, when introduced directly into the circulation, causes no inflammation, and even when swallowed produces at most a transient hyperæmia of the parts with which it comes in contact. "If its action be more intensified," he says, "it causes a rapid degeneration of the gastric mucous membrane, but no gastroenteritis." The same results have been obtained from veratria. Esche took half a grain of the acetate; and it produced "collapse, with a pale, cold, wet skin, pinched features, a rapid, thready, irregular pulse, violent vomiting, and marked muscular tremblings" (Wood).

It is not surprising, therefore, that when Hahnemann had to prescribe for Asiatic cholera on its first invasion of Europe, he should have placed Veratrum in the first rank of its remedies. In every epidemic since it has gained high commendation, especially in Russia and America. But Hahnemann perceived* that it met the disease less deeply than did Cuprum; and English physicians have observed the same thing as regards Arsenicum. Dr. Russell's remarks on this point are so valuable, that I will cite them here, especially as you may not have access to his treatise.† "As far as our experience goes, we feel at present inclined to trust to it more in cases of violent vomiting and purging, and all the other prominent phenomena of cholera, but which are destitute of what we should call the essential physiognomy of the disease. Such cases will pass for cholera in all reports, Homœopathic and Allopathic, and they will be cured: but to a practical eye there is something about them different from fatal cases, at the very outset. The disease seems to be going inwards, advancing towards the seat of life, not coming outwards from it. That they are often fatal, there is no doubt; and that

* *Lesser Writings*, p. 842.
† *On Epidemic Cholera* (p. 226).

Veratrum cures them, there is no doubt either : but still Veratrum is not sufficient in the worst type of the disease : and the reason of its great exaltation is, that it cures so many curable cases very like true cholera. . . . . We have found it most useful in cases where there was violent vomiting and purging, without that sudden deadly collapse which we have characterised as the indication for Arsenicum." It follows from this that it is precisely suited to choleraic diarrhœa. I used to give it in summer diarrhœa, but of late years have abandoned it in favour of China. As the autumn comes on, however, when vomiting is superadded to the purging, and when the intestinal evacuations are expelled in a forcible gush, with little or no griping, I give Veratrum instead of, or in alternation with, China, and with great advantage.

The colic and cramps of cholera add to the indications for Veratrum in its treatment, though the latter belong yet more to the action of Cuprum. The colic of Veratrum, however, is very well-marked. It is often associated with hiccough, and is apt to cause a sense of suffocation in the chest and stomach, which, as well as the abdomen, it affects. One of Hahnemann's earliest homœopathic cures was a case of recurring colicodynia of severe character and long standing, possibly— as the patient was a printer—due to the action of lead. Veratrum was given because of the similarity of the symptoms to those it causes ; and, though the dose was so large as at first to cause a painful aggravation, it effected a speedy and permanent cure.* Hahnemann also found it specific in the so-called "water-colic" which haunted some marshy parts of Brunswick and Lunenburg.† Dr. Bayes commends it highly in cases of pain after food and water-brash, with cold hands and face ; and it should be useful in spasmodic hiccough.

The spasms of veratria are found to be due to a direct action of the drug upon the muscular substance. They are the primary expression of a toxic influence exerted upon it which soon goes on to paralysis. The heart, as being itself a hollow muscle, shares in this effect ; and hence the weakening and retarding of its beats so marked in Veratrum-poisoning. This property has been turned to account in the use of the American species—Veratrum viride—as a cardiac depressant in fever and inflammation, as we shall see presently. We rather utilise it by giving Veratrum album as a "tonic" in cases of cardiac and general muscular debility. The "great weakness and exhaustion with cold sweat on the forehead" which is Dr.

* See *Lesser Writings*, p. 353.
† *Ibid.*, p. 605.

Guernsey's chief indication for it ; the intermitting heart, and "debility with blue hands and cold feet," in which Dr. Bayes finds it so useful, belong to this category. So also in all probability does the paralytic state of the rectum which it caused in one of Hahnemann's provers, and the constipation depending on this cause which it has often proved able to benefit.*

Veratrum album was the hellebore much used by the ancients in the treatment of chronic disease, and especially of insanity. A learned account of the practice is given by Hahnemann in the treatise *De Helleborismo Veterum* by which he gained his licence in Leipsic in 1812. It was used as a drastic emetic and purgative, and probably effected any good which came out of the evil by the shock and change it gave to the system. But Hahnemann thinks that it sometimes acted specifically ; and cites Aetius as saying—"it is not the vomiting whereby the Veratrum album is of use in chronic disease ; for many have taken and digested it with scarcely any evacuant action, and yet have experienced no less benefit from its use than those who have been worked by it." He says that at least one third of the cases of insanity occurring in lunatic asylums might be cured by it in such small doses as the twelfth dilution administered in the patient's drink. The pathogenesis of the drug hardly supports this strong statement. The marked symptoms of insanity which stand at the end of Hahnemann's list are all from Greding—that is, they were observed upon insane patients taking the drug, and are worse than worthless. Delirium, however, is sometimes caused by poisoning or overdosing ; and Hahnemann wrote in 1806—I know not on what authority—"it produces in its direct action a kind of mania, amounting from larger doses to hopelessness and despair ; small doses make indifferent things appear repulsive to the imagination, although they are not so in reality." In the preface to his proving he says it is useful in some cases of hypochondriasis.

The coldness which we have seen Veratrum causing is always a great indication for it in practice. Besides cholera, we have it sometimes in ague and in typhus ; and Hahnemann in the former, and Wurmb and Caspar in the latter instance, have testified to the value of the drug. In fact, where the general condition characteristic of Veratrum is present—tendency to copious diarrhœa and vomiting, with prostration, fainting, coldness and cold sweating, it will benefit almost every case, of whatever kind it may be.

* See Dr. Dunham's remarks in his *Homœopathy the Science of Therapeutics*, p. 127.

Aconite, Antimonium tartaricum, Colchicum and *Digitalis* are the chief analogues of Veratrum album.

The medium dilutions—from the third to the twelfth—have been those generally used. But in cholera practitioners have gone both higher and lower: the thirtieth has been in favour with many, while in the last epidemic in Liverpool Mr. Proctor got the best effects from the first decimal.

And now of the green or American hellebore

Veratrum viride.

The tincture is prepared from the root.

A proving of Veratrum viride by Dr. Burt, in substantial doses, is contained in the second edition of Dr. Hale's *New Remedies;* and the therapeutic portion of his fourth edition relates numerous cases of over-dosing with it, besides giving a full account of its clinical uses. Dr. Allen has collated these with other provings and poisonings.

The green hellebore shows its relationship to the white by occasionally causing a choleraic condition, as in a child of Dr. Burt's whose case is related by Dr. Hale. But, though vomiting is frequent and severe, there is rarely purging. The symptoms come on rapidly, and depart as soon. More frequently, however, the main action of the drug is expended on the circulation. Either the condition of nausea may be induced, with its usual phenomena, as we have seen them occurring from Tartar emetic and other drugs ; or there may be— as with the salt just named and with Digitalis—great slowing of pulse and respiration, without other symptoms ; or there may be from the first what always shows itself sooner or later, a great loss of muscular power in both heart and arteries, causing syncope and threatening death.

Veratrum viride has thus a three-fold sedative influence upon the circulation, which it can reduce like Tartar emetic through the medium of nausea, like Digitalis through the inhibitory influence of the vagi, and also by directly weakening the force of the heart. It is not surprising that, with such properties, it should be extensively used in the old school as an arterial sedative in fevers and inflammations. It is less natural that homœopathists should follow the example, seeing that the action is obviously one of a contrary rather than of a similar. I cannot recommend you to imitate them ; nor is our manna so scant for such needs that we should lust after the flesh-pots of Egypt. The only use of Veratrum viride of this kind which I can advise is a local one. There is evidence from many quarters* that the application of the pure tincture or a strong lotion will arrest erysipelas, synovitis, and other acute but superficial inflammations and congestions in a very rapid manner; and, if it is so, it would be a pity that we should not apply it for the purpose.

The real homœopathic use of Veratrum viride grows out of its action on the nervous centres. Dr. Ringer speaks of it as causing "dull, heavy, frontal headache, sometimes accompanied by shooting or stabbing pain over one or both brows." Dr. Burt had constant aching pains in the back of the neck and shoulders, so that it was almost impossible to hold the head up; and in his case of poisoning paroxysms of opisthotonos appeared. Dr. Wood shows that viridia causes convulsions, of cerebral origin; and Dr. Coe speaks of observing choreiform muscular contortions from the use of the "concentrated preparation," veratrin. Dr. Charles Adams, examining microscopically animals poisoned by the drug, found "intense capillary congestion of both the white fibrous structure and gray cineritious substance," more in the cerebellum and pons than in the cerebrum. We are thus led to see the probability of Veratrum viride acting as a true simile in erethistic and hyperæmic conditions of the brain and cord; and experience has proved it to be so. Dr. Hale esteems it very highly in such conditions, considering it to act somewhat like Aconite and Belladonna combined. His book contains numerous instances showing its value in cerebro-spinal meningitis, the acute cerebral irritations of childhood, and puerperal convulsions. Dr. Shuldham has lately published some cases illustrating the same power of the drug;† and Dr. Cooper comes in at the end of a long list of witnesses to testify to its virtues in chorea.‡ In all these affections it quiets nervous irritation and disposes to sleep; and, if fever be present, it disperses it in perspiration. Used in this way, Veratrum viride seems a really valuable addition to our store of remedies. It appears to be especially suited to the condition of the nervous system and the circulation which obtains in the puerperium, and is esteemed by many excellent practitioners—it is sufficient to instance Dr. Ludlam—the best initial remedy for the febrile and inflammatory states incident thereto. Dr. Hale considers it indicated in pyrexia by a full,

* *Brit. Journ. of Hom.*, xxii., 651; xxv,, 256; xxxiv., 281.
† *Monthly Hom. Review*, xiii., 597; xiv., 37.
‡ *Brit. Journ. of Hom.*, xxxiv., 272.

hard, bounding pulse, and a tongue yellow at the sides with a red streak, wide or narrow, in the middle.

I have already indicated the medicines most analogous to our present one. The first decimal dilution has been most frequently used.

I have now to say a few words about the great mullein, or high taper "—

Verbascum thapsus.

The tincture is prepared from the fresh herb.

There is a proving of Verbascum in the sixth volume of the *Materia Medica Pura,* containing 32 symptoms from Hahnemann, and 141 from four others. Dr. Hempel has (accidentally of course) omitted it from his translation.

I mention this medicine rather because it is one of Hahnemann's than because of any active virtues it possesses. The only applications to which its pathogenesis has led have been to prosopalgia and migraine on the one hand, and to hoarse dry night-coughs (like those of Sambucus) on the other. It once indeed, in Dr. Clotar Müller's hands, cured radically a migraine of twenty years' standing.[*] He was led to its choice by a " peculiar sympathetic affection of the ear on the side affected. At the height of the headache, which mainly consisted in pressure and pinching in the temple and zygoma, there commenced an intolerable drawing in the ear, with a sensation as if something stopped it up." Dr. Cretin esteems it highly in prosopalgia. Its symptoms, says Dr. Jousset, are —" pains by flashes, excited by the least movement, in closing the teeth and touching them with the tongue : face red, acid eructations."

Dr. Cushing, of Lynn, Massachusetts, tells us that he places implicit confidence in Verbascum as a remedy for incontinence of urine. He made a proving of the remedy ten years ago, and one of the most prominent symptoms was a constant dribbling from the bladder. " Since that time," he says, " I have treated many cases of enuresis, mostly nocturnal, some of which had resisted years of treatment by old school and new ; and I do not know of one thus treated that has not been cured."[†]

* *Brit. Journ. of Hom.,* xxi., 19. See also case of prosopalgia in vol. xi., p. 299.
† *Amer. Hom. Observer,* xiii., 563.

The mother-tincture (as recommended by Hahnemann himself) has generally been used; but Dr. Cushing gives the third attenuation.

We come next to two species of Viola. First, we have the sweet violet itself,

Viola odorata.

The tincture is prepared from the entire fresh plant.

There is a short pathogenesis of Viola odorata in the eighth volume of the *Archiv*, but without explanation as to its origin.

Our fullest information as to the clinical uses of the violet is given by Teste. He finds it particularly suitable in cases of spasmodic cough and dyspnœa occurring in lymphatico-nervous constitutions: the symptoms are more troublesome in the day time. In one of his cases the cough and dyspnœa were due to the retrocession of measles; and the eruption was restored by the medicine. In a note, Teste says:—"Petroz informs me that he has used Viola with success in various rheumatic affections of the upper limbs." Later, in the *Gazette Homœopathique de Paris*, Tessier published several cases of rheumatism affecting the carpal and metacarpal joints, in which striking results followed the administration of Viola odorata. Dr. Kitchen translated these for the first volume of the *Philadelphia Journal of Homœopathy*, adding some confirmatory cases of his own.[*] A curious point about them all is that the rheumatism was always on the right side of the body. In two cases where both wrists were affected, the right one soon got well, but the left remained *in statu quo*.

Teste thinks Viola is an analogue of *Chelidonium*.

The twelfth dilution in Tessier's hands and the first in Dr. Kitchen's seem to have acted equally well.

The other species of Viola is the pansy, or heartsease,

Viola tricolor.

Here also the entire plant is used for making the tincture.

The same volume of the *Archiv* contains a similar pathogenesis of this species of Viola also; and here again Teste is our therapeutic informant. His facts, however, are not of his

[*] See *Brit. Journ. of Hom.*, xxiv., 314.

own observing, but come from the older authors. They show that the pansy enjoyed at one time a high reputation in crusta lactea and other forms of impetigo.* One case he mentions is especially interesting, where it cured nervous paroxysms in a young girl which seemed to have been caused by the suppression of milk crust. For myself, I have rarely needed any other medicine for this plague of children ; and I have more than once given it in recent impetigo in adults with very satisfactory results. I have seen it act well even in the sixth dilution, which proved curative in a case recorded by Dr. Dudgeon : † but as a rule I give the first and second decimal. Dr. Guernsey recommends it where the hair is so matted by porrigo capitis as to resemble plica.

I have next another American medicine to introduce to you, the prickly ash,

Xanthoxylum fraxineum.

The tincture is prepared from the bark and berries, in equal proportions.

A good proving, on three men and three women, with clinical remarks, may be found in the second edition of Dr. Hale's *New Remedies*.

These provings, conducted with substantial doses, are not a little notable, and ought to prove fruitful. The only symptoms which have as yet led to practical results are those of the female generative organs. It caused in one woman the appearance of the menses a week before their usual time, and attended with much pain : in another, there seemed "an unnatural forcing of nature," the menses came on profusely, "with dreadful distress and pain, baffling description." It has accordingly been used to relieve dysmenorrhœa, and with success. Like all drugs which help dysmenorrhœa, it is applicable to after-pains : I have occasionally given it for these with good effect. Dr. Hale says that it is specially suitable to women of spare habit, nervous temperament, and delicate organisation ; and where the pain is neuralgic in character. Dr. Massy thinks the prolongation of such pain along the crural nerve an indication for it, which would sug-

---

* On this Hahnemann remarks :—" The pansy violet at first increases cutaneous eruptions, and thus shows its power to produce skin diseases, and consequently to cure the same effectually and permanently " (*Lesser Writings*, p. 328).

* *Brit. Journ. of Hom.*, xi., 355.

gest it in cases of ovarian origin. My own choice of it is determined by the concomitance of dysmenorrhœa with menorrhagia, which is rare.

The dilutions from the first to the third decimal have been used.

And now I come to the last medicine on my list, which is a metal of some therapeutical importance,

Zincum.

We use indifferently the metal itself, its oxide, or its sulphate —making triturations of each.

Hahnemann published a pathogenesis of metallic Zinc in the first edition of the *Chronic Diseases*, containing 743 symptoms, which from the preface we may gather to have been observed upon patients taking the 18th dilution. In the second edition the list has swollen to 1,375. Some of the additional symptoms (*i.e*, those of Franz, Hartmann, Haubold, Rückert, v. Gersdorff, and Stapf) are taken from a proving recorded in the sixth volume of the *Archiv*, in which the first trituration was mainly employed: the remainder are from "Ng." in Hartlaub and Trinks' *Arzneimittellehre*, and from four others. Some experiments with the oxide, from Wibmer's Toxicology and from the *Hygea*, are related by Hempel; and Dr. Allen gives pathogeneses of the chloride and the sulphate. A full study of Zinc—containing all recorded homœopathic cures by it existing in German literature—has been recently contributed by Dr. Gerstel to the *Internationale Homöopathische Presse* (vols. iii—v), and is translated in the *North American Journal of Homœopathy*.

It is very much the fashion to say that, save the emetic effects of the sulphate and the irritant properties of the chloride, the preparations of Zinc have no pathogenetic action on the system. But the high repute it has gained at various times in disorders of the nervous system—and especially in the form of the oxide—should have led to a doubt of such a negation. *Nil prodest quod non læditur idem.* The experiments of Wibmer show that the oxide has a marked effect on the nervous centres, causing vertigo, sleeplessness, formication, and oscillatory movements of the muscles of the extremities. Bouchut found it produce sleeplessness and restlessness by night; and on the other hand Orfila noted stupor and inactivity in the dogs he poisoned by it. These

3 L

last represent the ultimate effect of the drug in man. Wibmer says—"The action of small doses, if their use is continued beyond a certain period, may produce a general cachexia, with complete prostration of the nutritive functions : the intellectual faculties are likewise impaired, the beats of the heart are slow and feeble, and the power of locomotion and strength of body are enfeebled to a high degree." A good illustration is afforded by a case mentioned by Pereira, in which a gentleman, " for the cure of epilepsy, took daily, on an average, twenty grains of the oxide, till he had consumed 3,246 grains, which must have taken him about five months. At the end of this time he was found of a pale, earthy hue, wasted away, and almost idiotical ; his tongue was thickly coated, the bowels were constipated, the inferior extremities cold and œdematous, the abdomen tumid, the superior extremities cold and shrivelled, and their skin dry like parchment : the pulse was about 60, thready, and scarcely perceptible."

Dr. Headlam Greenhow has described an affection of those who are exposed to the fumes of deflagrating Zinc, as " brass-founders' ague." It is characterised by shivering, short hot stage, and profuse sweating : during the chill there is malaise, nausea, and constriction of the chest.* This closely corresponds with what Wibmer describes as the primary effect of the internal use of the oxide. "If small doses," he writes, " are continued for some time, the prover first experiences an uneasiness and pressure in the stomach, together with eructations and constipation, frequently also vertigo, headache, dulness and tightness of the head, spasmodically contracted pulse, palpitation of the heart, cold hands and feet, pains in the diaphragm, between the shoulder-blades, and down the spine as far as the sacrum, sleeplessness, languor, formication and drawing of the limbs. These symptoms generally abate after vomiting or a discharge from the bowels, and still more frequently after the bursting out of a general perspiration."

Dr. von Tunzelmann has communicated an instance in which water which had acted on the zinc of galvanized iron pipes proved prejudicial to three persons who drank of it.† The first suffered from paralysis of the sixth nerve, with diplopia and strabismus ; and had dark and turbid urine, with pain in the loins. Another had the latter symptoms ; and the urine, on being examined, was found loaded with

* *Med. Times and Gazette*, 1862, i., 227.
† *Brit. Journ. of Hom.*, xxxii., 610.

urate of ammonia and containing a small quantity of sugar. In the third subject there was severe rachialgia, with photophobia, insomnia, and total anorexia. The value of these observations is somewhat impaired by the fact that all the patients had not long before been the victims of lead-poisoning, which in each had affected the same parts that afterwards became troubled by the zinc. Dr. Boardman has shown that the minute quantity of the metal ordinarily present under such circumstances is hardly capable of causing bad effects in healthy persons.*

The uses of Zinc in all schools of medicine correspond with these pathogenetic effects. The erethistic condition it first sets up in the brain, medulla oblongata, and spinal cord finds its representative in the cerebral excitement without hyperæmia in which the followers of Rademacher so highly esteem the acetate; in the infantile convulsions for which Trinks and Madden commend the sulphate; and in the epilepsy and chorea in which it has traditional repute. Dr. Bayes has found our minute doses to act very well in several cases of the latter complaint. But the homœopathic use of the drug has been mainly as a remedy for states of cerebral depression. It has proved curative in chronic headaches† and in melancholia where this condition was present. Dr. Kidd thinks he has seen benefit from it in chronic atrophy of the brain,‡ and the late Dr. Elb of Dresden found it most useful in that threatened paralysis of the brain which sometimes occurs in scarlatina, whether before, during, or after the eruptive period.§ In hydrocephaloid it vies with Phosphorus. Dr. Marcet's recommendation of it (following Huss) in chronic alcoholism is of the same nature. The febrile attacks induced by the metal, moreover, have been unconsciously applied in the same way; for Pereira reckons the sulphate an anti-periodic, and he and Ringer concur in ascribing to the oxide a power of checking the sweats of phthisis.

We are yet within the sphere of the nervous system when we speak of the virtues of another preparation of Zinc—the phosphide—in neuralgia. It is supposed by Mr. Ashburton Thompson that it is solely in virtue of its Phosphorus that this compound acts. But he himself allows that it often proves emetic, which is a property of Zinc rather than Phosphorus. He also related in the eleventh volume of the *Practitioner* two

---

* See *London Medical Record*, vol. ii.
† See *Brit. Journ. of Hom.*, xii., 489.
‡ *Annals*, iii., 427.
§ *Brit. Journ. of Hom.*, vii., 40.

cases in which the Zinc phosphide, given for non-neuralgic complaints in doses of the seventy-second of a grain, after being taken a few times caused " severe frontal headache accompanied by frequent stabs of pain apparently darting from before backwards to the occipital region, but intracranial, and not attended by any disturbance of sensation in the scalp." These pains were removed by Phosphorus, which makes it very unlikely that it was that element of the Zinc phosphide which caused them ; and shows us that Zinc, in this form at least, is capable of causing neuralgic sufferings, as Mr. Thompson has shown it to be of curing them. In his book—of which I spoke when upon Phosphorus—he omits this illustration of the pathogenetic power of Zinc phosphide, while reiterating his confidence in it as curative. The same thing may be said of the power of the valerianate of Zinc in neuralgia, which Dr. Hale finds very effective in doses of from the tenth to the hundredth of a grain.[*] In the same direction points Dr. George Clifton's recent communication to the British Homœopathic Society[†] of the good he has got from the sulphate in migraine. The vomiting here is an important element in the homœopathicity of drug to disease ; and it is known that sulphate of Zinc excites it when introduced otherwise than by the stomach, i.e., by a direct impression on the nervous centre of the process, as in the malady itself.

There is some reason to think that the favour which Zinc has gained as a local application to the eyes arises from a specific action on this part, for Drs. Allen and Carroll Dunham have each recorded a case of pterygium crassum cured by it, and Dr. Leadam recommends it for granular lids remaining after ophthalmia neonatorum—the drug in all these cases being given internally.

The case I have cited from Pereira indicates Zinc as a suitable remedy for " tabes sicca," that primary atrophy without hectic which we sometimes see in adults. Teste, moreover, recommends it for cardialgia occurring in delicate and nervous females, and for disorders of the nerves, motor and sensory, which supply the heart and air-passages ; also of those which surround the joints and penetrate the bones.

Dr. Gerstel's view of the action of Zinc is in entire harmony with what has now been said. He regards it as a pure neurotic, related only to the cerebral complications of blood-diseases, and influencing the organs only through the nerves which supply them. Thus it relieves the brain from any depression caused

[*] See *Brit. Journ. of Hom.*, xxv, 163.
[†] *Ibid.*, xxxiv., 108.

by scarlatina or typhus, or occurring during dentition ; cures chronic headaches lying deep in the cerebral substance, and insomnia or drowsiness (as also vertigo) depending on anæmia of the brain ; and relieves nervous gastric and abdominal troubles occurring with a clean tongue. He mentions two cases in which involuntary fits of laughter were removed by it.

Dr. Guernsey recommends Zincum in constipation where there is remarkable dryness of the stools, which are insufficient and difficult of expulsion, as if the power of the rectum were lost ; also in painful states of the left ovary, when great relief occurs during the menstrual flow. This last circumstance of amelioration, and a fidgetty, restless state of the legs and feet, are his chief general indications for the drug.

Cuprum and *Plumbum* are somewhat analogous medicines. The lower triturations have generally been used.

LECTURE LVIII.

SUPPLEMENTARY.

With Zincum our main series of medicines terminates. There are yet, however, a good many which must not be passed over entirely without notice, though a brief notice is all that can be given to them. And before entering upon the consideration of these, I have a few words to say by way of addition to the lectures on general topics with which I commenced the present course, for the sake of bringing down their contents to the present time.

In my Introductory Lecture, I spoke (p. 9) of "the 'characteristics' and 'key-notes' which have been largely used in homœopathising of late, especially in America;" and mentioned Dr. H. N. Guernsey as foremost among their propounders. You have since heard me frequently citing this physician's authority for symptoms of the kind; and I should have told you at the outset whence I have obtained his observations. I did so at first from a series of notes of his lectures on Materia Medica, delivered at the Hahnemann Medical College of Philadelphia, which appeared as a supplement to the *American Journal of Homœopathic Materia Medica* some ten years ago. I have since drawn upon later and fuller materials in the third edition of his *Application of the principles and practice of Homœopathy to Obstetrics and the Disorders peculiar to Women and Young Children*. While upon this subject, moreover, I may commend to you a new *Text-Book of Materia Medica*, by Dr. Cowperthwait, Professor of Materia Medica in the Homœopathic Department of the University of Iowa, which applies (and indeed almost limits) itself to the special record of these characteristic symptoms.

In the same lecture, I mentioned (p. 11) among the books which might profitably be used in connection with my course "the *New and Comprehensive System of Materia Medica and Therapeutics* of our indefatigable American colleague, Dr. Hempel." Since I did so, this venerable physician, to whom Homœopathic literature owes so much, has left us for his well-earned rest. To mitigate our regret for his loss, however, he has been devoting the last years of his life to preparing—in conjunction with Dr. Arndt—a third edition of his *magnum opus;* and he had the pleasure, in the blindness which had fallen upon him, of hearing the proof-sheet of the preface read to him a few days before his death. The work has not yet appeared ; but I feel sure that it will display that " pruning of many redundancies and supplying of more deficiencies " which I ventured to desiderate in its previous editions, and will be a most valuable possession to the student.

In the second of my two lectures on the sources of our Materia Medica, I briefly mentioned as untrustworthy the pathogeneses supplied by Dr. Houat, of Réunion. The use of these in some recent American compilations (among which I regret to have to include the *Guiding Symptoms* of Dr. Hering) compels me to emphasise my condemnation of them. Dr. Allen, who has wavered as to their use, sometimes incorporating them with the rest of his symptomatology, but more frequently relegating them to an appendix, has recently published a paper in the *North American Journal of Homœopathy* (August, 1879) giving them up as genuine pathogenetic effects, but accounting for them as being collections of symptoms cured by the several drugs. In the *British Journal* for January of the present year, I have shown cause why even this plea for them should not be admitted, and have counselled their absolute rejection as falsehoods. The index to Dr. Allen's work, now in progress, will (I am glad to say) omit all reference to them.

Of Dr. Hale's *New Remedies* (p. 51) I should mention that a fifth edition of the therapeutic portion has appeared. I hope that when its companion volume follows it, it will be found to contain those detailed provings which enriched the second edition, and which continue to render it an indispensable possession for us.

The general principles of drug-action, of which I treated in my fourth and fifth lectures, have of late received much discussion in the French homœopathic journals, in connexion with attempts on the part of Drs. Jousset and Espanet in the direction of a reconstruction of our Materia Medica. The criticisms which their essays provoked in the bosom of the Société Médicale Homœopathique de France are recorded at length in its *Bulletin*, and the pages of *L'Art Médical* for the corresponding months contain several valuable papers on the subject. One of these, by Dr. Fredault, has been translated in the current number (April, 1880) of the *British Journal of Homœopathy ;* and is especially worthy of your attention.

While this has been going on in France, America has contributed much thought and observation to one of the questions raised in my seventh lecture, viz. : the effect of trituration on insoluble substances like gold-leaf and flint. Dr. Conrad Wesselhœft's microscopic examinations, to which I then briefly referred, have since been more fully carried out ; and the controversy they have excited is far from being settled. Dr. Wesselhœft inclines to the conclusion that very little reduction is effected in the size of particles after the first centesimal trituration, and that the only result of attenuating farther is to diminish the number present in any given specimen. The Materia Medica Bureau of the American Institute has taken up the question, and promises to report on it at this year's meeting; so I hope that we shall soon have materials for forming our own judgment. Further advance has also been made in the examination of the so-called " fluxion potencies," of which I have there spoken, and which purport to raise our attenuations to the millionth degree, and even higher. The tests of arithmetic on the one hand, and of the rate at which colour disappears on the other, have shown that dilution practised in this way falls very far short of Hahnemann's ; so that the mm (millionth) of Swan would only be the 443rd of the master's scale if carried out according to the method propounded, while as actually prepared it is found to be about equivalent to the 10th.* I was justified, therefore, in suggesting that the beneficial effects of using these preparations have been due to the fact that they were lower instead of higher than the potencies their employers had been accustomed to use.

I now begin upon the supplementary list of medicines. The first is the black spruce,

Abies nigra. A tincture made from the gum was proved by Dr. Seaman on himself and two girls† without much result. But Dr. St. Clair Smith, chewing the gum, found it produce a sensation as of an undigested hard-boiled egg in the stomach. This led Dr. Allen to give it in dyspeptic conditions so characterised, and both he and others have done so with great success.‡ A patient of my own, after a fall from a bicycle, vomited blood, and complained of a persistent sensation as if something were sticking in the œsophagus, towards

---

* See *The Organon* for April, 1880, and the *North Amer. Journ. of Hom.* for February of the same year.
† See *Ohio Medical and Surgical Reporter,* vol. **i.**
‡ See *Hahn. Monthly,* Oct., 1877.

its lower end. Arnica removed the hæmatemesis, but did not touch the morbid sensation. Under Abies nigra 3x it yielded immediately.

An Indian plant, the
Acalypha Indica, when taken by Dr. Tonnerre, of Calcutta, in the dose of ten drops of a tincture prepared from it, caused a severe fit of dry cough, followed by spitting of blood. Drs. Holcombe and Thomas have used it successfully in pulmonary hæmorrhage, and Mr. Clifton considers that in hæmoptysis from pulmonary tuberculosis there is no medicine equal to it in value.* The medium dilutions have been employed.

Ammoniacum is well known in ordinary practice as remedial in bronchorrhœa. It is supposed to be a "stimulant expectorant," but no physiological evidence of its action in this direction has been adduced. It has received a good homœopathic proving at the hands of Dr. Buchner, and Dr. Allen can give us a pathogenesis of 291 symptoms obtained by eight observers. S. 180 is "expectoration mucous, and more copious than usual," which suggests that any influence the drug may have upon bronchial fluxes conforms to the law of similars.

Aralia racemosa. This plant, the "spikenard," is in extensive domestic use in America for coughs of all kinds. Dr. Samuel Jones proved it on himself.† He is inclined to asthma, and an asthmatic paroxysm came on after taking it ; but it was, he says, very different from his usual attacks. It rather resembled hay-fever ; and in this complaint, and similar suffocative coughs, Dr. Jones has found it very beneficial.
A tincture is prepared from the fresh root.

Aranea diadema introduces us to the family of Spiders, and I shall speak of them all under its heading, as I have of the serpent-poisons under Lachesis.
The use of the spider's *web* in medicine is of very old date. Sir Thomas Watson cites many facts showing its undoubted efficacy in ague ; and Dr. Ozanam has suggested that it cures by means of the albuminous substance which it contains, and which Dr. Bence Jones discovered to be analogous to and isomeric with quinine.* In favour of this view is the fact

* See *Monthly Hom. Review,* xii., 399.
† His pathogenesis is given in the symptomatology of Hale's fourth edition, but is omitted by Allen.
‡ *Bull. de la Soc. Med. Hom. de France,* xvii., 454.

that the web—that of the black spider is commonly used—must not be too old, so as to have lost its glutinous feeling. Dr. Jones, who makes this statement, has collected in the *American Observer** a number of facts relative to the action, physiological and therapeutical, of cobweb, which well deserve attention. It seems to act as a general sedative, promoting quietness and sleep in cardiac affections, asthma, phthisis, and similar irritative conditions.

It is another thing to employ spiders themselves in medicine, to counteract morbid states analogous to those produced by their bites ; and I need not say that to do so is a peculiarity of the school of Hahnemann. Dr. Ozanam has here again contributed to our knowledge, in an *Etude sur le venin des Arachnides*, which—as reprinted from *L'Art Médical*—I lay before you. He brings together here all authentic observations as to the effects of spider bites, and indicates their therapeutic applications. Of the several members of the group he includes the Tarentula, the Theridion, and the Mygale, besides the Aranea, have taken their place in the Materia Medica of Homœopathy.

Aranea diadema is of the genus "epeira :" it is the "cross spider," "araignée a croix papale." Dr. Allen gives symptoms obtained from it by two provers, and some more (from two other provers) produced by the Aranea scinencia of Kentucky. The former has been a good deal used in homœopathic practice for intermittents, to which it has been thought appropriate when the cold stage is the most pronounced. The production, indeed, of coldness by spider bites, and the tendency their symptoms show towards periodical recurrence, are the facts which justify us in employing their venom in ague, which their mere empirical repute would hardly have warranted us in doing. Dr von Grauvogl seized upon the predominant chilliness of Aranea as indicating it in the subjects of his "hydrogenoid" constitution, who are always deficient in warmth as well as very susceptible to damp. He found it beneficial in many affections occurring in such persons. Dr. Chapman many years ago related a cure with it, in a very nervous woman, of a nightly sensation as of the hands and arms being enormously swollen, which had lasted for several years ; and von Grauvogl found a similar feeling indicative of it in toothache

Mygale. The venomous spiders of this genus are represented by the Mygale lasiodora of Cuba, and the Mygale avicularia. Allen gives some symptoms of the bite of the

* Jan , 1876. See *Brit. Journ. of Hom.*, xxxiv., 367.

latter, and a few resulting from the tincture of the former. M. avicularia has found some employment in chorea, but it is inferior here to the next spider I shall mention, the

Tarentula. This is the creature whose bite developes the peculiar nervous affections which music, in the measure called thereupon the tarentella, appears best able to remove. Much doubt has been cast, in modern times, upon the reality of this reputed disorder; but the records of Baglivi have been substantiated by later observers of unquestionable qualifications. It is true that the dancing mania frequently epidemic during the middle ages in Italy was wrongly ascribed to the bite of this spider, so that all "tarentism" is not "tarentulism;" but that certain unique nervous phenomena do result from the tarentula venom is indubitable.

Dr. Ozanam has devoted to this subject a considerable portion of that *Etude* of his which I have already mentioned. Homœopathic literature possesses also a monograph upon it from the pen of the late Marquis Nuñez, the protagonist of our method in Spain, whose translation into French by Dr. Perry, of Paris, I have here. It contains an exhaustive account of the history of tarentula-poisoning, and also the results of a proving instituted by the author on ten male and five female subjects.* That the experiments were made with the third, sixth, and twelfth attenuations is all the information we have about them; and some of the symptoms are such that we should like to have known a little more about their subjects and circumstances. Dr. Perry has still further impaired the value of the pathogenesis by interpolating a number of "clinical symptoms" of his own observation; and these, which in the French version are marked with his name, appear without any distinguishing sign in the translation into English contained in the twentieth volume of the *North American Journal of Homœopathy*. From this Dr. Allen has taken his symptoms,—with what misleading results may be imagined. He also uses all Baglivi's cases, of which Dr. Nuñez writes:—"in some, as in the first, it is unknown whether the bite was given by a scorpion or by a tarentula; the third, fourth, and fifth are due to scorpions; the seventh, copied from Epiphanio Fernando, is full of marvellous and incredible details; and the eighth is insignificant, so that the only ones which prove anything are the second and the sixth."

For the pathogenesis of Tarentula, therefore, we had better

* The Spanish species of tarentula was used; but it appears that this is of no less active character than its Apulian prototype.

go at present no further than the effects of the introduction of
the venom, as certified by the best observers. These consist,
at first, of phenomena like those of serpent-bites and of beestings. The affected part swells up, changes colour, and
becomes the seat of pain and itching : in the general system
is experienced depression, coldness, præcordial anxiety, and
vertigo. Instead, however, of going on to the local gangrene
and putrid infection of snake-bites, or proving only temporary
like the effects of the sting of the bee, the symptoms of tarentula-poisoning persist, but in the sphere of the nervous system
only. The prostration of strength and depression of spirits
increase, but with them there is an unappeasable restlessness :
the patient complains of neuralgiform pains in divers places :
respiration and circulation are embarrassed, and the muscles
are agitated with a convulsive trembling. Sexual excitement
is often present. The patients seem soothed by the sight of
bright colours, or by looking on smooth clear surfaces, as of
standing water ; but music of the kind I have mentioned is
their great solace. Their bodies move in part or as a whole
to its measure, and they are often led to execute a kind of
dance. Under the excitement thus produced they may be
early cured ; but otherwise their nervous system does not
ordinarily recover the shock it has received, and their malady
recurs from time to time, often at periodic intervals.

Dr. Ozanam perceived at once, from his study of the phenomena of tarentulism, how many applications of the morbific
agent were possible, upon the homœopathic principle. Besides
the " rebellious intermittent fevers " for which the other
arachnida are useful, he suggested its employment in hysteria,
hypochondriasis, chorea, satyriasis, nymphomania and other
affections. The cases given at the end of Dr. Nuñez's monograph show that in several of these it has not disappointed
expectation ; Dr. Jousset also commends it in chorea and convulsive hysteria.

Theridion curassavicum. Under this name Dr. Hering has
introduced into medicine, and proved on himself and others,
the " orange-spider " found in the West Indian island of
Curaçoa and elsewhere. He has given its pathogenesis in his
volume of Materia Medica, including also all existing observations as to its therapeutic use. It seems to have cured the
anthrax of sheep, to which of course—like all venomous
biters—it is sufficiently homœopathic. In the provers, it
caused a good deal of vertigo, with nausea even to vomiting;
also headache, preceded by flickering before the eyes. Dr.
Neidhard has reported the cure of some long-lasting sick

headaches with it; and it seems suitable to true migraine. The late Dr. Barlow esteemed it in infra-mammary pain, and Dr. Baruch speaks warmly of it as an intermediate, but deep-acting, remedy in scrofula.

All the spiders are prepared for medicinal use by trituration after death, or in a tincture consisting of the alcohol in which the living creature was drowned. The latter would seem the best procedure when the symptoms for which the spider is given are analogous to those excited by its bite.

Artemisia. In the first edition of my Pharmacodynamics I had a short article upon the Artemisia vulgaris—the common mug-wort. Our knowledge concerning it, I said, has been mainly contributed by Burdach, and is to be found in Hempel and the *New Materia Medica.* This shows that Artemisia has a decided influence upon the nervous system, enabling it to modify such disorders as epilepsy, chorea, somnambulism, &c. It has had quite a reputation among the common people as an anti-epileptic. The cases in which it is of most value, according to Burdach, are those in which the paroxysms recur several times daily. The curative effect is generally accompanied by profuse and fœtid perspirations. Burdach considers it also quite a specific for the epileptiform convulsion of children, as those of dentition.

I mentioned there a great improvement which it had wrought in my hands in a case of *petit mal.* This patient, however, soon relapsed; and as Artemisia had never been proved, and was not—so far as I knew—homœopathic to the nervous disorders it seemed to benefit, I omitted it from the second edition of my book, and have not since taken it up. Quite a new light, however, has been thrown on the subject by the observations made as to the effects of the excessive use of *absinthe,* a drink prepared from another Artemisia, the A. absinthium, wormwood. Besides general nervous disturbances analogous to those induced by alcohol, the victims of absinthe are liable to genuine epileptic attacks. A full account of the phenomena is given in Allen's appendix from a study of the subject by Dr. Challand, of Paris. This observer writes as follows:—"The effects observed from intoxication by absinthe are dependent upon disturbance of motility: they are convulsive phenomena. The epilepsy of absinthe developes itself in a relatively short time: it assumes at once and completely all the characteristics of that disease. . . . Sometimes the epilepsy of absinthe is not characterised by a complete attack, but has only vertigo or loss of consciousness,—symptoms which are found in true epilepsy. . . . Is the epilepsy of absinthe the effect of acute or chronic intoxication? We believe that it is an acute symptom manifested in the course of chronic intoxication, found more often in those who drink to excess habitually; its appearance is never delayed after the person has begun to drink absinthe to excess. After drinking for six months or a year, some day the person drinks to excess and the spasms come on. . . . A circumstance of great importance is the predisposition. We find a large number of drinkers who have never had spasms, or only slight symptoms. There are others, on the contrary, who are attacked at their first excess. . . . Dr. Voisin says that . . . the epilepsy of absinthe is usually characterised by the very large number of attacks in a very short space of time. I have reported a case of epilepsy from absinthe in which there were from one hundred and fifty to two hundred attacks in twenty-four hours."

These extracts are sufficient to show that the Artemisia absinthium, at any rate, is a true epileptifacient. Let us remember, then, that Cina is another variety of the same family—the A. semen contra, and that both it and its educt Santonine have caused convulsions when given in overdoses as worm-medicines; and we shall feel inclined to say that whatever any Artemisia can accomplish in epilepsy is an instance of homœopathic action. To the value of the A. vulgaris weighty testimony has lately been borne by Noth-nagel;* and we may get better results still by using the more potent A. absinthium.

The A. abrotanum has received a short proving from Dr. Gatchell on two persons, whose results you may see in Allen's first volume; but it does not appear to be possessed of any great activity.

Bufo is the common toad, the venomous character of the secretion from whose cutaneous glands has led to its employ-ment in medicine. It is not officinal in our Pharmacopœia, but Allen gives as its preparation, "trituration of the poison from the cutaneous glands, obtained by irritating the animal." His pathogenesis of Bufo is of little value, being made up mainly of a few apocryphal ancient reports of toad-poisoning, with the no less untrustworthy symptoms furnished by Houat.

Bufo also has obtained its reputation (such as it is) on the ground of its alleged anti-epileptic virtues. Dr. Laville re-ported some success with it at the Homœopathic Congress

* Ziemssen's *Cyclopædia*, xiv., 288.

held at Bordeaux in 1854; and Drs. Andrien, Leydet and Holcombe have confirmed his experience. You will find the reports of the two latter physicians in the fourth volume of the *American Journal of Homœopathic Materia Medica* (p. 139): the former gave the medium dilutions, the latter the 200th. I am not aware of any subsequent reports of the same kind; nor have I myself ever tried the remedy. Dr. Hale says he has done so without success.

Caladium seguinum. This is a plant of the Arum family, and is a native of India. It is in domestic use there for depressing the sexual passion; and Dr. Scholz, of Breslau, was hereby led to employ it for pruritus vulvæ in which he found it exercise a potent curative influence.* It has been proved in the homœopathic school by Hering and Schreter, and the former found his genital organs considerably puffed and irritated under its influence. It is in such conditions of the pudenda of the other sex that we have chiefly used it, and I can add my mite of confirmation to its value.

Carduus marianus. This plant, S. Mary's thistle, has a great popular reputation in Germany for jaundice and other bilious disturbances, and figures among Rademacher's "organ-remedies" as one acting on the liver. It has been proved by Reil,† and he found it to cause distension of the whole abdomen, but especially in the right side, the whole hepatic region being tender to pressure: the bile was deficient in the stools, while its colouring matter was found by chemical tests to be present in the urine. Carduus marianus is thus truly homœopathic to hyperæmia hepatis and simple jaundice, in which—and even in cirrhosis of the liver with dropsy—it has proved curative in the hands of practitioners of our system.‡

The tincture is directed to be prepared from equal parts of the root and seeds with the hull on.

Ceanothus Americanus is another organ-remedy; but the seat of its influence is not the liver but the *spleen*. In the third edition of his *New Remedies* Dr. Hale cited an old-school testimony to its value in inflammation and enlargement of this organ; and called attention to the statement made by its employer that "in chronic cases, when the organ is no

---

* See *Brit. Journ. of Hom.*, xiii., 509; xxvii., 592; xxix., 400.

† Translated from the *Vierteljahrschrift* in *N. Am. Journ. of Hom.*, iii., 379.

‡ See *Brit. Journ. of Hom.*, xxiv., 667; xxxvi., 369; and Hale, *sub voce*.

longer tender, under the use of the tincture it soon becomes painful and tender, and then sinks rapidly to its normal size." This was sufficient to suggest its homœopathicity, and led Dr. Burnett to give it in some cases of splenic disease which happened to come under his notice, and with most satisfactory results.* He recommends it to be given whenever there is complaint of deep-seated pain in the side, even when no tenderness or enlargement of the spleen can be made out; and has found consentaneous affections, such as leucorrhœa, disappear under its use with the pain itself.

Comocladia dentata. This is the "guao" of the West Indies. It belongs to the natural order Anacardiaceæ; and its effects on the skin closely resemble those of the Anacardium orientale and of Rhus, but are more intense than either. Dr. Navarro, of Cuba, describes deep hard-edged ulcers as resulting from the local application of the juice; and he uses the drug internally for similar conditions with success. Like Anacardium, it has some repute in true leprosy. We may not want it here, having its analogues at hand; but should any of us find his sphere of practice in one of the West Indian islands, he should bear it in mind. Dr. Allen gives a pathogenesis of it derived from several provers and observers. The tincture is prepared from the leaves and bark.

Equisetum hyemale. This remedy, like so many others, comes to us from domestic practice, in which (in America) it enjoys considerable repute as a remedy for urinary troubles. Dr. Hugh M. Smith made it the subject of the thesis for his degree at the New York Homœopathic Medical College in 1876; and, proving it on himself and three others, found it a decided irritant to the bladder. Its chief interest in our practice, however, has arisen from the usefulness it has been found to possess in that troublesome affection, the enuresis of childhood. Here Dr. Carmichael† and others have found it most effective; and Dr. G. A. Heath, of Newark, records a case of general paralysis in an old woman, in whom the control over the stools and urine, long completely lost, was rapidly restored under its influence.‡ A tincture or triturations are prepared from the whole plant, and the lowest attenuations have been those employed.

* See *Monthly Hom. Review,* March, 1879; and *Hom. World,* Jan. and March, 1880.
† *United States Med. Investigator,* vol. iii., No. 2.
‡ *Hahn. Monthly,* Sept., 1877.

Eryngium. Of this we have provings of two species, E. aquaticum and E. maritimum. Both seemed to depress the sexual instinct and energy, so that the aphrodisiac virtues popularly ascribed to the latter (the sea-holly) are probably to be homœopathically explained. E. aquaticum showed some power of irritating the respiratory and urinary mucous membranes, and has been found useful accordingly. Dr. Hale's fifth edition contains some experience suggesting a power on its part to dislodge urinary calculi. The root is the officinal part.

Eucalyptus. The "blue gum-tree" of Australia, thus named, has excited much interest of late by the anti-malarial properties it has displayed when planted in localities subject to intermittents. It is supposed to act mainly by its great power of draining the soil of moisture; but its balsamic exhalations also are active in the same direction, and its internal administration seems often to have proved effectual. It is also a powerful deodoriser and disinfectant, acting in this capacity even when given internally, as in malignant disease of the stomach and gangrene of the lungs.

Of its physiological action little is generally known, save that the essential oil it contains, eucalyptol, is somewhat intoxicating. It has been heroically proved, however, by one of our Australian practitioners, Dr. Fawcett. At his first experiment it produced an herpetic eruption, glandular enlargements, and the formation of foul indolent ulcers, with intestinal irritation even to hæmorrhage. On a second occasion he got rheumatic pains; and on a third the same eruption, with swellings in different parts of the body, one of which, under the right nipple, was of the size of a filbert, and the seat of stabbing and darting pains. He also records the case of a boy of 13, who ate largely of the gum and chewed the leaves, and who came under treatment with nodular swellings over the metacarpal and metatarsal joints, causing much pain on movement.

Eucalyptus may thus one day find a place in homœopathic therapeutics. Dr. Woodbury, of Boston, speaks highly of it, used locally as well as internally, in vascular tumours of the female urethra. In two most obstinate cases, he says, a perfect cure has been effected by this treatment without resort to any surgical measures whatever.

Gnaphalium. This plant, the "everlasting" of common nomenclature, has been proved in America in two forms, the

G. polycephalum by Drs. Banks and Fuller, the G. uliginosum by Dr. Woodbury. The first-named physician (who took the 1st and 2nd decimal triturations of the leaves and flowers) suffered from marked neuralgic pains in both face and lower extremities. In the former region the superior maxillary nerve of both sides was affected, and the pains were intermittent; in the latter, the seat of the suffering was the sciatic (which side not stated), and the pain was accompanied by cramps and sometimes replaced by numbness. This seems to show that in Gnaphalium polycephalum we have a true homœopathic anti-neuralgic; and Dr. Banks and Dr. Woodbury report each a cure of sciatica with it.

Grindelia. This is a genus of plants indigenous to California; and we have learned of late years something about two of its species, the G. robusta and the G. squarrosa. Both are strongly resinous, and the usual action of such balsamic substances may account for the virtues popularly ascribed to G. robusta in chronic affections of the mucous membranes. It appears to be especially beneficial in chronic bronchitic asthma. A lotion of one part of the tincture to ten of water is regarded by Dr. E. A. Gatchell as a sovereign application to itching eruptions. The G. squarrosa was proved by Dr. J. H. Bundy,* and produced acute pain, like that of rheumatic inflammation, in the eyeballs, which were injected, and were greatly distressed by movement. It also caused a sensation as if the respiration would cease as soon as the prover fell asleep, so that he had to rouse himself to avoid suffocation. Dr. Hale justly remarks that such a symptom is not uncommon in chronic cardiac disease, and Dr .C. Wesselhœft has reported a case of the kind in which the respiration was greatly liberated by the remedy.

Guaco is one of the "lianas" of South America, and is in much repute in its own country as an antidote to the bite of venomous serpents. It is applied locally and taken internally. The late Dr. Elb, of Dresden, was thus led to prove it, thinking it would display on the healthy body symptoms analogous to those of the snake-poisons. His results have never been published in full, but he gives some account of them in an article on spinal diseases contained in the sixty-first volume of the *Allgemeine Homöopathische Zeitung.* It seems to have produced (in doses of from five to twenty drops of the tincture) a good deal of burning and aching about the

* See Allen's Supplement, *sub voce.*

spine, especially its upper part ; and therewith some dysphagia, constriction in the larynx, and heaviness with difficulty of movement of the tongue. As the general condition was rather excited than depressed, and he often had headache and heat of the face, Dr. Elb inferred that the spine was in a state of active hyperæmia. He was thus led to give Guaco in spinal irritation occurring in robust and sanguine subjects, and found it almost specifically helpful to them. Herein it evidently resembles Naja. He also speaks highly of it to remove paralysis of the tongue and even of the extremities resulting from apoplectic effusion.

I have obtained this information from a communication made by Dr. Dunham to the fourth edition of the *New Remedies*, in whose " Symptomatology " it appears.

Guaræa is the " ball-wood " of the Antilles. It was proved in 1854 by Dr. Petroz,* and from its effects on the eyes he was led to give it in a severe case of conjunctivitis, with chemosis, occurring after cataract extraction, in which it proved rapidly curative. The remedy slumbered, however, for a long time ; and Allen does not even give its pathogenesis. Dr. Claude, however, has recently disinterred his countryman's discovery, and has recorded† several cases of the same kind in which it did everything that could be desired. We must not lose sight of it again. The presence of chemosis is the great indication for it ; and it has acted well in both the medium and the lowest attenuations.

* *Journal de la Soc. Gallicane*, v., 11.
† *N. Engl. Med. Gaz.*, Dec., 1876 ; and *L'Art Médical*, May, 1879.

LECTURE LIX.

SUPPLEMENTARY.

We will resume to-day our supplementary list of medicines. *Gymnocladus Canadensis* was introduced to us as far back as 1851, in an article contributed by Dr. Hering to the first volume of the *North American Journal of Homœopathy*, in which he relates several provings. It has caused an erysipelatoid swelling of the head, inflamed throat with a purple appearance of the right tonsil, and a violent cough (this last symptom, contained in Dr. Sellers' report, is omitted by Allen). The second of these effects has led to its only employment in homœopathic medicine, viz : for sore-throats with a bluish appearance or dark livid redness.

Hecla lava is, as its name imports, some of the matter which has issued from the well-known volcano of Iceland. Analysis shows it to consist of silica, alumina, lime and magnesia, with some oxide of iron. It was observed that the animals which fed in the pastures where the finer ashes of the mountain fall suffered from immense exostoses on the jaw-bones ; and in some the cranial and other bones swelled and bulged out. Dr. Garth Wilkinson, becoming acquainted with these results, saw the possibility of the lava becoming a homœopathic remedy in some affections of the teeth and jaws. He triturated some which he procured, and used it in toothache and in swellings about the jaws, "with magical effect in several cases ; also in gum abscess from decayed teeth, and with apparently good results in difficult teething." He communicated his experience to Dr. Holcombe, who gave it (30th dil.) with much benefit in neuralgic pains remaining after tooth extraction, and in osteitis affecting the lower maxilla. These facts were reported to the American Institute of Homœopathy in 1870.* Since then, Dr. Gilchrist has got good results from the remedy in exostosis and osteo-sarcoma,†

---

* See its Transactions for that year, p. 441.
† *United States Med. Investigator*, vol. ii., No. 1.

and Dr. Scales in whitlow and gumboil,[*] while Dr. Helmuth can speak of great relief to pain and arrest of growth as occurring in three out of four cases of exostosis in which he gave it.[†] It is a promising medicine.

Iberis. This is the Iberis amara, the "bitter candytuft" of our country, to which it is indigenous. Dr. Sylvester communicated to the South Eastern branch of the Provincial Medical and Surgical Association, in 1847, his experience with the seeds of this plant (which are the officinal portion), reporting it to be remarkably sedative to the heart's action, without displaying the retarding influence characteristic of Digitalis. Dr. Hale was thus led to prove it, and found three students in his class who undertook to do so.[‡] A marked cardiac action was displayed, showing itself in pain, palpitation, and even irregularity and intermission of the pulsations, which were sometimes weaker, but quite as often more forcible than usual.

Some doubt rested for a time on the validity of these experiments, as it was asserted that the provers were under the influence of expectant attention : Dr. Samuel Jones, too, found no effect from repeated and large doses in his own person. Dr. Hale, however, utterly denies that the provers were told of the drug's action on the heart ; and Dr. E. A. Gatchell, experimenting on frogs, found the plant to act very much as Digitalis does, prolonging and intensifying the systole, and retarding the circulation accordingly.[§] Iberis should therefore find a place in our treatment of cardiac maladies.

Jatropha. The seeds of the Jatropha curcas are very analogous to those of the croton tiglium ; and, like them, cause serous vomiting and purging. Hering, Thorer, Lembke and others have proved them, and their accidental ingestion has occasionally caused poisonous symptoms, so that Allen can give them a pathogenesis of 523 symptoms. Their effects led to their employment in choleraic conditions, but they have hardly taken place among the remedies for this state ; and they are only used in occasional cases of diarrhœa. Jatropha seems indicated when the stool is preceded and followed by much rumbling, and at times a noise as if a bottle were being

[*] *N. Engl. Med. Gazette,* June, 1876.
[†] *System of Surgery,* p. 436.
[‡] See *United States Med. and Surg. Journ.,* vol. vii.
[§] *N. Am. Journ. of Hom.,* Feb., 1877.

emptied ;* and also when the symptoms are ameliorated by
putting the hands into cold water.

Juglans. The walnut—Juglans regia—was proved many
years ago by Clotar Müller, in the form of a tincture of the
rind of the green fruit. He found it a specific cutaneous
irritant, developing itching eruptions of furuncular and eczematous character, lasting a long time, and leaving the affected
part of bluish-red colour and swollen appearance. Dr. Sook,
of Ohio, U.S., who made a subsequent proving, was relieved
permanently thereby of a burning itching eruption on the
lower extremities, always beginning to annoy him as soon as
he undressed. The allied butter-nut—Juglans cinerea—has
been proved in America, where it is indigenous, and found to
exert a similar action upon the skin, for whose eruptions it
has long been in domestic repute. Dr. Hale cites a series of
cases showing its efficacy in eczema, impetigo and ecthyma ;
and Dr. Burnett in this country reports† a similar experience,
calling it the "vegetable Arsenic." He has also found it both
cause and cure a suffocative post-sternal pain, occurring on
walking, and resembling in a mild way angina pectoris.

Lachnanthes tinctoria, the red-root, was proved by Dr.
Lippe (in the dilutions) nearly twenty years ago. It has,
however, come into little use, though it has been recommended
when one of its symptoms, "pain and stiffness in the neck,"
which may draw the head to one side, is present. Dr. Alabone,
of London, claims to have had striking success with it in
phthisis ; and Dr. H. Nankivell, in the paper on the therapeutics
of this disease read before the British Homœopathic Congress
of 1879, reported‡ some favourable experience with it in
" cases of the second and third stages, even when the amount
of lung destruction has been considerable, but where the
destructive process is for the time arrested, and the evening
temperature is not over 100½ or thereabouts." He gave the
mother-tincture, from 3 to 5 drops three times a day.

Lapis albus. This name was given by the late Dr. von
Grauvogl to a kind of gneiss found near the celebrated Gastein
springs. When on a visit to that place, he tells us, he observed
that the inhabitants of the valley of the Ache, who drank the
water of that torrent as it rushes through its bed of gneiss,

---

* See Allen's S. 279.
+ *Monthly Hom. Review,* xxii., 205
‡ *Ibid,* xxiii., 680.

are much affected with goitre. He drank the water himself, and his thyroid gland swelled. Dr. Bellows, of Boston, had previously maintained that the prevalence of bronchocele in Derbyshire is due to the presence of a similar gneiss in the drinking-water, and he describes it as a silico-fluoride of calcium.* Von Grauvogl, however, made a further observation, which was that the thermal waters which rise from the depths of the gneiss hill acted unfavourably in malignant growths and ulcerations ; and this led him to prove the gneiss itself. He triturated and diluted it up to the 6th decimal, which he gave to several men and women. The symptoms most frequently observed were burning and shooting pains in the cardia and pylorus, in the mammæ, and in the uterus. He administered it in a case where a cancerous ulcer of the cheek, in a woman of 50, had made an opening as large as half-a-crown, and rendered chewing and talking difficult. The hole filled up and healed,—the woman's complexion at the same time exchanging its yellowish and cachectic appearance for the hue of health. He thereupon gave it in uterine scirrhus, and reports five cases as completely and permanently cured by it. He also found it extremely beneficial in scrofulous ulcers, in diseases of the lymphatic glands, and in adenoid tumours growing in places where no glandular structure is normally found.†

This experience has hardly been confirmed by others ; but its source should prevent its being despised.

Melilotus. This is the sweet clover (M. officinalis), and might be supposed a very harmless flower. The tincture, however, is found to cause in sensitive people a very severe headache, which may be accompanied with determination of blood to the head and even with epistaxis. It has been found markedly beneficial in nervous headaches and conditions of cerebral oppression—one great advantage of it being that it acts so rapidly that five minutes have hardly elapsed ere its beneficial effects are experienced.‡ I value it much in nervous headaches, and always carry it in my pocket-case, in the form of the mother-tincture, which I administer by olfaction.

Mentha piperita. The peppermint is not used in our prac-

* See also Dr. Pease, in *United States Med. Investigator*, vol. i., No. 3.
† See *Allg. Hom. Zeitung*, June 15, 1874.
‡ See *United States Med. Investigator*, viii., **156**; *Bibl. Hom.*, ix., **29**.

tice as a " carminative," but it should be more largely employed
than it is in coughs. Dr. Demeures reported to the fourth
volume of the *Journal de la Société Gallicane* some symptoms
observed upon himself after taking one drop of the mother-
tincture, and among them was a very persistent dry irritative
cough, excited by drawing the least cold air into the larynx,
by reading aloud, by tobacco-smoke, or smoke of any kind.
He further says of it—" It is to dry cough, however caused,
what Arnica is to injuries, and Aconite to inflammatory complaints. It relieves even the cough of consumption. A single
dose (one globule of the 30th) was always sufficient whenever
there was dry cough ; however long it might have lasted, I
could safely promise a cure in twenty-four hours, provided
the affection corresponded with that caused by this agent."

Mentha piperita seems an analogue of Rumex crispus in
its relation to cough.

Myrica cerifera is the bayberry. It is in extensive use
among the herbalists, and is reputed by them a detergent to
the mucous membranes. It has been well proved in the
school of Hahnemann, by seven members of the Massachusetts Homœopathic Society on the one hand, and by Dr. G.
S. Walker on the other. The former set of provers did not
elicit much from it ; but Dr. Walker, who pushed it rather
more boldly, had on two occasions a decided attack of jaundice
from its use.* There was " bronze-yellow skin, fulness of the
hepatic region and abdomen ; scanty, yellow, frothy urine ;
loose, mushy, clay-coloured stools, destitute of bile ; much debility, and drowsiness almost amounting to stupor." This
jaundice resisted Podophyllum, Leptandra, Nux vomica and
Mercurius, but yielded promptly to Digitalis ; which would
suggest that it arose from catarrh of the bile-duct. Dr. Sharp,
wishing to see if in small doses the effect would be opposite
to that produced by large, got a friend to take a drop of the
first dilution night and morning for a week. During this time,
he reports, his bowels were rather more active than usual, and
the colour of the excreta much lighter, *i.e.*, of a lighter and
brighter yellow than usual.† This reminds us of Chamomilla ;
and suggests Myrica in icteric conditions similar to those
for which that remedy is suitable.

Nitri spiritus dulcis. This is the Latin form of the common
name ("sweet spirits of nitre") of the Spiritus ætheris nitrosi

---

* Hale, *New Remedies,* second edition.
† *Monthly Hom. Review,* xx., 748.

of the Pharmacopœia. Its interest in homœopathic practice is derived from a recommendation of it made by Hahnemann in his paper on the treatment of the fever of 1814, to which I have already more than once referred. " There sometimes," he writes there, " occurs a third state, a sort of a lethargy of the internal *sensorium commune*, a kind of half paralysis of the mental organs. The patient remains indolently lying, without sleeping or speaking ; he scarcely answers whatever we may do to induce him to do so, he appears to hear without understanding what is said, or without allowing it to make any impression upon him (the few words he says are whispered but not irrelevant); he appears to feel almost nothing, and to be almost immovable, and yet not quite paralysed. In this case a remedy is useful that previously used to be employed in large doses for purposes not very clearly defined ; I mean the *sweet spirits of nitre*. It must be so old, that is to say, so thoroughly sweetened that it no longer reddens the cork of the bottles. One drop of this is to be shaken up with an ounce of water, and given by teaspoonfuls to be consumed in the twenty-four hours. In the course of a few days this state passes into health and activity."*

The medicine has been proved by Lembke, as you may read in Allen ; who also gives effects of the inhalation of nitrous æther vapour. The late Dr. Liedbeck esteemed it highly as an antidote to the ill-effects of the excessive employment of salt.

Palladium. This rare metal was proved by Dr. Hering in 1850. Thirteen persons took part in his experiments, and the third trituration of the precipitated metal was employed. A full account of the proving, and of all that is known about the substance, is given by the venerable author in the *North American Journal of Homœopathy* for November, 1878. The alliance with Platina suggested by the natural history of Palladium came out manifestly in its proving ; and Dr. Hering suggested its trial in cases where Platina seemed to be indicated, but did not cure on account of its non-accordance with the mental symptoms. This advice has several times been acted on with success, especially in ovarian affections on the right side. Now that (for the first time) we have the full pathogenesis, we may make a larger use of the metal.

Piper methysticum. Under this its botanical name, the " kava-kava " of the Tahitian islands has been introduced into

* *Lesser Writings*, p. 715.

homœopathic practice by our Californian colleagues,—three of whom—Drs. Griswold, Hiller, and Wolff—have proved it on their own persons, with results which you may read in Allen. It has inebriating and aphrodisiac properties, for which it is used by the Pacific islanders : in the provers these were manifested in much dreaming, often of amorous nature, and in erethistic headache, with sense of fulness and enlargement. It also contains an oleo-resin, which acts upon the mucous membranes like the terebinthinates ; so that it has been used to some extent for gonorrhœa and gleet, as you may read in the fifth edition of Dr. Hale's book. Dr. Griswold has found two characteristics of its pains to be, " amelioration for a time from diverting the attention " and " restless desire to change the position." Guided by these features, both he * and Dr. Skinner† have given it with much advantage to relieve neuralgia and colic. The mother-tincture has generally been used.

Plantago. This is the common plantain—the " Plantago major " of Linnæus. Its virtues as an application to wounds and inflamed surfaces have been known from of old, and homœopathic practitioners have often used it for this purpose. Dr. Humphreys, of New York, published a monograph upon it in 1861, containing provings by eleven observers ; many symptoms have also been observed from it on his own person by one of our London chemists, Mr. Heath, of Ebury Street. All these you will find in Allen.

Plantago had (and has still in Switzerland) much repute as a local remedy for toothache, the root or leaves being put into the ear of the affected side. As it caused much pain in the teeth and jaws among its provers, it has been used in homœopathic practice as an internal remedy for odontalgia. Dr. Reutlinger says that with the 2x dilution of this medicine he cures seven-tenths of all cases of this kind in about fifteen minutes ; and Dr. Humphreys confirms the statement. Dr. Hale was at first inclined to doubt its efficacy, but acknowledges himself now obliged to admit its value, saying that of all homœopathic remedies for toothache, none can compare with the Plantago. I can say the same.

Some practitioners have found it useful in enuresis nocturna. It seems indicated here by the co-existence of diuresis, which is in a marked manner caused by it.

Prunus spinosa. An extensive list of symptoms, purporting

* Hale, *New Remedies*, 5th ed. p. 58. † *The Organon*, i., 298.

to be a pathogenesis of this plant, was furnished by Wahle to the fourteenth volume of the *Archiv*. There is the usual lack of information as to how the symptoms were obtained ; and Wahle is one of Hahnemann's disciples who has followed the later rather than the earlier manner of the master in their collection. I would not advise you to build much upon his pathogenesis ; but may tell you that two of its eye-symptoms have led to a very useful application of the medicine. They are—" A sharp pain beginning in the right side of the fore-head, shooting like lightning through the brain and coming out at the occiput," and " Pain in the right eyeball, as if the inner portion of the eye would be torn out." On these Drs. Allen and Norton remark : " as a remedy for ciliary neuralgia, whether originating from some diseased condition of the eye or not, there are few if any drugs more often called for than Prunus. The pains to which Prunus is adapted are especially found in disorders of the internal structures of the eye, there-fore it has been given in many of these cases and with marked benefit." They enumerate sclerotico-choroiditis posterior, chorio-retinitis, irido-choroiditis and irido-cyclitis among those deep-seated ocular inflammations which it has benefited. It not only relieves the pains, but checks the inflammation and clears the vision.

Senna is known in old-school therapeutics as a tolerably active purgative, influencing mainly the small intestines, and causing a good deal of colic in its operation. It may thus be homœopathically administered in some forms of diarrhœa. Its chief value for us, however, resides in the changes it induces in the urine, in which Martins ascertained that it always causes an increase in the amount of urea, chloride of sodium, earthy phosphates and urates, so that the specific gravity of the secretion is increased.* Dr. Drysdale has told us how to turn this action of the drug to good account, by recording a case of oxaluria with excess of urea (the specific gravity of the urine being 1035°), the stools also being diarrhœic, in which Senna φ, four drops twice a day, brought about rapid amendment.†

Sticta pulmonaria, the "lung-wort," is, as its name imports, in much repute for chest complaints. The few provings it has received did not develope any catarrhal or pulmonary symptoms ; and I can find nothing to warrant Dr. Hale's

* *Brit. Journ. of Hom.*, xvii., 555.
† *Ibid*, xxv., 657.

statement that "it was found to cause severe coryza with violent sneezing." Equally baseless seems his statement that these imaginary attacks "were preceded or followed by rheumatic pains *and swellings* of the small joints." Dr. Burdick, from whose experiences this picture appears to be drawn, had merely such pain and fulness in the ethmoid cells as might accompany coryza, and sharp dartings in many of the muscles and joints. However, there is no doubt of its being curative in hay-fever and influenza, and in harassing coughs accompanying these and allied disorders. It has also given rather rapid relief in acute but non-febrile rheumatism, which in one of the cases reported seems to have attacked the diaphragm. Dr. E. C. Price, of Baltimore, esteems it very highly in acute bursitis, as of the knee.*

The first and second decimal dilutions have been employed.

Stillingia sylvatica is a native of the Southern States of America ; and has some reputation as an "alterative" in syphilis, scrofula, and similar morbid diathetic states. It has been proved by several persons, but naturally has hardly elicited conditions answering to those it is able to benefit. Dr. Hale regards it as a periosteal remedy, like Phytolacca and Mezereum : he also esteems it in the cutaneous manifestations of syphilis. He reports a case of secondary nodes, with severe *dolores osteocopi*, in which striking benefit followed from its use. " It had a wonderful, and I might almost say instantaneous effect. The patient has slept well ever since he had it The immense nodes have gone from the head and legs ; and from the most deplorably down-hearted (sometimes almost raving), miserable, thin-looking object, he is changed into a buoyant, joking, rotund-looking fellow."

In the *New England Medical Gazette* for October, 1877, Dr. Hale has some remarks on the value of Stillingia in scrofula, which he has not transferred to the fifth edition of his *New Remedies*. He gives the following as a group of symptoms which, in the first to the third dilution, it is pretty safe to cure :—"Enlarged cervical glands ; moist, brownish, excoriating eruptions on the scalp ; muco-purulent discharge from the nose, with excoriation of the upper lip and alæ nasi ; a dull, pasty complexion ; capricious and unnatural appetite ; tumid and enlarged abdomen ; white, pasty stools, very fœtid ; dull red, soft, tubercular eruptions on the skin, ulcerating, and furnishing a large quantity of unhealthy pus ; a tendency to laryngeal cough."

* See *Hom. Times*, July, 1875 ; *United States Med. Investigator*, Jan. 1, 1878.

Symphytum is another plant which carries its reputation in its name. It was considered to promote the "growing together" of broken bones; and Homœopathy, here as in so many similar instances conserving the ancient traditions, has applied it for this purpose, and with eminently satisfactory results. It had hardly received any other use, however, till Dr. Cate, of Salem, U.S., conceiving that the action on bone thus displayed should not stand alone, gave it in a case of psoas abscess from disease of the vertebræ, and in another of inflammation of the inferior maxillary bone. In both instances a complete cure followed the steady administration of the second and third dilutions of the remedy.* Dr. Gerstel has since reported a rapid cure of traumatic periostitis with it.†

Titanium. The rare metal thus named was proved on himself in 1856 by Dr. Sharp, two grains of the first trituration being taken every day for a week. " I became," he says, "greatly disordered, and felt and looked wretchedly ill." Among other symptoms he experienced he mentions giddiness and vertical hemiopia. He gives one case, and refers to others, of general derangement of the system, with loss of strength and flesh, in which he has given smaller doses of the same potency with curative results.‡ It seems to promote sanguification.

Trillium, generally employed as trillin, a "concentrated preparation" made from the root of the Trillium pendulum, is in much favour among the American "eclectics" as a hæmostatic. It has not been proved; but Drs. Hale and Peterson's experience with it (as given by the former) in uterine hæmorrhage shows it effective in such small doses that we must suppose it to act homœopathically. We must remember it when Hamamelis and Millefolium fail us.

Vinca minor. This is the lesser periwinkle,—the plant so named, I mean; not the mollusc. We use a tincture prepared from the whole plant, which has been proved upon four persons in doses of from 20 to 60 drops, with little effect. "Excessive menstruation," however, is noted; and in my hands the medicine has four times availed to check passive uterine hæmorrhage occurring in women long past their cli-

* *New England Med. Gazette,* Oct., 1876; see also *Brit. Journ. of Hom.,* xxxiv., 378.
† *Ibid,* xxxvi, 101.
‡ *Essays in Medicine,* p. 394.

macteric. In three of these cases, indeed, the flow afterwards returned, and proved to have been the initial symptom of carcinoma; but the effect of the medicine was not less real for the time. I used the first decimal dilution. Vinca is said to be useful in such cutaneous affections as crusta lactea, and even to have cured the plica Polonica.

Viscum album. This plant—the familiar mistletoe—appears likely to find a place in therapeutics. Some cases of Dr. Huber's showing its virtue in several affections, especially rheumatism, sciatica, and metrorrhagia, were translated in the twenty-second volume of the *British Journal of Homœopathy.* Then Dr. Laville communicated some facts about it in relation to epilepsy, for which it has an old reputation.* He obtained two products from it,—an alkaloid which he calls viscine, and a resin. Two grains of the latter placed on the tongue of a large rabbit caused a violent fit of epilepsy, which lasted more than half an hour. He finds it of great value in the treatment of this disease in the lower animals, especially in herbivora. In the twelfth volume of the *Monthly Homœopathic Review* we have communications from Drs. Wilde and Belcher, showing the mistletoe to have a high and deserved repute among the common people in this country for the cure of chorea. A short pathogenesis of Viscum is given by Allen; but it deserves further proving and testing.

And now my remarks must end. Dr. Hale, our indefatigable purveyor of "new remedies," presents in his fifth edition many more which may yet be noteworthy. Such are the *bromide of camphor,* which he some time ago recommended in cholera infantum, and which has lately been reported† as very effective therein; the *Cornus florida,* which seems a true ague-remedy, and the *Cornus circinata,* which is valuable in aphthous mouths; the *Corydalis formosa,* which acts in secondary syphilis like Stillingia; *Cypripedium* and *Scutellaria,* which are "nervines" of some energy; *Erechthites* and *Erigeron,* possessing hæmostatic properties, and the latter relieving tympanites like Terebinthina; the *Geranium maculatum,* which causes ineffectual desire for stool, like Nux, and disorders the ocular accommodation like Conium; *Gossypium,* which acts on the female sexual organs; *Myositis* and *Silphium,* which seem good in bronchorrhœa; *Populus tremuloides,* a vesical irritant, and beneficial in tenesmus of the neck

* See an account of his book in *Brit. Journ. of Hom.,* xxv., 673.
† *Amer. Observer,* April, 1880.

of the bladder; *Robinia*, which has caused and cured gastric acidity; *Triosteum*, which seems not undeserving of its name " fever wort ";* *Ustilago maidis*, which is to maize what ergot is to rye, and has a similar influence on the uterus, controlling passive hæmorrhage therefrom; and the *Viburnum opulus*, which is a really valuable remedy for spasmodic dysmenorrhœa. For these, however, I must refer you to his book: my own list of medicines, primary and supplementary, has come to its close.

One remark only I will make in conclusion. It is now often admitted that there are some uses of medicines which seem consonant with the "homœopathic hypothesis," and that some of the remedies which have been arrived at by its employment are really useful agents. But it is always assumed that such instances constitute a small minority of the curative applications of drugs, and in no way warrant the adoption of the principle as a general method of treatment. Well; we have now considered together every important constituent of the Materia Medica. I have sought to bring before you as fully as possible the ascertained facts of the physiological and therapeutical action of each, and impartially to discuss the connection of the two. You will bear me out, I think, when I say that the result has been that nineteen-twentieths of the direct curative actions of drugs manifestly appear to be homœopathic in respect of *modus operandi*, and either have been or might have been arrived at by the application of the rule, " let likes be treated by likes." I venture to affirm that no other result can come of a fair survey of the facts of the case, conducted with this object in view. This is our position, and here we take our stand. Our opponents must meet us on the field of Materia Medica if they wish to convince us; and I think you will agree with me that they must retire, either vanquished or themselves convinced.

I have now merely to thank you for your attention, and to bid you farewell.

* See Transactions of N. York Hom. Med. Society, viii., 53.

LECTURE LX.

SUPPLEMENTARY.

Once more* we have to look back, and see what changes and what supplementings our former statements require. And this time it will be the whole course of lectures I have delivered which calls for and will receive such retrospect.

And in making it, I cannot begin without a sigh for the many names you have heard mentioned with honour which the last six years have transferred to our death-list. Quin, Black, Madden, Bayes, Chepmell, Hilbers, in this country ; Hering, Gray, Guernsey, in America ; Bähr, in Germany ; Nuñez, in Spain ; with many another of less note, have fallen out of our ranks to seek their well-earned repose. Peace to the souls of our heroes ! We grieve to lose them, but must seek to repair their loss by fresh devotion to our common cause.

The only additions I have to make to my first lecture relate to the books there recommended. I told you (p. 887) that a third and posthumous edition of Hempel's *Materia Medica*, edited by Dr. Arndt, might shortly be expected, and promised to be an improvement on its predecessors. I have now to say that this promise has been fulfilled, but only in the first volume of the re-issue. The second you will gain nothing by purchasing. To the collections of clinical experience I have indicated (p. 8) as available for the student, I may add one which I have often referred to, but never specified ; it is the *Clinical Therapeutics* of Dr. Hoyne, of Chicago. It includes under the head of each drug all the recommendations of it and instances of its successful use on which he can lay his hand ; and, though it often needs to be taken *cum grano*,† is full of suggestiveness and illumination. I may also note that Dr. Phillips' *Materia Medica* has now

---

* See Lecture LVIII. My readers will pardon me that, for the homogeneousness of the work, I put the modifications and additions required by the lapse of time in the form of an additional supplementary lecture.
† See *Brit. Journ. of Hom.*, xxxvii., 178.

been completed by a second volume embracing the mineral kingdom, and containing the result of very considerable research. Lastly, I would mention that our *British Homœopathic Pharmacopeia* has reached (1882) its third edition. Any noteworthy alterations it contains will receive attention as we speak of individual medicines.

In Lectures II. and III. we have spoken of the works, original and compiled, which constitute the "Materia Medica," technically so-called, of Homœopathy. I would note that the British translation of Hahnemann's *Reine Arzneimittellehre* has now been completed; though we still wait for America to furnish us with the *Chronischen Krankheiten* similarly rendered. But my chief remark here must be made on what was said at the close of Lecture III. (p. 52) on the compilations we possess, which from the primary sources of our Materia Medica draw a complete and orderly presentation of our knowledge. The latest and best of which I could then speak was Dr. Allen's *Encyclopædia;* and I find nothing to retract in the warm commendation which I then bestowed upon that monument of industry and devotion. Its critical examination, indeed, has shown it to require much emendation ;* but this its own editor is foremost in and best capable of giving.† I ended, however, by advising you not to content yourselves with any such secondary work as this, in which the symptoms produced by drugs are arranged in schema-form for ready reference. But in sending you to the detailed provings and poisonings I knew well that few would be able to make the journey, on account of the multiplicity and frequent inaccessibility of the points they would have to reach. I have now to tell you that an attempt is being made to place these primary records at the disposal of every student. The *Cyclopædia of Drug Pathogenesy*, now being issued under the auspices of the British Homœopathic Society and the American Institute of Homœopathy, is not only a critical revision of our Materia Medica, but also such a presentation of it as shall make it intelligible and interesting. It is a series of pathogenetic clinical cases, in which the real disease-producing powers of drugs are displayed to view as in no other way they can be. I may be partial; but I cherish the brightest hopes for the future of Homœopathy when it shall be in possession of such a Materia Medica as this.

My remarks in Lecture VII. on our homœopathic attenuations, brought down to a later date in Lecture LVIII. (p.

---

* See *Brit. Journ. of Hom.*, vols. xxxix.—xli., appendix.
† See *North Amer. Journ. of Hom.*, 1880—3.

888), would require considerable amplification were I to
re-write them now. You will find the subject fully discussed
in two articles on "Triturations" and "Dilutions" in the 38th
and 39th volumes respectively of the *British Journal of
Homœopathy,** and in Dr. Dake's communication to the International Convention of 1881, printed in its Transactions.
The conclusions to which these lead us differ little from those
to which Dr. Wesselhœft's first investigations pointed. In trituration, however well conducted, some proportion of the drug
undergoes nothing but coarse comminution; much of the
finest subdivision is already reached at the first step of the
process; and in the succeeding stages there is a progressive
diminution in the number of particles present, so that beyond
the 6th hardly any can remain. Dilution (or a suspension
equivalent thereto) here takes up the attenuating process;
but at its best cannot go farther than the divisibility of matter
permits, *i.e.* (as it would seem), to about our 12th potency.
Chemical, microscopic, and spectroscopic research cannot
follow the presence of the drug even thus far; and the only
quarter to which we can look for support in our clinical results
with the higher dilutions is that of pathogenesy. If Dr.
Jäger's "neural-analytic" experiments† are valid, this has
already pronounced unmistakably in their favour; but their
worth is as yet *sub judice.* More ordinary methods of proceeding have not taken us‡ beyond the 9× dilution as that
from which positive effects on the healthy human body can
be obtained; and Dr. Allen is so little satisfied with the
evidence here that he has, in a recent Presidential Address,
called on the American Institute of Homœopathy to examine
the subject. We shall look forward with much interest to
their results.

We come now to particular medicines, and have first some
additional remarks to make about *Carbolic acid.* The pretty
full pathogenesis in the *Cyclopædia* supports and illustrates
the account I have given of its physiological action. It adds
a curious symptom, occurring several times in those affected
by the vapour of the drug—increased olfactory sensibility;
and this I have found a valuable indication for it in practice.§
Of the results of experiments on animals, which I have
mentioned as not yet confirmed by occurrence in the human
subject, "pseudo-membranous and purulent inflammation of

---

* See also p. 111 of the latter volume.
† See *Brit. Journ. of Hom.,* xxxix., 23, 148.
‡ *Ibid.,* p. 17.
§ See *Knowledge of the Physician,* p. 233.

the bronchial tubes" must be put out of court altogether, as not warranted by the facts ; but simple bronchitis and pneumonia (lobar) have not infrequently been observed in human poisoning. The same may be said of albuminous nephritis ; but not of the hepatic and ocular symptoms specified, or of the convulsions.

Of *Fluoric acid* the symptoms I have cited as noteworthy must be read in their connexions, as you will find them in the *Cyclopædia*. In this light several of them look very differently from their appearance in the schema ; and some will not be found at all, as being unconfirmed results of dilutions higher than the 6th. Of fresh therapeutic applications I have a curious one to mention. In the *Lancet* for 1881 (i., 497), Dr. Woakes relates twenty cases of goitre treated by him with the acid, of which seventeen were cured. He explains his use of it by pointing to the analogy of fluorine with iodine and bromine, both of which have proved anti-goitrous remedies ; so that he was induced to try this their near relative. It may have been so ; but one cannot help suspecting that he had come across the facts I have related, of the production of bronchocele in a dog by fluoride of potassium in the hands of M. Maumené, and his ascription of the disease generally to the presence of fluorides in the drinking water. Anyhow, it is a pretty piece of homœopathic practice, and deserves imitation. Dr. Woakes gave ʒss—ʒij doses of a ½ per cent. solution.

Of *Nitric acid* I would say that you will find Scott's and Wunderlich's cases in full in the *Cyclopædia*, with some additional observations of its pathogenetic effects.

In speaking of *Phosphoric acid* as having " more than once proved curative of purpura and passive hæmorrhages," I should have used the " more than once " of the latter only. I know of but one case of purpura reported as cured by it, viz., that in Frank's *Magazin*, ii., 581 ; but there are cases of metrorrhagia and hæmoptysis in which it was the remedy in this and other parts of the same collection (ii., 581 ; iv., 737), and testimonies to its value in such affections are adduced by Marcy and Peters.

About *Aconite* I have several points to make. 1. As regards the preparation, the new edition of the *Pharmacopeia* directs that the ordinary tincture (to be dispensed unless the other is specified) shall be made from the freshly collected leaves and flowering tops only. The tincture of the root (fresh or dry) is to be made with proof spirit by percolation. 2. I am bound to say that the rendering of Schroff's experiments from the original (in the *Cyclopædia*) does not bear out the account of their febrile symptoms which I gave from the translation of them in *L'Union Médicale*. To compensate for this, however, we have in the detailed Austrian provings several beautiful pictures of the sthenic pyrexia induced by the drug.   3. I would direct attention to the valuable recasting of Dr. Dudgeon's arrangement of Aconite for the *Hahnemann Materia Medica*, contained in the volume of *Materia Medica, Physiological and Applied,* lately issued by the Hahnemann Publishing Society.   In its therapeutic section you will find him as enthusiastic as Gubler about the value of the remedy in neuralgia, to which it is so perfectly homœopathic.   4. I have said little of *Aconitine* as distinct from its parent plant.   Its splendid pathogenesis in the *Cyclopædia*, however, should bring it into some use among us, which indeed, for neuralgia, it has long enjoyed in my hands.   Our Pharmacopeia has not even yet made it officinal ; you will see that the preparation of the *Pharmacopeia Britannica* must be employed in preference to Morson's if you wish to have a homœopathic anti-neuralgic.

You will find some additional information relative to the action of *Æsculus* in piles in my commentary on Allen's *Encyclopædia* appended to the *British Journal of Homœopathy* for 1881—3 ; and will see it acting on these even when the nuts are carried in the breeches pockets.

I must withdraw the discouragement with which I have spoken of Dr. Dyce Brown's recommendation of *Agaricus* in the " douleurs fulgurantes " of locomotor ataxy.   If these were indeed directly dependent on the inflammatory induration present, my objection would hold good.   But further study of the subject has seemed to show that between this and the lightning pains intervenes an area of such spinal irritation as the drug can cause, and can therefore cure.   It may accordingly actually quiet these pains, as one of our German colleagues reports that he finds it do.*

Mr. S. H. Blake has confirmed Dr. Brown's suggestion of *Ailanthus* as a probable remedy for passive congestive headache.   You will find three cases treated by him with it in the 25th volume of the *Monthly Homœopathic Review* (p. 283).

Of *Aloes* I would say that Dr. Claude (who has given us a valuable study of its pathogenesis†) has contributed another case of rectal tenesmus (following catheterism) in which it was curative ; while Hempel's third edition supplies several

---

* See *Knowledge of the Physician,* p. 238.
† *Bull. de la Soc. Hom. Méd. de France,* vol. xxii.

confirmations of Dr. Guernsey's recommendation of it in passing of mucus by stool.

The result of the sifting of Hering's pathogenesis of *Alumen* which has been done for the *Cyclopædia* has left a residuum which seems to show the drug possessed of considerable power in attenuation. It deserves study ; for it looks quite homœopathic to the enteralgia for which (as I have mentioned) it is in repute in the old school, though the reversal of the usual conditions of dosage is not a little curious.

Of *Ammonium muriaticum* I have cited Böcker's observation that it greatly increases the elimination of urea. It is now more probable that the excess of urea is due to simple conversion of the ammoniacal salt itself.*

My statement under *Antimonium tartaricum* (p. 205, note) that Dr. Allen had omitted Molin's early provings of this drug was made before his tenth volume was issued. In the appendix contained therein it will be found *in extenso*.

The urethral irritation of *Argentum nitricum*, hitherto evidenced only in Dr. J. O. Müller (p. 223), is seen in the pathogenesis of the *Cyclopædia* in another experimenter (i., 9) ; and here seems to have involved the prostate.

From the list (p. 242) of instances in which intermittent fever seems to have been excited by *Arsenicum*, you must strike out the name of Clarus, as I find he is only the reporter of Delaharpe's observation ; but in its place you may put that of our own Massy, a case from whose pen you will find in the *Cyclopædia*. The value of this remedy in pernicious anæmia has been further substantiated in ordinary practice,† and is a beautiful instance of *similia similibus*. I should say that trituration is now recognised by our Pharmacopeia as an alternative mode of preparing Arsenicum. The iodide of arsenic has recently received much praise from Dr. Mackechnie in pericarditis and pleurisy,‡ and from Dr. Clarke in organic disease of the heart§ ; while in phthisis and malignant tumours it continues by general consent to play a remedial part of the first importance.

The experience of Dr. Flint with *Baryta* in aneurism (p. 283) has not been allowed to stand alone. Dr. Howitt, of Toronto, has reported ‖ a very satisfactory cure of one of the

* See *Cyclopædia*, i., 251, note †.
† See *Lancet*, 1885, i. 63 ; *Guy's Hosp. Rep.*, xxvi.
‡ *Monthly Hom. Review*, xxvi., 519 ; xxix. 35.
§ *Brit. Journ. of Hom.*, xlii., 303.
‖ *Monthly Hom. Rev.*, Nov., 1885.

descending aorta, where the 1 × of B. muriatica was given, which Dr. Torry Anderson has capped with another,* in which the patient became quite a new man under B. carbonica 3 ×. And in the *Homœopathic World* for January, 1885, may be read a case of Dr. Clarke's, in which the symptoms of aneurism of the thoracic and abdominal aorta, relieved by Lycopodium,† were still more markedly influenced by the same remedy.

Borax continues to win laurels in dysmenorrhœa and sterility.‡ A new field, moreover, has been opened for it by the observation of Dr. Gowers, warranted by three cases, of its power of causing psoriasis.§ It has since become my favourite remedy in recent cases of this malady, and the late Dr. McClatchey reported most favourably of it.‖

Bovista, too, has struck out a new line of action in the direction of parovarian cysts, cures with it being reported by Drs. Hawkes and E. Madden, and check to progress by Mr. S. H. Blake.¶

The compilers of the new edition of our *Pharmacopeia*, undismayed by the accidents to which I have adverted as produced by Rubini's saturated solution of *Camphor*, have adopted this as the φ. I would advise you not to use it, and to caution your patients against its employment. The 1 in 6 solution is strong enough for all ordinary purposes.

I have nothing fresh to say about Cina itself; but in my Boston lectures (p. 256) I have made something more of the undoubted cerebral action of *Santonine*, and have cited a case of occipital headaches cured by it in which its chromatic hallucinations were present. The fact that Cina is an Artemisia, and the relation of other members of this group (see p. 893) to epilepsy, indicate a connexion here which needs further working out.

Interest in *Coca* has been revived of late by the remarkable anesthetic power discovered to belong to its alkaloid, cocaine. The action, however, is mainly a local one; and nothing fresh has been ascertained as to the general influence of the drug, nothing, therefore, which can enhance its homœopathic usefulness.

The suggestion I made as to *Cuprum* being likely to prove an anti-squamosum has, in my own practice at least, proved

---

* *Annals*, x., 256.

† I have mentioned (p. 622) that this medicine has gained some credit in aneurism. I should have given a reference to the *Journ. de la Soc. Gall.*, i., 183.

‡ See *Hahn. Monthly*, Mar., 1880.

§ *Lancet*, Sept. 24, 1881.

‖ *Hahn. Monthly*, Feb., 1883.

¶ See *The Organon*, July, 1878; *Monthly Hom. Rev.*, xxv., 474, xxvii., 556.

a fruitful one. Its use, in conjunction with that of Carbolic acid (which does most for the irritation), has given me quite a fresh power over chronic psoriasis and lepra. I give the 3rd dilution of the acetate. Dr. Winterburn communicates a cure of vaginismus with it.*

The Transactions of the World's Homœopathic Convention of 1876 appeared at last in 1881, and we have the interesting communication of Dr. Pitet on *Curare*. His experience with it encourages the belief that in many paretic conditions, general and local, its homœopathicity to the functional disorder will suffice to give it curative power. It is especially in such state of the respiratory nerves that Dr. Pitet has found it useful. He gave the dilutions from the 4th to the 12th.†

In speaking of *Digitalis*, I have mentioned Dr. Black's study of its action. Before his lamented death he had expanded this into the exhaustive monograph on the drug which appears in the *Materia Medica, Physiological and Applied*, of which I have already spoken (p. 916). He agrees with me in looking to direct action on the muscular walls of the heart as explaining most of its cardiac phenomena ; though he points out that death of the organ in systole is by no means so common in the higher animals as in frogs. In my Boston Lectures I have called attention to it (p. 247) as a possible remedy for migraine, its visual disturbance being very like that with which the paroxysms of this malady often commence. Dr. Black cites (from Brunton) three favourable testimonies to its value here.

To the instructive bit of borrowing recorded under *Drosera* we can now add another from this side of the Channel. In 1880 Dr. Murrell reported in the *Lancet* the result of treatment of whooping-cough in an adult. He first took bromide of potassium for a fortnight without any benefit, whereupon he was given " five-drop doses of a 1 in 10 tincture of drosera rotundifolia." " He took this," says the narrative, "for a week, and then returned, saying that it had made him much worse. It increased the spasm and cough and made him whoop more ; he whooped as many as twelve times in one paroxysm." The dose was then reduced to half a drop of the same tincture, and at the end of the week he came back reporting great improvement, which in another fortnight resulted in complete cure.

---

* *Amer. Homœopath*, March, 1884.

† See also a case of cure by it in Dr. Allen's hands in *North Amer. Journ. of Hom.*, Aug., 1879; and a proving under Dr. C. Wesselhœft's auspices in *N. Engl. Med. Gaz.* for Dec., 1885.

A medical club in the United States, which has done me the honour of denoting itself by my name, published in 1883 a monograph on *Gelsemium*,* in which all the trustworthy pathogenetic effects of the drug are arranged in schema-form for reference, with a luminous commentary. I have only here to echo the general commendation this volume has received. You will do well to read with especial attention the analysis of the eye-symptoms, which brings out with much acumen the part played in them by congestion. The remark of the authors that certain symptoms " possibly indicate its use in writer's cramp" has been verified by the experience lately communicated by Dr. Galley Blackley and others to the British Homœopathic Society.† Drs. Ringer and Murrell were so struck by the mingling of spasmodic and paralytic phenomena in their experiments on animals, that they had suggested the probability of its containing two diversely acting alkaloids. It is just this complex action which makes it homœopathically useful in the present malady.

Glonoin has lately, under its common name of nitro-glycerine, become a favourite remedy in the hands of certain practitioners of the old school in the treatment of angina pectoris. Its analogy (which I have pointed out) to nitrite of amyl would naturally suggest it as a palliative here ; but Dr. Murrell finds it even curative. His brochure on the subject‡ should be consulted, though we must supplement his historical statements from our further knowledge. He uses a 1 per cent. solution (our 1st centesimal) in increasing doses. In the actual paroxysm it acts less rapidly than the amyl, but its effects seem much more lasting. Dr. Bartholomew thinks it of value for reducing the high arterial tension present in the subjects of contracted kidneys. In my comparison between glonoin and amyl nitrite you must strike out the statement that the pulse is not much affected by the latter. The observations cited in the *Cyclopædia* show great quickening of the pulse to be a constant and early symptom of its action. The first note on p. 262 there will also suggest that the influence of both drugs may possibly be exerted primarily on the nervous centres.

The Drs. Serrand, of Cauterets, have put on record, in the *Bulletin de la Société Médicale Homœopathique de France* (Feb.,

---

* *Gelsemium sempervirens.* A monograph by the Hughes Medical Club of Massachusetts. Otis Clapp & Son, Boston.

† *Annals*, x., 501.

‡ *Nitro-glycerine as a Remedy for Angina Pectoris.* By William Murrell, M.D. London, 1882.

1881), a number of cases illustrating the curative powers of *Hamamelis*. One of them is an instance of neuralgia of the internal saphenous nerve, which is a new application of the drug, but receives confirmation from another case reported in the *Bibliothèque Homœopathique* for June of the same year.

Dr. Franklin has cured four out of five cases of lupus non-exedens with *Hydrocotyle*.*

The repute of *Hypericum* in effects of injuries has increased of late. Dr. Gilchrist, from an experience of sixty-four operations, major and minor, asserts positively that its use, internally and locally (1 to 20), precludes any after-suffering ;† and Dr. Helmuth tells me that it quite supersedes the use of morphia after operations in his hands.

In qualification of what I have said of the relation of *Iodide of potassium* to tertiary syphilis, I am bound to cite Dr. Meyhoffer's statements.‡ "It has become the fashion, even among the disciples of Hahnemann, to exhibit the iodide of potassium in increasing doses ; we are convinced that this course is as useless as it is often injurious. From the moment the drug produces pathogenetic symptoms, it exaggerates the functions of the tissues, exhausts the already diminished vitality, and thence, instead of stimulating the organic cell in the direction of life, impairs or abolishes its power of contraction. We use, as a rule, the 1st dilution, from 6 to 20 drops a day ; if after a week no decided progress is visible, one drop of the tincture of iodine is added to each hundred of this 1st dil." In this way, he says, "the mucous tubercles, gummy deposits, and ulcerations resulting therefrom in the larynx undergo a favourable termination." (It is of laryngeal syphilis that he is speaking.)

The volume of *Materia Medica*, to which I have referred while speaking of Aconite and Digitalis, contains also a reproduction of Dr. Drysdale's arrangement of *Kali bichromicum*, originally published in the *Hahnemann Materia Medica*. Its physiological section has nothing that is new ; though it brings out more clearly than I have made it appear that the poison inflames the alimentary mucous membrane specifically, and not merely by local action. Therapeutically, this article is noteworthy for the confirmation it supplies from old-school sources of two of our chief applications of the drug, viz., to chronic gastric affections, and to syphilis. Vulpian is

* See *Monthly Hom. Rev.*, xxvi., 31.

† *N. Engl. Med. Gaz.*, April, 1880; *U. S. Med. Inv.*, March 15, 1881.

‡ *Chronic Diseases of Organs of Respiration*, i., 190.

the contributor in the first case, Güntz in the second. From the former are cited six cases of "very serious disorder of the stomach, simulating, indeed, malignant disease," in which striking amelioration if not cure followed the use of centi-gramme doses. Güntz has applied it in about half grain doses on a large scale in the treatment of syphilis, and finds it frequently abortive and constantly curative of constitutional symptoms; giving, on the whole, results more favourable than those of mercury.

The same volume contains a really exhaustive treatise on *Crotalus*, by Dr. Hayward, which in its therapeutic sections includes also Lachesis and the other serpent-poisons, so that it may read side by side with my lecture on these (XXXIX.), of which it makes kindly mention, and with which it is in entire accord. Dr. Hayward's great experience with Crotalus as a remedy gives us some valuable hints for its employment ; as (p. 255) in the delusions of cerebral decay, (p. 280) in spas-modic grinding of the teeth at night, (p. 301) in the local inflammatory and hæmorrhagic and the general icteric effects of wasp-sting, (p. 310) in hæmaturia, and (p. 327) in palpitation with feeling as if the heart tumbled over and trembled much. Still more important is his statement (p. 362) : "For the last ten years the present writer has used Crotalus in all cases of fever of all kinds when anything of a hæmorrhagic, or putres-cent, character has been exhibited, and with the most prompt and marked effect in removing the hæmorrhagic symptoms and checking the tendency to putrescence."

To the treatises we have on mercurial action I can now add the exhaustive memoir by Dr. Huber, translated as an appendix to the *North American Journal of Homœopathy* for 1882—4. The use to be made of this may be seen in my Boston Lectures (p. 177), where I am discussing the relation of Mercury to rheumatism and iritis. The conclusions I there reached do not differ from those I have previously advanced, but I am able to base them upon a wider range of *data*. As regards iritis, I may refer you to a discussion of its relation to Mercury in vol. x. of the *Annals* (p. 137), where I have reviewed the evidence in detail. The power of the cyanide over diphtheria has received fresh illustration of late, both in the old school[*] and the new.[†] In spite of this, when, after the death of our lamented Princess Alice from the disease, the German Empress

---

[*] See *Amer. Obs.*, Aug. 1882 (Annushat); *Brit. Journ. of Hom.*, xlii., 313; xxxix., 251; xl., 266 (Rothe).

[†] See *Brit. Journ. of Hom.*, xli., 336; xlii., 358; *Annals*, x., 231; *St. Louis Periscope*, Dec., 1885.

offered a prize for the best essay upon it, Dr. von Villers, the main introducer of the treatment, was not allowed to compete because of his homœopathic convictions! He has of course given us his essay, and you may read it in the 41st volume of the *British Journal*. Nothing can be more satisfactory; and you will observe that he still abides by his very minute doses. The old-school observers, and those among ourselves who use the low triturations, though they find it the best of remedies known to them, do not get such brilliant results as Dr. von Villers.

The Hahnemann Society's volume contains an article on *Nux vomica*, from the pen of Dr. Black. It is stronger on the physiological than on the therapeutic side. The latter section was indeed left unfinished when our colleague's death took the pen from his hands; but his study (§ 26—74) of the pathogenetic effects of the drug is very full and instructive.

Our knowledge of *Osmium* is increasing, and it bids fair to become an important remedy. Dr. Bojanus' essay in the *Internationale Homœopathische Presse* (vol. v.) should by all means be consulted; also Dr. Galley Blackley's observations on its effect upon the skin. Dr. Allen thinks it indicated in glaucoma, and Dr. Norton has given it in chronic cases with benefit; while in the old school some use is being made of osmic acid and osmate of potash in nervous diseases.*

The hint given under *Physostigma*, that myotics readily excite iritis, has been turned to good account in America, but rather with the analogous Jaborandi and its alkaloid pilocarpin.†

In the third edition of our *Pharmacopeia*, another change has been made in the preparation of *Phosphorus*. It is directed to be made in saturated solution with ether or absolute alcohol, the former being said to require 200 minims, the latter 550, for the grain. From these the 3 × potency can be made with absolute alcohol, and those above it with rectified spirit. The most important therapeutic application which this drug has of late years received has been the systematic treatment of rachitis with it, in minute doses, which has been carried out on a large scale in Germany, and with brilliant results.‡ The homœopathicity of the practice I have already suggested (p. 736), and the dosage employed points in the same direction.

The indications of *Plumbum* as a remedy for progressive

* See *North Amer. Journ. of Hom.*, Nov. 1884, p. 195.
† See *Trans. of Intern. Hom. Conv.* for 1881, p. 124.
‡ *North Amer. Journ. of Hom.*, xxxii., 487; and *Monthly Hom. Rev.*, xxviii., 402.

muscular atrophy have been further confirmed by two cases
published by Dr. Seutin, of Brussels, in the *Revue Hom.
Belge* for March, 1884. If you have not access to this
periodical, you will find an account of the case in the last
monograph of the *Materia Medica, Physiological and
Applied,* which is upon this metal, and proceeds from Dr.
Black's pen. As before, its account and discussion of the
pathogenetic effects of lead constitutes its chief and great
value. To the experience with Plumbum in kidney disease
collected by him may be added a case of desquamative
nephritis with dropsy recovering under its use (2 × trit. of the
acetate) in Wiel's hands.*

The value of *Pulsatilla* in orchitis has received repeated
attestations from the old school of late. In my own hands it
assumes a growing importance as a reducer of the prostatic
irritation which troubles so many elderly men ; but here I
find the 6th dilution most effective.

Dufresnoy's experience, that persons not constitutionally
susceptible to *Rhus* as a poisonous agent are not likely to
receive benefit from it if used as a medicine, has been supported by an observation of Dr. Edwards Smith's.† He treated
two patients presenting eczema under the same form and
characteristics, with Rhus ; one recovered quickly, the other
remained untouched by the remedy. On inquiry it was ascertained that the former was susceptible, the latter insusceptible,
to the poisonous influence of the plant. This, I should
say, is opposed to Hahnemann's dictum on the subject
(*Organon,* § 117).

The late Dr. H. Bernard, whose loss Belgian homœopathy
so much deplores, has put on record another case showing the
value of *Rumex crispus* in pruritus increased by exposure to
cool air.‡

To the bit of experience of Dr. H. C. Allen, as to *Sarsaparilla* causing herpes, I can now add one from Dr. Holcombe
as to its curative power in cutaneous disorder : "During the
very hot summer months," he writes,§ "a great many children,
and some grown persons, present themselves with cutaneous
affections—their name is legion. Last year I gave to all such
cases small doses, three times a day, of Sarsa, 3rd trit., and
never before have I practised among skin diseases with such
satisfaction and such triumph."

* *Brit. Journ. of Hom.,* xl., 367.
† *Clinical Review,* Dec., 1885, p. 59.
‡ *Hom. World,* Nov., 1880.
§ *U. S. Med. Inv.,* Aug. 15, 1879.

Of *Secale* we have a proving by students of the Michigan University, under Dr. H. C. Allen's superintendence, and published in the Transactions of the American Institute of Homœopathy for 1885. It was made with the potencies from 2 to 200. As of old, however, the phenomena of ergotism continue to be our richest store of information as to the action of this drug. Recently, in an epidemic observed by Tuczek, he observed that all the cases presented symptoms of a lesion of the posterior columns of the cord, and in some cases the complete picture of locomotor ataxy was developed. In four cases in which the cord was examined after death, it was found to present a symmetrical lesion of the columns of Burdach. This action has not yet been turned to account; but Dr. Jousset reports a case of diffuse myelitis in which it seems (2nd trit.) to have been the curative agent.* Dr. L. B. Wells has cured three cases of senile gangrene with it.†

I have perhaps been hypercritical in altering *Silicea* to "Silica." Mr. Wyborn calls my attention to the fact that "Calcarea" also is properly an adjective, whose substantive understood is "terra." I know of no drug which does such wonders in chronic disease as this. Two cases, one of hydrocephalus, one of ascites, in rachitic children, have lately recovered in a marvellous manner under its influence in my hands,—the potencies from 12 to 30 being those employed.

In speaking (under *Sulphur*) of Hahnemann as assigning seven-eighths of chronic disease to a psoric origin, I fell into a very common mistake. In my Hahnemannian Lecture‡ I have corrected it. You will see there (p. 75) that he excludes from the category of the maladies he so affiliates those which arise from unhealthy surroundings, noxious habits, and depressing influences, and also the medicinal affections which the heroic treatment of his day made so common.

To the description of the otitis caused by *Tellurium* in Dr. Dunham, it should be added that Dr. Houghton subsequently examined his tympanum, and found it "irregular, thickened in parts, thin in other portions, the result of perforation and cicatrisation."

Dr. C. W. Wolf, some twenty-five years ago, propounded a theory that mankind were being radically poisoned by vaccination; that the virus thus conveyed to the system was Hahnemann's sycosis; and that for its ill-effects the great

---

* *L' Art Médical*, Jan., 1885.

† *U. S. Med. Inv.*, Oct. 1, 1880.

‡ *Hahnemann as a Medical Philosopher—The Organon.* Gould & Son, 1882.

remedy was *Thuja*.* Dr. Burnett, unaware (as he tells us) of these ideas of his predecessor, has arrived at a somewhat similar conclusion as to the morbid condition resulting from vaccination ; and from a remark of Dr. Goullon's was led to Thuja as a probable homœopathic remedy for the same. His views and practice are set forth in his brochure entitled "Vaccinosis and Homœo-prophylaxis"; and, whatever may be thought of his pathology, he certainly makes a good case for his therapeutics. I have hitherto been accustomed (following Hering) to rely on Silicea for the few troubles I have regarded as truly *propter* (and not merely *post*) *vaccinationem ;* but Dr. Burnett's experience gives another string to one's bow.

I do not know whether the use of *Verbascum* in phthisis, lately communicated by an Irish physician, is an application of the dynamic virtues of the drug. At any rate the emulsion described by him seems worth substituting for cod liver oil in some cases.

You will find some further experience with *Viola tricolor* as a remedy for infantile eczema from Dr. Bigler in the *Hahnemannian Monthly* for Jan., 1880, and from Dr. Piffard in the *Homœopathic World* for October, 1882 ; and some fresh provings of *Xanthoxylum* in the eighth volume of the Proceedings of the Massachusetts State Homœopathic Society.

And now of the minor or newer medicines discussed in my two supplementary lectures (LVIII. and LIX.).

Drs. Burnett, Maffey and Lloyd Tuckey† have had very good effects from *Aralia,* 1 × to 3 ×, in night cough following the first sleep ; and Dr. J. Foster confirms the homœopathic applicability of *Ammoniacum,* in all dilutions, to bronchitic cough with sticky phlegm.‡

Guaco forms the subject of an interesting communication addressed by Dr. Talbot to the Boston Homœopathic Medical Society.§ He tells us that an attempt was made to prove it in 1853 by the Massachusetts State Society, but with few decisive results. One of these, however, was a choleriform diarrhœa, with aching in sacrum and loins, and he has been led thereby to employ it in diarrhœa and dysentery so characterised, and with very good effect, so that he constantly carries it in his pocket-case. He also confirms Elb's recommendation of it in the paralysis following apoplexy.

---

* See *Brit. Journ. of Hom.,* xviii., 459.
† *Hom. World,* April, 1881; July and Aug., 1882; July, 1883.
‡ *Ibid.,* Nov., 1883.
§ See *New England Med. Gazette* for Aug., 1884.

Last, of new candidates for favour—new, at least, to these lectures.

Convallaria majalis, the lily of the valley, has lately come into much repute as a cardiac remedy, acting very much like Digitalis; as also does the *Adonis vernalis*.* The former has received a proving, which you will find in the *North American Journal of Homœopathy* for May, 1883. It is rather for inducing the physiological action of such remedies (of which I have spoken when on their prototype) that either is likely to be useful than in more strictly homœopathic applications.

The *Lathyrus sativus*, a vetch which grows in India, has long been known to cause a peculiar kind of paralysis in those who live too much on flour made from its bean. An account of its effects is given in the 5th edition of Aitken's *Science and Practice of Medicine* (i., 860). "The paralysis," he writes, "is observed most frequently during the rainy season in India —cold and wet being perhaps an exciting cause—so that the first lameness may be a mixture of palsy and rheumatism. Men who had gone to bed quite well awake in the morning feeling their legs stiff, especially at the knees, their loins weak, and their gait unsteady. Fever does not seem to attend the accession of the phenomena ; but pain gets worse, and eventually the lower limbs are quite paralysed. The patient walks with great difficulty, the toes turn inwards, the legs waste, and the great toe-nail scrapes the ground, till in persons who go bare-footed the nail has been known to get rubbed down to the quick. Males are said to be more often affected than females." A recent epidemic of lathyrism occurring among the Kabyles of Algeria, and proceeding from the L. cicera, presented similar features, ascribed to an acute transverse myelitis, with sexual and vesical paralysis, as well as loss of motor and sensory power in the legs.† Dr. Clarke has recently brought before the British Homœopathic Society a series of five cases of spinal paralysis treated by it with much amelioration.‡

Naphthalin, one of the carbon compounds, $C_{10}H_8$, a crystalline substance prepared from tar, is known in old-school practice as an antiseptic only. Its sole physiological action, so far as observed, is irritation of the periphery of the urinary apparatus (violent desire to urinate, reddening and tumefaction of external urethral orifice, and œdema of prepuce), and an intoxication somewhat like that of carbolic

* See *Med. Era*, Oct., 1884.
† See *Med. Advance*, Jan., 1886, p. 411.
‡ See *Monthly Hom. Rev.*, Dec., 1885.

acid—face assuming a pale-yellowish hue, and patient growing restless, or lying as if stupefied by a narcotic. But it is
acquiring, given in the lower triturations, quite a reputation
in the hands of some homœopathists against whooping-cough
and asthma.* For the former it was recommended by von
Grauvogl.

Of *Propylamine* (more properly, trimethylamine) I have
given some account in my Boston Lectures (p. 155). It really
appears to be homœopathic to the acute rheumatic conditions
in which at one time it gained so much repute, and has been
unduly neglected.

The *Syzygium jambolanum,* also an Indian plant, is coming
into use as an anti-diabetic, and one apparently of great
power. Banatvala first called attention to it, having witnessed
its popular employment ;† and Dr. Dudgeon soon after turned
it to excellent account in the 1 × dilution.‡ Dr. Burt has had
similarly favourable experience with it, but he gives five-grain
doses of the powdered seeds.§

With this I again take leave of the subject for the present.

* See *Brit. Journ. of Hom.,* xxxvii., 377; xxxix., 66, 84.
† *Lond. Med. Record,* Feb. 15, 1883.
‡ *Hom. World,* May, 1885.
§ *Med. Era,* Nov., 1885.

CLINICAL INDEX TO LECTURE LX.

APPENDIX.

HAHNEMANN'S DOSAGE.[*]

In the discussions about dose which from time to time arise in the school of Hahnemann, the practice of the master is frequently cited by either side, and statements made on the point by one party are frequently contradicted by the other, so that the would-be learner is left in confusion. It has seemed to me that it would be a useful contribution to the controversy if a chronological account were given—taken from the original documents—of all that Hahnemann wrote on this subject from his first promulgation of the homœopathic method until his death. I am not unmindful of the valuable materials brought together by Dr. Dudgeon in relation to Hahnemann's dosage in his *Lectures on Homœopathy*. But at the time of their publication it is obvious that my esteemed colleague had not at his command several of the most important sources of information on this score :—I refer to the first edition of the *Reine Arzneimittellehre* and the *Chronischen Krankheiten*, and the second edition of the first and second volumes of the former work. With these now before me, I am able to fill up certain gaps in his statement, and to present a complete account of the facts.

1796—1798.

It was in 1796 that, in his essay entitled " A new principle for ascertaining the curative power of drugs, with a few glances at those hitherto employed," Hahneman first propounded the homœopathic method. In this paper he several times speaks of " small doses " as being necessary when similarly-acting medicines are given, the context showing (and, indeed, sometimes stating) that he means doses too small to produce the physiological effects of the drugs. That such smallness did not, in the case of most medicines, mean their use in even fractional quantities, appears from his recorded practice during the next two years. In 1797 we find him reporting a case of colic in which he gave Veratrum album in four-grain doses, and another of asthma treated by Nux vomica in the same quantities. In 1798 he relates a series of cases of continued and remittent fevers occurring in that year, in which he gave " a few grains of Arnica root," Ignatia in doses of two or three grains to children from seven to twelve, from one-fifth to half a grain of Opium, thirty to forty grains of Camphor, six to seven grains of Ledum. In another paper " On some periodical and hebdomadal diseases," appearing in the same year, he speaks of giving eight grains of Ignatia and half-drachm and drachm doses of Cinchona.

[*] Reprinted from the *British Journal of Homœopathy* for April, 1878.

1799.

To this year belongs the introduction, sudden and without explanation, of what are now known as infinitesimal doses. In a pamphlet "On the cure and prevention of Scarlet Fever," published in 1801, Hahnemann relates his treatment of an epidemic of this disease commencing in the summer of 1799. He mentions the use of four medicines only—Ipecacuanha, Opium, Belladonna, and Chamomilla, and speaks of all as given in quantities of a minuteness hitherto unknown in medical practice. His tincture of Ipecacuanha was to contain one part of the drug in two thousand of alcohol; of this from one to ten drops were to be taken, according to the age of the patient. Opium was so diluted that a drop should represent only the five-millionth of a grain, and children below four were to have even this dose broken up. Belladonna was given in a dose of the 432,000th part of a grain of the extract ; and for prophylactic purposes a solution was made containing only a twenty-four millionth part of a grain of the same, of which from one to forty drops, according to age, were to be taken every third day. The tincture of Chamomilla was to contain the 800,000th part of a grain of the dry extract, of which one, two, or more drops were to be given.

1801.

In the second part of *Hufeland's Journal* for this year Hahnemann answers the question aroused by his pamphlet—What effect can these minute doses of Belladonna have ? I am not now concerned with his defence of them ; I have only to note that he speaks several times of the effects of a millionth part of the ordinary dose, and says,—" Those who are satisfied with these general hints will believe me when I assert, that I have removed various paralytic affections by employing for some weeks a quantity of diluted solution of Belladonna, where for the whole treatment not quite a hundred-thousandth part of a grain of the extract was required ; and that I have cured some periodical nervous diseases, tendency to boils, &c., by not quite a millionth of a grain for the whole treatment."

1806.

Hahnemann says nothing more upon the subject of dose (not even in his *Fragmenta de viribus medicamentorum positivis*, published in 1805) until his essay on " The Medicine of Experience," which appeared in *Hufeland's Journal* in 1806. Nor, indeed, does he advance here beyond the point he seems to have reached in 1799—1801. He speaks of the "smallest possible dose " sufficing, of its being of little or no importance how small the dose is ; but whenever he comes to particulars, he mentions only the hundredths, thousandths, and millionths of an ordinary dose with which we are already familiar.

1809.

I find no further mention of dose (beyond such general statements about smallness as those cited above) until we come to 1809. In a paper entitled "Observations on the three current methods of treatment," published in *Hufeland's Journal* of that year, we meet with a paragraph stating that in certain so-called " bilious conditions " " a single drop of the tincture of arnica-root will often remove, in the course of a couple of hours, all the fever, all the bilious taste, all the tormina ; the tongue becomes clean, and the strength is restored before night."* But in another communication belonging to the same year we find that in the case of two potent poisons Hahnemann had come to attenuate much farther than three years back. For a fever which had prevailed for a twelvemonth past in Germany, and which he describes in the *Allg. Anzeiger der Deutschen* for 1809, he names as remedies Nux vomica and Arsenicum, according to the symptoms, recommending the former to be given in doses of a trillionth, the latter in those of a sextillionth of a grain, *i.e.* in the 9th and 18th dilutions respectively.

1810.

In this year appeared the first edition of the *Organon* ; and we naturally expect to find in that section of it devoted to the subject of dose some more detailed exposition of Hahnemann's views upon the point than had as yet been vouchsafed. Little is said, however, beyond what we have already seen in the " Medicine of Experience." In a note to § 247, he writes :—" When I speak of the dose employed in homœopathic practice being the smallest possible, I cannot, on account of the difference in the power of medicines, give a table of the right measure and weight of the medicines."

1814.

In 1814, in an article " On the treatment of the typhus or hospital fever at present prevailing " (it was the time of the uprising of Germany against Napoleon which followed his retreat from Russia), we have further insight into Hahnemann's posology. The medicines he recommends, according to the symptoms, are Bryonia, Rhus, and Hyoscyamus. The first two are to be given in the twelfth dilution, and the third in the eighth, of a scale different from the centesimal, in that six drachms instead of a hundred drops of alcohol are to be used at each advance in attenuation. This would (as Dr. Dudgeon says†) make the 12th dilution correspond to something between our 15th and 16th, and the 8th to our 10th. Sweet spirit of nitre is also directed to be given under certain circumstances, and a drop of it is to be shaken up with an ounce of water, the mixture to be consumed by teaspoonfuls in the course of the twenty-four hours.

1816.

This year is an important epoch in the history of Hahnemann's dosage, or at least in our knowledge of it. In the first volume of the *Reine Arzneimittellehre*, published in 1811, he had not said a word, in his prefatory remarks to the several pathogeneses, as to the doses of

* *Lesser Writings*, translated by Dudgeon, p. 599.
† *Lectures*, p. 401.

the medicines he thought most suitable to be given. We thus know nothing of his views at that time regarding the dosage of Belladonna, Dulcamara, Cina, Cannabis, Cocculus, Nux vomica, Opium, Moschus, Oleander, Mercurius, Aconite, and Arnica. Now, however, this reserve is abandoned ; and in the second volume (published in 1816) and its successors, nearly every medicine is given its appropriate dose. In that now before us we find the following recommendations :—

Of Causticum a drop of the original preparation is to be given for a dose.

Arsenicum is to be administered in the 12th, 18th, or 30th dilution, preferably the last.

Of Ferrum the $\frac{1}{100}$th, $\frac{1}{10000}$th, or $\frac{1}{50000}$th of a grain is mentioned as appropriate.

Ignatia is recommended in the 9th or 12th potency; and Rheum, in acute affections, in the 9th.

As to Pulsatilla, Rhus, and Bryonia, very similar directions are given. If the patient be robust, and his malady of some standing, a drop of the pure juice will be an appropriate dose. But in delicate subjects and acute affections attenuations are to be given—the 12th being specified for the first medicine, the 12th or 15th for the second, the 18th for the third.

These views are well illustrated by the two celebrated cases published at this time by Hahnemann as examples of homœopathic treatment, and which are given in the preface to the present volume. The first was one of gastralgia, with water-brash, of three weeks' standing, occurring in a robust woman otherwise in good health. She received a drop of the juice of the root of Bryonia. The second was one of spoiled stomach, which had existed five days, and whose subject was a weakly and delicate man. His remedy was half a drop of the twelfth dilution of Pulsatilla. Both these cases were treated towards the end of 1815.

From the same preface, moreover, we learn that Hahnemann had now adopted the centesimal scale of attenuation,—great care being taken (in which later homœopathic pharmacy has not followed him) to make each potency what it professes to be. Dry plants are to be treated with twenty parts of alcohol, and each drop of this tincture to be reckoned as containing a twentieth part of medicinal power (Arzneikraft) in making the dilutions. Correspondingly, the tinctures prepared from fresh plants by mixing their expressed juice with equal parts of spirit are to be considered as of half-strength, so that two drops are to be added to 98 of alcohol to make the first centesimal dilution.

1817.

This year brings us a third volume of the *Reine Arzneimittellehre*, and in it we find the following recommendations as to dose.

China is to be given in the 12th dilution,
Asarum in the 12th or 15th,
Ipecacuanha in the 3rd,
Scilla in the 15th or 18th,
Stramonium in the 9th,
Veratrum in the 12th.

Nothing is said on this score as to Chamomilla and Helleborus. In the preface Hahnemann speaks of a drop of the thirtieth dilution of Arsenicum as being sometimes " altogether too large a dose."

1818.

A fourth volume of the *R.A.M.L.* now appears, containing twelve medicines. The following are the statements and recommendations about dose to be found in it.

Of Hyoscyamus, it is said in the preface to the medicine, that a dose which contains the trillionth part of a drop of the juice (*i.e.* of the 9th dilution) is more than sufficient for homœopathic purposes; and in a note to one of the symptoms, suggesting its use in hydrophobia, and warning against giving it in too large doses, the 12th, 15th, and 18th dilutions are mentioned as most suitable.

Digitalis is recommended, with the qualification as to "often more than enough," in the 15th dilution.

About Aurum he gives no definite advice, but speaks of using the first and and second triturations of gold-leaf (this mode of preparation is now introduced for the first time), and the 15th and 18th dilutions of the muriate.

Of Guaiacum a drop of the mother-tincture is said to be a full dose.

Camphor is to be given in drop doses of the primary solution, which is in the proportion of one part in eight.

Ledum is recommended in the :5th dilution ;

Ruta in a dilution containing one part of the juice in 100,000, *i.e.* what we should now call the 5th decimal ;

Sarsaparilla in drop doses of the mother-tincture ;

Sulphur, Hepar Sulphuris and Argentum in grain doses of the second trituration.

1819.

This year gives us several expressions of Hahnemann's views on the subject of dose.

1. The fifth volume of his *Materia Medica Pura* bears its date. In this we find him making the following recommendations :—

Of Euphrasia, Menyanthes, and Sambucus, "the smallest part of a drop of the juice " is mentioned as a sufficient dose.

Cyclamen is to be administered in the same proportion of the third dilution.

Of Calcarea acetica a drop of the saturated solution is advised ;

Of Muriatic acid, the smallest part of a drop of the thousand-fold dilution, *i.e.* our 3rd decimal ;

Of Thuja a similar quantity of the 30th.

A single drop of the juice of Taraxacum is to be given ,

A small part of a drop of Phosphoric acid in the second dilution ;

Of Spigelia and Staphisagria the smallest part of a drop of the 30th.

2. In this year was published the second edition of the *Organon*. The paragraphs on the subject of dose are very differently worded from the corresponding ones in the first edition, and are identical with those of the fifth, which we all have in our hands. In a note to one of them Hahnemann refers to the prefaces to the several medicines in his *Reine Arzneimitiellehre* for the appropriate dilution of each, but says that further experience has shown that it is better to go still " lower " than the doses there indicated. By " lower " he evidently means what we understand by " higher."

3. In the same year we have a short communication to a popular

Journal " On uncharitableness towards suicides," in which he states that " this most unnatural of all human purposes, this disorder of the mind that renders them aweary of life, might always with certainty be cured if the medicinal powers of pure *gold* for the cure of this sad condition were known." For this purpose he recommends an attenuation to the billionth degree, *i.e.*, the sixth potency. In the previous year he had spoken of effecting cures by using altogether from three to nine grains of the first trituration.

1821.

In this year was published the sixth and last volume of the first edition of the *Reine Arzneimittellehre*. The phrase " the smallest part of a drop," which we have so often encountered in the fifth volume, is now constantly used, and seems to imply the regular employment of globules as the form of administration. Understanding this, I may briefly state Hahnemann's recommendations as to the suitable dilutions of each medicine.

Of Angustura he mentions the 6th ;
Of Manganum aceticum the 24th ;
Of Capsicum the 9th ;
Of Colocynth the 18th and 21st.
Of Verbascum the pure juice is to be given ;
Of Spongia the mother-tincture for goitre ; for other purposes higher attenuations (the range not specified) ;
Of Drosera the 9th dilution ;
Of Bismuth the 2nd trituration ;
Of Stannum the 6th.

In a note to one of the symptoms of Cicuta Hahnemann speaks of giving a small part of a drop of the juice for a dose in impetigo.

In the same year Aconite and Coffea are recommended as the remedies for " purpura miliaris." The former is to be given in the 24th, the latter in the 3rd dilution.

1822.

Hahnemann now began to issue a second edition of his *Materia Medica Pura*, the first volume appearing in the present year. As in the corresponding volume of the first edition nothing was said about dose, I must limit myself to stating the dilutions now mentioned.

Of Belladonna the 30th is recommended ;
Of Dulcamara the 24th ;
Of Cina the 9th ;
Of Cannabis the pure juice ;
Of Cocculus the 12th ;
Of Nux vomica the 30th ;
Of Opium the 6th ;
Of Moschus the 3rd decimal (1000 *facher*) ;
Of Oleander the 6th ;
Of Mercurius solubilis the 12th (trituration) ;
Of Mercurius corrosivus the 15th ;
Of Aconite the 24th ;
Of Arnica the 6th.

The phrase " small " or " smallest part of a drop " is used for each of these, save that of Mercurius solubilis "a grain or less" is to be given.

1824.

The second volume of this edition, appearing in 1824, can have its recommendations as to dose compared with its fellow in the former issue. Making such comparison, accordingly, we find that the only material change which has occurred relates to Rhus and Bryonia. Of Pulsatilla it is still allowed to give a drop of the pure juice in a suitable case ; but of the two other drugs, about which formerly the same direction was given, it is now said that the juice is never required, the 30th dilution answering equally well for all cases. Arsenicum, Ferrum, Ignatia, and Rheum are to be given as in 1816 ; and of Causticum the original solution is still prescribed, in doses of "a drop or less."

1825.

Two volumes—the third and fourth—of the second edition of the *Reine Arzneimittellehre* appeared during this year. In the third the recommendations as to China, Asarum, Ipecacuanha, Scilla, Stramonium, and Veratrum remain unchanged ; and the twelfth is for the first time specified as the appropriate dilution for Chamomilla. In the fourth the doses of Guaiacum, Camphor, Ledum, Ruta, Sarsaparilla, Sulphur and Argentum remain as they were in the first edition. Hyoscyamus is raised from the 9th to the 12th dilution ; and in the note about hydrophobia the 24th and 30th are substituted for the 12th, 15th, and 18th, as the most appropriate potencies. Of Digitalis the 30th is said to be still better than the 15th ; and of Aurum he states that he now gives the 12th dilution instead of the 1st and 2nd triturations. Hepar sulphuris is raised from the 2nd to the 3rd.

1826.

In the fifth volume, published in this year, the only changes which occur are as to Muriatic and Phosphoric acids. Ths former is now to be given in a "millionfache" instead of a "tausendfache" solution, *i.e.*, in the 3rd potency ; the latter in the 9th attenuation instead of, as hitherto, in the second.

There also occurs, in this volume, one of the few notices given by Hahnemann of those potencies above the 30th which afterwards played so large a part in homœopathic posology. He says that, in sycosic gonorrhœa, he finds Thuja more potent in the 60th than in the 30th dilution. It would seem, however, that he did not attach much importance to this observation, as subsequently, in both editions of the *Chronischen Krankheiten*, the appropriate dose for Thuja in sycosis is said to be the 30th.

1827.

In the sixth volume, Angustura, Capsicum, Verbascum and Bismuth

remain as they were in respect of dose. Manganum is raised to the
30th, Colocynth to the 24th or 30th, and Drosera also to the latter point.
Cicuta, of whose dosage in Hahnemann's hands the only trace hitherto
was his use of the pure juice in a case mentioned, is now recommended in the 30th; and this dilution is specified as the one most
appropriate for Spongia in all affections save goitre. On the other
hand, Ambra, Carbo animalis and Carbo vegetabilis—here introduced
for the first time—are all to be given in a small part of a grain of the
third trituration ; and of Stannum he says that he has hitherto used the
6th, but now finds the 3rd to answer every purpose. We shall see
directly that this last exhibits his usual practice somewhere about this
time with all drugs prepared by trituration and given in chronic
disease.

1828.

This year brings us a very important addition to our knowledge of
Hahnemann's posology at the time which we have reached. It is
the first edition of the *Chronischen Krankheiten*, of which the first
three volumes now appeared. I will give all the statements about dose
which they contain.

In the introductory essay, speaking of the "antipsoric" medicines
generally, he says that he began by giving a small portion of a grain
of the 2nd or 3rd trituration (by which process all then recognized were
prepared); but that later, feeling this to be an uncertain quantity, he
prepared and used the subsequent attenuations. In accordance with
this statement we find him mentioning in a note cases of itch which he
had treated with half-grain doses of the third trituration of Carbo
vegetabilis and Sepia respectively. In speaking of the treatment of
the three miasmatic diseases he describes, he recommends—for sycosis,
Thuja 30 and Nitric acid 6 ; for syphilis, Mercurius solubilis 6 ; and for
recent itch, three globules saturated with a tincture made by treating
five grains of Sulphur with a hundred drops of alcohol. If a second
dose is required, he advises the 6th dilution to be used, as prepared in
the usual way ; and if Carbo animalis or vegetabilis should be required,
they are to be given in the 12th. Recommending Antimonium
crudum where a spoiled stomach was annoying the patient, he mentions
the 6th potency as appropriate ; and in a letter dated April, 1829, we
find him using the medicine at this strength in certain intermittent
fevers.*

In the prefaces to the several medicines the following recommendations are made as to dose :—

For Ammonium carbonicum and Baryta carbonica the 18th is said to
be most suitable ;

For Calcarea carbonica, Graphites, and Lycopodium the potencies
from the 18th to the 30th.

For Iodium the 30th.

Of Magnesia carbonica he says that he has long employed the 12th,
but now prefers the 24th and 30th.

For Magnesia muriatica he mentions the 6th as the most generally
suitable, but says that we may at times go with advantage to the 12th
and 18th.

Natrum carbonicum he at first employed in an aqueous solution to
the 3rd degree : but now recommends the 12th potency prepared from
the third trituration.

* See *Brit. Journ. of Hom.*, xi., 64.

Nitric acid, as an antipsoric, should be given in the dilutions from the
18th to the 30th ;
Petroleum in the 18th ;
Phosphorus and Sepia in the 30th ;
Silica and Zincum from the 18th to the 30th.

1829—1843.

We have now tracked Hahnemann through the whole course of his
posology from 1796 to 1828. We have seen him diligently following his
experience in whatever direction it led him, on the whole advancing
from lower to higher attenuations, but never hesitating (as in the case
of Stannum) to take the opposite step when the facts seemed to require
it. We have found him recognising throughout the great difference
between medicines as regards their dose, so that his latest instructions
fix this for one and the other at all points of the scale of dilution from
the mother-tincture to the 30th. All has hitherto shown life and
progress, and the history is worthy of our best attention. But at
the point we have now reached a chilling blast sweeps over the scene,
and stiffens it to a rigid and monotonous blankness. At some time
in the course of 1829 Hahnemann determined to fix the dose of all
medicines indiscriminately at the 30th dilution. The thing was done
solely, as he himself says, for the sake of uniformity. The "medicine
of experience" had nothing to say to it, for we are told in the fifth
edition of the *Organon*, published in 1833, tha it "holds good, and will
continue to hold good, as a homœopathic ther peutic maxim, *not to be
refuted by any experience in the world*, that tue best dose of the properly selected remedy is always the very smallest one in one of the high
dynamisations (x)," which last is his sign for the 30th. Accordingly,
in the fourth volume of the first edition of the *Chronischen Krankheiten* (1830), in the first and second of the third edition of the *Reine
Arzneimittellehre* (1830-3), and throughout the second edition of the
later work (1835-39), every medicine whose pathogenesis is given is
directed to be employed in the 30th dilution.

Not that Hahnemann himself rigidly observed the uniformity he in-
culcated. Without laying any stress on the cases which Dr. Dudgeon
has cited, as treated by him in 1842-3, where the language is obscure ;
or on the contents of his pocket-case found after death, in which all
dilutions from the 3rd to the 30th were present, it is sufficient to refer to
the second edition of the *Chronic Diseases*. In the introductory essay
thereto (1835) Nitric acid is still recommended for sycosis in the 6th ;
and in the preface to the third part (1837) he states that if, after the
30th potency has exhausted its action, the medicine is still indicated,
it should be given in a lower potency, suggesting the 24th. At the
end of this preface he speaks of giving, where the same medicine had
to be continued several days, a dose daily each time in a lower degree
of potency. On the other hand, there are indications of a tendency to
look beyond the limit of the 30th ; for we read in the *Organon* of 1833
—" The higher we carry the attenuations accompanied by dynamisation,
with so much the more rapid and penetrating action does the preparation seem to affect the vital force and to alter the health, with but
slight diminution of strength even when this operation is carried very
far—in place, as is usual (and generally sufficient) to X, when it is
carried up to XX, L. C, and higher ; only that then the action always

appears to last a shorter time." By these figures he meant what we should call the 60th, 150th, and 300th potencies. In the preface to the fifth volume (1839) he speaks of " obtaining, even in the fiftieth potency, medicines of the most penetrating efficacy;" and von Bönninghausen tell us, that in his last years he not uncommonly employed the 60th.

On the basis of this survey of the facts of the case it is not unfair to argue that the truest disciples of Hahnemann in the matter of dose are those who follow him as he was in the years from 1796 to 1828, rather than those who count the 30th itself a low potency, and dwell habitually in an exalted region far above that which the master but looked into and himself but seldom entered.

ALPHABETICAL LIST OF THE MEDICINES TREATED OF IN THIS MANUAL.

N.B.—The different types indicate the relative importance of the medicines, and may afford useful hints as to order of study.

CLINICAL INDEX.